Chelation Therapy in the Treatment of Metal Intoxication

Chelation Therapy in the Treatment of Metal Intoxication

Jan Aaseth
Department of Public Health
Hedmark University College, Elverum
Department of Internal Medicine
Innlandet Hospital, Kongsvinger
Hedmark, Norway

Guido Crisponi
Department of Chemical and Geological Sciences
University of Cagliari
Cagliari, Italy

Ole Andersen
Department of Science and Environment
Roskilde University
Roskilde, Denmark

ELSEVIER

AMSTERDAM • BOSTON • HEIDELBERG • LONDON
NEW YORK • OXFORD • PARIS • SAN DIEGO
SAN FRANCISCO • SINGAPORE • SYDNEY • TOKYO
Academic Press is an Imprint of Elsevier

Academic Press is an imprint of Elsevier
125 London Wall, London EC2Y 5AS, UK
525 B Street, Suite 1800, San Diego, CA 92101-4495, USA
50 Hampshire Street, 5th Floor, Cambridge, MA 02139, USA
The Boulevard, Langford Lane, Kidlington, Oxford OX5 1GB, UK

British Library Cataloguing-in-Publication Data

A catalogue record for this book is available from the British Library

Library of Congress Cataloging-in-Publication Data

A catalog record for this book is available from the Library of Congress

ISBN: 978-0-12-803072-1

Typeset by Thomson Digital

Contents

Contributors

Jan Aaseth, Department of Public Health, Hedmark University College, Elverum; Department of Internal Medicine, Innlandet Hospital, Kongsvinger, Hedmark, Norway

Jan Alexander, Norwegian Institute of Public Health, Oslo; Norwegian University of Life Sciences, Akershus, Norway

Ole Andersen, Department of Science and Environment, Roskilde University, Roskilde, Denmark

Guido Crisponi, Department of Chemical and Geological Sciences, University of Cagliari, Monserrato, Cagliari, Italy

Petr Dusek, Department of Neurology and Center of Clinical Neuroscience, Charles University in Prague, 1st Faculty of Medicine and General University Hospital, Prague, Czech Republic

Lars Gerhardsson, Occupational and Environmental Medicine, Sahlgrenska Academy and University Hospital, Gothenburg, Sweden

Valeria Marina Nurchi, Department of Chemical and Geological Sciences, University of Cagliari, Monserrato, Cagliari, Italy

Marit Aralt Skaug, Faculty of Public Health, Hedmark University College, Elverum, Norway

Preface

The idea of writing an interdisciplinary book on the clinical uses of chelating agents in genetic diseases and various metal overexposures was conceived around 2011–13 and developed during the 10th Nordic Trace Element Society Conference in Loen, Norway in 2013. The author group organized symposia on metal chelation during this conference, as well as during the conferences in Belek, Turkey, in 2011, and in Dubrovnik, Croatia, in 2015, both of which were organized by ISTERH (The International Society of Trace Element Research in Humans).

The history of chelating agents was initiated during World War II. And during the subsequent decades important advances in chemistry, molecular biology, and the molecular understanding of roles of metals in health and diseases have taken place. During World War II, BAL (2,3-dimercaptopropanol) was developed as an antidote to the war gas dichlorovinyl arsine (Lewisite). Lewisite was, however, never used, so the first clinical use of BAL was to treat intoxications due to the use of organic drugs against syphilis. Later, BAL was recommended as a therapeutic antidote against inorganic mercury, lead, and copper. And during a five-year-period from 1951 intramuscular injections of BAL was even used in the treatment of Wilson's disease.

The next chelator to come into clinical use was calcium-EDTA (ethylenediaminetetraacetic acid), initially to combat lead intoxication and for decorporation of radionuclides, the latter role presently played more efficiently by the calcium–sodium and zinc–sodium salts of diethylenetriaminepentaacetic acid (DTPA). Military, industrial, and medicinal production and uses of radionuclides also gave a boost to studies from the viewpoint of assessing hazards, protection, and decorporation of radionuclides, the classical chelators here being DTPA and Prussian blue (PB).

An important development in chelation treatment was the introduction of desferal (desferrioxamine, DFO) for treatment of transfusional iron overload in thalassemias and sickle cell anemia, preventing disability and early death for hundreds of thousands of individuals in Southern Europe, Africa, and Asia. DFO has also saved the lives of numerous children acutely poisoned by ingesting their mothers' iron supplements. In recent years, the development of deferiprone and deferasirox as orally active chelating agents has extensively eased the treatment of pathological iron deposits resulting from blood transfusions and hemolytic processes accompanying thalassemia and sickle cell anemia, resulting in better treatment compliance and improved life quality for these patients.

As is well known for our readers, from basic lessons in biochemistry, iron as Fe(II) or Fe(III) is an oxygen-seeking or oxygen-carrying metal, with affinity to nitrogen also, as is illustrated by the function and structure of heme in hemoglobin. And the therapeutic iron chelators, as well, bind and detoxify Fe-cations from tissue deposits by use of the same ligand groups, oxygen, and nitrogen.

In contrast, several toxic heavy metals, such as arsenic, mercury, copper, and lead may be referred to as sulfur-seekers, having higher affinity to endogenous sulfur than oxygen groups. These metal cations may be bound and inactivated by the two vicinal thiol groups on the therapeutic agent BAL. However, today, the clinical use of BAL is limited due to its own high toxicity. Its less toxic derivatives, meso-2,3-dimercaptosuccinic acid (DMSA) and D,L-2,3-dimercapto-1-propanesulfonic acid (DMPS), have now entered the clinical arena and superseded dimercaprol in most cases of heavy metal poisonings. These latter dithiols are nowadays available for oral administration, as tablets, as well as for parenteral administration.

The present book also gives guidelines for clinicians who are responsible for diagnosis and treatment of metal poisonings and overload diseases. In addition, some guidelines for further research are precipitated in the last chapter.

Jan Aaseth
Guido Crisponi
Ole Andersen
December 2015

List of Abbreviations

Recommended name	IUPAC name	Recommended acronym	Further names	Trade name
D-penicillamine	(2S)-2-amino-3-methyl-3-sulfanylbutanoic acid	DPA	Dimethyl-cysteine, H_2Pen, PSH	Cuprimine
DMSA	*meso*-2,3-Dimercaptosuccinic acid	DMSA	Succimer	Chemet
DMPS	D,L-2,3-dimercapto-1-propanesulfonic acid	DMPS		Unithiol, Unitiol, Dimaval
Deferiprone	3-Hydroxy-1,2-dimethylpyridin-4(1H)-one	DFP	L1	Ferriprox
Deferoxamine	*N*′-{5-[Acetyl(hydroxy)amino]pentyl}-*N*-[5-({4-[(5-aminopentyl)(hydroxy)amino]-4-oxobutanoyl}amino)pentyl]-*N*-hydroxysuccinamide	DFO	Desferri-oxamine, DFOA	Desferal
Deferasirox	4-[(3Z,5E)-3,5-bis(6-oxo-1-cyclohexa-2,4-dienylidene)-1,2,4-triazolidin-1-yl]benzoic acid	DFX		Exjade
Trientine hydrochloride	*N*,*N*′-Bis(2-aminoethyl)ethane-1,2-diamine	Trien	Trieth-ylene tetramine, TETA	Syprine
BAL	2,3-Dimercaptopropan-1-ol	BAL		Dimercap-rol
Calcium disodium edetate	calciumdisodium-2-({2-[Bis(carboxymethyl)amino]ethyl}(carboxymethyl)amino)acetate	$CaNa_2EDTA$		Calcium-disodium-versenate

(*Continued*)

Recommended name	IUPAC name	Recommended acronym	Further names	Trade name
Calcium diethylenetriaminepentaacetate	2-[Bis[2-[bis(carboxymethyl)amino]ethyl]amino]acetic acid, calcium trisodium salt	Ca-DTPA	Calcium trisodium pentetate	Ditripentat-Heyl
Zinc diethylenetriaminepentaacetate	2-[Bis[2-[bis(carboxymethyl)amino]ethyl]amino]acetic acid, zinc trisodium salt	Zn-DTPA	Zinc trisodium pentetate	
Prussian blue	Iron(II,III) hexacyanoferrate(II,III)	PB		Radiogardase, Antidot Thallii-Heyl
Disodium edatate	disodium-2-({2-[Bis(carboxymethyl)amino]ethyl}(carboxymethyl)amino) acetate	Na-EDTA		Endrate Chelest B Komplexon III

Note: The abbreviations used are also explained in each chapter.

Chapter 1

General Chemistry of Metal Toxicity and Basis for Metal Complexation

Jan Aaseth, Lars Gerhardsson, Marit Aralt Skaug, Jan Alexander

Chapter Outline

1.1 GENERAL CHEMISTRY OF METALS

About 60% of the adult human body is water, and most of the biochemical interactions take place in the aqueous environment, either extra- or intracellularly. In small children, the amount of water is larger, about 75% of the body weight.

A useful definition of metals from a biological or toxicological viewpoint is based on the properties of their ions in aqueous solutions, for example, in the human body. A metal is an element, which under biologically significant

Chelation Therapy in the Treatment of Metal Intoxication. http://dx.doi.org/10.1016/B978-0-12-803072-1.00001-8

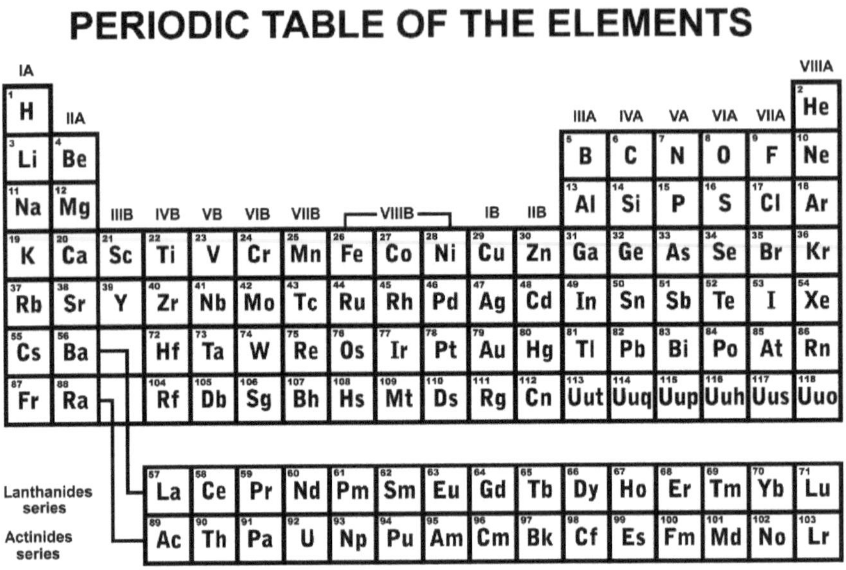

FIGURE 1.1 Elements in the periodic table. The groups from IA to VIIIA may also be numbered successively from 1 to 18, including the 10 elements in the intermediate B-series. It should be noted that most of the transition metals in the first row (Mn^{2+}, Fe^{2+}, Co^{2+}, Ni^{2+}, Cu^{2+}, Zn^{2+}) have electronegativities in the range 1.6–1.8 on the Pauling scale, and these cations are classified as "intermediate" according to the theory of Pearson (1963) implying that they have high affinity to electron donor groups containing nitrogen. This is illustrated by the structures of hemoglobin and cobalamine, where Fe^{2+} and Co^{2+}, respectively, are coordinated between four nitrogens. These elements might also bind oxygen, for example, the oxygen-carrying function of hemoglobin. Metals on the left side of the periodic table, for example, Be^{2+}, Ca^{2+}, and Sr^{2+} have lower electronegativities on the Pauling scale, and will consequently be prone to form ionic bonds, for example, to oxygen in the phosphate or carboxylic groups. These elements are often referred to as "hard" or oxygen seeking. On the other hand, metals on the right side of the periodic table, for example, Ag^+, Au^+, Hg^{2+}, CH_3Hg^+, Pd^{2+}, Cd^{2+}, Pt^{2+}, and As^{3+} are "soft" sulfur-seeking metals and will more easily establish bonds to thiols or selenol groups.

conditions may exist as a solvated cation (M), that is, the element has lost one or more electrons. Elements with electronegativity below 2.0–2.5 on the Pauling scale may loose electrons and exist as cations in aqueous solutions and may thus be classified as metals (Aaseth, Skaug, Cao, & Andersen, 2015). The electronegativities of the transition metals (vanadium, chromium, manganese, iron, and copper) are about 1.6–1.8, whereas mercury, lead, and arsenic have higher electronegativities, namely around 2.0. Elements on the left side in the periodic table (Fig. 1.1) have lower electronegativities and are classified as metals. It should be noted, however, that the distinction between metals and nonmetals is not a sharp one.

In some groups of the periodic table, such as in group IVA (alternatively numbered group 14), there is a gradual transition of properties from nonmetals to metals as we descend from the lighter to the heavier elements, in the order

C, Si, Ge, Sn, and Pb. Borderline elements such as As, Ge, Sb, Se, and Te are sometimes referred to as metalloids.

1.2 ESSENTIAL AND NONESSENTIAL ELEMENTS

At present, 20 of the elements in the periodic table are defined as essential for humans, with certainty. First, these are the four organic elements H, C, N, and O. In addition seven "macro-minerals" are essential, namely Na, K, Ca, Mg, Cl, P, and S.

Furthermore, nine trace elements are defined as essential, namely Fe, Mn, Cu, Zn, Se, Co, Ni, Mo, and I. At present, some other elements are under discussion to be included in the category as essential, such as F, B, Si, and As.

To be categorized as an essential, however, an element must satisfy all of the following conditions:

1. It must be present in the human tissues.
2. It's dietary deficiency must result in a reduction of a biological function from optimal to suboptimal.
3. The reduction in physiological function can be normalized by appropriate supplementation of the element (Mertz, 1974).

Oxygen and hydrogen: A human body of 70 kg contains about 46 and 7 kg, respectively, of oxygen and hydrogen. These elements are predominantly bound in water, which makes up 60–65% of the body weight of an adult individual. While intracellular water makes up about two-third of this amount of water, the extracellular compartment makes up the remaining one-third. In aerobic organisms, continuous supply of molecular oxygen is a prerequisite for the controlled combustion to generate chemical energy in mitochondria.

Carbon: This element makes up the principal organic constituent of endogenous molecules of living organisms, for example, carbohydrates and fat as well as proteins. The content of carbon in an adult human body is about 13 kg, since elemental carbon cannot be utilized by the human body, it must be ingested as organic carbon in reduced form in carbohydrates, fat, and/or proteins.

Nitrogen: This element is also essential in organic form. It is particularly found in amino acids, in proteins, and as constituents of nucleic acids. The amount of nitrogen in an adult human body is almost 2 kg.

Calcium: This is the most abundant inorganic constituent of the human body, accounting for about 1.2 kg of the body weight. As hydroxyapatite, $Ca_5(PO_4)_3(OH)_2$, calcium is a major component of normal bone and teeth. Hydroxyapatite makes up the bone mineral and the matrix of teeth, and this calcium compound gives bones and teeth their rigidity.

Calcium is cofactor for numerous enzymes and is also important for intracellular functions as a messenger in cascade signaling reactions, for example, muscle and nerve function, and for blood coagulation. The blood plasma levels of total calcium are kept fairly constant, within narrow limits, 2.2–2.6 mmol/L

(9–10.5 mg/dL). However, about 50% of this blood plasma calcium is bound to albumin, and measurements of "ionized" calcium (1.1–1.4 mmol/L or 4.5–5.6 mg/dL) may be the recommended analysis, since the amount of total calcium varies with the level of albumin.

If the diet provides insufficient amounts of this element, the organism will mobilize calcium from bone, through a process that is brought about by increased circulating levels of the parathyroid hormone (PTH).

Hypercalcemia: It is a disorder commonly encountered by primary care physicians. The diagnosis often is made incidentally in asymptomatic patients. Clinical manifestations affect the neuromuscular, gastrointestinal, renal, skeletal, and cardiovascular systems. The most common causes of hypercalcemia are primary hyperparathyroidism and malignancy. Some other important causes of hypercalcemia include overdoses of vitamin D. An initial diagnostic workup should include measurement of intact PTH, and any medications that are likely to be causative should be discontinued. PTH is suppressed in malignancy-associated hypercalcemia and elevated in primary hyperparathyroidism. It is essential to exclude other causes before considering parathyroid surgery, and patients should be referred for parathyroidectomy only if they meet certain criteria. Many patients with primary hyperparathyroidism have a benign course and do not need surgery. Hypercalcemic crisis with total Ca above 14 mg/dL (or above 3.5 mmol/L) is a life-threatening emergency, often precipitated by malignancy. Aggressive intravenous rehydration is the mainstay of management in severe hypercalcemia, and an intravenously administered bisphosphonate (pamidronate or zoledronate) can usually alleviate the clinical manifestations of hypercalcemic disorders. Whereas bisphosphonates have Ca-chelating properties, the previous use of another chelator, disodium-EDTA, in hypercalcemia is considered obsolete today. In hypercalcemia mediated by vitamin D and in hematologic malignancies, for example, myeloma, glucocorticoids may be the first line of therapy after fluids.

Hypocalcemia: It may occur due to hypoparathyroidism, acute or chronic kidney failure, low vitamin D intake, genetic anomalies, or iatrogenic causes related to some antiosteoporosis or chelation drugs. In chronic hypocalcemia bone mineralization may be compromised, whereas acute cases may present by convulsions, tetany, or numbness.

Phosphorus: This essential element exists in the human body as phosphate groups (PO_4^{3-}), not only in bone and blood, but also in organic compounds such as ATP and in DNA and other nucleotides (Fig. 1.2). Phosphorus has important regulatory functions in intracellular processes via kinase-catalyzed phosphorylation and dephosphorylations that activate and deactivate a large number of key enzymes in internal metabolism. Chemically, arsenate and phosphate have similarities, and arsenic compounds may interfere with the organic binding of phosphates in DNA. The total amount of phosphorus in a human body is about 700 g. At physiological pH, phosphate in blood exists predominantly as a mixture of the buffering anion pair HPO_4^{2-} and $H_2PO_4^{-}$. Average

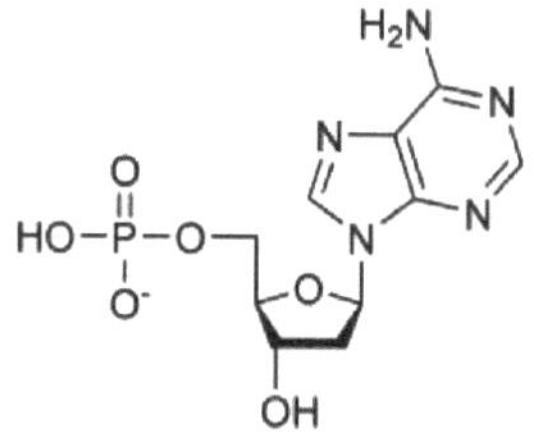

FIGURE 1.2 A nucleotide containing the sugar deoxyribose covalently bond to adenine and a phosphate group. This structure is named a deoxyribonucleotide, and is a constituent of DNA. The oxygen in the phosphate group can bind magnesium and other metals with low electronegativity by complexation through a predominantly ionic bond.

phosphate levels in blood plasma are 0.8−1.5 mmol/L. Increased phosphate levels in blood may result from renal insufficiency. Patients with end-stage renal disease in dialysis with blood phosphate values above 1.8 mmol/L should be treated with a phosphate binder. Nowadays, lanthanum carbonate (Fosrenol, Shire Pharmaceutical) is a commonly used phosphate binder. Whereas dietary phosphate restriction and removal of phosphate by dialysis is often insufficient to prevent hyperphosphatemia, administration of lanthanum carbonate as chewable 500, 750, or 1000 mg tablets, three times a day, combined with dialysis, is usually efficient to avoid severe hyperphosphatemia with secondary hyperparathyroidism.

Sulfur: This essential element for the human body must be ingested in an organic form. The sulfur amino acid methionine is the sulfur species classified as essential in the human diet. Another important sulfur amino acid, cysteine, can be synthesized by the human body if sufficient quantities of methionine are available. The sulfur in cysteine exists as a thiol group. Due to the ability of thiols to undergo redox reactions, cysteine has antioxidant properties. These properties are typically expressed in the tripeptide glutathione, which occurs intracellularly in millimolar concentrations in humans as well as in other organisms. The bioavailability of orally given glutathione (GSH) as such is negligible; it is degraded in the intestine so it must be synthesized intracellularly from its constituent amino acids, namely cysteine, glycine, and glutamic acid. GSH is an important endogenous detoxifying agent both for reactive organic electrophilic compounds and for metals. It is a necessary cofactor of the selenium-enzyme family of glutathione peroxidases that detoxifies intracellular peroxides. Cysteine and methionine play important roles in protein structure. The thiol group also has a high affinity for heavy metals, so that proteins containing cysteine may be targets in heavy metal poisonings. The low molecular weight thiol-rich protein, metallothionein, has a particularly high ability to bind metals such as zinc, copper, mercury, lead, and cadmium.

Potassium: This cation occurs predominantly intracellularly and contributes significantly to the intracellular osmolality. The body contains about 105 g of potassium. The electrochemical potential in nerves depends on the physiological presence of potassium, and thus it is of importance for the signaling in nerves. In the intracardial pathways of signaling and regulation of heart rhythm, it is of particular significance. Some other elements such as lithium, cesium, and thallium have chemical similarities with potassium, and may displace potassium from important intracellular locations.

Sodium: This is the extracellular counterpart of potassium. It regulates the amount of water in the extracellular space via osmotic homeostatic processes together with other electrolytes and macromolecules, and together with potassium it regulates the total amount of water in the body. In nerves it is fundamental for the electrical signaling. Unphysiologically high intakes of sodium as table salt may increase the blood pressure. Ordinarily, the body contains about 90 g of sodium.

Chlorine: In the form of the chloride anion this element is important for balancing the cations in the body, in particular the sodium cation extracellularly and the potassium cation intracellularly. The human body contains about 115 g of chlorine. Extracellularly, the important anions are chloride (about 100 mmol/L) and bicarbonate (normally about 25 mmol/L). Since the physiological extracellular amount of cations (sodium plus potassium) is about 140 mmol/L, there are a so called "anion gap" of about 140–125 mmol/L, that predominantly is made up of negatively charged proteins.

Magnesium: It is important in more than 300 metabolic reactions, many of these are related to energy production and consumption. A crucial substrate in these reactions is the Mg-ATP complex. One example of a magnesium-dependent energy-consuming process is the import of potassium into cells that is coupled to the export of sodium out of cells and catalyzed by the Na-K-ATPase. Magnesium is also important in the structure of skeleton and muscles. The amount of magnesium in an adult human body is about 30 g.

Iron: It is implied in at least hundred enzymatic reactions, and Fe^{2+} represents the oxygen-carrying core of hemoglobin. The extracellular amounts of the toxic "ionized iron" are negligible, since the plasma protein transferrin has extremely high affinity for Fe^{3+}. Extracellular hemoglobin may also act as a prooxidant, but intracellularly it is shielded not only by the red cell membrane, but also by intracellular glutathione (about 3 mmol/L) and the antioxidative enzyme glutathione peroxidase. In sickle cell anemia, thalassemia, and/or transfusional siderosis, toxic amounts of iron are deposited in liver, heart, and other organs.

Zinc: It takes part in the enzymatic action of more than 300 proteins and has important functions in organizing the tertiary structure of proteins via zinc fingers. Many zinc finger proteins function via interactions with nucleic acids, for example, regulation of gene expression by transcription factors interacting with DNA responsive elements through zinc fingers. Zinc deficiency in developing countries leads to decreased resistance against infection, particularly in children, and in severe cases, it may lead to hypogonadism and dwarfism. Abundant intakes of zinc induce synthesis of a metal-binding protein, metallothionein, also in gut mucosal cells, and may thereby protect against toxic actions of copper, for example, in Wilson's disease.

Copper: It is important in various enzymatic reactions, particularly as an electron donor. In the respiratory chain in mitochondria, the copper enzyme cytochrome c oxidase operates as an electron transporter. High intakes of copper may lead to toxic effects. In the hereditary defect in copper excretion known as Wilson's disease, physiological intakes are also toxic.

Iodine: It is required for the biosynthesis of the thyroid hormones, thyroxin, and triiodothyronine. Iodine deficiency is an important health problem throughout the world, leading to goiter, decreased synthesis of thyroid hormones, hypothyreosis, and children with impaired brain development and cretinism.

Selenium: It is essential for a variety of enzymes including several antioxidants. Unlike sulfur that has to be ingested in organic form, predominantly as methionine, inorganic selenium as selenite is incorporated into the amino acid selenocysteine and further into selenoenzymes by a specific genetic machinery that is unique and different from that of "ordinary" amino acids in the human organism.

Chromium: In its trivalent state, chromium apparently contributes to regulate blood glucose levels and the transport of glucose into cells, presumably by some interaction with the insulin action. The exact mechanism of this interaction is however not fully understood.

Manganese: It is essential in a number of enzymes, of which the manganese superoxide dismutase (MnSOD) is of particular importance, since it protects mitochondria from toxic oxidants. Overexposure to manganese, for example, exposure at the work place, may give rise to "manganism" with symptoms as in Parkinsonism.

Molybdenum: It is considered to have several functions. In the gut microbiome, it is important for the transformation of inorganic nitrogen by nitrogen-fixing bacteria, into organic forms.

Cobalt: It is essential as a component of vitamin B_{12} (cobalamin), that is vital for several biological processes, especially for the transfer of methyl groups, for example, into DNA. Whereas iron can be introduced into the resembling porphyrin ring in the human body by an enzyme ferrochelatase, the entire cobalamin molecule must be supplied by the diet.

1.3 EFFECTS OF TOXIC EXPOSURE OF AN ESSENTIAL OR NONESSENTIAL METAL

1.3.1 Basic Concepts in Chemical Toxicity Testing

Both essential and nonessential metals may exert toxic effects if the dose of ingestion or exposure exceeds certain levels (Mertz, 1981), often referred to as *critical levels*. The effects induced at these levels by a toxic agent may be referred to as critical effects. These effects arises from the so-called *critical organ* (Nordberg, 2004). For example, the central nervous system is the critical organ in cases of elemental mercury vapor exposure. When discussing metal

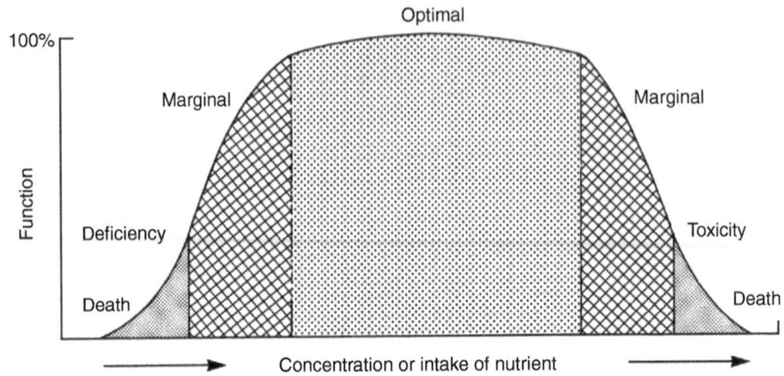

FIGURE 1.3 Schematic picture illustrating an optimal plateau of intake of an essential trace element. Apparently, unphysiologically low or high intakes lead to pathological processes. *(Source: Adapted from Mertz, 1981.)*

toxicity it should be emphasized that not only concentration range, but also speciation and oxidation state are crucial factors that affect the poisoning aspects of a metal in question.

Dose-effect and dose-response relationships are fundamental concepts in toxicology. A dose-effect relationship exists if an increase in the dose of a chemical (here: of a metal compound) causes a quantifiable increase in the toxic effect observed or if additional undesirable effects occur (may be illustrated as in the right half of Fig. 1.3). On the other hand, if an observed effect is not quantifiable in single individuals, but is either present or not present (often called all-or-none effect), a *dose-response* relationship exists if the percentage of a population responding with that effect depends on the dose of the chemical. A schematic dose-response relationship is shown in Fig. 1.4. It is also possible to depict a quantifiable effect on a dose-response curve, by illustrating the percentage of the population with the value of a biomarker above a certain level, for example, beta-2-microglobulin in urine above a certain threshold.

The goal of chemical toxicity testing, and toxicological research is to identify potential adverse health effects that can be caused by low doses of unintentional exposure to environmental toxicants, for example, toxic metal compounds.

One basic principle of the framework provided by National Research Council in the analysis of the dose-response curve (Fig. 1.4) is to define a window of interest in the lower part of the curve (Barnes & Dourson, 1988). This is the window between the lowest observed adverse effect level (LOAEL) and the no observed adverse effect level (NOAEL). Thus, the LOAEL is the lowest dose tested with a statistically significant effect, whereas the NOAEL is identified as the highest dose tested without a statistically significant effect. The LOAEL identifies the more frequently used term "critical dose." A more frequently used approach nowadays is to model the dose-response relationship

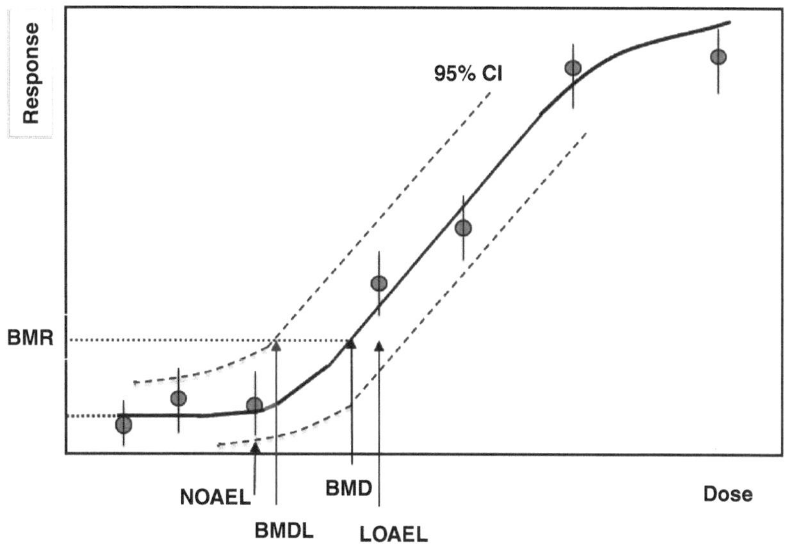

FIGURE 1.4 Schematic dose-response curve, illustrating the no adverse effect level (NOAEL) and the lowest adverse effect level (LOAEL) of a toxic substance. Confidence interval *(CI)*, benchmark response *(BMR)*, benchmark dose *(BMD)*, and benchmark dose lower confidence interval *(BMDL)* are also indicated. A risk assessor would choose the study displaying the most sensitive endpoint when identifying the LOAEL or the critical dose.

with confidence limits and based on a defined benchmark response (BMR), usually 5 or 10%, determine the benchmark dose (BMD) and a benchmark dose lower confidence limit (BMDL) associated with the BMR. In this way not only information on the tested doses are used, but the whole dose response (EFSA, 2009).

The identification of a critical exposure, that is, a benchmark dose or LOAEL in an individual does not constitute an indication for institution of chelation therapy. Thus, in the case of lead, for instance in an analysis of several epidemiological studies, EFSA identified a BMDL01 (1% change, benchmark response) for neurocognitive effect in children of 12 μg/L in blood (Alexander et al., 2010). The US Centers for Disease Control and Prevention (CDC) use a reference value of 50 μg/L (0.24 μmol/L) in blood. This reference value is based on the 97.5 percentile of the National Health and Nutrition Examination Survey (NHANES) blood lead distribution in children. The present guidelines (AAP, 1995, 2005) involve that monitoring and removal of environmental lead is the action of choice at blood Pb levels in the range 50–450 μg/L (0.24–2.2 μmol/L), whereas chelation treatment is indicated only at blood Pb levels exceeding 450 μg/L (2.2 μmol/L). In these cases, chelation with DMSA (Succimer) is recommended (see chapter: Chelation Treatment During Acute and Chronic Metal Overexposures—Experimental and Clinical Studies for details).

1.3.2 Exposure Patterns and Mechanisms of Metal Toxicity

Various factors act as determinants of a clinical effect after exposure to a toxic metal. Such factors include route of absorption; the dose and the chemical and physical form of the metal concerned; genetic variation manifested through racial, familial, and individual susceptibility; nutritional status; immunological status; and presence of intercurrent disease. The exposure pattern, in terms of concentration, time, and route of exposure, is an important determinant of clinical effects that requires further consideration here.

The effects of *ingestion* of a toxic metal may be seen in the domestic or general environment rather than in an industrial setting. Short-term, high-level exposure by ingestion may follow the accidental, suicidal, or homicidal ingestion of a toxic metal compound, giving rise to well-recognized acute syndromes, usually involving the gastrointestinal tract and possibly involving secondarily the renal, cardiovascular, nervous, and hematopoietic systems.

Long-term, low-level exposure by ingestion is seen increasingly in the general environment as a result of the contamination of food and drink by metals that have cumulative properties in the organism, for example, arsenic. Clinical effects may involve any organ system in the body, but the gastrointestinal tract is not primarily involved.

A short-term *inhalation* exposure may produce a clinical effect very different from that produced by a long-term exposure—similar in terms of total dose over a longer period of time. Short-term, high-level inhalation exposure is most often occupational in origin. It may not only give rise to acute respiratory effects but may also involve the cardiovascular, central nervous, renal, and hematopoietic systems. Long-term, low-level inhalation exposure is usually also occupational in origin, and control measures form a large part of industrial hygiene practice. However, long-term, low-level inhalation exposure to certain toxic metals may also occur in the general environment and from smoking cigarettes. The effects may involve any organ system in the body and may spare the respiratory system.

Mercury: It offers a good example of the extreme variation in clinical effects that may be produced, depending on the pattern of exposure and the chemical form of the metal (Kazantzis, 1980). After short-term high-level inhalation exposure to mercury vapor (Hg^0), the lung initially is the critical organ resulting in pneumonitis and respiratory failure, whereas the CNS is the critical organ after long-term low-level exposure to the same mercury vapor. Upon distribution to the vulnerable sites, the lipophilic elementary Hg^0 is converted to the toxic species, Hg^{2+} that binds to and intoxicates thiol groups on proteins and also selenol groups in selenoenzymes, for example, in the brain.

After the ingestion of an inorganic soluble mercuric salt, for example, $HgCl_2$, the kidney becomes the critical organ, manifesting with anuria resulting from tubular necrosis. As a result of the long-term ingestion of methylmercury (CH_3Hg^+) as a food contaminant, nervous system effects may develop, but with a clinical picture that differs from that seen after the long-term inhalation of inorganic mercury vapor. The variability in clinical effects produced by the toxic metals is further illustrated in the following section. Adverse effects that result from exposure to the individual metals are described in succeeding chapters of this handbook.

Mechanisms of metal toxicity may also be illustrated by effect of mercury on cellular and subcellular constituents, as the various mercury compounds penetrates to and intoxicates various functional thiol and selenol groups of proteins in cellular compartments in various organs. As ions of inorganic or organic mercury are electrophilic, they have high affinity to electron donor groups, particularly to sulfur and selenium groups. Thus, proteins containing the sulfur amino acid cysteine or the selenoamino acid selenocysteine may constitute sensitive sites in cases of mercury exposure.

1.3.3 Gastrointestinal Effects of Metal Exposure

Acute gastroenteritis follows the ingestion of a toxic quantity of most metals in the form of soluble salts. A common occurrence is precipitated by contamination of foods or drinks, especially if acidic, by dissolution of metal from food containers. Symptoms develop a short time after ingestion, often involving a number of people, and may be mistaken as "viral food poisoning." Vomiting and diarrhea may be followed by circulatory collapse and involvement of other systems, depending on the poison absorbed. Poisonings with soluble compounds of copper, antimony, cadmium, lead, tin, and zinc have occurred in this way. Acute gastroenteritis with collapse may be the predominant feature after the ingestion of rodenticides containing thallium, arsenic, yellow phosphorus, or zinc phosphide. Similar symptoms may follow the ingestion of soluble compounds of bismuth, chromium, iron, silver, and vanadium. The ingestion of a soluble mercuric salt gives rise to gastroenteritis with a bloody diarrhea that may resemble fulminating ulcerative colitis. Lead colic, which may occur as an acute effect after prolonged exposure to lead, has on some occasions simulated an acute surgical emergency.

Long-lasting gastrointestinal symptoms have occurred in people drinking canned juice contaminated with high concentrations of tin or zinc, or drinking water contaminated with copper. Such intake of copper may disturb the intestinal microbiome. Intestinal colic has been observed in children or industrial workers with relatively low-level lead exposure. Anorexia, vomiting, diarrhea, and stomatitis have resulted from occupational exposure to thallium compounds.

1.3.4 Respiratory Effects of Metal Exposure

Acute chemical pneumonitis, which may be accompanied by pulmonary edema, follows the inhalation of a number of freshly formed metal fumes. Particularly toxic in this respect is the inhalation of freshly formed cadmium oxide fume, with acute symptoms developing some hours after an apparently innocuous exposure (Beton, Andrews, Davies, Howells, & Smith, 1966). The inhalation of antimony pentachloride, arsine, beryllium fume, iron pentacarbonyl, lithium hydride, nickel carbonyl, titanium tetrachloride, selenium dioxide, hydrogen selenide, vanadium pentoxide, or zinc chloride can give rise to a similarly acute picture with pulmonary edema. The inhalation of high concentrations of mercury vapor or dust or inorganic mercury compounds can also give rise to pneumonitis before other symptoms of mercurialism develop. Respiratory symptoms with rigors and fever resembling an acute respiratory infection may follow the inhalation of freshly formed zinc fume, brass fume, or other metallic oxides, giving rise to metal-fume fever. Pneumonic consolidation has followed the inhalation of manganese dust. In some cases of chemical pneumonitis steroid inhalations may reduce the symptoms, and administration by CaEDTA via nebulizer may also alleviate the condition.

An inflammatory response with granuloma formation may result from exposure to beryllium with a latency of several years (Stoeckle, Hardy, & Weber, 1969). Progressive dyspnea with the clinical and radiological characteristics of emphysema is seen in workers exposed to cadmium oxide fume. A rather benignant fibrosis referred to as Shaver's disease has followed occupational exposure to aluminum dust. Vanadium pentoxide dust has given rise to an illness resembling asthmatic bronchitis. Pulmonary fibrosis has occurred in workers exposed to dusts of tungsten and titanium carbides. Chronic asthma can occur after long-term inhalation of chromate dust.

1.3.5 Hepatic and Renal Effects

Renal damage, manifesting as acute oliguria or anuria caused by acute tubular necrosis, is another way in which metal poisoning may present, although this feature often follows an initial presentation with acute gastrointestinal, circulatory, or respiratory effects. Oliguria and anuria caused by tubular necrosis are common occurrences, especially in children, after the ingestion of soluble mercuric or iron salts. Hemodialysis combined with administration of appropriate chelator may be beneficial in such cases. Renal failure may also follow pneumonitis resulting from cadmium fume inhalation, and acute oliguria has also been a sequel to the absorption of a number of soluble metal compounds, including antimony, arsine, bismuth, copper, uranium, and vanadium salts.

Chronic renal disorders may also follow exposure to toxic metals. Proximal tubular dysfunction with tubular proteinuria may develop after cumulative exposure to cadmium or other metal compounds. Hypercalciuria has also occurred in long-term cadmium exposure as a further manifestation of tubular dysfunction. This has been associated with osteomalacia in a few cases after industrial exposure (Kazantzis, 1979). Osteomalacia has been observed in a Japanese population environmentally exposed to cadmium (Friberg, 1984), and it was presumed that this so-called itai-itai disease was precipitated by renal tubular dysfunction.

Impairment in renal functions terminating in renal failure has been observed after childhood lead poisoning. And heavy proteinuria as in nephrotic syndrome has followed exposure to inorganic mercury, gold, and bismuth preparations. The previous use of gold salts in the treatment of rheumatoid arthritis could give rise to tubular dysfunction. And the platinum compounds particularly *cis*-diamine-dichloroplatinum used in the treatment of testicular cancer may also give rise to such side effects.

Several metals are also hepatotoxic, giving rise to effects ranging from abnormalities in enzyme levels to clinical jaundice. Such effects have been reported after exposure to copper, arsenic, antimony, bismuth, iron, and other metal compounds.

1.3.6 Effects on the Nervous System

Metal poisoning may present with an acute illness involving the CNS. Most important, because unfortunately still not uncommon in children, are convulsive attacks that may terminate in coma or lead to death as a result of acute lead poisoning. A successful therapeutic outcome in such cases depends on early diagnosis and treatment. Convulsions may also follow the absorption of iron, barium, lithium, thallium, and organic tin compounds. Acute psychosis may also be the presenting feature in metal poisoning. After heavy exposure to tetraethyl lead, a patient may present with delusions, hallucinations, and hyperactivity that may precede coma and death (Beattie, Moore, & Goldberg, 1972).

Peripheral neuropathy may develop in the recovery stage of acute arsenic intoxication, about 1–3 weeks after exposure. It is a mixed motor and sensory neuropathy, with a "glove and stocking" distribution. Neuropathy develops in those who survive the acute gastrointestinal effects of thallium poisoning, and it may lead to a later fatal termination. With both these metals, skin changes occur at a later stage, with the former metal, arsenical pigmentation results, and with the latter, hair loss. A motor neuropathy involving predominantly the upper limbs with wrist drop and extensor weakness of the fingers is seen in chronic lead poisoning. By contrast, antimony salts of organic acids give rise to a sensory neuropathy that may involve the trigeminal nerve. Bismuth and copper have also given rise to peripheral neuropathy.

Permanent brain damage with cerebral cortical atrophy or hydrocephalus may be the sequel to acute lead encephalopathy. Convulsions may recur over a long period, and idiocy may develop.

The use of lead paints and leaded gasoline has given rise to the widespread occurrence of lead in the environment. Elevated blood lead levels after long-term exposure to house dust with decaying fragments of leaded paint has been shown in epidemiological studies to affect cognitive development in children (Bellinger, Stiles, & Needleman, 1992; Needleman, Schell, Bellinger, Leviton, & Allred, 1990).

Degenerative changes in the nerve cells of the basal ganglia giving rise to a Parkinsonian syndrome were considered to result from the absorption of manganese after long-term occupational exposure, so called "manganism" (Mena, Court, Fuenzalida, Papavasiliou, & Cotzias, 1970). Parkinson's disease, not an uncommon disorder, is characterized by muscular rigidity, akinesia, tremor, and postural deformities. In a case-control study to determine whether welding-related Parkinsonism in welders exposed to manganese differs from idiopathic Parkinson's disease, welders had a significantly younger age of onset of Parkinsonism, suggesting welding as a risk factor for this condition (Racette et al., 2001). Degenerative changes affecting in particular the granular cells in the cerebellum and neurons in the calcarine, precentral, and postcentral cortex, follow the absorption of alkyl mercury compounds and present with a characteristic neurological syndrome whose principal features are paresthesia of extremities and face, ataxia, dysarthria, and concentric constriction of the fields of vision. Pyramidal signs may also occur. Another characteristic neurological disorder consisting principally of intention tremor of the hands, tremor of the eyelids and tongue, and a combination of behavioral and personality changes known as erethism develops after chronic exposure to mercury vapor.

1.3.7 Hematological Effects

Acute hemolytic anemia often accompanied by renal failure may be the presenting feature after the inhalation of arsine (AsH_3) or stibine (SbH_3) gases (Jenkins, Ind, Kazantzis, & Owen, 1965). Thus, arsine toxicity is distinct from that of other arsenic compounds. Apparently, arsine as well as stibine attack hemoglobin, causing the red cells to be destroyed by the body (Hatlelid, Brailsford, & Carter, 1996). Signs of exposure, which can take several hours to become apparent, are the symptoms of hemolytic anemia, hemoglobinuria and nephropathy. In severe cases, the damage to the kidneys can be long lasting. Chelating agents are considered to be contraindicated and exchange transfusion is the treatment of choice in arsine and stibine poisonings.

Acute hemolysis has also followed the ingestion of large doses of soluble copper salts, when copper ions are absorbed into the circulation. Similarly, hemolysis may also be an early sign of Wilson's disease, resulting from the release of copper ions from liver tissue. Cases of copper-induced hemolysis have been successfully treated with chelation. D-penicillamine has often been used in these cases. Hemolytic anemia might also be a clinical trait of thalassaemia and other hemoglobinopathies.

Chronic arsenic poisoning is associated with an anemia caused by decreased formation and increased destruction of red cells. Arsenic also suppresses the formation of white blood cells, and its compounds apparently have a therapeutic potential in the treatment of certain types of leukemia. Thus, complete remission of acute promyelocytic leukemia has been reported after treatment with arsenic trioxide (Soignet et al., 1998). The anemia of chronic lead poisoning also results from decreased hematopoiesis combined with increased red cell destruction (Goyer & Rhyne, 1973). In contrast, cobalt increases hematopoiesis and has given rise to polycythemia, but not to increased production of other cellular elements in the blood.

1.3.8 Cardiovascular Effects

A number of metallic ions interfere with the normal function of myocardial cells, giving rise to arrhythmias, including ventricular fibrillation. Ventricular fibrillation may be responsible for a fatal outcome in cases of poisoning by antimony, barium, or lithium salts. Cobalt can give rise to cardiomyopathy (Alexander, 1972). Some metals have been shown to have a hypotensive effect. These include antimony, cadmium, cobalt, copper, iron, and vanadium, a state of shock being a common presenting feature in poisoning with these metals.

1.3.9 Metal Allergies

Many metal compounds by their binding to proteins act as haptens that induce allergic reactions. Nickel allergy is the most common form of cutaneous hypersensitivity. Many commonly used alloys contain nickel, often in combination with palladium or cobalt that may also induce allergy. In a study of Norwegian school children, the highest frequency of positive metal patch tests was found among girls with a combination of atopy and ear piercing (Dotterud & Falk, 1994).

Coronary in-stent restenosis may be triggered by contact allergy to nickel or chromate ions released from stainless-steel stents (Koster et al., 2000). Leather products, especially leather shoes, are common sources of chromium exposure and dermatitis, since chromium is used for leather tanning (Hansen, Johansen, & Menne, 2003). Mercury amalgam is probably the dental alloy mostly associated with oral mucosal changes such as oral lichen planus. Mercury exposure may also cause cutaneous lichen planus and palmoplantar pustulosis (Fardal, Johannessen, & Morken, 2005). There are limited documentation of possible effects of ointments containing steroids and/or chelating agents.

1.3.10 Carcinogenic Effects

Arsenic, cadmium, chromium, nickel, and beryllium compounds have been shown to be carcinogenic to humans (Wild, Bourgkard, & Paris, 2009). Most of the data have been collected from retrospective studies of humans with an occupational exposure to these metals. For arsenic an increased risk of lung and skin cancer has been reported (Lundstrom, Englyst, Gerhardsson, Jin, & Nordberg, 2006). For cadmium, the overall cancer risk is increased, particularly for lung cancer (Sorahan & Lancashire, 1997). Increased lung cancer risk has also been found among workers exposed to chromium(VI) (Langard, Andersen,

& Ravnestad, 1990). A significant excess of lung cancer as well of as cancer of the nasal sinuses has been observed in nickel refinery and welding workers (Langard, 1994). Exposure to beryllium has also been found to cause an excess in lung cancer mortality (Ward, Okun, Ruder, Fingerhut, & Steenland, 1992). To the knowledge of the authors, no studies have shown any anticarcinogenic potential of chelation therapy of metal exposed groups.

1.4 BASIS FOR METAL COMPLEX FORMATION WITH ENDOGENOUS AND EXOGENOUS LIGANDS

In clinical medicine, treatment with a chelating agent (Fig. 1.5) aims at the removal of toxic metal ions from the sensitive tissue sites in the critical organs. This can be achieved when the chemical affinity of the complexing agent for the metal ions is higher than the affinity of the metal for the sensitive biological molecules. An example of a widely used copper-chelating agent in clinical toxicology is D-penicillamine (dimethyl cysteine) that also has relatively high affinity for mercury (Strand, Lund, & Aaseth, 1983).

Chemical assessments of *the stability constants* of the metal-complexes formed may give a first indication of the effectiveness of a chelating agent in clinical metal poisonings. In simple cases of formation of a metal complex (ML), the interaction can be described by the equilibrium shown later, where M represents the solvated metal ion and L represents a chelator with electron pair–donating groups. The stability constant, K_1, for a mononuclear 1-to-1-complex is then given by a simple equation, as follows:

$$K_1 = \frac{[ML]}{[M][L]} \qquad (1.1)$$

The square brackets in Eq. (1.1) denote concentrations (or activities) of interacting species at equilibrium. Since chelating agents may contain several coordination groups, such as, for example, the classical chelating agent EDTA (ethylenediamine tetraacetate), the complexity of the calculations of equilibrium concentrations, even in simple aqueous solutions, may be much more complicated, as can be illustrated by listing some other oligonuclear complexes,

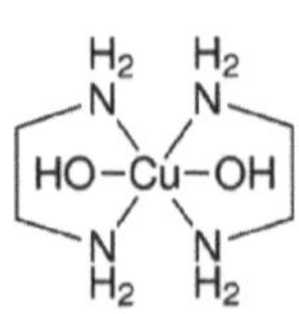

FIGURE 1.5 The bis(ethylenediamine) copper(II) hydroxide complex is an example of a chelate. Ethylenediamine contains two donor nitrogen atoms and acts as a bidentate ligand. A heteroatomic ring is formed. This process of ring formation is called chelation, and ligands such as ethylenediamine may be referred to as chelating agents.

such as M_2L, ML_2, and M_2L_2. In addition, when complexation occurs in body fluids, M and L enter into several side reactions, involving that the free concentrations of L and M in the body fluids and tissues may be much smaller than the total concentrations ($[L_t]$ and $[M_t]$) of the interacting species. This has been taken into account by introducing the so-called conditional stability constant (Ringbom & Harju, 1972) or effective stability constant, K_{eff} (Aaseth, 1983). Theoretically, the chelated, or mobilized metal fraction, [ML], will be determined by the effective stability constant, K_{eff} and the tissue concentration $[L_t]$ of the chelating agent, as is seen by rearranging Eq. (1.1):

$$\frac{[ML]}{M_t} = K_{eff} \times [L_t] \tag{1.2}$$

It should be emphasized here that a high tissue concentration $[L_t]$ can only be obtained by using chelators with relatively low toxicity. Furthermore, to achieve an efficient chelation treatment, the chelation reaction should never reach equilibrium, that is, the chelate formed, [ML], should be continuously removed from the equilibrium, for instance via urine.

Some crucial qualities of a chelator to deduce its clinical effectiveness may be summarized as follows:

- appropriate pharmacokinetics;
- high affinity toward the toxic metal;
- low toxicity;
- formation of chelate with rapid elimination (detoxification).

It is apparent from Table 1.1 that the antidote BAL (British AntiLewisite) is much more toxic than other dithiol antidotes (Aposhian et al., 1984; Zvirblis & Ellin, 1976) or D-penicillamine (Cantilena & Klaassen, 1981). Also other metal antidotes, such as trientine, deferoxamine, or deferiprone, have relatively low toxicity compared to BAL (Ciba-Geygy, 1994; Kontoghiorghes, 1995; Lewis & Tatken, 1980). With regard to the chemical stability of a therapeutic chelate, it is of interest that the first approximation of the affinity of a ligand (L) toward a toxic metal can be deduced from the Hard-Soft-Acid-Base (HSAB) concept, as discussed earlier (Aaseth, 1983; Andersen & Aaseth, 2002).

Lewis (1938) defined an acid as an electron pair acceptor, and a base as an electron pair donor. According to this terminology, all the positively charged metal ions can be classified as acids, since they may act as electron acceptors. The formation of a solvated (hydrated) metal ion is in fact the formation of a complex. Here, the water molecule acts as an electron donor, and H_2O can thus be described as a Lewis base. Many other oxygen-containing agents can be described as Lewis bases as well. In aqueous solutions, metal ions exist in solvated forms, and chelation or complexation involves that water in the solvated shell is replaced by another ligand (another Lewis base) to give a metal complex.

Lewis acids and bases can be classified as hard or soft ones. A hard metal ion is one that retains its valence electrons very strongly and has small size and high

TABLE 1.1 Clinically Important Chelating Agents

Compound	Species	Administration route	LD_{50}	References
$CaNa_2EDTA$	Mouse, rat	ip	4–6 g/kg	(Catsch & Harmuth-Hoene, 1976)
BAL	Mouse	ip	90–180 mg/kg	(Zvirblis & Ellin, 1976)
DMSA	Mouse	ip	2.48 g/kg	(Aposhian et al., 1984)
DMPS	Mouse, rat	ip	1.1–1.4 g/kg	(Aposhian et al., 1984)
Trientine	Mouse, rat	oral	1.6–2.5 g/kg	(Lewis & Tatken, 1980)
D-penicillamine	Mouse	ip	337 mg/kg	(Cantilena & Klaassen, 1981)
Deferoxamine	Rat	iv	520 mg/kg	(Ciba-Geygy, 1994)
Deferiprone	Mouse, rat	ip	0.6–1 g/kg	(Kontoghiorghes, 1995)

The acute toxicity is illustrated by representative LD_{50}-values selected from the large published database.
Modified from Andersen (1999).

charge. In contrast, a soft ion is relatively large and does not retain its valence electrons firmly. Examples of hard metal ions are Li^+, Mg^{2+}, and Fe^{3+}. Soft metals include copper(I), mercury(II), arsenic, polonium(II) and platinum(II) (Lippard, Berg, & Garner, 1995).

The hardness/softness characteristics of the electron donor ligands and the metal ions determine the stability of metal complexes and chelates, as discussed by Pearson in his works on the HSAB theory (Pearson, 1963). As a rule, the formation of stable complexes results from the interaction of hard bases with hard acids, or soft bases with soft acids. Typical examples of hard bases contain oxygen as donor atom, whereas nitrogen can be classified as a hard-to-intermediate donor atom. Thus, Fe(II) as well as Fe(III) will interact with oxygen or nitrogen in biological fluids, for example, in the synthesis or formation of molecules such as heme or hemoglobin. On the other hand, easily polarized ligands containing sulfur or selenium are classified as soft groups, forming stable complexes with mercury, polonium, arsenic, and with copper(I) and lead. Thus, the monothiols D-penicillamine and cysteine (Fig. 1.6) have high affinity to copper and lead. The bonding in hard–hard complexes is largely electrostatic, for example, the

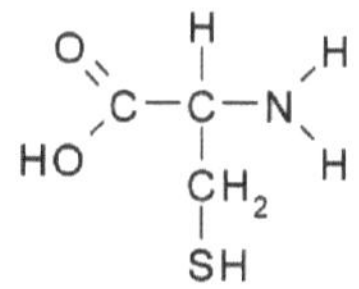

FIGURE 1.6 Chemical structure of the amino acid cysteine that is a monothiol. Cysteine is a constituent of the tripeptide glutathione and of several proteins, for example, the low molecular weight protein family of metallothioneins. Both glutathione and metallothioneins have high affinity to sulfur-seeking metals such as mercury and arsenic.

iron-oxygen bond, whereas soft–soft complexes have bonds with a predominantly covalent nature, for example, the mercury-thiol bond. Mercury, as well as arsenic, has strikingly high electronegativity, namely about 2.0 in Pauling units, and consequently high tendency to be engaged in covalent bonding to carbon as well as to sulfur, compared to other metals. This explains the existence of a large number of organomercurials and organoarsenicals.

Because of the availability of numerous small biological ligands in living organisms, the concentrations of "free" toxic metals are often very low. Thus, endogenous low molecular weight compounds such as cysteine, arginine, glutamate, citrate, and glutathione, as well as proteins are metal-binding agents. An example of an endogenous multidentate structure of great biological significance is the porphyrin core of hemoglobin, which encapsulates Fe^{2+}, and thereby presents this toxic ion as the vital carrier of oxygen (Fig. 1.7).

The iron-porphyrin chelate can be referred to as a *robust* complex, involving that iron cannot be removed rapidly from its binding sites by an exogenous chelator. Therapeutic chelation of toxic metal ions in vivo may also proceed slowly, as the removal of the metal from endogenous multidentate molecules may involve several steps. Even if the equilibrium (stability) constant of the complex with a therapeutic agent is favorable, complex formation in vivo may be limited because of exchange rate effects and transport kinetics of the chelator (Andersen & Aaseth, 2002). The ability of a chelator to penetrate into the particular compartment of the metal deposits and thus reach the critical molecular sites may constitute important determinants for its clinical efficacy. For instance, the removal of iron, copper, or lead deposits from the central nervous

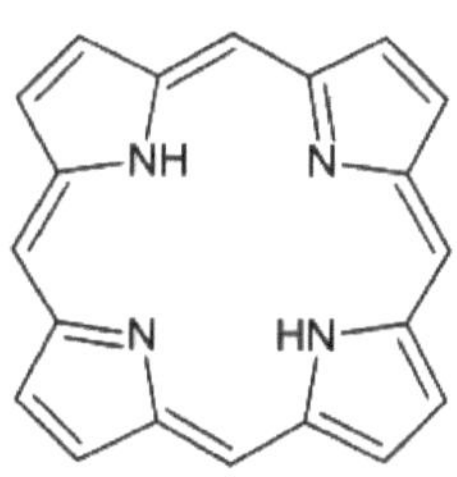

FIGURE 1.7 The porphyrin structure of hemoglobin uses nitrogen groups as chelating ligands resulting in high affinity for iron.

system usually proceeds slowly, because the penetration of chelators or chelates across the blood–brain barrier in most cases is limited.

Due to the complexity of biological systems, effects of antidotal agents are usually better quantitatively characterized by animal experiments (or clinical trials) than by theoretical calculations, as discussed extensively by Catsch and Harmuth-Hoene (1976). Because of the difficulty of conducting clinical trials, animal studies are indispensable. In such studies, new agents can be compared with traditional ones, for example, in delayed versus immediate treatment, as well as on dose-effect relationships, and on the toxicity of the agents. LD_{50}-values of clinically used chelators determined in animal experiments are given in Table 1.1. Although extrapolations from animals to humans may be difficult, it is crucial to assess the toxicity and efficiency of a new agent in the experimental studies before using it clinically. Some new approaches in the treatment of metal intoxications are outlined in the following sections, and further details may be found in the recent review by Crisponi, Nurchi, Crespo-Alonso, and Toso (2012).

1.5 ENDOGENOUS COMPLEXING AND DETOXIFICATION COMPOUNDS

Metallothioneins (MTs) and glutathione are examples of metal-complexing proteins or peptides in biological systems. But many other complexing agents exist and play a role in metal metabolism and detoxification. Other thiol-containing proteins, such as serum albumin, are important in the binding and transport of toxic metals. Proteins such as transferrin and ferritin ensure that the redox-active essential metal Fe does not create oxidative stress. The ability to sequester potentially toxic metals in an inert, preferably chelated form, is an essential trait of living organisms. Here, we will briefly discuss some of these endogenous metal-binding agents.

1.5.1 Albumin

Albumin is the most abundant protein in human blood plasma. The physiological reference range for albumin concentrations in serum is approximately 35–50 g/L (about 0.5–0.75 mmol/L). Its molecular weight is 66.5 kDa. Albumin is produced in the liver as proalbumin, which is cleaved in the Golgi vesicles to the circulating albumin. It has a serum half-life of approximately 20 days.

It binds metal cations such as Ca^{2+} and Mg^{2+}. It also contains a cysteine residue with a free thiol group that can bind and transport heavy metals such as copper, mercury, and cadmium. In addition, albumin binds and transports hormones, fatty acids, and drugs, and maintains the colloid-osmotic pressure of blood.

The gene for albumin is located on chromosome 4 and mutations in this gene can result in anomalous proteins. However, mutations causing hypoalbuminemia are rare. Pathologically low albumin, hypoalbuminemia, usually have other causes, for example, reduced production due to liver cirrhosis, or excessive losses, for example, due to nephrotic syndrome or protein-losing enteropathy. A down-regulation of albumin levels are also seen in acute inflammatory states as it is a negative acute phase protein.

Since about 50% of the blood plasma calcium is bound to albumin, the plasma level of total calcium of 2.2−2.6 mmol/L (9−10.5 mg/dL), is about twofold higher than the "ionized" calcium of 1.1−1.4 mmol/L (4.5−5.6 mg/dL).

1.5.2 Transferrin and Ferritin

Transferrin is a glycoprotein that binds iron very tightly, but reversibly. Although iron bound to transferrin is less than 0.1% (4 mg) of the total body iron, it is the most important iron pool, with the highest rate of turnover (25 mg/24 h). Transferrin has a molecular weight of around 80 kDa and contains two specific high-affinity Fe^{3+} binding sites. The affinity of transferrin for Fe^{3+} is extremely high with a stability constant of 10^{23} M^{-1} at pH 7.4 (Aisen, Leibman, & Zweier, 1978) but decreases progressively with decreasing pH below neutrality. When not bound to iron, the protein is referred to as apotransferrin.

When iron loaded transferrin encounters a transferrin receptor on the surface of a cell, for example, on an erythroid precursor cell in the bone marrow, it binds to it and, as a consequence, is transported into the cell in a vesicle by receptor-mediated endocytosis. The pH of the vesicle is reduced by to about 5.5 by a hydrogen ion pump, causing transferrin to release its iron ions. The receptor with its ligand, transferrin, is then transported back to the cell surface, ready for another round of iron uptake. Each transferrin molecule has the ability to carry two iron ions in the ferric form.

The gene coding for transferrin in humans is located in the chromosome band 3q21 (Yang et al., 1984). The liver is the main site of transferrin synthesis, but other tissues and organs, such as the brain, also produce it. In humans, transferrin consists of a polypeptide chain containing 679 amino acids. The N- and C- terminal sequences of the protein are represented by globular lobes and between the two lobes are the iron-binding sites.

The amino acids which bind the iron ion to the transferrin are identical for both lobes; two tyrosines, one histidine, and one aspartic acid. However, since iron ions have six coordinative binding valences, additional anions are required; preferably carbonate (CO_3^{2-}).

The main role of transferrin is to deliver iron from absorption centers in the duodenum and macrophages to all tissues. Transferrin plays a key role where erythropoiesis and active cell division occur (Macedo & de Sousa, 2008). The receptor helps maintain iron homeostasis in the cells by controlling iron concentrations. The transferrin binding receptor is a disulfide-linked dimer. In humans, each monomer consists of 760 amino acids. It enables ligand binding to the transferrin, and each monomer can bind to one or two molecules of iron. Each monomer consists of three domains: the protease, the helical, and the apical domains. The shape of transferrin receptor resembles a butterfly-like complex, due to the three clearly shaped domains.

Transferrin is also associated with the innate immune system. It is found in the mucosa, of the gut and binds iron, thus creating an environment low in free iron that impedes bacterial survival in a process called iron withholding. The level of transferrin decreases in inflammation (Ritchie et al., 1999). Most recently, transferrin and its receptor have been shown to diminish tumor cells in experimental models (Macedo & de Sousa, 2008). The metal-binding properties of transferrin have influence on the transport and metabolism of several other metals, including Ti^{4+}, Cr^{3+}, Bi^{3+}, Al^{3+}, and Pu^{4+} (Vincent & Love, 2012).

Carbohydrate deficient transferrin (CDT) increases in the blood with heavy ethanol consumption and can be monitored via laboratory testing.

The physiological reference range for transferrin is about 200–350 mg/dL. Laboratory test results should always be interpreted using the reference range provided by the laboratory that performed the test. An increased plasma transferrin level is often seen in patients suffering from iron deficiency anemia. Levels of serum iron and total iron binding capacity (TIBC) are used in conjunction with transferrin in diagnostics of iron deficiency or overload. A decreased plasma transferrin level can occur in iron overload diseases and protein malnutrition.

Ferritin is principally an intracellular iron-complexing protein, in contrast to transferrin that has an exclusively extracellular distribution. Ferritin stores iron and releases it in a controlled fashion. The protein is produced by almost all living organisms, including algae, bacteria, higher plants, and animals. In humans, it acts as a buffer against iron deficiency and iron overload (Wang, Knovich, Coffman, Torti, & Torti, 2010). Ferritin is found in most tissues as a cytosolic protein, but small amounts are secreted into the serum where it functions as an iron carrier. Ferritin keeps iron in a soluble and nontoxic form. Free iron is toxic to cells as it acts as a catalyst in the formation of free radicals from reactive oxygen species via the Fenton reaction. Hence vertebrates evolve an elaborate set of protective mechanisms and chaperones to bind iron in various tissue compartments. Within cells, iron is stored as ferritin or hemosiderin. As ferritin accumulates within cells of the reticuloendothelial system, protein aggregates are formed as hemosiderin. Iron in ferritin or hemosiderin can be extracted for release by the same cells although hemosiderin iron is less readily available. Under steady state conditions, the serum ferritin level correlates with total body iron stores; thus, the serum ferritin is the most convenient laboratory test to estimate iron stores.

Horse-spleen ferritin, a protein of 450 kDa, traditionally considered as a mammalian ferritin model, consists of a protein shell composed of 24 polypeptide subunits, with a hollow core capable of containing several thousand Fe atoms as trivalent ferrihydrite (Carmona et al., 2013). The polypeptide components are classified as heavy (H) or light (L) subunits, where the H-unit is associated with rapid detoxification of Fe(II), due to its content of ferroxidase, while the L-unit is associated with mineralization and long term storage in the cavity. It is assumed that Fe(II) moves through hydrophilic channels until oxidized by a ferroxidase center in the H-subunit. It has been shown that other elements than Fe can interact with ferritin, thus disturbing its function as a Fe detoxifier. Cadmium is competing with Fe for the same sites within the cavity but also on the external shell surface, particularly around the entry of the hydrophilic channels. This may hinder the entry of Fe. Zinc can also bind at the channel entrances, and its binding to ferroxidase site may reduce its oxidation capability. Copper is also known to interact with the ferritin molecule. Given the similarities between the transition elements Mn and Fe, it is also reasonable to assume that Mn(III) can interact with ferritin.

Ferritin genes are highly conserved between species. All vertebrate ferritin genes have three introns and four exons (Torti & Torti, 2002).

The exact function and structure of the expressed ferritin protein varies in different cell types. This is controlled primarily by the amount and stability of mRNA. mRNA concentration is further tweaked by changes to how it is stored and how efficiently it is transcribed (Theil, 1987). The presence of iron itself is a major trigger for the production of ferritin.

All subunits of bacterial ferritin are H-type and have ferroxidase activity, which carries out the conversion of iron from the ferrous (Fe^{2+}) to ferric (Fe^{3+}) forms. This limits the deleterious Fenton reaction, which occurs between ferrous iron and hydrogen peroxide producing the highly toxic hydroxyl radical. The ferroxidase activity occurs in the middle of each H-type subunits (Ebrahimi, Bill, Hagedoorn, & Hagen, 2012). After oxidation the Fe(III) product stays metastable in the ferroxidase center being displaced only by entering Fe(II), a mechanism that appears to be common among ferritins of all three kingdoms of life. The light chain of ferritin has no ferroxidase activity, but may be responsible for electron transfer across the protein cage (Carmona, Li, Zhang, & Knez, 2014).

Ferritin concentrations increase drastically in the presence of an infection or cancer. Endotoxin is also an upregulator of the gene coding for ferritin, thus causing the concentration of ferritin to rise. The concentration of ferritin has been shown to increase in response to stresses such as anoxia. This implies that it is an acute phase protein. A mitochondrial fraction of ferritin has many roles pertaining to molecular function. It participates in ferroxidase activity, ferrous and ferric iron binding, oxidoreductase activity, as well as transition metal binding, and iron ion transport across membranes.

Serum ferritin levels are measured in medical laboratories as part of the iron studies workup for iron deficiency or iron overload. The ferritin levels measured usually have a direct correlation with the total amount of iron stored in the body. However, ferritin levels may also be increased due to its capacity as an acute phase protein.

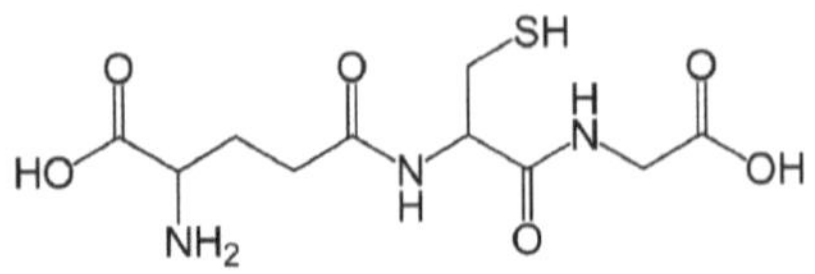

FIGURE 1.8 Chemical structure of the tripeptide glutathione.

The reference ranges for ferritin can vary between laboratories but are usually between 20 and 300 μg/L for males, and 15–150 μg/L for females.

If the ferritin level is low, there is a risk for lack of iron, which could lead to anemia. If ferritin is high, there is iron in excess or there is an acute inflammatory reaction in which ferritin is mobilized without iron excess. Ferritin is used as a marker for iron overload disorders, such as hemochromatosis or hemosiderosis. As ferritin is also an acute-phase reactant, its level is often elevated in the course of an inflammatory disease, but a normal C-reactive protein level excludes that elevated ferritin is caused by acute phase reactions.

1.5.3 Glutathione

GSH is an important antioxidant in animals, plants, fungi, and some bacteria, preventing damage to important cellular components caused by reactive oxygen species such as free radicals and peroxides. It is a tripeptide, that may be referred to as gamma-glutamyl-cysteinyl-glycine, as it has a gamma peptide linkage between the carboxyl group of the glutamate side-chain and the amino group of cysteine, which is attached by normal peptide linkage to a glycine (Fig. 1.8).

In general, thiols are reducing agents, and GSH is the crucial reducing agent intracellularly, existing at a concentration of about 3 mmol/L or more in animal cells.

Glutathione is not an essential nutrient, as it is biosynthesized in the body from its amino acid constituents. The thiol group (SH) of cysteine serves as an electron donor and is responsible for its biological activity. Cysteine is the rate-limiting factor in cellular glutathione biosynthesis, since this amino acid is relatively rare in foods.

The cellular biosynthesis of glutathione involves two ATP-dependent steps: First, gamma-glutamylcysteine is synthesized from L-glutamate and cysteine via the enzyme gamma-glutamyl-cysteine synthetase. This reaction is the rate-limiting step in glutathione synthesis. Second, glycine is added to the C-terminal of gamma-glutamylcysteine via the enzyme glutathione synthetase.

Glutathione exists in both reduced (GSH) and oxidized (GSSG) states. In the reduced state, the thiol group of cysteine is able to donate a reducing equivalent (H^++ e^-) to unstable molecules, such as reactive oxygen species. In donating an electron, glutathione itself becomes reactive, but readily reacts with another reactive glutathione to form glutathione disulfide (GSSG). Such a reaction is probably due to the relatively high concentration of glutathione in cells (3–5 mmol/L in the liver). Glutathione also reduces disulfide bonds formed within cytoplasmic proteins to cysteines by serving as an electron donor. In the process, glutathione is converted to its oxidized form, GSSG (Pompella, Visvikis, Paolicchi, De Tata, & Casini, 2003). Oxidized GSSG is, however, rapidly reduced back by glutathione reductase, using NADPH as an electron donor (Couto, Malys, Gaskell, & Barber, 2013).

Glutathione has multiple functions, as follows:

1. It is the major endogenous antioxidant produced by the cells, participating directly in the neutralization of free radicals and reactive oxygen compounds, as well as maintaining exogenous antioxidants such as vitamins C and E in their reduced (active) forms (Scholz, Graham, Gumpricht, & Reddy, 1989). In addition, GSH acts as an antioxidant through its role as a cofactor for the seleno-enzyme glutathione peroxidase.
2. GSH is used in metabolic and biochemical reactions such as DNA synthesis and repair, protein synthesis, prostaglandin synthesis, amino acid transport, and enzyme activation, involving that every organ system in the body can be affected by the state of the glutathione cycle, especially the immune system, the nervous system, the gastrointestinal/liver system, and the lungs.
3. GSH is an important substrate for conjugation reactions, catalyzed by the glutathione-S-transferase enzyme. Thus, in the case of the reactive metabolite formed by a paracetamol overdose, glutathione or its precursor acetylcysteine are efficient antidotes.
4. Glutathione is needed for the detoxification of methylglyoxal, a toxin produced as a by-product of the carbohydrate metabolism. Thus, the glyoxalase enzyme system catalyzes the conversion of methylglyoxal and reduced glutathione to S-D-lactoyl-glutathione, and the subsequent hydrolysis of S-D-lactoyl-glutathione to glutathione and lactic acid.
5. GSH is able to bind, transport, and store several metals, thus affecting metal homeostasis in biological systems.

Here, we will concentrate on its ability to bind toxic metals. Metals reported to bind to GSH is copper, selenium, zinc, chromium, mercury, cadmium, arsenic, silver, and lead (Aaseth, Alexander, & Norseth, 1982; Alexander, Aaseth, & Refsyik, 1981; Ballatori, 1994; Ballatori & Clarkson, 1985; Cherian & Vostal, 1977; Wang & Ballatori, 1998). In general, the metal-GSH complexes are kinetically labile, and GSH-bound metals can exchange with other ligands, leading to rapid redistribution of metals in the body. The bile appears to be a main excretory pathway for some metal-GSH complexes (Cherian & Vostal, 1977), which was earlier indicated for the methylmercury-GSH conjugate (Refsvik, 1978).

When GSH reacts with a metal, two main outcomes are possible: the metal can be stabilized in a nonreactive conjugate (Refsvik, 1978), or the metal, for example, copper can undergo a redox reaction paralleled by oxidation of GSH and formation of reactive oxygen species (ROS) resulting in increased toxicity (Aaseth, Skaug, & Alexander, 1984; Sivertsen, 1980). More often, GSH can bind to metals and prevent their toxic effects. Thus, GSH has been shown to protect against Hg^{2+}-mediated toxicity in isolated proximal tubule fragments from rabbits and proximal tubular cells from rats (Burton et al., 1995). Also, GSH-metal complexes can serve as source of metals during the synthesis of metalloproteins, such as superoxide dismutase and metallothionein.

Overall, GSH can chelate metals and reduce their toxicity, but GSH can also facilitate the transport of some metals across biological membranes and thereby increase their toxicity in target organs.

In healthy cells and tissue, more than 90% of the total glutathione pool is in the reduced form (GSH) and less than 10% exists in the disulfide form (GSSG). An increased GSSG-to-GSH ratio is considered indicative of oxidative stress (Halprin & Ohkawara, 1967). Calcitriol (1,25-dihydroxyvitamin D_3), the active metabolite of vitamin D_3, increases GSH levels in the brain and appears to be a catalyst for glutathione production (Garcion, Wion-Barbot, Montero-Menei, Berger, & Wion, 2002). *S*-adenosylmethionine has also been shown to increase cellular glutathione content in persons suffering from a disease-related glutathione deficiency (Lieber, 2002).

Low glutathione is commonly observed in negative nitrogen balance, as seen in cancer, HIV/AIDS, sepsis, and trauma (Droge & Holm, 1997).

1.5.4 Metallothionein

MTs are a family of cysteine-rich, low molecular weight proteins (molecular weight ranging from about 1000–14000 kDa). They are localized intracellularly, usually to the membrane of the Golgi apparatus. MTs have the capacity to bind both essential and nonessential heavy metals, for example, zinc and copper, cadmium, mercury, silver and arsenic, through the thiol group of its cysteine residues, which represent nearly 30% of their constituent amino acids (Nordberg & Nordberg, 2000). MTs are present in prokaryotes, plants, yeast, invertebrates, and vertebrates including humans.

MT was discovered by Margoshes and Vallee (1957) from purification of a Cd-binding protein from equine renal cortex (Margoshes & Vallee, 1957). The functions of MTs are yet not fully understood, but experimental data suggest that MTs provide protection against toxic metals, in addition to being involved in regulation of the physiological metals Zn and Cu (Capdevila, Bofill, Palacios, & Atrian, 2012). MT also provides protection against oxidative stress (Felizola et al., 2014). There are four main isoforms expressed in humans: MT1 (with various subtypes), MT2, MT3, and MT4. All these isoforms are intracellular proteins containing an array of 20 conserved cysteines and polynuclear metal–sulfur coordination sites. The most widely detected isoforms in mammals,

MT-1 and MT-2, are rapidly induced in the liver by a wide range of metals, in particular by zinc ions, but also by drugs and inflammatory mediators (Coyle, Philcox, Carey, & Rofe, 2002). In addition to MT-1 and MT-2, two tissue-specific MTs have been reported in mammals, MT-3 in the central nervous system and MT-4 in the epithelial cells (Palmiter, 1998). The CNS-specific isoform, MT-3, has been reported to exert a growth inhibitory as well as a protective action against oxidative stress on neuron cells (Coyle et al., 2002; Lee & Koh, 2010).

The production of MT-1 and MT-2 in liver and kidney cells is apparently dependent on the availability of the dietary zinc and copper, and the amino acids histidine and cysteine. The metal content of MTs can vary, depending on the stability constants of different metals. And one MT does not have to contain only one type of metal. MT has been documented to bind a wide range of metals including cadmium, zinc, mercury, copper, arsenic, and silver (Freisinger & Vasak, 2013).

Most likely, MTs have an important role in the uptake, transport, and regulation of zinc homeostasis in biological systems, including in mammalians (Richards & Cousins, 1976). Mammalian MT binds three Zn(II) ions in its beta domain and four in the alpha domain. In some MTs, mostly bacterial, histidine participates in zinc binding. By binding and releasing zinc, metallothioneins (MTs) may regulate zinc levels within the body. Based on MT affinity constants, a number of toxic metal ions including Hg^{2+}, Ag^{+}, Cu^{+}, Cd^{2+}, Pb^{2+}, and Bi^{2+}, should be able to displace Zn^{2+} from MT (Nath, Kambadur, Gulati, Paliwal, & Sharma, 1988). The free zinc, in turn, is a key element for the activation and binding of transcription factors, in particular the metal regulatory transcription factor 1 (MTF-1) and thereby the released zinc induces synthesis of more MT (Huang, Shaw, & Petering, 2004).

Cysteine residues from MTs can also capture harmful oxidant radicals like the superoxide and hydroxyl radicals (Kumari, Hiramatsu, & Ebadi, 1998). In this reaction, cysteine is oxidized to cystine, and the metal ions, for example, zinc ions, which were bound to cysteine, are liberated to the media. Since free Zn can activate the synthesis of more MTs, this mechanism has been proposed to be an important mechanism in the control by MTs of oxidative stress.

Metallothionein gene expression is induced by a high variety of stimuli, including metal exposure, oxidative stress, glucocorticoids, hydric stress, etc. The level of the response to these inducers depends on the MT gene.

Metallothionein also carries zinc ions from one part of the cell to another. When zinc enters a cell, it can be picked up by thionein and carried to another part of the cell where it is released to another organelle or protein. In this way the thionein-metallothionein interactions become a key component of the zinc signaling system within cells. This system is particularly important in the brain, where zinc signaling is presumed to be prominent both between and within nerve cells. The same signaling also seems to be important for the regulation of the tumor suppressor protein p53.

Because MTs play an important role in transcription factor regulation, problems with MT function or expression may lead to malignant transformation of cells and ultimately to cancer (Cherian, Jayasurya, & Bay, 2003).

1.5.5 Selenoproteins

Selenium is an essential trace element. It is placed below sulfur in the periodic table with approximately similar Pauling electronegativity. The selenol group may similarly to the thiol group serve as a soft ligand for complexation with soft metals. Because of its lower pKa (5.4) the selenol group in selenocysteine is, in contrast to the thiol group in cysteine (pKa 8.2) ionized at physiological pH (Byun & Kang, 2011). Endogenous selenols may occur both as low molecular weight compounds and in selenospecific proteins. Low molecular weight selenol compounds are selenocysteine where sulfur has been replaced by selenium, labile glutathione selenopersulfide (GSSeH) and methylselenol occurring in the intermediary metabolism of selenium. The human selenoproteom consists of 25 selenoproteins that, with the exception of selenoprotein P, contain one selenocysteine (Hatfield, Tsuji, Carlson, & Gladyshev, 2014). Many of the selenoproteins are enzymes taking part in the removal of peroxides, redox regulation, and thyroxin metabolism. The selenol group is usually found in the catalytic site. Soft metals, in particular Hg^{2+}, $MeHg^{+}$, Cd^{2+}, may bind to selenoproteins and inactivate the enzymatic activity. Full length selenoprotein P contains 10 selenocysteins of which two takes place in seleno–sulfur bridges. It is synthesized in the liver and excreted to plasma and serves as a vehicle for transportation of selenium from the liver to other tissues. Its concentration in plasma is approximately 0.8 μM (Burk & Hill, 2009). Metals such as Hg^{2+}, Cd^{2+}, Ag^{+}, and Cu^{2+} bind to selenoprotein P.

1.6 CONCLUSIONS

In the present chapter, the general chemistry of metal toxicity has been briefly outlined. Essential as well as nonessential metals may give rise to toxic effects if the doses of exposure are high and exceeds the critical dose. Short-term high- or long-term low-level exposure by ingestion may be seen in the domestic environment, while exposure by inhalation may be occupational in origin. Acute or chronic effects of metal toxicity may be manifested in different organs, including respiratory, cardiovascular, renal, and central nervous systems.

Metal accumulation and poisoning may also occur in the absence of environmental exposure, as, for example, in transfusional siderosis, for example, in the thalassemias. Therapeutic chelating agents compete for toxic metals with ligands essential for physiological function. Chelating agents possess high affinity for the metal to be removed, releasing the metal ions from vulnerable endogenous structures by forming a nontoxic chelate. Chelation is indicated in the treatment of metal poisonings and metal storage diseases, and to aid the elimination of metallic radionuclides. General principles of chelation have been outlined. Endogenous protective molecules such as complexing proteins, peptides, and chaperones including metallothionein, selenoproteins, and ferritin, have been discussed in the present chapter.

REFERENCES

AAP. (1995). Treatment guidelines for lead exposure in children. *Pediatrics, 96*, 155–160.

AAP. (2005). Lead exposure in children: prevention, detection and management. *Pediatrics, 116*, 1036–1046.

Aaseth, J. (1983). Recent advance in the therapy of metal poisonings with chelating agents. *Human Toxicology, 2*(2), 257–272.

Aaseth, J., Alexander, J., & Norseth, T. (1982). Uptake of Cr-51-labeled chromate by human-erythrocytes—a Role of Glutathione. *Acta Pharmacologica Et Toxicologica, 50*(4), 310–315.

Aaseth, J., Skaug, M. A., Cao, Y., & Andersen, O. (2015). Chelation in metal intoxication—principles and paradigms. *Journal of Trace Elements in Medicine and Biology, 31*, 260–266.

Aaseth, J., Skaug, V., & Alexander, J. (1984). Haemolytic activity of copper as influenced by chelating agents, albumine and chromium. *Acta Pharmacologica Et Toxicologica, 54*(4), 304–310.

Aisen, P., Leibman, A., & Zweier, J. (1978). Stoichiometric and site characteristics of binding of iron to human transferrin. *Journal of Biological Chemistry, 253*(6), 1930–1937.

Alexander, C. (1972). Cobalt-beer cardiomyopathy. A clinical and pathologic study of twenty-eight cases. *American Journal of Medicine, 53*(4), 395–417.

Alexander, J., Aaseth, J., & Refsyik, T. (1981). Excretion of zinc in rat bile—a role of glutathione. *Acta Pharmacologica Et Toxicologica, 49*(3), 190–194.

Alexander, J., Benford, D., Boobis, A., Ceccatelli, S., Cravedi, J., Di Domenico, A., & van Leeuwen F. R. (2010). Scientific opinion on lead in food. *The EFSA Journal, 8*(4), 1–147.

Andersen, O. (1999). Principles and recent developments in chelation treatment of metal intoxication. *Chemical Reviews, 99*(9), 2683–2710.

Andersen, O., & Aaseth, J. (2002). Molecular mechanisms of in vivo metal chelation: implications for clinical treatment of metal intoxications. *Environmental Health Perspectives, 110 Suppl.*(5), 887–890.

Aposhian, H., Carter, D., Hoover, T., Hsu, C., Maiorino, R., & Stine, E. (1984). DMSA, DMPS, and DMPA—as arsenic antidotes. *Fundamental and Applied Toxicology, 4*, S58–S70 (2 Pt 2).

Ballatori, N. (1994). Glutathione mercaptides as transport forms of metals. *Advances in Pharmacology, 27*, 271–298.

Ballatori, N., & Clarkson, T. (1985). Biliary-secretion of glutathione and of glutathione metal-complexes. *Fundamental and Applied Toxicology, 5*(5), 816–831.

Barnes, D., & Dourson, M. (1988). Reference dose (RfD): description and use in health risk assessments. *Regulatory Toxicology and Pharmacology, 8*(4), 471–486.

Beattie, A., Moore, M., & Goldberg, A. (1972). Tetraethyl-lead poisoning. *Lancet, 2*(7766), 12–15.

Bellinger, D., Stiles, K., & Needleman, H. (1992). Low-level lead exposure, intelligence and academic achievement: a long-term follow-up study. *Pediatrics, 90*(6), 855–861.

Beton, D., Andrews, G., Davies, H., Howells, L., & Smith, G. (1966). Acute cadmium fume poisoning: five cases with one death from renal necrosis. *British Journal of Industrial Medicine, 23*(4), 292–301.

Burk, R., & Hill, K. (2009). Selenoprotein P—expression, functions, and roles in mammals. *Biochimica Et Biophysica Acta, 1790*(11), 1441–1447.

Burton, C., Hatlelid, K., Divine, K., Carter, D., Fernando, Q., Brendel, K., & Gandolfi, A. (1995). Glutathione effects on toxicity and uptake of mercuric chloride and sodium arsenite in rabbit renal cortical slices. *Environmental Health Perspectives, 103*(Suppl. 1), 81–84.

Byun, B., & Kang, Y. (2011). Conformational preferences and pKa value of selenocysteine residue. *Biopolymers, 95*(5), 345–353.

Cantilena, L., & Klaassen, C. (1981). Comparison of the effectiveness of several chelators after single administration on the toxicity, excretion, and distribution of cadmium. *Toxicology and Applied Pharmacology, 58*(3), 452–460.

Capdevila, M., Bofill, R., Palacios, Ò., & Atrian, S. (2012). State-of-the-art of metallothioneins at the beginning of the 21st century. *Coordination Chemistry Review, 256*(1–2), 46–62.

Carmona, F., Palacios, O., Galvez, N., Cuesta, R., Atrian, S., Capdevila, & Dominguez-Vera, J. (2013). Ferritin iron uptake and release in the presence of metals and metalloproteins: chemical implications in the brain. *Coordination Chemistry Reviews, 257*(19–20), 2752–2764.

Carmona, U., Li, L., Zhang, L., & Knez, M. (2014). Ferritin light-chain subunits: key elements for the electron transfer across the protein cage. *Chemical Communications, 50*(97), 15358–15361.

Catsch, A., & Harmuth-Hoene, A. (1976). Pharmacology and therapeutic applications of agents used in heavy-metal poisoning. *Pharmacology & Therapeutics Part A Chemotherapy Toxicology and Metabolic Inhibitors, 1*(1), 1–118.

Cherian, M., Jayasurya, A., & Bay, B. (2003). Metallothioneins in human tumors and potential roles in carcinogenesis. *Mutation Research, 533*(1–2), 201–209.

Cherian, M., & Vostal, J. (1977). Biliary-excretion of cadmium in rat .1. Dose-dependent biliary-excretion and form of cadmium in bile. *Journal of Toxicology and Environmental Health, 2*(4), 945–954.

Ciba-Geygy. (1994). Product Monograph on Desferrioxamine.

Couto, N., Malys, N., Gaskell, S., & Barber, J. (2013). Partition and turnover of glutathione reductase from saccharomyces cerevisiae: a proteomic approach. *Journal of Proteome Research, 12*(6), 2885–2894.

Coyle, P., Philcox, J., Carey, L., & Rofe, A. (2002). Metallothionein: the multipurpose protein. *Cellular and Molecular Life Sciences, 59*(4), 627–647.

Crisponi, G., Nurchi, V., Crespo-Alonso, M., & Toso, L. (2012). Chelating agents for metal intoxication. *Current Medicinal Chemistry, 19*(17), 2794–2815.

Dotterud, L., & Falk, E. (1994). Metal allergy in north Norwegian schoolchildren and its relationship with ear piercing and atopy. *Contact Dermatitis, 31*(5), 308–313.

Droge, W., & Holm, E. (1997). Role of cysteine and glutathione in HIV infection and other diseases associated with muscle wasting and immunological dysfunction. *FASEB Journal : The Official Publication of the Federation of American Societies for Experimental Biology, 11*(13), 1077–1089.

Ebrahimi, K., Bill, E., Hagedoorn, P., & Hagen, W. (2012). The catalytic center of ferritin regulates iron storage via Fe(II)-Fe(III) displacement. *Nature Chemical Biology, 8*(11), 941–948.

EFSA (2009). Guidance of the scientific committee on a request from EFSA on the use of the benchmark dose approach in risk assessment European. *EFSA Journal, 1150*, 1151–1172.

Fardal, O., Johannessen, A., & Morken, T. (2005). Gingivo-mucosal and cutaneous reactions to amalgam fillings. *Journal of Clinical Periodontology, 32*(4), 430–433.

Felizola, S., Nakamura, Y., Arata, Y., Ise, K., Satoh, F., Rainey, W., & Sasano, H. (2014). Metallothionein-3 (MT-3) in the human adrenal cortex and its disorders. *Endocrine Pathology, 25*(3), 229–235.

Freisinger, E., & Vasak, M. (2013). Cadmium in metallothioneins. *Metal Ions in Life Sciences, 11*, 339–371.

Friberg, L. (1984). Cadmium and the kidney. *Environmental Health Perspectives, 54*, 1–11.

Garcion, E., Wion-Barbot, N., Montero-Menei, C., Berger, F., & Wion, D. (2002). New clues about vitamin D functions in the nervous system. *Trends in Endocrinology and Metabolism, 13*(3), 100–105.

Goyer, R., & Rhyne, B. (1973). Pathological effects of lead. *International Review of Experimental Pathology, 12*, 1–77.

Halprin, K., & Ohkawara, A. (1967). The measurement of glutathione in human epidermis using glutathione reductase. *The Journal of Investigative Dermatology, 48*(2), 149–152.

Hansen, M., Johansen, J., & Menne, T. (2003). Chromium allergy: significance of both Cr(III) and Cr(VI). *Contact Dermatitis, 49*(4), 206–212.

Hatfield, D., Tsuji, P., Carlson, B., & Gladyshev, V. (2014). Selenium and selenocysteine: roles in cancer, health, and development. *Trends in Biochemical Sciences, 39*(3), 112–120.

Hatlelid, K., Brailsford, C., & Carter, D. (1996). Reactions of arsine with hemoglobin. *Journal of Toxicology & Environmental Health, 47*(2), 145–157.

Huang, M., Shaw, I. C., & Petering, D. (2004). Interprotein metal exchange between transcription factor IIIa and apo-metallothionein. *Journal of Inorganic Biochemistry, 98*(4), 639–648.

Jenkins, G., Ind, J., Kazantzis, G., & Owen, R. (1965). Arsine poisoning: massive haemolysis with minimal impairment of renal function. *British Medical Journal, 2*(5453), 78–80.

Kazantzis, G. (1979). Renal tubular dysfunction and abnormalities of calcium metabolism in cadmium workers. *Environmental Health Perspectives, 28*, 155–159.

Kazantzis, G. (1980). Mercury. In H. Waldron (Ed.), *Metals in the environment* (pp. 221–261). London: Academic Press.

Kontoghiorghes, G. (1995). Comparative efficacy and toxicity of desferrioxamine deferiprone and other iron and aluminum chelating drugs. *Toxicology Letters, 80*(1–3), 1–18.

Koster, R., Vieluf, D., Kiehn, M., Sommerauer, M., Kahler, J., Baldus, S., & Hamm, C. (2000). Nickel and molybdenum contact allergies in patients with coronary in-stent restenosis. *Lancet, 356*(9245), 1895–1897.

Kumari, M., Hiramatsu, M., & Ebadi, M. (1998). Free radical scavenging actions of metallothionein isoforms I and II. *Free Radical Research, 29*(2), 93–101.

Langard, S. (1994). Nickel-related cancer in welders. *The Science of the Total Environment, 148*(2–3), 303–309.

Langard, S., Andersen, A., & Ravnestad, J. (1990). Incidence of cancer among ferrochromium and ferrosilicon workers: an extended observation period. *British Journal of Industrial Medicine, 47*(1), 14–19.

Lee, S., & Koh, J. (2010). Roles of zinc and metallothionein-3 in oxidative stress-induced lysosomal dysfunction, cell death, and autophagy in neurons and astrocytes. *Molecular Brain, 3*(1), 30.

Lewis, G. (1938). Acids and bases. *Journal of the Franklin Institute, 226*(3), 293–313.

Lewis, R., & Tatken, R. (1980). *Registry of toxic effects of chemical substances* (2nd ed.) (p. 762). United States: US Department of Health and Human Services.

Lieber, C. (2002). S-adenosyl-L-methionine: its role in the treatment of liver disorders. *The American Journal of Clinical Nutrition, 76*(5), 1183S–1187S.

Lippard, S., Berg, J., & Garner, C. (1995). Principles of bioinorganic chemistry. *Natural Product Reports, 12*(4), 443.

Lundstrom, N., Englyst, V., Gerhardsson, L., Jin, T., & Nordberg, G. (2006). Lung cancer development in primary smelter workers: a nested case-referent study. *Journal of Occupational & Environmental Medicine, 48*(4), 376–380.

Macedo, M., & de Sousa, M. (2008). Transferrin and the transferrin receptor: of magic bullets and other concerns. *Inflammation & Allergy Drug Targets, 7*(1), 41–52.

Margoshes, M., & Vallee, B. (1957). A cadmium protein from equine kidney cortex. *Journal of the American Chemical Society, 79*(17), 4813–4814.

Mena, I., Court, J., Fuenzalida, S., Papavasiliou, P., & Cotzias, G. (1970). Modification of chronic manganese poisoning. Treatment with L-dopa or 5-OH tryptophane. *New England Journal of Medicine*, *282*(1), 5–10.

Mertz, W. (1974). The newer essential trace elements, chromium, tin, nickel, vanadium and silicon. *The Proceedings of the Nutrition Society*, *33*(3), 307–313.

Mertz, W. (1981). The essential trace elements. *Science*, *213*(4514), 1332–1338.

Nath, R., Kambadur, R., Gulati, S., Paliwal, V., & Sharma, M. (1988). Molecular aspects, physiological function, and clinical significance of metallothioneins. *Critical Reviews in Food Science and Nutrition*, *27*(1), 41–85.

Needleman, H., Schell, A., Bellinger, D., Leviton, A., & Allred, E. (1990). The long-term effects of exposure to low-doses of lead in childhood—an 11-year follow-up report. *New England Journal of Medicine*, *322*(2), 83–88.

Nordberg, G. (2004). Cadmium and health in the 21st century—historical remarks and trends for the future. *Biometals*, *17*(5), 485–489.

Nordberg, M., & Nordberg, G. (2000). Toxicological aspects of metallothionein. *Cellular and Molecular Biology*, *46*(2), 451–463.

Palmiter, R. (1998). The elusive function of metallothioneins. *Proceedings of the National Academy of Sciences of the United States of America*, *95*(15), 8428–8430.

Pearson, R. (1963). Hard and soft acids and bases. *Journal of American Chemical Society*, *85*(22), 3533–3539.

Pompella, A., Visvikis, A., Paolicchi, A., De Tata, V., & Casini, A. (2003). The changing faces of glutathione, a cellular protagonist. *Biochemical Pharmacology*, *66*(8), 1499–1503.

Racette, B., McGee-Minnich, L., Moerlein, S., Mink, J., Videen, T., & Perlmutter, J. (2001). Welding-related parkinsonism: clinical features, treatment, and pathophysiology. *Neurology*, *56*(1), 8–13.

Refsvik, T. (1978). Excretion of methyl mercury in rat bile: the effect of diethylmaleate, cyclohexene oxide and acrylamide. *Acta Pharmacologica Et Toxicologica*, *42*(2), 135–141.

Richards, M., & Cousins, R. (1976). Metallothionein and its relationship to the metabolism of dietary zinc in rats. *The Journal of Nutrition*, *106*(11), 1591–1599.

Ringbom, A., & Harju, L. (1972). Determination of stability constants of chelate complexes: part I. Theory. *Analytica Chimica Acta*, *59*(1), 33–47.

Ritchie, R., Palomaki, G., Neveux, L., Navolotskaia, O., Ledue, T., & Craig, W. (1999). Reference distributions for the negative acute-phase serum proteins, albumin, transferrin and transthyretin: a practical, simple and clinically relevant approach in a large cohort. *Journal of Clinical Laboratory Analysis*, *13*(6), 273–279.

Scholz, R., Graham, K., Gumpricht, E., & Reddy, C. (1989). Mechanism of interaction of vitamin-E and glutathione in the protection against membrane lipid-peroxidation. *Annals of the New York Academy of Sciences*, *570*, 514–517.

Sivertsen, T. (1980). Copper-induced GSH depletion and methaemoglobin formation in vitro in erythrocytes of some domestic animals and man. A comparative study. *Acta Pharmacologica Et Toxicologica*, *46*(2), 121–126.

Soignet, S., Maslak, P., Wang, Z., Jhanwar, S., Calleja, E., Dardashti, L., & Warrell, R. J. (1998). Complete remission after treatment of acute promyelocytic leukemia with arsenic trioxide. *New England Journal of Medicine*, *339*(19), 1341–1348.

Sorahan, T., & Lancashire, R. (1997). Lung cancer mortality in a cohort of workers employed at a cadmium recovery plant in the United States: an analysis with detailed job histories. *Occupational & Environmental Medicine*, *54*(3), 194–201.

Stoeckle, J., Hardy, H., & Weber, A. (1969). Chronic beryllium disease. Long-term follow-up of sixty cases and selective review of the literature. *American Journal of Medicine*, *46*(4), 545–561.

Strand, R., Lund, W., & Aaseth, J. (1983). Complex-formation of zinc, cadmium, and mercury with penicillamine. *Journal of Inorganic Biochemistry, 19*(4), 301–309.

Theil, E. (1987). Ferritin—structure, gene-regulation, and cellular function in animals, plants, and microorganisms. *Annual Review of Biochemistry, 56*, 289–315.

Torti, F., & Torti, S. (2002). Regulation of ferritin genes and protein. *Blood, 99*(10), 3505–3516.

Vincent, J., & Love, S. (2012). The binding and transport of alternative metals by transferrin. *Biochimica Et Biophysica Acta, 1820*(3), 362–378.

Wang, W., & Ballatori, N. (1998). Endogenous glutathione conjugates: occurrence and biological functions. *Pharmacological Reviews, 50*(3), 335–356.

Wang, W., Knovich, M., Coffman, L., Torti, F., & Torti, S. (2010). Serum ferritin: past, present and future. *Biochimica Et Biophysica Acta, 1800*(8), 760–769.

Ward, E., Okun, A., Ruder, A., Fingerhut, M., & Steenland, K. (1992). A mortality study of workers at seven beryllium processing plants. *American Journal of Industrial Medicine, 22*(6), 885–904.

Wild, P., Bourgkard, E., & Paris, C. (2009). Lung cancer and exposure to metals: The epidemiological evidence. In M. Verma (Ed.), *Cancer Epidemiology: Vol. 472* (pp. 139–167). Totowa, New Jersey: Humana Press.

Yang, F., Lum, J., McGill, J., Moore, C., Naylor, S., van Bragt, P., & Bowman, B. (1984). Human transferrin: cDNA characterization and chromosomal localization. *Proceedings of the National Academy of Sciences of the United States of America, 81*(9), 2752–2756.

Zvirblis, P., & Ellin, R. (1976). Acute systemic toxicity of pure dimercaprol and trimercaptopropane. *Toxicology and Applied Pharmacology*, 36(2), 297–299.

Chapter 2

Chelating Agents as Therapeutic Compounds—Basic Principles

Guido Crisponi, Valeria Marina Nurchi

Chapter Outline

2.1 CHEMICAL AND BIOLOGICAL PRINCIPLES FOR IN VIVO CHELATION

Chelation therapy has the intent of scavenging toxic metal ions from the organism, or of attenuating their toxicity by converting them in less toxic compounds, or of transferring them from the site where they exert their toxic action to a compartment where this cannot be executed.

The essential properties of a chelating agent, based on chemical and biomedical considerations, have been better defined through the years. These requisites that are briefly outlined in chapter: General Chemistry of Metal Toxicity and Basis for Metal Complexation will be schematically recapitulated and then discussed in major details here, pointing out the interconnections between them:

1. high stability of the formed complexes, not less than that with endogenous ligands; high stability at physiological pH and at acidic pH of urine;
2. selectivity toward the target metal ion; the chelating agent must not perturb the essential metal status;

Chelation Therapy in the Treatment of Metal Intoxication. http://dx.doi.org/10.1016/B978-0-12-803072-1.00002-X

3. high exchange rate of metal between endogenous ligands and chelating agents;
4. the pharmacokinetics of chelating agent in vivo;
5. slow biochemical metabolism of the chelating agent, once entered into the body;
6. favorable toxicity profile of chelating agent and its complexes;
   a. be as tolerable as possible for administration at doses as high as possible;
   b. no fetotoxicity, no teratogenicity;
7. good intestinal absorption, so that the drug can be orally administered, but:
   a. be available for both oral and parenteral administration;
   b. be soluble in water and physiological medium for parenteral administration;
8. good bioavailability properties;
9. easy excretion of the toxic metal ion in the complexed form, via kidneys or via bile;
10. the chelating agent should reduce absorption of toxic metal ion from gastrointestinal tract.

In the following some of the earlier traced requirements will be discussed in some detail.

2.1.1 Stability

The stability of the formed complex is the true necessary requisite, though not sufficient, so that the metal ion can be completely transformed into the chelated species to be excreted. Chelators can be classified as bidentate, tridentate, and so on, according to the number of coordinating groups in the molecule able to bind the target metal ion. Ligand denticity describes the number and the stoichiometry of the formed complexes. Ligands with low denticity form multiple complexes whose speciation depends both on total ligand concentration and on metal/ligand ratio; hexadentate chelators, on the contrary, form only one kind of complex. The stability constant of a complex $Me_pL_qH_r$, related to its formation equilibrium pMe + qL + rH = $Me_pL_qH_r$, is generally expressed as follows:

$$\beta = \frac{[Me_pL_qH_r]}{([M_e]^p[L]^q[H]^r)} \quad (1.1)$$

where L is the completely deprotonated form of the ligand, with charges omitted for simplicity (Rossotti & Rossotti, 1961). It is apparent from this expression that Eq. (1.1) in chapter: General Chemistry of Metal Toxicity and Basis for Metal Complexation, represents a simplified description, valid only for a mononuclear 1:1 complex. The protonation constants should also be taken into account, since the complex formation depends on the competition between proton and metal ion for the same basic sites on ligand. Extracellularly these interactions takes place at pH 7.4, whereas the intracellular pH is about 6.8 and in the gastrointestinal spaces at pH 1–2 and 6. In addition to the stability constants, other factors too, such as solubility of the formed complex, the stoichiometry of the complex, proton competition, and so on, contribute to the binding efficiency of a ligand toward a given metal ion. Side reaction coefficients for M and L and conditional constants were discussed in early studies by Ringbom (1963), Ringbom and Harju (1972a,b) and Ringbom and Still (1972). In vivo, both reactants, L and M, enter into numerous side reactions. The methods for quantifying the ligand effectiveness toward a target metal ion have been recently reviewed by Bazzicalupi, Bianchi, Giorgi, Clares, and García-Espana (2012). In the present chapter we will make use of the pM parameter, as it was used in 1981 by the group of Raymond (Harris, Raymond, and Weitl, 1981), as—$\log[M_f]$ at $[M_T]= 1\times10^{-6}$ M and $[L_T] = 1\times10^{-5}$ M at pH 7.4, where $[M_f]$ is the concentration of free metal ion and $[M_T]$ and $[L_T]$ are the total concentrations of metal and ligand respectively. The higher the stability of the formed complex the less metal ion remains unchelated in solution (free metal ion), determining a higher pM value. The stability requisites earlier discussed largely depend on the hard/soft nature of the metal ion, and of the coordinating groups on the ligand (Pearson, 2005). For this reason a schematic hard-intermediate-soft classification of a number of toxic metal ions, and of the main coordinating groups, is reported in Table 2.1.

Other factors, discussed in different chapters of this book, are of great importance in determining the stability of formed complexes, as the structure and denticity of the ligand that induce the preorganization of the complex (Pearson, 1963), and the favorable entropic contribution related to the chelate effect (Schwarzenbach, 1952). In addition, empirical correlations between a number of properties both of the ligands and of the metal ions and the stability of the formed complexes have been suggested in literature; these can be of great efficacy in the design of the most appropriate chelating agents for a target metal ion (Hancock & Martell, 1989).

TABLE 2.1 Grouping of Metal Ions, and of Coordinating Groups, as a Function of Their Hard, Soft, or Intermediate Nature

Metal ions			Coordinating groups		
Hard	Intermediate	Soft	Hard	Intermediate	Soft
(Li^+, Na^+, K^+), Be^{2+}, Mg^{2+}, Ca^{2+}, Sr^{2+},Mn^{2+}, Al^{3+}, Ga^{3+}, Cr^{3+}, Fe^{3+}, Sn^{4+}, $(CH_3)_2Sn^{2+}$, UO_2^{2+}, VO^{2+}	Fe^{2+}, Co^{2+}, Ni^{2+}, Cu^{2+}, Zn^{2+}, Pb^{2+}, Sn^{2+}, (Sb^{3+}, Bi^{3+})	Cu^+, Ag^+, Au^+, Hg^+, Pd^{2+}, Cd^{2+}, Pt^{2+}, Hg^{2+}, CH_3Hg^+, Pt^{4+}	H_2O, OH^-, F^-, $RCOO^-$, Cl^-, RO^-, (NH_3, RNH_2)	RNH_2	R_2S, RSH, RS^-

2.1.2 Selectivity

Ideally, a metal chelator should possess high enough selectivity to remove the target metal ion without any interference by the other metal ions in biological fluids, basically by those essential metal ions which are present in significant concentration. Selectivity depends on the thermodynamic stability of the complexes formed by the chelating agent with the target metal ion in comparison with the stability of those formed with the essential metal ions, taking into account that the concentrations of these can be several orders of magnitude higher than that of the toxic metal ion. The selective behavior of a chelating agent for a given toxic ion can be correctly evaluated by means of available speciation programs, as Hyss (Alderighi et al., 1999), when the thermodynamic parameters (protonation constants of the chelating agent, and complex formation constants with the target and with the essential metal ions) are known and a reliable evaluation of the concentrations of all the involved metal ions and of the chelating agent can be achieved. The knowledge of the pharmacokinetic properties of the chelating agent is relevant, since its concentration varies with the time after administration reaching a maximum, and then declining with a characteristic trend. The selectivity is therefore a value that varies with the time elapsed from administration. A numerical example will allow clarification of this statement, even though it does not represent a general treatment. We assume a diprotic chelating agent characterized by the protonation constants $\log K_1 = 8.0$ and $\log K_2 = 5.0$ ($\log \beta_2 = 13.0$), and two metal ions, the target toxic metal ion M_T and an interfering essential metal ion M_E; both form a single 1:1 complex with the chelating agent, the target metal ion with a complex formation constant $\log \beta_{MTL} = 18.0$ three order of magnitude higher than that of the essential metal ion $\log \beta_{MEL} = 15.0$. These constants allow to calculate a $pM_T = 18.3$ and a $pM_E = 15.3$. Taking into account these values, we calculate the concentrations at physiological pH of the formed M_TL and M_EL complexes for different sets of concentration of the three independent species M_T, M_E, and L:

- M_T concentration was assumed always as 1×10^{-3} M;
- M_E concentration was assumed equal to that of M_T, and 10, 100, and 1000 times greater respectively;
- L concentration was assumed equal to that of the target metal ion, and 10 and 100 times in excess, respectively.

The percent concentrations of M_TL and M_EL with respect to the total assumed concentrations of M_T, M_E, respectively, for all the above 12 sets of M_T, M_E, and L, are reported graphically in Fig. 2.1.

The plot on the left of Fig. 2.1 allows to remark that when the ligand concentration is 1 x 10^{-3} M, that is, equal to that of the target metal ion, the ligand is not selective and increasing concentrations of the interfering essential metal ion hinder the complete chelation of the target metal ion (only about 40% is

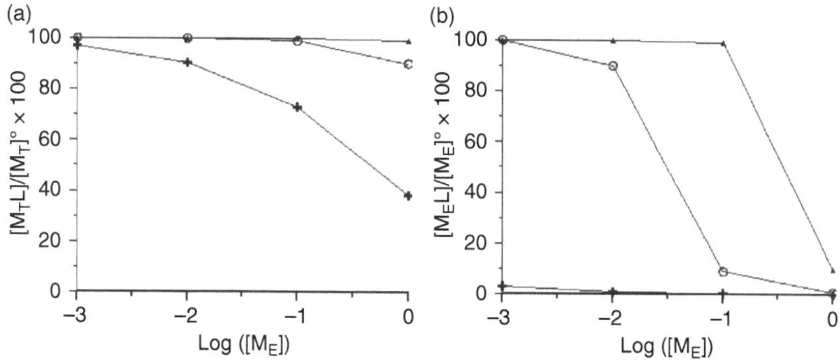

FIGURE 2.1 (a) Percent concentration of M_TL versus the log of concentration of the interfering metal ion at different total ligand concentration (+) 0.001 M, (o) 0.01 M and (*) 0.1 M; (b) Percent concentration of M_EL vs the log of concentration of the interfering metal ion at different total ligand concentration (+) 0.001 M, (o) 0.01 M, and (*) 0.1 M.

chelated when the essential metal ion is 1000 times in excess). A 10-fold excess of the ligand (1×10^{-2} M) protects chelation of the target metal ion from the interfering essential metal ion up to a 100 times excess. When a 100 fold excess of the ligand (1×10^{-1} M) is used the target metal ion is completely chelated without any interference of the essential metal ion.

A completely different aspect is depicted in the right plot in Fig. 2.1, that presents the behavior of the essential metal ion. When there is a stoichiometric amount of ligand with respect to the target metal ion only a very low percent of the essential metal ion is chelated, but at higher ligand concentrations the percent of chelated essential metal ion also reaches 100%, then decreases according to the essential metal ion/ligand concentration ratios. This gives evidence of a potentially dangerous effect of chelation therapy, the depletion of essential metal ions. Two conflicting effects of increasing concentrations of chelating agent have therefore to be remarked, while from one side this favors the complete coordination of the target metal ion even in presence of large amounts of interfering essential metal ions, from the other side it leads to essential metal ion depletion.

As illustrated in the previous example, these two effects basically depend on the thermodynamic properties of the interaction of the ligand with the involved metal ions (Nurchi et al., 2014), but the kinetic properties of these interactions can play an important role as well.

2.1.3 Kinetic Aspects of Chelation

The thermodynamic aspects of chelation earlier discussed are the preliminary requisites for the activity of any chelating agent. Nevertheless, even if the thermodynamic aspects are favorable, kinetic factors can strongly influence and interfere on the behavior of the chelating agent.

At least three kinetic factors can be identified (Jones & May, 1987):

1. the pharmacokinetic behavior of the chelating agent. This has been generally studied for the main chelating agents in use, and can be found in literature;
2. the kinetic behavior of the toxic metal ion in the organism, which depends on the rate of its distribution in the organs once entered in blood circulation from the site of adsorption, and on the rate of transfer from the organs to blood circulation when plasma is depleted by chelation courses;
3. the rate of interaction between the chelating agent and the toxic metal ion, free or bound to plasma transport proteins, or to proteins on which it exerts its toxic action.

The pharmacokinetics of a drug determines its daily administration and in some cases the way of administration. The three drugs in use for the treatment of iron overload can be assumed as paradigm: they present totally different pharmacokinetics, different intestinal absorption, and require a completely different administration. Desferal (DFO) is not orally adsorbed, and due to its very short half-life in plasma (5–10 min) has to be administered as continuous subcutaneous infusion (Crisponi, Nurchi, Crespo-Alonso, & Toso, 2012). The concentration in plasma of deferiprone (DFP), assumed orally, reaches a maximum 2 h after its administration, then declines to a very low value after about 6 h, mainly by its glucuronidation on the —OH group that completely hinders iron chelation. This determines the partitioning of the daily dose in three administrations, one every 8 h. Deferasirox (DFX) instead has a pharmacokinetic trend that allows a single daily administration, which permits a good coverage along the 24 h.

The chelating agent generally reaches its maximum concentration in plasma in a time determined by the kind of delivery, by the absorption, and by other minor factors. It then disappears from plasma because of metabolism, excretion, and transfer to the tissues, each one of these causes being predominant according to the chelating agent. Many chelating agents are metabolized in the body to species that loose the chelating properties of the parent molecule. These reactions can be very different, as the glucuronidation of hydroxypyridinones, the acetylation of triethylenetetramine (trien), or the formation of —S—S bonds between 2,3 dimercaptopropan-1-ol (BAL) and SH-containing ligands. The correct choice of drug administration becomes of vital importance when this kind of metabolic transformation is rapid as, for example, the subcutaneous infusion of desferal. All these processes, by reducing the amount of chelating agent in plasma, reduce the efficacy of its action. Therefore, when comparing the efficacy of two chelating agents, in addition to the thermodynamic properties, also the kinetic behavior has to be considered. A second process to be examined is the rate of disappearance of the toxic metal ion from the plasma. If this rate is high, the effect of whichever chelating agent is reduced, limiting its time of action; the best chelating agent in such a situation is that able to follow the metal ion into the tissues exploiting there its action.

A further point is the rate of interaction of the chelating agent with the target metal ion in the biological fluids, generally bound to transport constituents or to molecules on which it exerts its toxic action. If this rate is rapid enough with respect to the disappearance of the chelating agent from plasma, this will act successfully, otherwise its success will be completely compromised by the kinetic factors.

A first insight on the exchange rate can be obtained from the exchange rates of coordinated water, which, being a peculiarity of each single metal ion, is normally assumed as an index of the metal ion lability (Basolo & Pearson, 1967). The structural characteristics of the binding site on the proteins, as well as the denticity of the chelating agent furthermore largely influence the rate of interaction of the chelating agent with the target metal ion.

All these kinetic aspects have to be carefully examined when evaluating the behavior of any chelating agent in a given biological environment.

2.1.4 Absorption and Bioavailability of Chelating Agents

The chemical requisites regarding the absorption and the bioavailability have been pointed out by Ma, Zhou, Kong, and Hider (2012). Three key parameters regulate diffusion through biological membranes: molecular size, lipophilicity, and net charge (Hider & Liu, 2003). Specifically the cut off molecular weight for drugs to be absorbed in the human intestine is approximately 500 g/mol. Lipophilicity is generally estimated by the water–octanol partition coefficient (P). These general properties have been used by Lipinski, Lombardo, Dominy, and Feeney (1997), adopting a four parameter analysis, to predict membrane permeability. Their guidelines state that a poor absorption is likely when:

- molecular weight > 500 g/mol;
- log P > 5;
- more than 10 hydrogen bond donors are present in the molecule (expressed as a sum of OH and NH groups);
- more than 10 hydrogen bond acceptors are present in the molecule (expressed as a sum of O and N atoms).

The same parameters also determine the absorption of the chelating agent into cells, and the excretion of the formed metal complex. In this last case the formation of a neutral complex is of paramount importance: in the case of iron(III) complexes it is more appropriate to use a chelating agent bearing coordinating groups as —CO—COH or —CO—NOH (like in hydroxypyridinones or in hydroxamates) than —COH—COH or COH—COOH (as in catechol or in salicylate), since the first ones lead to easily extractable uncharged complexes, and the second ones to negatively charged complexes.

2.2 CHELATING AGENTS: CHEMISTRY, KINETICS, AND TOXICOLOGY

In the following the main chelating agents in use will be illustrated singularly, reporting basic information as the IUPAC name, the acronym, the trade name, the chemical and the structural formulae, the molecular weight, the protonation constants and the speciation plot, and the main characteristics reported on New Drug Application (NDA) data sheets. Recent literature reports will be furthermore reviewed.

2.2.1 BAL, DMPS, DMSA

2,3 Dimercaptopropan-1-ol, British Anti-Lewisite (BAL), dimercaprol, $C_3H_8OS_2$, molecular weight 124.23 g/mol, is characterized by the protonation constants log K_1 10.8 and log K_2 8.7, mean values of all the values at 25°C and 0.1 M ionic strength reported on the IUPAC Stability Constant Data Base (Pettit & Powell, 2001). This ligand was synthesized at Oxford on Jul. 1940 under the guidance of Sir Rudolph Peters as an answer to the war chemical agent Lewisite (Ord & Stocken, 2000). It was disclosed to the scientific community only at the end of the war in 1945 (Peters, Stocken, & Thompson, 1945), and it was the first chelating agent used for the treatment of heavy metal toxicity (Vilensky & Redman, 2003). As can be found in NDA 5-939/S-007, Rev. 10/06, dimercaprol is a colorless or almost colorless liquid having a disagreeable, mercaptan-like odor. Each milliliter of sterile BAL in oil contains 100 mg dimercaprol dissolved in 200 mg benzyl benzoate and 700 mg peanut oil. Due to its lipophilicity it is administered only by intramuscular injection, after local anesthesia. The speciation plot of BAL (Fig. 2.2) shows that the neutral form is the only species existing in the pH range 6.0–7.4 (Nugent, Kumar, Rampton, & Evans, 2001; Faa et al., 2008). Its lipophilicity explains its ability to penetrate intracellularly.

BAL was previously used in the treatment of arsenic, gold, and mercury poisoning, and in acute lead poisoning in combination with calcium disodium edetate. It is effective in acute poisoning by inorganic mercury salts if therapy is begun within 1–2 h following ingestion, while it is not effective for chronic

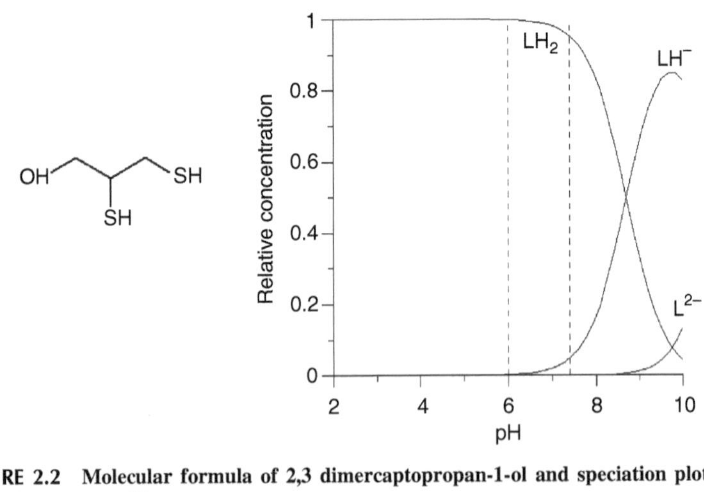

FIGURE 2.2 Molecular formula of 2,3 dimercaptopropan-1-ol and speciation plots of its variously protonated forms.

mercury poisoning. It is of uncertain value in the treatment of poisoning by other toxic elements such as antimony and bismuth. The chelating action of BAL is carried out by its vicinal sulfhydryl groups that by forming complexes with arsenic, gold, and mercury prevent, or reverse, their binding to vital sulfhydryl groups on enzymes. These complexes are excreted mainly in the urine. BAL has been used in combination with calcium disodium edetate to promote lead excretion. It should not be used against iron, cadmium, cobalt or selenium poisoning since the formed metal complexes are more toxic than the free metal ions. Further, BAL increases the brain deposition of arsenic and several other metals. Today, the clinical use of BAL is limited to the initial treatment of some acute intoxications, due to its high toxicity (LD_{50} 90–180 mg/kg) (Zvirblis & Ellin, 1976; Stine, Hsu, Hoover, Aposhian, & Carter, 1984). The most usual response to BAL is a rise in blood pressure, with tachycardia. Additional symptoms, in order of frequency, are nausea and vomiting, headache, a burning sensation in lips, mouth and throat, conjunctivitis, lacrimation, blepharal spasm, rhinorrhea, and salivation. BAL chelation is contraindicated in patients affected by glucose-6-phosphate dehydrogenase deficiency due to risk of hemolysis (Gerr, Frumkin, & Hodgins, 1994). In animal experiments, BAL administration increased the brain deposition of organic and inorganic mercury (Berlin & Ullberg, 1963; Aaseth, 1973) and increased the toxicity of lead (Germuth & Eagle, 1948). The less toxic derivatives of BAL, meso-2,3-dimercaptosuccinic acid (DMSA) and D,L-2,3-dimercapto-1-propanesulfonic acid (DMPS), have now superseded dimercaprol in most cases of heavy metal poisonings. These latter dithiols are nowadays available for oral administration, as tablets, as well as for parenteral administration. They are long-time stable at room temperature.

Meso-2,3-dimercaptosuccinic acid, DMSA, Succimer, Chemet, $C_4H_6O_4S_2$, molecular weight 182.22 g/mol, is characterized by four protonation constants, $\log K_1 = 12.05$, $\log K_2 = 9.65$, $\log K_3 = 3.43$, $\log K_4 = 2.71$, the first two relative to the mercapto groups, and the last two to the carboxylic groups (Aragoni et al., 1996). Its formula and the speciation plots are presented in Fig. 2.3.

In China, DMSA has been administered to hundreds of patients (Ding & Liang, 1991). DMSA is an orally active chelating agent for heavy metal ions. After an oral dose more than 95% of the blood content of DMSA is covalently bound to proteins, mainly to albumin, and more than 90% of urinary DMSA is excreted as the DMSA-cysteine mixed disulfide (Maiorino, Akins, Blaha, Carter, & Aposhian, 1990). It appears as a white crystalline powder with unpleasant mercaptan odor and taste. At physiological pH it exists as a highly soluble double negatively charged species (Fig. 2.3). DMSA is approved by FDA as lead chelator; it increases the urinary excretion of lead by forming water soluble lead complexes. This chelating agent and its metal chelates are hydrophilic, and they do not redistribute the toxic metals into the brain. About 50% of an oral dose is intestinally absorbed (Wiedemann, Fichtl, & Szinicz, 1982; Dart, Hurlbut,

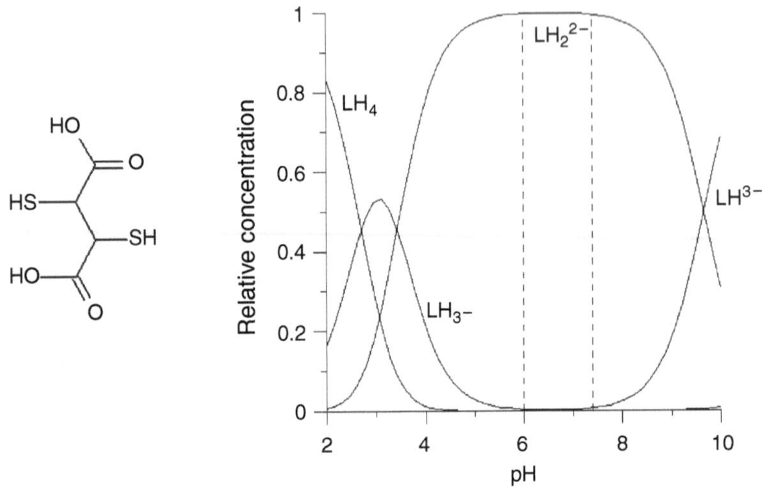

FIGURE 2.3 Molecular formula of DMSA and speciation plots of its variously protonated forms.

Maiorino, Mayersohn, & Aposhian, 1994). The distribution volume is predominantly extracellular, and the primary excretion route is urinary. Here, it is of interest that its ^{99m}Tc-chelate is routinely used as an imaging agent in nuclear medicine to visualize renal structure and function (Groshar, Embon, Frenkel, & Front, 1991). The NDA 19-998/S-013, Rev. Jul. 2007 presents detailed information on DMSA toxicity in rodents and dogs, as well as a pharmacokinetic study performed in healthy adult volunteers. About 25% of the administered dose was excreted in the urine; the peak blood level and the urinary excretion occurred between 2 and 4 h (Maiorino et al., 1990). Roughly 90% of the total amount eliminated in the urine was found as mixed DMSA-cysteine disulfides, remaining 10% unchanged. Pharmacodynamic studies were performed on 18 patients with lead levels in blood ranging between 44 and 96 μg/dL. Divided in three groups they received, respectively 10.0, 6.7, or 3.3 mg/kg of DMSA orally every 8 h for 5 days. The mean blood level decrease in the three groups after 5 days was 72.5, 58.3, and 35.5% respectively, and the mean urinary lead excretion in the first 24 h was 28.6, 18.6, and 12.3 times greater than the excretion measured in the pretreatment. During the five-day course at the higher dosage (30 mg/kg/day) a mean of 19 mg of lead was excreted. Three patients with lead levels of similar severity were treated as a control with $CaNa_2EDTA$ intravenously at a dose of 50 mg/kg/day for 5 days: the mean blood lead level decreased 47.4% and the mean urinary lead excretion was 21 mg. Urinary excretion of iron, calcium, and magnesium was not significantly affected by DMSA, which instead doubled that of zinc. The depletion of essential metal ions induced by DMSA was anyway small compared to that induced by $CaNa_2EDTA$ that provoked a 10-fold increase in urinary excretion of zinc, and doubled that of copper and iron. As observed with other chelators, a rebound in blood lead levels occurred both in adult and pediatric patients after discontinuation of DMSA treatment. Two serious adverse reactions to DMSA have been reported: a strong mucocutaneous reaction (Grandjean, Jacobsen, & Jorgensen, 1991), and a case of hemolytic anemia during the treatment for occupational lead intoxication. Also in this last case the patient suffered of glucose-6-phosphate dehydrogenase deficiency, the same genetic disease previously discussed for BAL chelation (Gerr et al., 1994).

Esters of DMSA have been reported as more effective than DMSA in scavenging intracellular mercury and cadmium, their better chelating properties probably being due to higher lipophilicity, which allows them to enter into the cells, as has been suggested for monoisoamyl-DMSA (Flora, Bhadauria, Pachauri, & Yadav, 2012). However, esterification of carboxylic groups may not sensibly decrease the net charge at pH 7.4, which remained almost equal to that of the parent molecule for the increased acidity of mercapto groups following esterification of the DMSA carboxylic groups with methanol (Fig. 2.4) (Aragoni et al., 1996).

2,3-dimercapto-1-propanesulfonic acid, DMPS, Unithiol or Dimaval, $C_3H_8O_3S_3$, molecular weight 188.29 g/mol, is characterized by two protonation constants, $\log K_1 = 11.62$, $\log K_2 = 8.53$, the sulfonic group behaving as a strong acid (Pettit & Powell, 2001). It was originally synthesized by Petrunkin in the previous Soviet Union (Petrunkin, 1956).

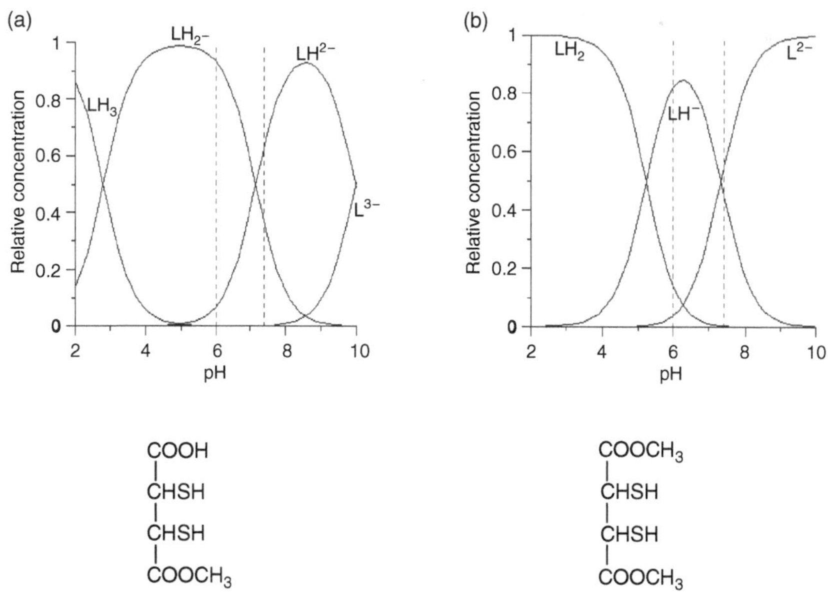

FIGURE 2.4 Molecular formula of methyl-DMSA (a) and dimethyl-DMSA (b) and speciation plots of their variously protonated forms.

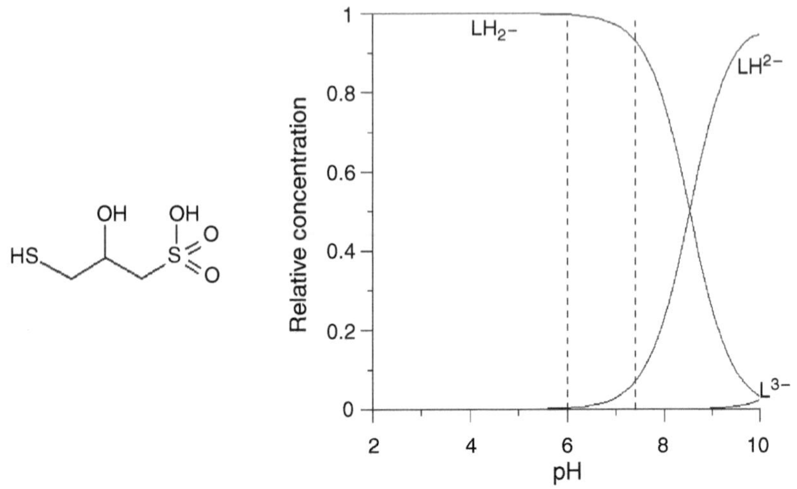

FIGURE 2.5 **Molecular formula of DMPS and speciation plots of its variously protonated forms.**

Its formula and the distribution curves are presented in Fig. 2.5.

This chelator is not licensed by FDA, but available in Europe. As DMSA, it is available for oral administration as a dry preparation, as well as for parenteral administration. It is absorbed to some extent, up to 50%, in the intestinal tract (Wiedemann et al., 1982; Dart et al., 1994). The primary route of excretion of DMPS is urinary, with blood half-life and urinary elimination half-time of less than 9–10 h (Maiorino, Dart, Carter, & Aposhian, 1991). DMPS is mainly bound to albumin in serum and its urinary excretion products are constituted by various acyclic and cyclic homopolymers, the mixed disulfide DMPS-cysteine being almost absent (Maiorino, Xu, & Aposhian, 1996). Its toxicity is low, and up to now the frequency of toxic side effects has been very low in a large number of treated patients. Possible adverse reactions have been gastrointestinal discomfort, skin reactions, mild neutropenia, and elevated liver enzymes (McNeill Consumers Products Company, 1994; Heyl, 1990). Similarly to DMSA, Unithiol is mainly bound to albumin in serum after oral administration; on the contrary polymeric products of DMPS were found in urinary excretion of the agent, mixed disulfides with cysteine being almost completely absent (Andersen, 1999). DMPS generally presents side effects analogous to those of DMSA; nevertheless it is better tolerated as regards the gastrointestinal symptoms, and causes hypotension (Andersen, 1999).

2.2.2 D-penicillamine

(2S)-2-amino-3-methyl-3-sulfanyl-butanoic acid, D-penicillamine, H_2Pen, Cuprimine, $C_5H_{11}NO_2S$, molecular weight 149,212 g/mol, is characterized by three protonation constants (log K_1 10.8, log K_2 8.1, and log K_3 2.2) ascribable

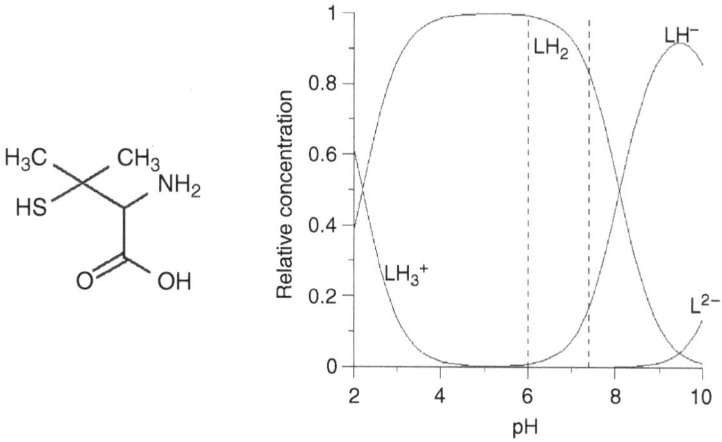

FIGURE 2.6 Molecular formula of D-penicillamine and speciation plots of its variously protonated forms.

to the —SH, —NH_3^+, and —COOH groups, respectively, obtained as the mean values among the cases reported at 25°C and 0.1 M ionic strength in the IUPAC Stability Constant Data Base (Pettit and Powell, 2001). The formula of D-penicillamine (β,β-dimethylcysteine) shows that it is an analog of the amino acid cysteine, thus containing a thiol group. It should be noted that the thiol group of D-penicillamine is relatively resistant to autooxidation since it is surrounded by two bulky methyl groups. The predominant species in 6.0–7.4 pH range is the zwitterionic form CH_2SH—$CHNH_3^+$—COO^- (Fig. 2.6). According to NDA 19-853 Cuprimine/S-012 & 014, D-penicillamine is a chelating agent recommended for the removal of excess copper in patients with Wilson's disease. In vitro studies indicate that one atom of copper combines with two molecules of D-penicillamine, so one gram of D-penicillamine should provoke the excretion of about 200 mg of copper; actually, the excreted amount is about 1% of this. D-penicillamine is generally simply reported as a copper chelating agent. In reality its mechanism of action is somewhat more complex: Peisach and Blumberg (1969) pointed out for the first time that the chelating properties of H_2Pen alone cannot be responsible for the mobilization of toxic copper in patients with Wilson's disease. They proposed a mechanism, called reductive chelation, in which unstable Cu^{II} complexes are formed that evolve to yield Cu^I and an oxidized form of the chelator. One year later this redox/complexation reaction between Cu^{II} and D-penicillamine was clarified by Sugiura and Tanaka (1970) by means of spectrophotometric and potentiometric measurements. They gave evidence that in excess of Cu^{II} a red–violet complex is produced whose absorptivity, more intense than that commonly found in cupric or cuprous complexes, was attributed to a mixed valence complex. In excess of H_2Pen, a yellow Cu^I complex is formed. They also remarked that only those compounds, which have a strong copper excretion activity, such as H_2Pen and

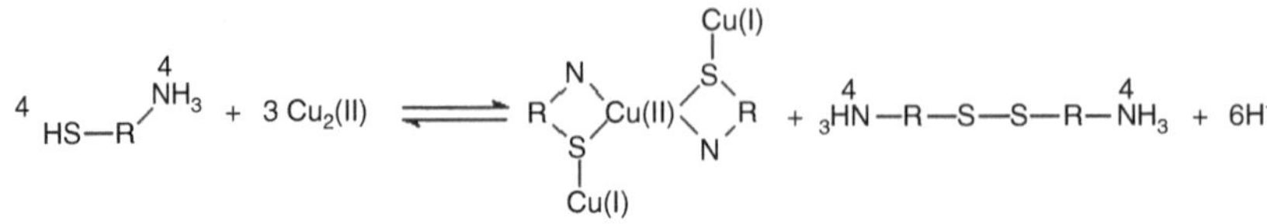

SCHEME 2.1 Red–violet complex formation as reported by Sugiura and Tanaka (1970).

β-methyl-β-ethylcysteine, form red–violet complexes, differently from the compounds that are not effective in copper excretion (N-acetylpenicillamine or cysteine). They proposed the reaction of formation of the red–violet complex reported in Scheme 2.1. They suggested that this mixed valence complex was implied in copper elimination by D-penicillamine. The same authors in a successive work (Sugiura & Tanaka, 1972) proposed a mechanism for copper transfer from the albumin–Cu^{II} complex to D-penicillamine and explained the reductive chelating action of H_2Pen.

Successively Birker and Freeman (1977) isolated the purple mixed valence cluster complex $[Cu^{II}_6Cu^{I}_8Pen_{12}Cl]^{5-}$, obtained crystals and determined the structure of $Tl_5[Cu^{II}_6Cu^{I}_8Pen_{12}Cl]^{5-}\cdot nH_2O$ by X-ray diffraction. This complex is stable for a long period at physiological conditions of pH and saline concentration, and decomposes in urine under aerobic conditions. The known stoichiometry of the crystal allowed to summarize its formation reactions in the form

$$14\,Cu^{II} + 20\,H_2Pen + Cl^- = [Cu_6{}^{II}Cu_8{}^{I}Pen_{12}Cl]^{5-} + 4(HPen)_2 + 32H^+$$

that accounts for the reaction proposed in Scheme 2.1. The structure determination gave some insights into the chelating action of D-penicillamine:

1. Cu^{II} is in equilibrium with the aqueous medium strongly coordinated by N and S atoms, while Cu^{I} is removed from equilibrium;
2. methyl groups of H_2Pen are essential in preventing Cu^{I} oxidation;
3. the 12 charged COO^- on the cluster surface determine its high aqueous solubility;
4. Cl^- is essential for the formation of the red–violet complex playing an important structural role.

Kato, Nakamura, and Uchiyama (1999) studied by ^1H NMR spectroscopy the reaction of Cu^{I} and Cu^{II} with H_2Pen in absence and in presence of glutathione, under aerobic and anaerobic conditions. They confirmed the previous observations of Birker and Freeman (1977), and indicated that the cluster is always the final product under aerobic conditions, regardless the presence of other thiols such as glutathione, that is, although the cluster is reductively decomposed by thiols, it is reproduced under oxidative conditions. This has been ascribed to the extremely high stability of the cluster with respect to that of any other copper complex with H_2Pen or with other thiols, accounting for the efficacy of D-penicillamine as a drug for Wilson's disease.

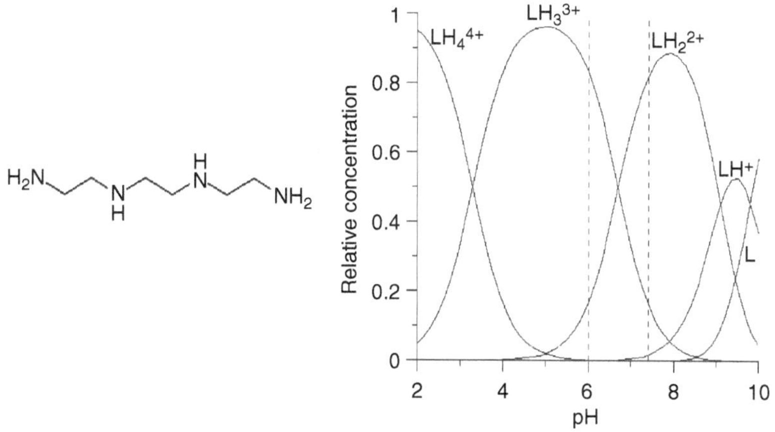

FIGURE 2.7 Molecular formula of trien and speciation plots of its variously protonated forms.

2.2.3 Triethylenetetramine

Triethylenetetramine, in its dihydrochloride form trien 2HCl was introduced in clinical use by Walshe (1969), as an alternative for the patients presenting intolerance toward D-penicillamine. Trien 2HCl, also known as Syprine, or Trientine, has the formula $C_6H_{18}N_4$ 2HCl, and a molecular weight 219.2 g/mol. It is characterized by four protonation constants [log K_1 9.79(5), log K_2 9.11(4), log K_3 6.68(2), log K_4 3.28(2)] (Nurchi et al., 2013). A very poor intestinal absorption of trien was reported by Walshe and Gibbs (1986). In Fig. 2.7 the speciation plot of trien as a function of pH is presented. The high positive charge of trien, from +2 to +3 in the gut pH range 6–7.4 (Nugent et al., 2001), explains its poor intestinal absorption according to Lipinski criteria (Lipinski et al., 1997). An oral LD_{50} of 17.1 mmol/kg in rat (Sweet, 1986) is reported. Gibbs and Walshe (1986) showed that only 6–18% of orally administered trien was systemically absorbed, in line with Kodama et al. (1997) (about 10% of the orally administered trien can be found in urines, ~1% as trien and ~8% as acetyltrien) and with the more recent results of Lu et al. (2007), who found urinary recovery between 0.03 and 13.4% in healthy volunteers and between 3.7 and 14.6% in diabetic patients. According to Siegemund, Lossner, Gunther, Kuhn, and Bachmann (1991) and Fox and Schilsky (2008), the amount of trien which remains unabsorbed in the gut decreases the intestinal copper absorption by complex formation. Trien is a very strong chelator toward Cu^{II}. Its complex formation equilibria have been extensively studied since the work of Schwarzenbach (1950), and the stability constant relative to a $[CuL]^{2+}$ complex reported by different authors (Martell, Chaberek, Courtney, Westerback, & Hyytiainen, 1957; Sacconi, Paoletti, & Ciampolini, 1961; Anderegg & Blauenstein, 1982) agree on a log K value 20.3 at 25°C and ionic strength 0.1 M; minor species of different stoichiometries, proposed by Laurie and Sarkar (1977) and by Delgado, Quintino, Teixeira, and Zhang (1997), are present only in a limited amount at pH 7.4. A pCu^{II} of 17.1 can be calculated from the protonation constants and the stability constant of the 1:1 complexes (Nurchi et al., 2013). Trien forms chelates also with other essential metal ions as Zn^{II} (Nurchi et al., 2013) and Fe^{II} (Sacconi et al., 1961), even if the stabilities of complexes with these essential metal ions are much lower than that with Cu^{II}. Chelation treatment with trien can induce zinc depletion when the ligand is in excess with respect to the amount required to chelate the target copper metal ion. Walshe (1973) after discussing the results of a 4 year treatment on the first Wilson's disease patient successfully handled with trien, presented a comparison of the ability of H_2Pen and trien to mobilize copper in a group of 18 patients. In those who had no previous treatment with H_2Pen both agents induced a very large cupruresis, while in patients effectively decoppered by prolonged treatment, the cupruretic response was lower. The different trend of copper serum concentration associated with cupruresis induced by chelating agents (H_2Pen causes a fall, while with trien a rise that returns to the base line at 5 h is observed) is attributed by Walshe to the mobilization of copper from different body compartments.

2.2.4 Deferoxamine, Deferiprone, and Deferasirox

N'-{5-[Acetyl(hydroxy)amino]pentyl}-N-[5-({4-[(5-aminopentyl)(hydroxy) amino]-4-oxobutanoyl} amino)pentyl]-N-hydroxysuccinimide, known as desferrioxamine or desferal, (DFO), was the first drug for treatment of iron overload. It is a siderophore produced by *Streptomyces pilosus*, discovered by the team of Prelog and his coworkers Keberle and Zahner (Keberle, 1964). It is a trihydroxamic acid with three residues of 1-amino-5-N-hydroxy aminopentane, two of succinic acid and one of acetic acid organized in a linear array; the free amino group determines its very high water solubility. Although it has been also obtained by synthesis, the use of the natural product is more economic. Initially used in the therapy of acute iron poisoning (Moeschlin & Schnider, 1963), deferoxamine was later introduced in thalassemia treatment. It is a hexadentate iron chelator, $C_{25}H_{48}N_6O_8$ (chemical structure in Fig. 2.8), molecular weight 560.68 g/mol, characterized by four protonation constants (log K_1 = 10.84, log K_2 = 9.46, log K_3 = 9.00, and log K_4 = 8.30, the first attributed to the terminal amine group, the other to the hydroxamic groups). At pH 7.4 it is mainly in the fully protonated positively charged LH_4^+ form.

The molecular weight > 500 g/mol in fact excludes it as an orally active chelator. Once entered into blood circulation clearance is rapid with a half life of 5–10 min. A small part of DFO is inactivated within plasma, and the major part is up taken by hepatocytes. The rapid loss of circulating activity explains the more efficient chelation obtained by prolonged infusion (Crisponi et al., 2012). Actually, DFO is usually administered by subcutaneous infusion, 8–12 h per night, 5–7 nights a week, with a dosage between 20 and 40 mg/kg body weight.

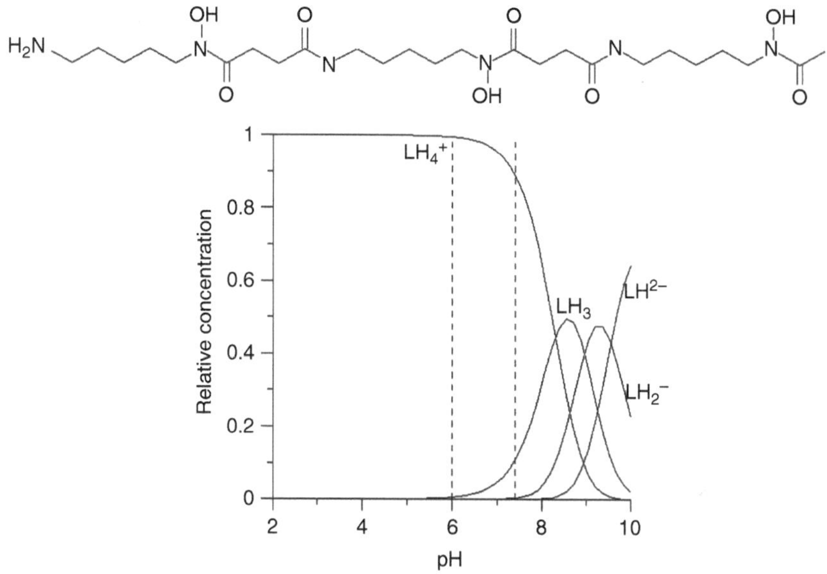

FIGURE 2.8 Molecular formula of deferoxamine and speciation plots of its variously protonated forms.

Iron is excreted in feces and, more than 60%, in urine. Frequent adverse effects of DFO are local reactions at the site of infusion and, associated with high doses, sensory-neural hypoacusia, ocular toxicity, retarded growth, skeletal changes, and infections. Moreover, although DFO has been demonstrated to be safe when administered in the presence of high iron overload, intensive therapy in young patients with low liver body iron stores may result in serious neurotoxicity, abnormalities of cartilage formation and other serious adverse effects (Ma et al., 2012). These important side effects, joined to the fastidious way of administration, lead to an important percentage of noncompliant patients. These difficulties prompted the search for oral drugs. Two agents became available: deferiprone and deferasirox.

3-hydroxy-1,2-dimethylpyridin-4(1H)-one, deferiprone (DFP) or Ferriprox, $C_7H_9N_2O_2$ (Fig. 2.9), molecular weight 139.152 g/mol, is characterized by two protonation constants (log K_1 = 9.64 and log K_2 = 3.56) and at pH 7.4 is found in its neutral form (Nurchi, Crisponi, Pivetta, Donatoni, & Remelli, 2008). By virtue of its low molecular weight, it is efficiently absorbed in the intestinal tract. DFP was synthesized by the Hider team at Essex University and patented in 1982 (Hider & Silver, 1982). DFP gives a 3:1 complex with iron, and likely removes Fe^{III} from ferritin and even from hemosiderin, lactoferrin, and transferrin.

This ligand undergoes metabolic glucuronidation leading to an inactive species. This determines the pharmacokinetic trend of DFP: its concentration in plasma reaches a maximum 2 h after its administration and then slowly

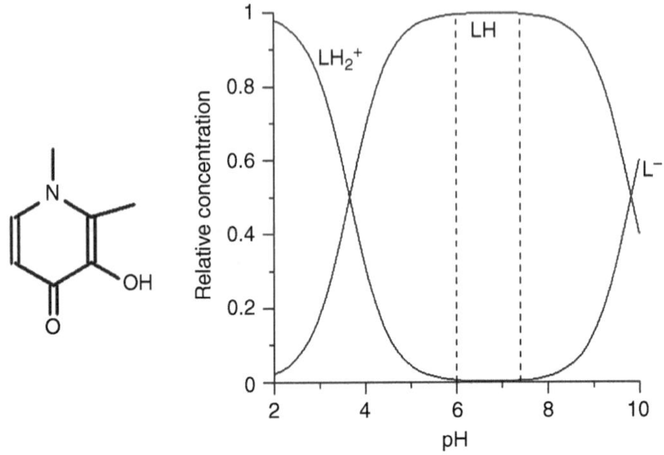

FIGURE 2.9 Molecular formula of deferiprone and speciation plots of its variously protonated forms.

declines to very low values in about 6 h. This behavior requires the partitioning of the daily dose in three administrations, one every 8 h. The majority of DFP–iron complex is excreted in the urine (70%). DFP has the clear advantage over DFO of being orally active, and, at doses of 75–100 mg/kg/day, it may be as effective as DFO in removing iron (Crisponi et al., 2012; Galanello, 2003). DFP therapy is significantly more effective than DFO in decreasing myocardial siderosis (Anderson et al., 2002; Pennell et al., 2006; Ceci et al., 2006). Agranulocytosis is the most serious side effect, occurring in about 1% of the patients (Galanello, 2003). Less severe common side effects are gastrointestinal symptoms, arthralgia, zinc deficiency, and fluctuating liver enzymes. Combined DFO–DFP therapy allows achievement of levels of iron excretion, achievable by either drug alone only at doses which cause serious toxicity effects (Wonke, Wright, & Hoffbrand, 1998; Origa et al., 2005).

Deferasirox (DFX, Exjade), $C_{21}H_{15}N_3O_4$ (Fig. 2.10), molecular weight 373.36 g/mol, synthesized by the Nick team at Novartis (Nick et al., 2003), is characterized by three protonation constants ($\log K_1 = 10.6$, $\log K_2 = 9.0$, and $\log K_3 = 3.7$, this last ascribed to the carboxylic group), and at pH 7.4 is found as the negatively charged form LH_2^-.

The plasma half-life after a single oral dose in humans is about 10 h allowing a once a day dosing (Galanello et al., 2003). Deferasirox and its chelates are excreted mainly via bile into feces. The agent can be combined with deferoxamine (Totadri et al., 2015) and it can mobilize iron from the heart (Pennell et al., 2010).

It received EU authorization in 2002 and in most countries in 2006. It is once-daily oral iron chelator effective in adults and children (Galanello, 2008). At the recommended dose 20–40 mg/kg/ day, its most frequent adverse events

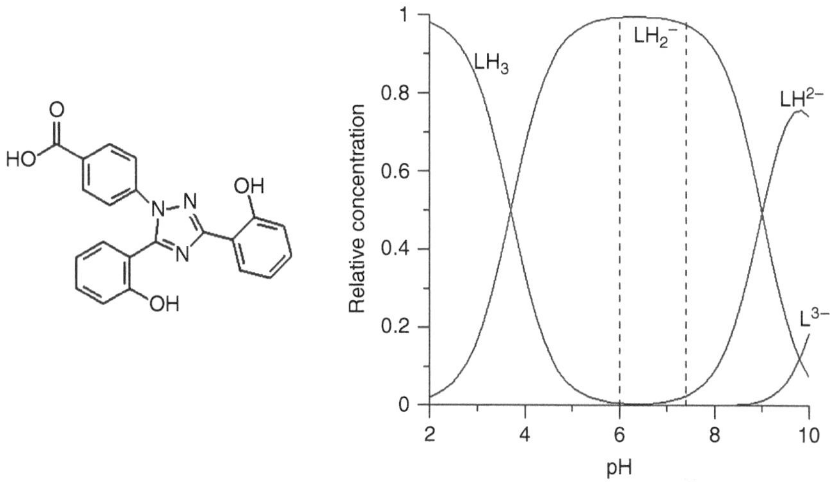

FIGURE 2.10 **Molecular formula of exjade and speciation plots of its variously protonated forms.**

include transient gastrointestinal disturbances and skin rash. Mild, usually nonprogressive increase of serum creatinine level, observed in approximately one third of patients, spontaneously returns to baseline in the majority of cases (Cappellini & Taher, 2008). Renal failure, reported following postmarketing use, is an important complication (www.pharma.us.novartis.com/info/products/brands/Exjade.jsp). According to Hider (2010) a possible role in the origin of this complication is played by the formation of zinc polymeric complexes.

2.2.5 EDTA and DTPA

Ethylenediaminetetraacetic acid, EDTA, $C_{10}H_{16}N_2O_8$, molecular weight 292.25 g/mol, is the most used polyaminocarboxylic acid in metal chelation. EDTA is characterized by four protonation constants ($\log K_1 = 10.1$, $\log K_2 = 6.1$, $\log K_3 = 2.8$, and $\log K_4 = 2.0$, obtained as the mean values among the values at 25°C and 0.1 M ionic strength reported in the IUPAC Stability Constant Data Base (Pettit & Powell, 2001). Information at the FDA site http://www.fda.gov/Drugs/DrugSafety/PostmarketDrugSafetyInformationforPatientsandProviders/ucm113738.htm (Feb. 18th, 2015) refers on the confusing term "EDTA" used for both two different drugs " *There are two drugs approved by the FDA that have similar names and are easily confused. To add to the confusion, both drugs are commonly referred to only as the abbreviation, "EDTA." One drug is named "Calcium Disodium Versenate" and is also known by the chemical name of edetate calcium disodium. This drug is approved by the FDA to lower blood lead levels among patients with lead poisoning. The other drug is marketed as "Endrate" and is also known by the chemical name of edetate disodium.*

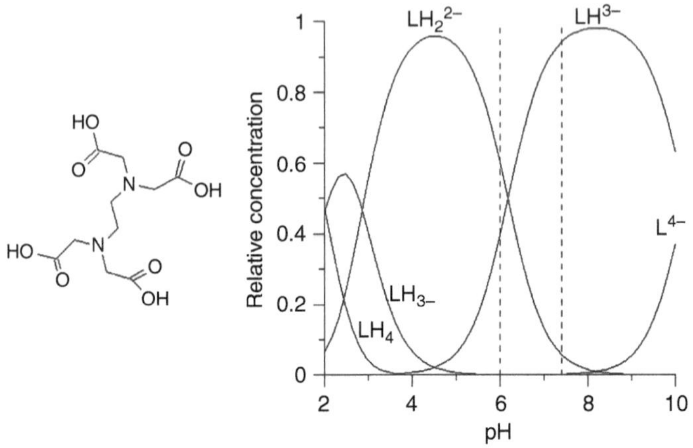

FIGURE 2.11 **Molecular formula of EDTA and speciation plots of its variously protonated forms.**

This drug is approved by the FDA for use in selected patients with high blood calcium levels (hypercalcemia) as well as for use among patients with heart rhythm problems due to intoxication with the drug digitalis".(Fig. 2.11)

Calcium disodium edetate ($CaNa_2EDTA$) is indicated in acute and chronic lead poisoning and in lead encephalopathy for reducing blood levels and stores of the toxic metal ion, in both pediatrics and adult populations. The pharmacologic action of calcium disodium edetate depends on the formation of chelates with all divalent and trivalent metals that displace calcium from the molecule, as lead, zinc, cadmium, manganese, iron, and mercury. Really mercury is unavailable for EDTA chelation being too tightly bound to body ligands. Among the essential metal ions whose homeostatic equilibria can be perturbed by $CaNa_2EDTA$ chelation, copper is not mobilized, manganese and iron excretion is not important, and that of zinc is greatly increased. Calcium disodium edetate is poorly absorbed from the gut and does not pass cellular membranes. In blood all the drug is found in plasma, being distributed primarily in the extracellular fluid. The half life of calcium disodium edetate is between 20 and 60 min. The main excretion is through the kidneys, with 50% excreted in 1 h and 95% within 24 h. Almost none of the compound is metabolized. The lead chelated by calcium disodium edetate derives mainly from bones, some reduction in lead levels taking place also in kidneys. When chelation is stopped, lead in soft tissues is redistributed to bone. Evidence has been given from animal studies that after a single dose of calcium disodium edentate there is an increase of urinary lead and a concomitant decrease of blood lead concentration; brain lead is significantly increased due to a redistribution of the toxic metal ion.

As far as the second EDTA drug, disodium edetate, is concerned, FDA is withdrawing the approval of the related NDAs due to the connected dangerous effects (Federal Register: Jun. 12, 2008 (Volume 73, Number 114)).

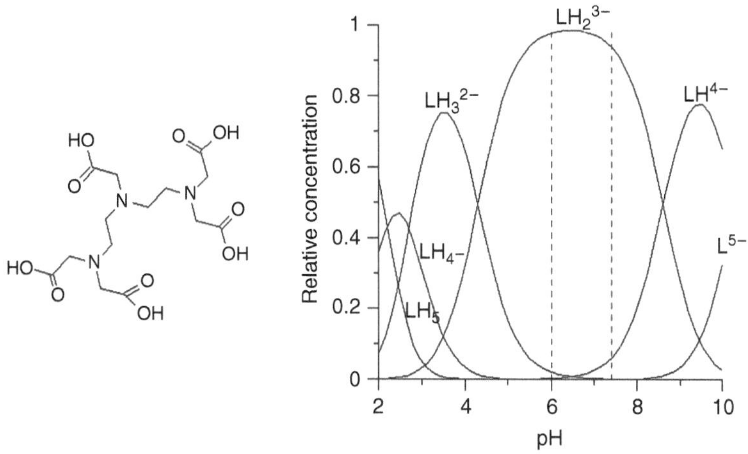

FIGURE 2.12 Molecular formula of DTPA and speciation plots of its variously protonated forms.

Diethylenetriaminepentaacetic acid, DTPA, $C_{14}H_{23}N_3O_{10}$, molecular weight 393.35 g/mol, is characterized by five protonation constants (log K_1 10.3, log K_2 8.6, log K_3 4.3, log K_4 2.7, and log K_5 2.2) obtained as the mean values among the cases reported at 25°C and 0.1 M ionic strength in the IUPAC Stability Constant Data Base (Pettit & Powell, 2001). The related speciation plot is presented in Fig. 2.12.

This drug is available in two different forms, as the sodium salt of calcium diethylenetriaminepentaacetate, Ca-DTPA, molecular weight of 497.4, or as the sodium salt of zinc diethylenetriaminepentaacetate, Zn-DTPA, molecular weight of 522.7 g/mol, both for intravenous or inhalation administration. Both forms are approved for the treatment of individuals with known or suspected internal contamination with plutonium, americium, or curium to increase the rates of their elimination. All clinical data were derived from the treatment of 286 individuals who were accidentally contaminated. Observational data were maintained in a US Registry of individuals with internal radiation contamination mainly deriving from acute occupational contamination with plutonium, americium, and curium. Zn-DTPA and Ca-DTPA form stable chelates with metal ions by exchanging zinc, or calcium, for a metal of greater binding capacity. In the case of plutonium, americium, or curium, the radioactive chelates are then excreted by glomerular filtration into the urine. Zn-DTPA and Ca-DTPA form less stable chelates with uranium and neptunium in vivo, thus resulting in deposition of these elements in tissues including bones. For these reasons DTPA treatments are not predictable as effective for scavenging uranium and neptunium.

Following intravenous administration, Zn-DTPA and Ca-DTPA are rapidly distributed throughout the extracellular fluid space. No significant amount of Zn-DTPA and Ca-DTPA penetrates into erythrocytes or other cells. No accumulation of Zn-DTPA and Ca-DTPA in specific organs has been observed. Ca-DTPA has the greatest chelating capacity immediately after internal contamination and up to 24 h, that is, when the radio-toxic element is still circulating and easily accessible for chelation. After the first dose of Ca-DTPA, a maintenance treatment with either Ca-DTPA or Zn-DTPA produces a similar elimination of radioactivity. At equivalent doses, Zn-DTPA present a lower toxicity (eg, less depletion of essential metal ions, lower mortality occurrence, absence of small bowel hemorrhagic lesions and kidney and liver vacuolization).

2.2.6 Prussian Blue

Ferric hexacyanoferrate(II), known as Prussian blue, has the empirical formula $Fe_4[Fe(CN)_6]_3$. It was probably synthesized for the first time by the paint maker Diesbach in Berlin in 1704, and it was one of the first synthetic pigments. A number of different, even if chemically related compounds, are named *Prussian blue*. Here this term refers only to insoluble ferric hexacyanoferrate(II). Prussian blue is available as Radiogardase® in USA http://www.google.it/url?sa=t&rct=j&q=&esrc=s&source=web&cd=1&ved=0CCEQFjAA&url=http%3A%2F%2Fwww.accessdata.fda.gov%2Fdrugsatfda_docs%2Flabel%2F2008%2F021626s007lbl.pdf&ei=VzrfVOCbMsnTaKb2guAM&usg=AFQjCNH7bM0BOG0n5M0hGh1BT4tkkVQ0TQ&sig2=S7bAt4pKhnEWGH9U2TeiqQ&bvm=bv.85970519,d.d2s and Antidotum Thallii-Heyl® distributed by Heyl Chemisch-pharmazeutische Fabrik GmbH, Berlin, Germany. The use of Prussian blue against thallium poisoning and as a decorporation agent for ^{134}cesium and ^{137}cesium has been investigated since the 1960s. It was recommended in the treatment of thallium intoxication in the 1970s and it is now normally used. The disaster at the Chernobyl nuclear reactor in 1986 led to further studies on the elimination of radioactive cesium. In 1987, following Goiania accident in Brazil (International Atomic Energy Agency, 1988), Prussian blue was used in the management of a large scale radiation calamity (Faustino et al., 2008). It is used as an orally ingested drug to enhance the excretion of isotopes of cesium and thallium from the body by means of ion exchange: thallium ions are excreted into the intestine and reabsorbed mainly in the colon into blood to be excreted again into the intestinal tract while cesium is excreted into the intestinal tract in the bile to be reabsorbed into portal blood and transported to the liver to again be excreted via bile (enterohepatic circulation). Therefore, orally administered Prussian blue is able to take over these two toxic metal ions in the intestine, stopping the reabsorption from the gastrointestinal tract and favoring their fecal excretion. Cesium and thallium adsorption by hexacyanoferrate(II) involves chemical ion exchange: the affinity of Prussian blue for a given metal ion increases as the ionic radius (i.r.) increases, so it will bind preferentially cesium (i.r. 0.169 nm) and thallium (i.r. 0.147 nm) respect to the essential metal ions potassium (i.r. 0.133 nm) and sodium (i.r. 0.116nm) (Nielsen et al., 1987). Therefore, a depletion of potassium and sodium is not likely (Nigrović, Bohne, & Madshus, 1966). Also rubidium (i.r. 0.148 nm) binds to Prussian blue (Hoffman, 2006). Prussian blue is not intestinally absorbed in significant amounts, and can be considered safe and effective for the treatment of internal contamination with radioactive or nonradioactive thallium, and with radioactive cesium.

REFERENCES

Aaseth, J. (1973). The effect of mercaptodextran on the toxicity of mercury in mice. *Acta Pharmacology Toxicology, 32*(6), 430–441.

Alderighi, L., Gans, P., Ienco, A., Peters, D., Sabatini, A., & Vacca, A. (1999). Hyperquad simulation and speciation (HySS): a utility program for the investigation of equilibria involving soluble and partially soluble species. *Coordination Chemistry Reviews, 184*, 311–318.

Anderegg, G., & Blauenstein, P (1982). Polyamines XIV. Protonation equilibria of linear tetraamines containing two ethylenediamine residues. *Helvetica Chimica Acta, 65*, 162–169.

Andersen, O. (1999). Principles and recent developments in chelation treatment of metal intoxication. *Chemical Review, 99*, 2683–2710.

Andersen, O., & Aaseth, J. (2002). Molecular mechanisms of in vivo metal chelation: implications for clinical treatment of metal intoxications. *Environmental Health Perspectives, 110*(S 5), 887–890.

Anderson, L. J., Wonke, B., Prescott, E., Holden, S., Walker, J. M., & Pennell, D. J. (2002). Comparison of effects of oral deferiprone and subcutaneous desferrioxamine on myocardial iron concentrations and ventricular function in beta-thalassaemia. *Lancet, 360*, 516–520.

Aragoni, M. C., Arca, M., Crisponi, G., Cristiani, F., Isaia, F., & Nurchi, V. M. (1996). Characterization of the ionization and spectral properties of mercapto-carboxylic acids. Correlation with substituents and structural features. *Talanta, 43*, 1357–1366.

Basolo, F., & Pearson, R. G. (1967). *Mechanisms of inorganic reactions*. New York: John Wiley and Son.

Bazzicalupi, C., Bianchi, A., Giorgi, C., Clares, M. P., & García-Espana, E. (2012). Addressing selectivity criteria in binding equilibria. *Coordination Chemistry Reviews, 256*, 13–27.

Berlin, M., & Ullberg, S (1963). Increased uptake of mercury in mouse brain caused by 2,3-dimercaptopropanol. *Nature, 197*, 84–85.

Birker, P. J., & Freeman, H. C. (1977). Structure, properties, and function of a copper-copper^{II} complex of D-penicillamine: pentathallium(I) μ8-chloro-dodeca(D-penicillaminato)-octacuprate(I) hexacuprate(II) n-hydrate. *Journal of the American Chemical Society, 99*(21), 6890–6899.

Cappellini, M. D., & Taher, A. (2008). Long-term experience with deferasirox (ICL670), a once-daily oral iron chelator, in the treatment of transfusional iron overload. *Expert Opinion on Pharmacotherapy, 9*, 2391–2402.

Ceci, A., Baiardi, P., Catapano, M., Felisi, M., Cianciulli, P., De Sanctis, V., Del Vecchio, G. C., Magnano, C., Meo, A., & Maggio A (2006). Risk factors for death in patients with beta-thalassemia major: results of a case-control study. *Haematologica, 91*, 1420–1421.

Crisponi, G., Nurchi, V. M., Crespo-Alonso, M., & Toso, L. (2012). Chelating agents for metal intoxication. *Current Medicinal Chemistry, 19*, 2794–2815.

Dart, R. C., Hurlbut, K. M., Maiorino, R. M., Mayersohn, M., Aposhian, H. V., & Hassen, L. V. (1994). Pharmacokinetics of meso-2,3-dimercaptosuccinic acid in patients with lead poisoning and in healthy adults. *Journal of Pediatrics, 25*(2), 309–316.

Delgado, R., Quintino, S., Teixeira, M., & Zhang, A. (1997). Metal complexes of a 12-membered tetraaza macrocycle containing pyridine and N-carboxymethyl groups. *Journal of the Chemical Society Dalton Transactions*, 55–64.

Ding, G. S., & Liang, Y. Y. (1991). Antidotal effects of dimercaptosuccinic acid. *Journal of Applied Toxicology*, *11*, 7–14.

Faa, G., Nurchi, V. M., Ravarino, A., Fanni, D., Nemolato, S., Gerosa, C., Van Eyken, P., & Geboes K (2008). Zinc in gastrointestinal and liver disease. *Coordination Chemistry Reviews*, *252*, 1257–1269.

Faustino, P. J., Yongsheng, Y., Progar, J. J., Brownell, C. R., Sadrieh, N., May, J. C., Leutzinger, E., Place, D. A., Duffy, E. P., Houn, F., Loewke, S. A., Mecozzi, V. J., Ellison, C. D., Khan, M. A., Hussain, A. S., & Lyon, R. C. (2008). Quantitative determination of cesium binding to ferric hexacyanoferrate: Prussian blue. *Journal of Pharmaceutical and Biomedical Analysis*, *47*(1), 114–125.

Flora, S. J. S., Bhadauria, S., Pachauri, V., & Yadav, A (2012). Monoisoamyl 2,3 dimercaptosuccinic acid (MiADMSA) demonstrates higher efficacy by oral route in reversing arsenic toxicity: a pharmacokinetic approach. *Basic & Clinical Pharmacology & Toxicology*, *110*(5), 449–459.

Fox, A. N., & Schilsky, M. (2008). Once daily trientine for maintenance therapy of Wilson disease. *The American Journal of Gastroenterology*, *103*, 494–495.

Galanello, R. (2003). Deferiprone in the treatment of transfusion-dependent thalassemia: a review and perspective. *Therapeutics and Clinical Risk Management*, *3*, 795–805.

Galanello, R., Piga, A., Alberti, D., Rouan, M. C., Bigler, H., & Séchaud, R. (2003). Safety, tolerability, and pharmacokinetics of ICL670, a new orally active iron-chelating agent in patients with transfusion-dependent iron overload due to beta-thalassemia. *The Journal of Clinical Pharmacology*, *43*, 565–572.

Galanello, R. (2008). Once-daily oral deferasirox for the treatment of transfusional iron overload. *Expert Review of Clinical Pharmacology*, *1*, 231–240.

Germuth, F. G., Jr., & Eagle, H. (1948). The efficacy of BAL (2,3-dimercaptopropanol) in the treatment of experimental lead poisoning in rabbits. *Journal of Pharmacology Experimental Therapeutics*, *92*, 397–410.

Gerr, F., Frumkin, H., & Hodgins, P. (1994). Hemolytic anemia following succimer administration in a glucose-6-phosphate dehydrogenase deficient patient. *Clinical Toxicology*, *32*, 569–575.

Gibbs, K.R., Walshe, J.M. (1986). *The metabolism of trientine: animal studies, in: orphan diseases, orphan drugs.* In I. Scheimberg & J.M. Walshe (Eds.), Manchester, UK:Manchester University Press.

Grandjean, P., Jacobsen, I. A., & Jorgensen, P. J. (1991). Chronic lead poisoning treated with dimercaptosuccinic acid. *Pharmacology Toxicology*, *68*, 266–269.

Groshar, D., Embon, O. M., Frenkel, A., & Front, D. (1991). Renal function and technetium-99m-dimercaptosuccinic acid uptake in single kidneys: the value of in vivo SPECT quantitation. *Journal of Nuclear Medicine*, *32*(5), 766–768.

Hancock, R. D., & Martell, A. E. (1989). Ligand design for the selective complexation of metal ions in aqueous solution. *Chemical Reviews*, *89*, 1875–1914.

Harris, W. R., Raymond, K. N., & Weitl, F. L. (1981). Ferric ion sequestering agents 6. The spectrophotometric and potentiometric evaluation of sulfonated tricatecholate ligands. *Journal of the American Chemical Society*, *103*, 2667–2675.

Heyl GmbH. Fachinformation: Dimaval (DMPS). HEYL Chemish-pharmazeutische Fabrik GmbH & Co, KG, Berlin, 1990.

Hider, R.C., Silver, J. (1982). KU patent GB-2118176.

Hider, R. C., & Liu, Z. D. (2003). Emerging understanding of the advantage of small molecules such as hydroxypyridinones in the treatment of iron overload. *Current Medicinal Chemistry*, *10*, 1051–1064.

Hider, R. C. (2010). Charge states of deferasirox-ferric iron complexes. *American Journal of Kidney Diseases*, *55*, 614–615.

Hoffman, R.S. (2006). Prussian blue. In N.E. Flomenbaum, M.A. Howland, L.R. Goldfrank, N.A. Lewin, R.S. Hoffman, L.S. Nelson (Eds.). *Goldfrank's Toxicologic Emergencies* (8th ed.). New York:McGraw Hill.

Kato, N., Nakamura, M., & Uchiyama, T. (1999). ^{1}H NMR studies of the reactions of copper(I) and copper(II) with D-penicillamine and glutathione. *Journal of Inorganic Biochemistry*, *75*, 117–121.

Keberle, H. (1964). The biochemistry of desferrioxamine and its relation to iron metabolism. *Annals of the New York Academy of Sciences*, *119*, 758–768.

Kodama, H., Murata, Y., Iitsuka, T., & Abe, T. (1997). Metabolism of administered triethylene tetramine dihydrochloride in humans. *Life Sciences*, *61*, 899–907.

International Atomic Energy Agency (1988). The Radiological accident in Goiânia. Vienna: ISBN 92-0-129088-8.

Jones, M. M., & May, P. M. (1987). The effect of kinetic factors on the thermodynamic evaluations of therapeutic chelating agents. *Inorganica Chimica Acta*, *138*, 67–73.

Laurie, S. H., & Sarkar, B. (1977). Potentiometric and spectroscopic study of the equilibria in the aqueous copper(II)–3,6-diazaoctane-1,8-diamine system and an equilibrium-dialysis examination of the ternary system of human serum albumin–copper(II)–3,6-diazaoctane-1,8-diamine. *Journal of the Chemical Society, Dalton Transactions*, 1822–1827.

Lipinski, C. A., Lombardo, F., Dominy, B. W., & Feeney, P. J. (1997). Experimental computational approaches to estimate solubility and permeability in drug discovery and development settings. *Advanced Drug Delivery Reviews*, *23*, 3–25.

Lu, J., Chan, Y., Gamble, G. D., Poppitt, S. D., Othman, A. A., & Cooper, G. J. S. (2007). Triethylenetetramine and metabolites: levels in relation to copper and zinc excretion in urine of healthy volunteers and type 2 diabetic patients. *Drug Metabolism and Disposition*, *35*, 221–227.

Ma, Y., Zhou, T., Kong, X., & Hider, R. C. (2012). Chelating agents for the treatment of systemic iron overload. *Current Medicinal Chemistry*, *19*, 2816–2827.

Maiorino, R. M., Akins, J. M., Blaha, K., Carter, D. E., & Aposhian, H. V. (1990). Determination and metabolism of dithiol chelating agents X. In humans, meso-2,3-dimercaptosuccinic acid is bound to plasma proteins via mixed disulfide formation. *Journal of Pharmacology and Experimental Therapeutics*, *254*, 570–577.

Maiorino, R. M., Dart, R. C., Carter, D. E., & Aposhian, H. V. (1991). Determination and metabolism of dithiol chelating agents XII. Metabolism and pharmacokinetics of sodium 2,3-dimercaptopropane-1-sulfonate in humans. *Journal of Pharmacology and Experimental Therapeutics*, *259*, 808–814.

Maiorino, R. M., Xu, Z. F., & Aposhian, H. V. (1996). Determination and metabolism of dithiol chelating agents XVII. In humans, sodium 2,3-dimercapto-1-propanesulfonate is bound to plasma albumin via mixed disulfide formation and is found in the urine as cyclic polymeric disulfides. *Journal of Pharmacology and Experimental Therapeutics*, *277*, 375–384.

Martell, A. E., Chaberek, S., Courtney, R., Westerback, S., & Hyytiainen, H. (1957). Hydrolytic tendencies of metal chelate compounds I. Cu(II) chelates. *Journal of the American Chemical Society*, *79*, 3036–3041.

McNeill Consumer Products Company (1994). Chemet product information; McNeill Consumer Products Co.: Fort Washington, PA.

Moeschlin, S., & Schnider, U. (1963). Treatment of primary and secondary hemochromatosis and acute iron poisoning with a new potent iron-eliminating agent (desferrioxamine-B). *The New England Journal of Medicine*, *269*, 57–66.

Nick, H., Acklin, P., Lattmann, R., Buehlmayer, P., Hauffe, S., Schupp, J., & Alberti, D. (2003). Development of tridentate iron chelators: from desferrithiocin to ICL670. *Current Medicinal Chemistry*, *10*, 1065–1076.

Nielsen, P., Dresow, B., & Heinrich, H. C. (1987). In vitro study of ^{137}Cs sorption by hexacyanoferrates (II). *Z Naturforsch*, *42B*, 1451–1460.

Nigrovic´, V., Bohne, F., & Madshus, K. (1966). Decorporation of radionuclide: research on radiocesium. *Strahlentherapie*, *130*, 413–419 (German).

Nugent, S. G., Kumar, D., Rampton, D. S., & Evans, D. F. (2001). Intestinal luminal pH in inflammatory bowel disease: possible determinants and implications for therapy with aminosalicylates and other drugs. *Gut*, *48*, 571–577.

Nurchi, V. M., Crisponi, G., Pivetta, T., Donatoni, M., & Remelli, M. (2008). Potentiometric, spectrophotometric and calorimetric study on iron(III) and copper(II) complexes with 1,2-dimethyl-3-hydroxy-4-pyridinone. *Journal of Inorganic Biochemistry*, *102*, 684–692.

Nurchi, V. M., Crisponi, G., Crespo-Alonso, M., Lachowicz, J. I., Szewczuk, Z., & Cooper GJS (2013). Complex formation equilibria of Cu^{II} and Zn^{II} with triethylenetetramine and its mono- and di-acetyl metabolites. *Dalton Transactions*, *42*, 6161–6170.

Nurchi, V. M., Crisponi, G., Arca, M., Crespo-Alonso, M., Lachowicz, J. I., Mansoori, D., Toso, L., Pichiri, G., Santos, M. A., Marques, S. M., Niclós-Gutiérrez, J., González-Pérez, J. M., Domínguez-Martín, A., Choquesillo-Lazarte, D., Szewczuk, Z., Zoroddu, M. A., & Peana, M. (2014). A new bis-3-hydroxy-4-pyrone as a potential therapeutic iron chelating agent. Effect of connecting and side chains on the complex structures and metal ion selectivity. *Journal of Inorganic Biochemistry*, *141*, 132–143.

Ord, M., & Stocken, L. (2000). A contribution of chemical defence in World War II. *Trends in Biochemical Sciences*, *25*, 253–256.

Origa, R., Bina, P., Agus, A., Crobu, G., Defraia, E., Dessì, C., Leoni, G., Muroni, P. P., & Galanello, R. (2005). Combined therapy with deferiprone and desferrioxamine in thalassemia major. *Haematologica*, *90*, 1309–1314.

Pearson, R. G. (1963). Hard and soft acids and bases. *Journal of the American Chemical Society*, *85*, 3533–3539.

Pearson, R. G. (2005). Chemical hardness and density functional theory. *Journal of Chemical Sciences*, *117*, 369–377.

Peisach, J., & Blumberg, W. E. (1969). A mechanism for the action of D-penicillamine in the treatment of Wilson's disease. *Molecular Pharmacology*, *5*, 200–209.

Pennell, D. J., Berdoukas, V., Karagiorga, M., Ladis, V., Piga, A., Aessopos, A., Gotsis, E. D., Tanner, M. A., Smith, G. C., Westwood, M. A., Wonke, B., & Galanello, R. (2006). Randomized controlled trial of deferiprone or deferoxamine in beta-thalassemia major patients with asymptomatic myocardial siderosis. *Blood*, *107*, 3738–3744.

Pennell, D. J., Porter, J. B., Cappellini, M. D., El-Beshlawy, A., Chan, L. L., Aydinok, Y., Elalfy, M. S., Sutcharitchan, P., Li, C. K., Ibrahim, H., Viprakasit, V., Kattamis, A., Smith, G., Habr, D., Domokos, G., Roubert, B., & Taher, A. (2010). Efficacy of deferasirox in reducing and preventing cardiac iron overload in beta-thalassemia. *Blood*, *115*, 2364–2371.

Peters, R., Stocken, L., & Thompson, R. (1945). British anti-Lewisite (BAL). *Nature*, *156*, 616–619.

Petrunkin, V. E. (1956). Synthesis and properties of dimercapto derivatives of alkylsulfonic acids. 1: Synthesis of sodium 2,3-dimercaptopropylsulfonate (unithiol) and sodium 2-mercaptoethylsulfonate. *Ukrainsky Khemichisky Zhurnal*, *22*, 603–607.

Pettit, L.D., Powell, K.J. (2001). The IUPAC Stability Constants Database, ver. 5.7, Academic Software and IUPAC, Otley, U.K.

Ringbom, A. (1963). *Complexation in analytical chemistry*. New York: Wiley-Interscience.

Ringbom, A., & Harju, L. (1972a). Determination of stability constants of chelate complexes. Part I. Theory. *Analytica Chimica Acta*, *59*(1), 33–47.

Ringbom, A., & Harju, L. (1972b). Determination of stability constants of chelate complexes. Part II. Applications. *Analytica Chimica Acta*, *59*(1), 49–58.

Ringbom, A., & Still, E. (1972). The calculation and use of a coefficients. *Analytica Chimica Acta*, *59*(1), 143–146.

Rossotti, F. J., & Rossotti, H (1961). *The determination of stability constants*. New York: McGraw Hill.

Sacconi, L., Paoletti, P., & Ciampolini, M. (1961). Thermochemical studies Part VI. Heats and entropies of reaction of transition-metal ions with triethylenetetramine. *Journal of Chemical Society*, 5115–5120.

Schwarzenbach, G. (1950). Metallkomplexe mit polyaminen III: mit triäthylen-tetramin = "trien". *Helvetica Chimica Acta, 33*, 974–985.

Schwarzenbach, G. (1952). Der Chelateffekt. *Helvetica Chimica Acta, 35*, 2344–2359.

Siegemund, R., Lossner, J., Gunther, K., Kuhn, H. J., & Bachmann, H. (1991). Mode of action of triethylenetetramine dihydrochloride on copper metabolism in Wilson's disease. *Acta Neurologica Scandinavica, 83*, 364–366.

Stine, E. R., Hsu, C. A., Hoover, T. D., Aposhian, H. V., & Carter, D. E. (1984). N-(2,3-dimercaptopropyl) phthalamidic acid: protection, in vivo and in vitro, against arsenic intoxication. *Toxicology and Applied Pharmacology, 75*, 329–336.

Sugiura, Y., & Tanaka, H. (1970). Studies on the sulfur-containing chelating agents XXV. Chelate formation of penicillamine and related compounds with copper(II). *Chemical and Pharmaceutical Bulletin, 18*, 368–373.

Sugiura, Y., & Tanaka, H. (1972). Evidence for a ternary complex containing albumin, copper, and penicillamine. *Molecular Pharmacology, 8*, 249–255.

Sweet, D.V. (1986). Registry of Toxic Effects of Chemical Substances, Dep. of Health and Human Services, Washington, DC.

Totadri, S., Bansal, D., Bhatia, P., Attri, S. V., Trehan, A., & Marwaha, R. K. (2015). The deferiprone and deferasirox combination is efficacious in iron overloaded patients with β-thalassemia major: a prospective, single center, open-label study. *Pediatric Blood and Cancer, 62*(9), 1592–1596.

Vilensky, J. A., & Redman, K. (2003). British anti-Lewisite (dimercaprol): an amazing history. *Annals of Emergency Medicine, 41*, 378–383.

Walshe, J. M. (1969). Management of penicillamine nephropathy in Wilson's disease: a new chelating agent. *Lancet, 2*, 1401–1402.

Walshe, J. M. (1973). Copper chelation in patients with Wilson's Disease: a comparison of penicillamine and triethylene tetramine dihydrochloride. *Quarterly Journal of Medicine, 42*, 441–452.

Walshe, J. M., & Gibbs, K. (1986). The metabolism of triethylene tetramine (trientine). *Pilzen medical reports. Charles University*.

Wiedemann, P., Fichtl, B., & Szinicz, L. (1982). Pharmacokinetics of ^{14}C-DMPS (sodium-1,3 ^{14}C-2,3-dimercaptopropane-1-sulphonate) in beagle dogs. *Biopharmaceutics & Drug Disposition, 3*, 267–274.

Wonke, B., Wright, C., & Hoffbrand, A. (1998). Combined therapy with deferiprone and desferrioxamine. *British Journal of Haematology, 103*, 361–364.

Zvirblis, P., & Ellin, R. I. (1976). Acute systemic toxicity of pure dimercaprol and trimercaptopropane. *Toxicology and Applied Pharmacology, 36*, 297–299.

Chapter 3

Diagnosis and Evaluation of Metal Poisonings and Chelation Therapy

Petr Dusek, Jan Aaseth

Chapter Outline

3.1 INTRODUCTION

Endogenous or exogenous metal poisoning may affect any of the organ systems of the body and give rise to a variety of effects. The most commonly involved organ systems include the nervous, gastrointestinal, hematopoietic, and renal systems. Metal intoxications are uncommon and their presenting features may be entirely nonspecific, the clinical examination giving no lead on the cause of the illness. Consequently, clinicians will rarely be alerted to the possibility of metal poisoning and making correct timely diagnosis can be very difficult. The principal features that should be considered in arriving at a correct diagnosis are elaborated in the following chapter.

3.2 HISTORY OF SYMPTOMS AND EXPOSURE

In many cases, a history of the work or environmental exposure will give the clue to the diagnosis. In an industrial situation, there may be a clear history of exposure that may be obtained from the patient, a relative, or a coworker. The clinician should not fail to take a full and accurate occupational history when a poisoning case of presumed occupational origin is under examination. It may

Chelation Therapy in the Treatment of Metal Intoxication. http://dx.doi.org/10.1016/B978-0-12-803072-1.00003-1

be necessary to seek additional information from the employer or his agent, or from an occupational hygienist or a health and safety representative. Exposure to a toxic metal may, however, occur without this being suspected by any of the persons questioned, and this can only be inferred by an adequate knowledge of the work processes involved. An example may be given with exposure to arsine gas, which usually presents as an acute medical emergency. Arsenic may be a contaminant in scrap metals or dusts from metals. And arsine may then be formed when arsenic dust is mixed with an acid, or when arsenide and acidic water is mixed (Romeo, Apostoli, Kovacic, Martini, & Brugnone, 1997). The condition of arsenic intoxication should be suspected if a scrap-metal worker is presenting with signs on hemolysis and other appropriate clinical symptoms, namely drowsiness and confusion. In general, a dusty, poorly ventilated workplace should raise concern, since poor ventilation increases hazards of occupational origin of symptoms. As another example, manganese intoxication should be suspected in workers in mining, welding, and smelting industries who gradually develop typical neurological symptoms of "manganism," that is dystonia, levodopa unresponsive parkinsonism with predominant gait disturbance, cognitive dysfunction and psychiatric symptoms (Long et al., 2014; Mena, Marin, Fuenzalida, & Cotzias, 1967; Mergler et al., 1994).

Similarly, if exposure is suspected in the domestic environment, a careful examination and history is of crucial importance, and may disclose inappropriate intake of drugs or dietary supplements such as iron pills, lithium tablets, or household chemicals. Usage of traditional Asian medicine may be a source of lead or arsenic poisoning (Barber & Jacyna, 2011; Lin et al., 2012; Zhou, Zhou, Liu, Wang, & Wang, 2015). Here, relatives of the poisoned patient may give valuable information. Unlabeled pills or chemicals should, of course, be kept for analysis. Voluntary suicidal or homicidal metal poisonings, for example, by arsenic, copper or mercury compounds, are rare, and although a careful history and clinical examination may give a diagnostic hint, specific treatment are often delayed in such cases (Franchitto et al., 2008; Massey, Wold, & Heyman, 1984; Sarikaya et al., 2010; Takeda, Yukioka, & Shimazaki, 2000). Homicidal metal poisonings may be particularly difficult to diagnose, as exemplified by a case story when a thallium salt was mixed into the tea of a poisoned victim (Cavanagh, Fuller, Johnson, & Rudge, 1974). Another example is the murder of the former Russian spy, Alexander Litvinenko in 2006 with ^{210}Po that illustrates the difficulty in diagnostics when an isolated case of a metal or radioactivity poisoning occurs. Specialized health personnel is of utmost importance in such cases (Nemhauser, 2010).

When exposure takes place in the general environment, diagnosis of metal poisoning, especially if caused by long-term absorption, can be very difficult. Complete dietary and drug history should be taken. Methylmercury poisoning after the eating of contaminated bread in Iraq was diagnosed at the beginning of the outbreak in 1972, because the medical officers had previous experience

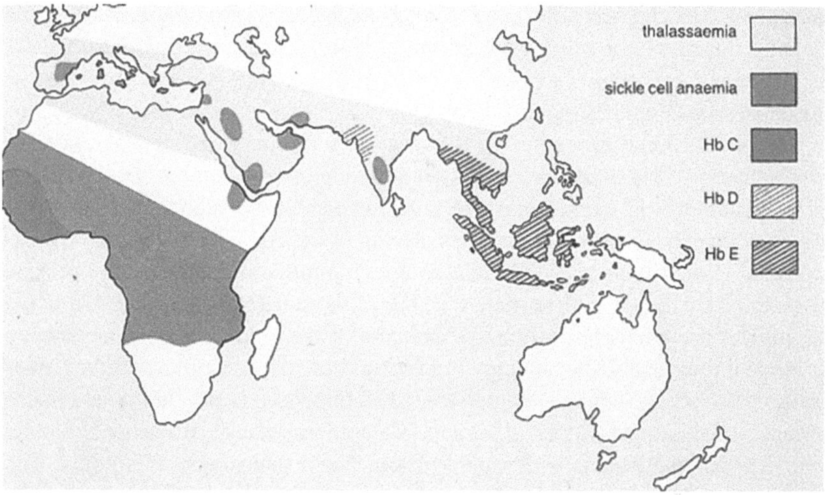

FIGURE 3.1 Geographic distribution of thalassaemia, sickle cell anemia, and other hemoglobinopathies. Due to migration during recent years the number of cases is increasing in Europe and Northern America.

of the condition (Bakir et al., 1973). Chelation treatment regimens, that is, with D-penicillamine could therefore be tried out during the Iraq disaster. In contrast, the earlier outbreak of methylmercury poisoning, that was precipitated by consumption of contaminated fish in the Minamata bay in Japan in 1953, was not officially recognized as a poisoning before 1956 (Ekino, Susa, Ninomiya, Imamura, & Kitamura, 2007). Manganese poisonings in methcathinone (ephedron) abusers, frequently described in eastern European countries, has been connected with the use of potassium permanganate for the synthesis of the drug (de Bie, Gladstone, Strafella, Ko, & Lang, 2007; Sikk et al., 2010; Stepens et al., 2008).

Metal intoxication may be also a side effect of medical treatment. Iatrogenic iron accumulation can occur after multiple blood transfusions, for example, in cases of myelodysplastic syndrome with sideroblastic anemia or in thalassemic diseases. The thalassemias are a heterogeneous group of genetic disorders of hemoglobin synthesis with prevalence following specific geographical distribution (Fig. 3.1). Symptomatic treatment of anemia in thalassemias as well as in sickle cell anemia requires regular blood transfusions, already from childhood. It is important to realize that pathological iron deposition in tissues may be seen after only about ten transfusions. For the prevention and treatment of resulting transfusional siderosis, chelation treatment is required. Parenterally administered deferoxamine combined with oral deferiprone has been a recommended choice (Kolnagou, Kleanthous, & Kontoghiorghes, 2011), although other oral agents are also available today that are well suited for long-term treatment (see chapter: Chelating Therapy in Metal Storage Diseases). While hepatic damage is a crucial symptom in hemochromatosis, cardiac disease is the most important cause of death in thalassaemia patients (Westwood, Anderson, & Pennell, 2003).

Iatrogenic metal exposures with symptoms of toxicity can also be related to chemotherapy with cisplatin (*cis*-diammoniumdichloro-platinum) that frequently is accompanied by renal side effects and in some cases also by polyneuropathy (see chapter: Chelation Treatment During Acute and Chronic Metal Overexposures—Experimental and Clinical Studies). Similar side effects may be seen during the treatment with arsenic trioxide in the postremission phase of acute promyelocytic leukemia, which is a variant of acute myeloid leukemia. Arsenic trioxide is now established therapy in this disorder after the initial anthracycline-induced remission (Muchtar et al., 2013). Lithium, used in psychiatry as a maintenance treatment of bipolar disorder, is a common cause of iatrogenic metal intoxication manifested with gastrointestinal and neurologic symptoms. The relatively high prevalence of lithium poisoning is due to its narrow therapeutic range and usage in population with a high likelihood of overdose. Also, the previously extensive use of gold salts in the treatment of rheumatoid arthritis frequently resulted in nephropathy (Aaseth, Haugen, & Forre, 1998; Jellum, Munthe, Guldal, & Aaseth, 1980) while bismuth compounds used as wound healing promoting agents may cause myoclonic encephalopathy (Bridgeman & Smith, 1994; Ovaska et al., 2008).

3.3 CLINICAL FINDINGS

The presenting clinical features, especially in acute poisoning, are usually quite nonspecific (Table 3.1). Signs of gastroenteritis such as nausea, vomiting, diarrhea, fever, and abdominal pain followed by oliguria or anuria due to renal tubular necrosis are common after ingestion of inorganic mercuric or cupric compounds, and also after ingestion of other metal salts. In severe cases of such acute metal salt poisonings, the gastroenteritis may be hemorrhagic and accompanied by hypovolemia and hypotension. Neurologic symptoms of encephalopathy ranging from headache, irritability, and mild drowsiness to more severe dysfunction including confusion, hallucinations, seizures, and coma have been described after lead intoxication and inhalation of mercury, nickel, or arsenic fumes. Hemolytic anemia, metabolic acidosis, and arrhythmias due to cardiomyopathy are also fairly common signs of metal intoxication (Gunay et al., 2006).

These early signs are unspecific, and in the absence of a careful ascertainment of history, the diagnosis of acute metal poisoning may be missed. For example, lead colic has been mistaken for the acute surgical abdomen (Janin, Couinaud, Stone, & Wise, 1985), which illustrates the importance of combining clinical findings with a careful exposure history. However, there are certain clinical sequences that should alert the physician to the possibility of metal

TABLE 3.1 Causes and Symptoms of Metal Intoxications

Metal	Acute presentation	Chronic presentation	Typical sources of intoxication	Results of paraclinical examinations
Lead	Abdominal pain Encephalopathy Motor neuropathy	Motor neuropathy, encephalopathy (parkinsonism) Abdominal pain and cramps, constipation(lead colic) Tubulointersticial nephropathy Gingival Burton'sline Arterial hypertension Anemia, gout, arthralgia	Old lead-containing paint Battery industry Lead smelting Food or beverage stored in leaded containers Retained bullets Traditional Asian medicine	Anemia, basophilic stippling in erythrocytes Increased urine δ-aminolaevulinic acid and zinc protoporphyrin in the blood Hyperintense lesion in T2w MR images in putamen and white matter predominantly in insula Dense metaphyseal band in long growing bones on X-ray
Arsenic	Sialorrhea, gastroenteritis polyneuropathy, encephalopathy MODS	Sensori-motor polyneuropathy, Encephalopathy Mees' lines on finger nails Skin lesions (pigmentation, leukodermic spots, palmar and solar keratoses) Hepatopathy Lung, liver, skin and other cancers	Contaminated well water Traditional Asian medicine Suicidal, homicidal, accidental	Pancytopenia, basophilic stippling in erythrocytes Increased LE
Thallium	Gastroenteritis Perioral erythematous skin lesions MODS	Polyneuropathy, hyperalgesia, encephalopathy, visual disturbances Alopecia, Mees' lines on finger nails	Suicidal, homicidal, accidental	

(*Continued*)

TABLE 3.1 Causes and Symptoms of Metal Intoxications (*cont.*)

Metal	Acute presentation	Chronic presentation	Typical sources of intoxication	Results of paraclinical examinations
Mercury	Pneumonitis (inhalation) Gastroenteritis (ingestion) Encephalopathy Fever, skin rash	Polyneuropathy, encephalopathy (tremor), visual and hearing disturbances Acrodynia, gingivo-stomatitis Hypertension Nephrotic syndrome	Thermometers and manometers Contaminated fish Skin ointments Gold mining Religious practices Dental amalgams	Increased epinephrine, norepinephrine in plasma/urine
Cadmium	Pneumonitis (inhalation) Gastroenteritis (ingestion) Renal tubular damage	Nephropathy, Osteoporosis Pulmonary fibrosis, lung cancer Yellow seam on dental necks	Cadmium alloy industry, welding	Proteinuria Patchy infiltrations on chest X-ray
Manganese	Metal fume fever (inhalation)	Dystonia-parkinsonism, depression, psychosis	Manganese alloy industry, welding Dry-cell battery industry Manganese mines Parenteral nutrition Potassium permanganate ingestion Methcatinone abuse	Hyperintense signal of globus pallidus, brainstem white matter and striatum in T1w MR images
Copper	Gastroenteritis(ingestion) Hemolytic anemia Rhabdomyolysis Renal tubular damage Acute hepatic failure	Liver cirrhosis	Contaminated water Suicidal, accidental High alimentary intake	Increased LE, bilirubin methemoglobinemia, hemoglobinuria

Iron	Gastroenteritis Encephalopathy Coagulopathy, metabolic acidosis Renal tubular damage	Liver cirrhosis	Iron supplements overdose Suicidal, accidental	
Silver	Gastroenteritis (ingestion) Bone marrow suppression, Pneumonitis	blue-gray coloration of skin, nails, mucosae, and conjunctivae	Battery industry Iatrogenic—silver coated prostheses	
Chromium	Gastroenteritis Hemolytic anemia Renal tubular damage	Rhinitis, septum perforation Pulmonary fibrosis, lung cancer (inhalation)	Chromium alloy industry, smelting Leather tanning	Septum perforation and nodular thickening of mucosa in paranasal sinuses on CT
Nickel	Gastroenteritis Pneumonitis, myocarditis, Dermatitis Encephalopathy Hepatopathy	Pulmonary fibrosis, lung, and nasopharyngeal cancer (inhalation)	Petroleum, plastic, and rubber production	Patchy infiltrations on chest X-ray Leucocytosis Increased LE
Zinc	Metal fume fever (inhalation) Gastroenteritis (ingestion)	Copper deficiency (pancytopenia, myelopathy)	Welding Contaminated water	Decreased ceruloplasmin
Bismuth	Renal tubular damage Myoclonic encephalopathy (tremor)	Cognitive disorder Shoulder arthropathy Gingivo-stomatitis, Gingival black Bismuth line	Iatrogenic—bismuth paste, bismuth salts overdose	Methemoglobinemia

Abbreviations: MODS, multiorgan dysfunction syndrome; LE, liver enzymes; CT, computed tomography; MR, magnetic resonance.

poisoning. Gastroenteritis followed by acute peripheral neuropathy characterizes several metal poisonings, mainly with lead, arsenic, and mercury. If hair loss is also observed, thallium poisoning is an obvious diagnostic possibility (Cavanagh et al., 1974; Pelclova et al., 2009).

Common syndrome associated with the inhalation of metal oxide fumes, usually as occupational exposure to zinc or manganese, is metal fume fever characterized by self-limiting fever, headache, fatigue, and sings of respiratory system irritation such as dyspnea and cough occurring within several hours after exposure (Bergstrom, 1977). Pneumonitis may manifest as acute pulmonary edema, which in a subject free of heart disease should raise the suspicion of a toxic inhalation exposure. Here, one toxic candidate is nitrogen dioxide if the patient has worked with silage. However, acute cadmium fume poisoning should be suspected, especially if soldering or welding had been performed, since iron and steel may be plated with cadmium (Beton, Andrews, Davies, Howells, & Smith, 1966; Yates & Goldman, 1990). Other fairly common cause of pneumonitis is nickel carbonyl inhalation (Sunderman, 1989). Serious metal poisoning, for example, with arsenic or bismuth salts, should also be considered among the differential diagnoses of oliguria or anuria of unknown etiology.

Several metals give rise to renal tubular dysfunction, in particular cadmium, mercury, copper, platinum, uranium, and lead (Chugh, Sharma, Singhal, Das, & Datta, 1977; Vacca, Hines, & Hall, 1986). With lead, this condition is seen more often in children. Thus, lead poisoning should be also considered in cases of glycosuria or albuminuria in childhood (Brewster & Perazella, 2004).

During acute or chronic intoxications, metals are taken up by bones, which is usually an asymptomatic process. Chronic cadmium intoxication is fairly specific by causing intractable bone pain, osteoporosis, and pathological fractures in association with chronic nephropathy, known as itai-itai disease (Gil et al., 2011; Noda, Yasuda, & Kitagawa, 1991).

Several metal compounds may give rise to peripheral neuropathy, but causes of motor or sensory polyneuropathy are often obscure, and many cases remain undiagnosed. Metal poisoning by lead, arsenic, thallium, or other compounds should be considered in the differential diagnosis of "idiopathic" polyneuropathy. In acute and chronic lead poisoning multiple mononeuropathy with lesion of radial and peroneal nerves leading to hand and foot drop has been described (Cullen, Robins, & Eskenazi, 1983; Dedeken et al., 2006). Rarely, chronic lead or mercury poisoning may even mimic motor neuron disease (Barber, 1978; Campbell & Williams, 1968; Livesley & Sissons, 1968). Acute arsenic intoxication often manifests with ascending weakness resembling acute inflammatory demyelinating polyneuropathy (Donofrio et al., 1987; Goebel et al., 1990; Ratnaike, 2003; Stenehjem et al., 2007).

Few of the signs described in this chapter are specific to metal poisoning. There are, however, certain specific signs indicative of metal exposure, although not necessarily of poisoning. Among these, the following should be mentioned: the characteristic garlic smell in the breath of selenium workers, the green tongue of the vanadium worker, blue-grey skin and mucosae discoloration of silver workers, and the pigmented Burton's line, a thin gray-blueish line visible along the margin of the gums at the base of the teeth, caused by the deposition of insoluble lead sulfide in lead workers (Pearce, 2007).

A mottled brown pigmentation of the skin, with verrucous hyperplasia and leukodermic spots, affecting the neck is seen in people exposed to arsenicals (Chakraborti et al., 2015). Also, palmar and solar skin keratosis as well as white transverse striae on the fingernails (Mees' lines) are indicative of exposure to arsenic, although the latter sign can occur in carbon monoxide poisoning, or after chemotherapy (Zhou et al., 2015). Erythematous rash followed by skin desquamation and acrodynia affecting hands and feet is described in mercury poisoning, particularly in children (Brannan, Su, & Alverson, 2012; Celebi, Canbay, Aycan, Sahin, & Aypar, 2008). Ulceration and perforation of the nasal septum should alert the clinician to consider previous long-term exposure to chromates (Kim et al., 1989).

3.4 GENETIC DISORDERS WITH SYSTEMIC METAL ACCUMULATION

Metal accumulation may also occur in the absence of environmental exposure as a result of genetic disorder affecting metabolic pathways of trace metals. Hereditary hemochromatosis is an autosomal recessive disorder most commonly caused by mutations in the *HFE* gene, but rarely also in other genes (Table 3.2), resulting in excessive absorption and storage of iron (Bacon et al., 2011). Deposition of iron in organs and tissues causes fibrotic changes and functional impairment, in particular liver cirrhosis, arthropathy, diabetes mellitus, hypogonadism, cardiac arrhythmias, and a bronze-like skin pigmentation caused by melanin and hemosiderin deposition (Flaten, Aaseth, Andersen, & Kontoghiorghes, 2012). Other genetic disorders with systemic iron accumulation are aceruloplasminemia caused by mutation in *ceruloplasmin* gene and hereditary ferritinopathy caused by mutation in *ferritin light chain (FTL)* gene. Contrary to hereditary hemochromatosis, neurological symptoms typically dominate in these disorders. Impaired iron metabolism in aceruloplasminemia affects erythropoiesis, pancreatic endocrine cells and brain leading to diabetes mellitus, microcytic anemia unresponsive to iron supplements, retinal degeneration and neuropsychiatric symptoms such as dystonia, Parkinsonism, and cognitive dysfunction (Kono, 2013). Hereditary ferritinopathy is manifested by neurological symptoms including choreo-dystonia, Parkinsonism, ataxia, and cognitive dysfunction (Devos et al., 2009; Chinnery et al., 2007). Iron accumulation in liver and other tissues is variable and usually is not a cause

TABLE 3.2 Hereditary Disorders with Systemic Metal Accumulation

Disease	Gene	Clinical symptoms	Typicalfindings
Aceruloplasminemia	Ceruloplasmin (CPL)	Anemia, diabetes, retinal degeneration, neurological disorders (ataxia, parkinsonism, choreodystonia, cognitive decline)	Absent serum ceruloplasmin Decreased serum Fe and incerased ferritin T2* hypointensities on brain MRI in basal ganglia, thalamus, dentatenucleus, and cortex Hypointense signal of liver on T2*w MR images
Hereditary ferritinopathy	Ferritinlightchain (FTL)	Neurological disorder (choreodystonia, ataxia, parkinsonims, cognitivedecline), hepatopathy	Decreased serum ferritin T2* hypointensities along with cystic caviations on brain MRI in basal ganglia, thalamus, dentatenucleus, and cortex
Hereditary hemochromatosis	Common: HFE Rare: Hemojuvelin (HJV), Transferrin receptor-2 (TfR2), Ferroportin (SLC40A1), Hepcidin (HAMP)	Hepatopathy, cardiomyopathy, diabetes, skin pigmentation, arthritis, sexual dysfunction	Increased serum ferritin Hypointense signal of liver on T2*w MR Increased iron concentration in liver biopsy
Wilson's disease	ATPase, Cu^{2+}transporting, beta polypeptide (ATP7B)	Hepatopathy, neurological disorders (tremor, ataxia, parkinsonism, dystonia), hemolysis, renal tubular damage	Brownish (Keyser-Fleischer) ring at corneal rim Decreased serum ceruloplasmin Increased serum nonceruloplasmin-bound copper, increased 24-h urine copper excretion Increased copper concentration in liver biopsy T2 hyperintenstities on brain MRI in basal ganglia, thalamus, and brain stem
Manganese transporter deficiency	Manganese transporter (SLC30A10)	Hepatopathy, neurological disorder (parkinsonism-dystonia)	Increased serum manganese Polycythemia T1 hyperintensities on brain MRI in globus pallidus, brain stem, and putamen

of significant impairment (Ory-Magne et al., 2009; Vidal, Delisle, Rascol, & Ghetti, 2003).

Manganese transporter deficiency due to recessive mutation in *SLC30A10* gene is a rare cause of genetic hypermanganesemia leading to manganese accumulation in many organs, particularly in brain and liver. It manifests as hepatic dysfunction, polycythemia, and neurological symptoms such as dystonia with a characteristic high-stepping (cock-walk) gait, spastic paraparesis, Parkinsonism and motor neuropathy (Quadri et al., 2012; Tuschl et al., 2012).

The recessively inherited metabolic disorder, Wilson's disease (formerly known as hepatolenticular degeneration), caused by mutation in copper transporter *ATP7B* is manifested by symptoms of copper toxicosis. This disease is characterized by a failure to excrete copper into bile, resulting in copper accumulation first in the liver, then in the brain, cornea, kidneys, and other organs (Walshe, 1984). It may be complicated by acute hepatic necrosis leading to the release of copper into the circulation, causing damage to muscle fibers, erythrocyte membranes, and renal parenchyma leading to hemolytic anemia, rhabdomyolysis, and renal failure (Meyer & Zalusky, 1977; Propst et al., 1995). Chronic copper accumulation results in widespread neurological disturbances including tremor, dysarthria, Parkinsonism, dystonia and psychiatric disturbances, and pigmented rings at the corneal rims of the eye referred to as Kayser-Fleischer rings (Dusek, Litwin, & Czlonkowska, 2015).

3.5 TOXICOLOGICAL ANALYSES

The diagnosis of metal poisoning can be confirmed in the acute stage and often in the chronic stage by finding an increased concentration of the suspected metal in the appropriate sample. In general blood is the most useful sample in case of acute or continuous intoxication while urine or hair are more appropriate for detection of chronic stage of poisoning, that is, from weeks to months. Whole blood examination is preferred over serum since metals tend to accumulate in erythrocytes (Blisard, Standefer, & Davis, 1989; Ho et al., 2011). The monitoring of the effect of chelation therapy makes use of metal determinations in blood and/or urine. However, the techniques involved in trace metal analyses in body fluids and tissues present certain difficulties, and such analyses should only be performed in laboratories that are equipped for this purpose and that participate in external quality control. Environmental sampling may need to be performed on air, water, or food. Pills or drug residues in bottles may require analysis after an acute poisoning incident, as may blood, urine, feces or tissue samples from the patient. In particular, examination of blood and urine samples for metal concentration can be considered a routine procedure in the diagnostics.

Also the diagnosis and follow-up of hereditary metal overload diseases require analyses of blood, urine, and sometimes other tissues. The diagnosis of Wilson's disease depends on analyses of nonceruloplasmin bound serum copper, 24 h urine copper excretion and copper concentration in liver biopsy specimen (Table 3.2). Penicillamine challenge test, that is, increase of urine copper excretion after a dose of D-penicillamine, may be helpful in case of borderline results, but its validity is not universally accepted (Muller et al., 2007). Treatment to produce a negative copper balance is effective with the chelating agents D-penicillamine or triethylenetetramine (trientine) that both increase urinary copper excretion substantially (Aaseth, Skaug, Cao, & Andersen, 2015). Monitoring of 24 h urine copper excretion has to be performed on regular basis to guide chelation treatment dosage and check for patients' compliance (Dusek et al., 2015).

The increased iron deposition characterizing transfusional siderosis and hemochromatosis is accompanied by increased serum iron values with increased saturation of serum transferrin (>30%), and serum ferritin values above reference range. In aceruloplasminemia, the laboratory findings in serum include decreased iron and increased ferritin (Miyajima, 2015) while serum ferritin is decreased in hereditary ferritinopathy (Keogh, Morris, & Chinnery, 2013). Long-term chelation treatment with deferiprone or deferasirox may be beneficial in aceruloplasminemia but its efficacy is variable, particularly with respect to neurological symptoms (Badat, Kaya, & Telfer, 2015; Lindner et al., 2015; Pan, Tang, Chen, Song, & Shang, 2011; Tai et al., 2014).

In the SLC30A10 manganese transporter deficiency syndrome serum manganese levels are typically several times increased (Tuschl et al., 2012). Chelation treatment with intravenous disodium calcium edetate ($CaNa_2$-EDTA) improves clinical symptoms and leads to significantly increased 24 h urinary manganese levels and reduced serum manganese levels (Stamelou et al., 2012). Chelation with $CaNa_2$-EDTA may be helpful also in manganism caused by environmental exposure provided it is started very early (Herrero Hernandez et al., 2006).

In some cases, the interpretation of toxicological analyses in blood or urine is difficult. Thus, arsenic in urine may be increased also after consumption of nontoxic compounds in seafood. In arsenic, manganese, or thallium poisonings, for example, the diagnosis can be confirmed by taking hair and nail clippings for analysis at a stage when blood and urine concentrations are not reliable or helpful. Evidence of methylmercury absorption can also be obtained from analysis of hair samples even when blood levels have fallen into the reference range. In the diagnosis of lead poisoning, difficulty may arise when exposure had ceased some time ago and much of the lead has been translocated from blood to bone. In such cases, blood lead levels may have returned to the reference interval when diagnosis is attempted. In vivo determination of lead in bone, preferably in finger bone, by X-ray fluorescence, has been used for biological monitoring of deposited lead (Skerfving, Gerhardsson, Schutz, & Stromberg, 1998). A $CaNa_2$-EDTA provocation test has also been used to estimate body burden of lead. A standard $CaNa_2$-EDTA dose will increase the urinary excretion of stored lead. However, reference values are not defined for this test, and the justification of using the EDTA-test has been questioned (Aaseth et al., 2015; Andersen, 1999).

A case report illustrates the importance of an early and correct diagnosis of lead poisoning (Amundsen, Naess, Hammerstrom, Brudevolt, & Bjerve, 2002). A 54-year-old woman was admitted to hospital with anemia and unspecific gastrointestinal symptoms. Peripheral blood smears and bone marrow aspirate showed basophilic stippling of erythrocytes suggestive of lead poisoning, which was confirmed by high concentrations (>3 μmol/L) of lead in blood. The lead source was the glazing of a ceramic wine jug. Chelating therapy with dimercaptosuccinic acid (DMSA) was started. Monitoring of lead in blood and urine verified the clinical efficacy of DMSA. The initially low hemoglobin became normalized. And the patient returned to work after several months. In contrast, an attempt to treat an arsenic poisoned patient with the same agent, DMSA, was not very successful, as judged from clinical follow-up and repetitive urine analyses (Stenehjem et al., 2007). Trials in Bangladesh have verified that DMSA was practically without effect in arsenic overexposure, whereas dimercaptopropane sulfonate (DMPS) effectively increased urinary arsenic excretion (Guha Mazumder et al., 2001). It is apparent, also from these cases, that routine monitoring of the effect of chelating agents makes use of determinations of metal concentrations in blood and/or urine, in addition to the careful clinical follow-up.

3.6 BIOCHEMICAL MEASUREMENTS

For most metal poisonings, biochemical investigation is required in addition to the determinations of metal concentrations in body fluids. In general, biochemical tests of renal and hepatic function are always required, to assess possible impairments of these organs. Renal tubular dysfunction characterizing overexposure with cadmium, mercury, lead or platinum salts, may be disclosed by determinations of urine β_2-microglobulin, microalbuminuria and/or glycosuria. Poisonings with lead, copper and other metals may give rise to raised levels of liver enzymes in blood (Table 3.1). Combined poisonings with a metal salt and paracetamol may accentuate impairments of hepatic or renal functions. Complete blood count with peripheral smear should be also performed routinely. Anemia with erythrocytes containing basophilic stippling may point toward lead intoxication. As indicated in Table 3.1, mercury poisoning may be accompanied by increased levels of epinephrine in urine (Torres, Rai, & Hardiek, 2000).

In iatrogenic or hereditary siderosis and in Wilson's disease the monitoring of liver function tests and liver enzymes are of particular importance in the evaluation of the disease, and also in the evaluation of the therapy. Low ceruloplasmin is an important marker of Wilson's disease and aceruloplasminemia. In hereditary hemochromatosis, repeated phlebotomy has been effective in reducing serum ferritin and normalizing liver enzymes as well as alleviation of derangements of other organs. In some cases of hemochromatosis with excessive iron deposits, phlebotomy has been combined with an iron-chelating agent, in particular with deferoxamine (Flaten et al., 2012). Because early diagnosis is essential for the successful treatment of these conditions, relatives of patients with primary hemochromatosis, Wilson's disease and other hereditary metal disorders are candidates for genetic screening. It follows that biochemical data are essential for the specific diagnosis of certain metal poisonings. But medical biochemistry may not be particularly helpful in others. For example, in the diagnosis of lead poisoning, it is useful to estimate δ-aminolevulinic acid and coproporphyrin in the urine, as well as erythrocyte zinc protoporphyrin in the blood, in addition to the determinations of lead concentrations in the blood. In contrast, the diagnosis of poisoning by metallic mercury vapor is essentially clinical, although monitoring of metal concentrations in urine should be done as well. The diagnosis of alkylmercury poisoning is also essentially clinical together with the determination of mercury in blood.

3.7 PHYSIOLOGICAL, RADIOLOGICAL, AND ULTRASONOGRAPHIC INVESTIGATIONS

Electrocardiography, echocardiography, respiratory function tests, electroencephalography, and nerve conduction studies provide examples of possible ancillary investigations for the diagnosis—and for the determination of the extent of functional damage caused by poisoning—by certain metals. After exposure to elemental mercury vapor and some other metal compounds, the possible cerebral harm is routinely quantified by neuropsychological tests (Mathiesen, Ellingsen, & Kjuus, 1999). Disturbances of physiological functions after metal exposures are further outlined in the sections on individual metals in chapter: Chelation Treatment During Acute and Chronic Metal Overexposure—Experimental and Clinical Studies.

Targeted X-ray may be helpful in case when foreign metallic body, for example, retained projectile, is suspected (St Clair & Benjamin, 2008). After prolonged metal exposure, dense bands develop at the metaphyseal ends of growing bones. They are referred to as "lead bands" despite not being specific for lead intoxication (Beck, Krafchik, Traubici, & Jacobson, 2004; Blickman, Wilkinson, & Graef, 1986). Urgent abdominal X-ray is recommended after presumed ingestion of metal or signs of metal poisoning of unknown origin (Gustavsson & Gerhardsson, 2005; Tan, Chen, Hsu, & Lai, 2015). Detection of metallic radiopacities should prompt measures to eliminate further absorption of metal such as prokinetic drugs, gastrointestinal lavage, or surgical procedure.

Neuroimaging, particularly MRI, cannot only depict effects of metal toxicity that can be helpful in diagnosis but also quantify the concentration of metal that can be helpful in treatment monitoring. Due to its high concentration in tissues, iron has the highest influence on MRI contrast among metals. MRI techniques most sensitive for paramagnetic iron effects are T2*-weighted and susceptibility weighted imaging. Both are also validated for iron quantification using T2* relaxation time calculation and quantitative susceptibility mapping (Dusek, Dezortova, & Wuerfel, 2013). In T2 and T2*-weighted imaging iron deposits are depicted as low signal, dark (hypointense) regions. In hemochromatosis, MRI may be useful in monitoring iron deposits in liver, joints, or pituitary (Eustace et al., 1994; Gandon et al., 1994).

Since cardiomyopathy and cardiac death are the most serious complications of transfusional siderosis, echocardiographic monitoring is usually done in the follow-up. However, reduced ejection fraction, as demonstrated by echocardiography, is a late finding in this disease. Therefore, estimation of cardiac deposits of iron by quantitative MRI is of particular importance in the evaluation of these cases (Pepe et al., 2011).

Brain MRI showing diffuse symmetric hyposintensity in basal ganglia, thalamus, cerebral cortex, and cerebellar dentate nuclei in T2 and T2*-weighted imaging is virtually pathognomonic for aceruloplasminemia (Miyajima, 2015). Manganese deposits have quite distinct MRI picture that can be distinguished from iron accumulation, that is, symmetric hyperintensity particularly in globus pallidus, periaqueductal grey matter, cerebral pedunculi, and less pronounced in putamen and white matter on T1-weighted MRI images (Fig. 3.2) (Fitsanakis et al., 2006). This abnormality reflects recent exposure to manganese, and

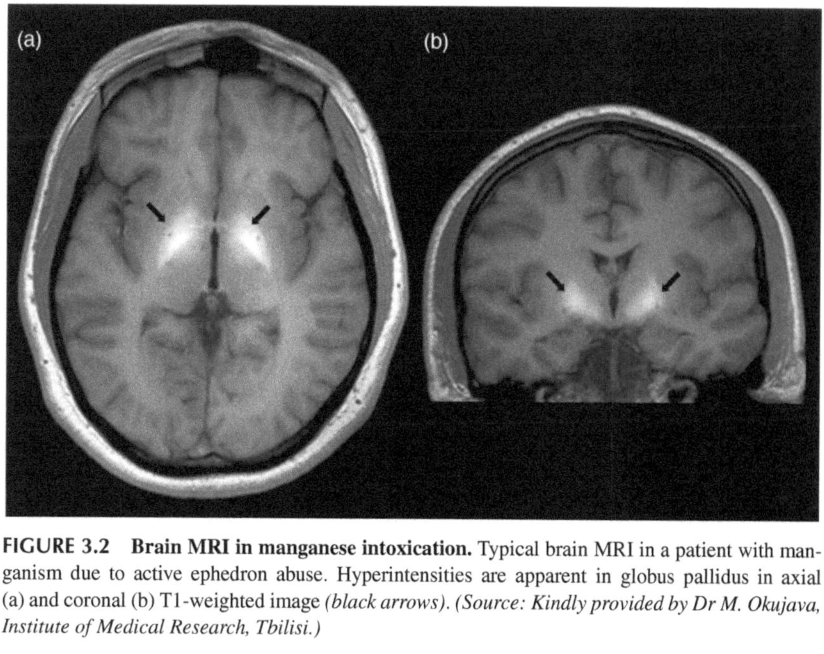

FIGURE 3.2 Brain MRI in manganese intoxication. Typical brain MRI in a patient with manganism due to active ephedron abuse. Hyperintensities are apparent in globus pallidus in axial (a) and coronal (b) T1-weighted image *(black arrows). (Source: Kindly provided by Dr M. Okujava, Institute of Medical Research, Tbilisi.)*

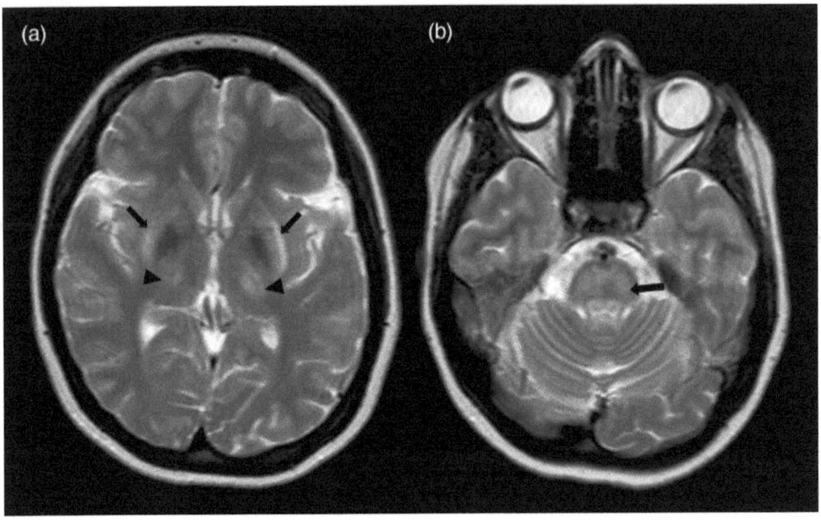

FIGURE 3.3 Brain MRI in Wilson's disease. Typical brain MRI in a patient with Wilson's disease. (a) Symmetrically increased signal intensity in putamen *(black arrows)* and thalamus *(arrowheads)* in T2-weighted image representing demyelination, cavitation and edema. (b) Increased signal in pontine white matter in T2-weighted image *(black arrow)* reflecting demyelination. *(Source: Kindly provided by Dr A. Burgetova, Department of Radiology, 1.LFUK a VFN, Prague.)*

usually disappears within 1 year after the withdrawal from exposure (Sikk et al., 2013). MRI is less specific in poisonings of other metals, usually showing only consequence of tissue damage. Brain MRI in lead, mercury, or copper intoxication shows signs of encephalopathy, that is, hyperintensities in basal ganglia and white matter on T2-weighted imaging probably reflecting tissue edema, demyelination, and cavitations (Fig. 3.3) (Atre et al., 2006; Benz, Lee, Kellner, Dohlemann, & Berweck, 2011; Sinha et al., 2006; Tuzun, Tuzun, Salan, & Hekimoglu, 2002).

REFERENCES

Aaseth, J., Haugen, M., & Forre, O. (1998). Rheumatoid arthritis and metal compounds—perspectives on the role of oxygen radical detoxification. *Analyst, 123*(6), 3–6.

Aaseth, J., Skaug, M. A., Cao, Y., & Andersen, O. (2015). Chelation in metal intoxication—principles and paradigms. *Journal of Trace Elements in Medicine and Biology, 31*, 260–266.

Amundsen, T., Naess, I. A., Hammerstrom, J., Brudevolt, R., & Bjerve, K. S. (2002). Blyforgiftningen kasuistikk. *Tidskr Nor Laegeforen, 122*(6), 1471–1472.

Andersen, O. (1999). Principles and recent developments in chelation treatment of metal intoxication. *Chemical Reviews, 99*(6), 2683–2710.

Atre, A. L., Shinde, P. R., Shinde, S. N., Wadia, R. S., Nanivadekar, A. A., Vaid, S. J., & Shinde, R. S. (2006). Pre- and posttreatment MR imaging findings in lead encephalopathy. *American Journal of Neuroradiology, 27*(6), 902–903.

Bacon, B. R., Adams, P. C., Kowdley, K. V., Powell, L. W., & Tavill, A. S. American Association for the Study of Liver Diseases. (2011). Diagnosis and management of hemochromatosis: 2011 practice guideline by the American Association for the Study of Liver Diseases. *Hepatology*, *54*(6), 328–343.

Badat, M., Kaya, B., & Telfer, P. (2015). Combination-therapy with concurrent deferoxamine and deferiprone is effective in treating resistant cardiac iron-loading in aceruloplasminaemia. *British Journal of Haematology*, *171*(3), 430–432.

Bakir, F., Damluji, S. F., Amin-Zaki, L., Murtadha, M., Khalidi, A., al-Rawi, N. Y., & Doherty, R. A. (1973). Methylmercury poisoning in Iraq. *Science*, *181*(6), 230–241.

Barber, T., & Jacyna, M. (2011). Acute lead intoxication from medications purchased online presenting with recurrent abdominal pain and encephalopathy. *Journal of the Royal Society of Medicine*, *104*(6), 120–123.

Barber, T. E. (1978). Inorganic mercury intoxication reminiscent of amyotrophic lateral sclerosis. *Journal of Occupational Medicine*, *20*(6), 667–669.

Beck, C., Krafchik, B., Traubici, J., & Jacobson, S. (2004). Mercury intoxication: it still exists. *Pediatric Dermatology*, *21*(6), 254–259.

Benz, M. R., Lee, S. H., Kellner, L., Dohlemann, C., & Berweck, S. (2011). Hyperintense lesions in brain MRI after exposure to a mercuric chloride-containing skin whitening cream. *European Journal of Pediatrics*, *170*(6), 747–750.

Bergstrom, R. (1977). Acute pulmonary toxicity of manganese dioxide. *Scandinavian Journal of Work, Environment & Health*, *3*(Suppl. 1), 1–41.

Beton, D. C., Andrews, G. S., Davies, H. J., Howells, L., & Smith, G. F. (1966). Acute cadmium fume poisoning. Five cases with one death from renal necrosis. *British Journal of Industrial Medicine*, *23*(6), 292–301.

Blickman, J. G., Wilkinson, R. H., & Graef, J. W. (1986). The radiologic "lead band" revisited. *AJR Americal Journal of Roentgenology*, *146*(6), 245–247.

Blisard, K. S., Standefer, J. C., & Davis, L. E. (1989). Diagnosing heavy-metal intoxication in patients with neurologic signs. *Western Journal of Medicine*, *150*(6), 573.

Brannan, E. H., Su, S., & Alverson, B. K. (2012). Elemental mercury poisoning presenting as hypertension in a young child. *Pediatric Emergency Care*, *28*(6), 812–814.

Brewster, U. C., & Perazella, M. A. (2004). A review of chronic lead intoxication: an unrecognized cause of chronic kidney disease. *The American Journal of the Medical Sciences*, *327*(6), 341–347.

Bridgeman, A. M., & Smith, A. C. (1994). Iatrogenic bismuth poisoning. Case report. *Australian Dental Journal*, *39*(6), 279–281.

Campbell, A. M., & Williams, E. R. (1968). Chronic lead intoxication mimicking motor neurone disease. *British Medical Journal*, *4*(6), 582.

Cavanagh, J. B., Fuller, N. H., Johnson, H. R., & Rudge, P. (1974). The effects of thallium salts, with particular reference to the nervous system changes. A report of three cases. *Quarterly Journal of Medicine*, *43*(6), 293–319.

Celebi, N., Canbay, O., Aycan, I. O., Sahin, A., & Aypar, U. (2008). Mercury intoxication and neuropathic pain. *Paediatric Anaesthesia*, *18*(6), 440–442.

Cullen, M. R., Robins, J. M., & Eskenazi, B. (1983). Adult inorganic lead intoxication: presentation of 31 new cases and a review of recent advances in the literature. *Medicine*, *62*(6), 221–247.

de Bie, R. M., Gladstone, R. M., Strafella, A. P., Ko, J. H., & Lang, A. E. (2007). Manganese-induced Parkinsonism associated with methcathinone (Ephedrone) abuse. *Archives of Neurology*, *64*(6), 886–889.

Dedeken, P., Louw, V., Vandooren, A. K., Verstegen, G., Goossens, W., & Dubois, B. (2006). Plumbism or lead intoxication mimicking an abdominal tumor. *Journal of General Internal Medicine*, *21*(6), C1–C3.

Devos, D., Tchofo, P. J., Vuillaume, I., Destee, A., Batey, S., Burn, J., & Chinnery, P. F. (2009). Clinical features and natural history of neuroferritinopathy caused by the 458dupA FTL mutation. *Brain*, *132*(Pt 6), e109.

Donofrio, P. D., Wilbourn, A. J., Albers, J. W., Rogers, L., Salanga, V., & Greenberg, H. S. (1987). Acute arsenic intoxication presenting as Guillain-Barre-like syndrome. *Muscle & Nerve*, *10*(6), 114–120.

Dusek, P., Dezortova, M., & Wuerfel, J. (2013). Imaging of iron. *International Review of Neurobiology*, *110*, 195–239.

Dusek, P., Litwin, T., & Czlonkowska, A. (2015). Wilson disease and other neurodegenerations with metal accumulations. *Neurologic Clinics*, *33*(6), 175–204.

Ekino, S., Susa, M., Ninomiya, T., Imamura, K., & Kitamura, T. (2007). Minamata disease revisited: an update on the acute and chronic manifestations of methyl mercury poisoning. *Journal of Neurological Sciences*, *262*(1–2), 131–144.

Eustace, S., Buff, B., McCarthy, C., MacMathuana, P., Gilligan, P., & Ennis, J. T. (1994). Magnetic resonance imaging of hemochromatosis arthropathy. *Skeletal Radiology*, *23*(6), 547–549.

Fitsanakis, V. A., Zhang, N., Avison, M. J., Gore, J. C., Aschner, J. L., & Aschner, M. (2006). The use of magnetic resonance imaging (MRI) in the study of manganese neurotoxicity. *Neurotoxicology*, *27*(6), 798–806.

Flaten, T. P., Aaseth, J., Andersen, O., & Kontoghiorghes, G. J. (2012). Iron mobilization using chelation and phlebotomy. *Journal of Trace Elements in Medicine and Biology*, *26*(2–3), 127–130.

Franchitto, N., Gandia-Mailly, P., Georges, B., Galinier, A., Telmon, N., Ducasse, J. L., & Rouge, D. (2008). Acute copper sulphate poisoning: a case report and literature review. *Resuscitation*, *78*(6), 92–96.

Gandon, Y., Guyader, D., Heautot, J. F., Reda, M. I., Yaouanq, J., Buhe, T., & Deugnier, Y. (1994). Hemochromatosis: diagnosis and quantification of liver iron with gradient-echo MR imaging. *Radiology*, *193*(6), 533–538.

Gil, H. W., Kang, E. J., Lee, K. H., Yang, J. O., Lee, E. Y., & Hong, S. Y. (2011). Effect of glutathione on the cadmium chelation of EDTA in a patient with cadmium intoxication. *Human & Experimental Toxicology*, *30*(6), 79–83.

Goebel, H. H., Schmidt, P. F., Bohl, J., Tettenborn, B., Kramer, G., & Gutmann, L. (1990). Polyneuropathy due to acute arsenic intoxication: biopsy studies. *Journal of Neuropathology & Experimental Neurology*, *49*(6), 137–149.

Guha Mazumder, D. N., De, B. K., Santra, A., Ghosh, N., Das, S., Lahiri, S., & Das, T. (2001). Randomized placebo-controlled trial of 2,3-dimercapto-1-propanesulfonate (DMPS) in therapy of chronic arsenicosis due to drinking arsenic-contaminated water. *Journal of Toxicology: Clinical Toxicology*, *39*(6), 665–674.

Gunay, N., Yildirim, C., Karcioglu, O., Gunay, N. E., Yilmaz, M., Usalan, C., & Togun, I. (2006). A series of patients in the emergency department diagnosed with copper poisoning: recognition equals treatment. *Tohoku Journal of Experimental Medicine*, *209*(6), 243–248.

Gustavsson, P., & Gerhardsson, L. (2005). Intoxication from an accidentally ingested lead shot retained in the gastrointestinal tract. *Environmental Health Perspectives*, *113*(6), 491–493.

Herrero Hernandez, E., Discalzi, G., Valentini, C., Venturi, F., Chio, A., Carmellino, C., & Pira, E. (2006). Follow-up of patients affected by manganese-induced Parkinsonism after treatment with CaNa2EDTA. *Neurotoxicology*, *27*(6), 333–339.

Ho, G., Keutgens, A., Schoofs, R., Kotolenko, S., Denooz, R., & Charlier, C. (2011). Blood, urine, and hair kinetic analysis following an acute lead intoxication. *Journal of Analytical Toxicology*, *35*(6), 60–64.

Chakraborti, D., Rahman, M. M., Mukherjee, A., Alauddin, M., Hassan, M., Dutta, R. N., & Hossain, M. M. (2015). Groundwater arsenic contamination in Bangladesh-21 years of research. *Journal of Trace Elements in Medicine and Biology*, *31*, 237–248.

Chinnery, P. F., Crompton, D. E., Birchall, D., Jackson, M. J., Coulthard, A., Lombes, A., & Burn, J. (2007). Clinical features and natural history of neuroferritinopathy caused by the FTL1 460InsA mutation. *Brain*, *130*(Pt 1), 110–119.

Chugh, K. S., Sharma, B. K., Singhal, P. C., Das, K. C., & Datta, B. N. (1977). Acute renal failure following copper sulphate intoxication. *Postgraduate Medical Journals*, *53*(6), 18–23.

Janin, Y., Couinaud, C., Stone, A., & Wise, L. (1985). The "lead-induced colic" syndrome in lead intoxication. *Surgery Annuals*, *17*, 287–307.

Jellum, E., Munthe, E., Guldal, G., & Aaseth, J. (1980). Fate of the gold and the thiomalate part after intramuscular administration of aurothiomalate to mice. *Annals of the Rheumatic Diseases*, *39*(6), 155–158.

Keogh, M. J., Morris, C. M., & Chinnery, P. F. (2013). Neuroferritinopathy. *International Review of Neurobiology*, *110*, 91–123.

Kim, M. J., Lee, J. D., Choi, H. S., Kim, D. I., Chung, T. S., Suh, J. H., & Roh, J. H. (1989). CT findings of the nose and paranasal sinuses in chromium intoxication. *Yonsei Medical Journal*, *30*(6), 305–309.

Kolnagou, A., Kleanthous, M., & Kontoghiorghes, G. J. (2011). Efficacy, compliance and toxicity factors are affecting the rate of normalization of body iron stores in thalassemia patients using the deferiprone and deferoxamine combination therapy. *Hemoglobin*, *35*(6), 186–198.

Kono, S. (2013). Aceruloplasminemia: an update. *International Review of Neurobiology*, *110*, 125–151.

Lin, W. H., Wang, M. C., Cheng, W. C., Yen, C. J., Cheng, M. F., & Cheng, H. C. (2012). Lead intoxication caused by traditional Chinese herbal medicine. *The American Journal of Medicine*, *125*(6), e7–e8.

Lindner, U., Schuppan, D., Schleithoff, L., Habeck, J. O., Grodde, T., Kirchhof, K., & Stoelzel, U. (2015). Aceruloplasminaemia: a family with a novel mutation and long-term therapy with deferasirox. *Hormone and Metabolic Research*, *47*(6), 303–308.

Livesley, B., & Sissons, C. E. (1968). Chronic lead intoxication mimicking motor neurone disease. *British Medical Journals*, *4*(6), 387–388.

Long, Z., Jiang, Y. M., Li, X. R., Fadel, W., Xu, J., Yeh, C. L., & Dydak, U. (2014). Vulnerability of welders to manganese exposure—a neuroimaging study. *Neurotoxicology*, *45*, 285–292.

Massey, E. W., Wold, D., & Heyman, A. (1984). Arsenic: homicidal intoxication. *Southern Medical Journals*, *77*(6), 848–851.

Mathiesen, T., Ellingsen, D. G., & Kjuus, H. (1999). Neuropsychological effects associated with exposure to mercury vapor among former chloralkali workers. *Scandinavian Journal of Work, Environment & Health*, *25*(6), 342–350.

Mena, I., Marin, O., Fuenzalida, S., & Cotzias, G. C. (1967). Chronic manganese poisoning. Clinical picture and manganese turnover. *Neurology*, *17*(6), 128–136.

Mergler, D., Huel, G., Bowler, R., Iregren, A., Belanger, S., Baldwin, M., & Martin, L. (1994). Nervous system dysfunction among workers with long-term exposure to manganese. *Environmental Research*, *64*(6), 151–180.

Meyer, R. J., & Zalusky, R. (1977). The mechanisms of hemolysis in Wilson's disease: study of a case and review of the literature. *Mount Sinai Journal of Medicine*, *44*(6), 530–538.

Miyajima, H. (2015). Aceruloplasminemia. *Neuropathology*, *35*(6), 83–90.

Muchtar, E., Vidal, L., Ram, R., Gafter-Gvili, A., Shpilberg, O., & Raanani, P. (2013). The role of maintenance therapy in acute promyelocytic leukemia in the first complete remission. *Cochrane Database of Systematic Reviews*, *3*, CD009594.

Muller, T., Koppikar, S., Taylor, R. M., Carragher, F., Schlenck, B., Heinz-Erian, P., & Dhawan, A. (2007). Re-evaluation of the penicillamine challenge test in the diagnosis of Wilson's disease in children. *Journal of Hepatology*, *47*(6), 270–276.

Nemhauser, J. B. (2010). The polonium-210 public health assessment: the need for medical toxicology expertise in radiation terrorism events. *Journal of Medical Toxicology*, *6*(6), 355–359.

Noda, M., Yasuda, M., & Kitagawa, M. (1991). Iron as a possible aggravating factor for osteopathy in itai-itai disease, a disease associated with chronic cadmium intoxication. *Journal of Bone and Mineral Research*, *6*(6), 245–255.

Ory-Magne, F., Brefel-Courbon, C., Payoux, P., Debruxelles, S., Sibon, I., Goizet, C., & Rascol, O. (2009). Clinical phenotype and neuroimaging findings in a French family with hereditary ferritinopathy (FTL498-499InsTC). *Movement Disorder*, *24*(6), 1676–1683.

Ovaska, H., Wood, D. M., House, I., Dargan, P. I., Jones, A. L., & Murray, S. (2008). Severe iatrogenic bismuth poisoning with bismuth iodoform paraffin paste treated with DMPS chelation. *Clinical Toxicology*, *46*(6), 855–857.

Pan, P. L., Tang, H. H., Chen, Q., Song, W., & Shang, H. F. (2011). Desferrioxamine treatment of aceruloplasminemia: long-term follow-up. *Movement Disorder*, *26*(6), 2142–2144.

Pearce, J. M. S. (2007). Burton's line in lead poisoning. *European Neurology*, *57*(6), 118–119.

Pelclova, D., Urban, P., Ridzon, P., Senholdova, Z., Lukas, E., Diblik, P., & Lacina, L. (2009). Two-year follow-up of two patients after severe thallium intoxication. *Human & Experimental Toxicology*, *28*(6), 263–272.

Pepe, A., Meloni, A., Capra, M., Cianciulli, P., Prossomariti, L., Malaventura, C., & Maggio, A. (2011). Deferasirox, deferiprone and desferrioxamine treatment in thalassemia major patients: cardiac iron and function comparison determined by quantitative magnetic resonance imaging. *Haematologica*, *96*(6), 41–47.

Propst, A., Propst, T., Feichtinger, H., Judmaier, G., Willeit, J., & Vogel, W. (1995). Copper-induced acute rhabdomyolysis in Wilson's disease. *Gastroenterology*, *108*(6), 885–887.

Quadri, M., Federico, A., Zhao, T., Breedveld, G. J., Battisti, C., Delnooz, C., & Bonifati, V. (2012). Mutations in SLC30A10 cause parkinsonism and dystonia with hypermanganesemia, polycythemia, and chronic liver disease. *The American Journal of Human Genetics*, *90*(6), 467–477.

Ratnaike, R. N. (2003). Acute and chronic arsenic toxicity. *Postgraduate Medical Journals*, *79*(6), 391–396.

Romeo, L., Apostoli, P., Kovacic, M., Martini, S., & Brugnone, F. (1997). Acute arsine intoxication as a consequence of metal burnishing operations. *American Journal of Industrial Medicine*, *32*(6), 211–216.

Sarikaya, S., Karcioglu, O., Ay, D., Cetin, A., Aktas, C., & Serinken, M. (2010). Acute mercury poisoning: a case report. *BMC Emergency Medicine*, *10*, 7.

Sikk, K., Haldre, S., Aquilonius, S. M., Asser, A., Paris, M., Roose, A., & Taba, P. (2013). Manganese-induced parkinsonism in methcathinone abusers: bio-markers of exposure and follow-up. *European Journal of Neurology*, *20*(6), 915–920.

Sikk, K., Taba, P., Haldre, S., Bergquist, J., Nyholm, D., Askmark, H., & Aquilonius, S. M. (2010). Clinical, neuroimaging and neurophysiological features in addicts with manganese-ephedrone exposure. *Acta Neurologica Scandinavica*, *121*(6), 237–243.

Sinha, S., Taly, A. B., Ravishankar, S., Prashanth, L. K., Venugopal, K. S., Arunodaya, G. R., & Swamy, H. S. (2006). Wilson's disease: cranial MRI observations and clinical correlation. *Neuroradiology*, *48*(6), 613–621.

Skerfving, S., Gerhardsson, L., Schutz, A., & Stromberg, U. (1998). Lead—biological monitoring of exposure and effects. *Journal of Trace Elements in Experimental Medicine*, *11*(2–3), 289–301.

St Clair, W. S., & Benjamin, J. (2008). Lead intoxication from ingestion of fishing sinkers: a case study and review of the literature. *Clinical Pediatrics*, *47*(6), 66–70.

Stamelou, M., Tuschl, K., Chong, W. K., Burroughs, A. K., Mills, P. B., Bhatia, K. P., & Clayton, P. T. (2012). Dystonia with brain manganese accumulation resulting from SLC30A10 mutations: a new treatable disorder. *Movment Disorder*, *27*(6), 1317–1322.

Stenehjem, A. E., Vahter, M., Nermell, B., Aasen, J., Lierhagen, S., Morland, J., & Jacobsen, D. (2007). Slow recovery from severe inorganic arsenic poisoning despite treatment with DMSA (2.3-dimercaptosuccinic acid). *Clinical Toxicology*, *45*(6), 424–428.

Stepens, A., Logina, I., Liguts, V., Aldins, P., Eksteina, I., Platkajis, A., & Donaghy, M. (2008). A Parkinsonian syndrome in methcathinone users and the role of manganese. *The New England Journal of Medicine*, *358*(6), 1009–1017.

Sunderman, F. W. (1989). A pilgrimage into the archives of nickel toxicology. *Annals of Clinical & Laboratory Science*, *19*(6), 1–16.

Tai, M., Matsuhashi, N., Ichii, O., Suzuki, T., Ejiri, Y., Kono, S., & Harada, M. (2014). Case of presymptomatic aceruloplasminemia treated with deferasirox. *Hepatology Research*, *44*(6), 1253–1258.

Takeda, T., Yukioka, T., & Shimazaki, S. (2000). Cupric sulfate intoxication with rhabdomyolysis, treated with chelating agents and blood purification. *Internal Medicine*, *39*(6), 253–255.

Tan, T. H., Chen, Y. H., Hsu, C. C., & Lai, C. C. (2015). Intra-abdominal radiopacities after arsenic intoxication. *The Journal of Emergency Medicine*, *49*(5), e159–e160.

Torres, A. D., Rai, A. N., & Hardiek, M. L. (2000). Mercury intoxication and arterial hypertension: report of two patients and review of the literature. *Pediatrics*, *105*(6), E34.

Tuschl, K., Clayton, P. T., Gospe, S. M., Jr., Gulab, S., Ibrahim, S., Singhi, P., & Mills, P. B. (2012). Syndrome of hepatic cirrhosis, dystonia, polycythemia, and hypermanganesemia caused by mutations in SLC30A10, a manganese transporter in man. *The American Journal of Human Genetics*, *90*(6), 457–466.

Tuzun, M., Tuzun, D., Salan, A., & Hekimoglu, B. (2002). Lead encephalopathy: CT and MR findings. *Journal of Computer Assisted Tomography*, *26*(6), 479–481.

Vacca, C. V., Hines, J. D., & Hall, P. W., 3rd. (1986). The proteinuria of industrial lead intoxication. *Environmental Research*, *41*(6), 440–446.

Vidal, R., Delisle, M. B., Rascol, O., & Ghetti, B. (2003). Hereditary ferritinopathy. *Journal of the Neurological Sciences*, *207*(1–2), 110–111.

Walshe, J. M. (1984). Copper: its role in the pathogenesis of liver disease. *Seminar in Liver Diseases*, *4*(6), 252–263.

Westwood, M., Anderson, L. J., & Pennell, D. J. (2003). Treatment of cardiac iron overload in thalassemia major. *Haematologica*, *88*(6), 481–482.

Yates, D. H., & Goldman, K. P. (1990). Acute cadmium poisoning in a foreman plater welder. *British Journal of industrial Medicine*, *47*(6), 429–431.

Zhou, S., Zhou, J., Liu, S., Wang, R., & Wang, Z. (2015). Arsenical keratosis caused by medication: a case report and literature. *International Journal of Clinical & Experimental Medicine*, *8*(6), 1487–1490.

Chapter 4

Chelation Treatment During Acute and Chronic Metal Overexposures—Experimental and Clinical Studies

Ole Andersen

Chapter Outline

Chelation Therapy in the Treatment of Metal Intoxication. http://dx.doi.org/10.1016/B978-0-12-803072-1.00004-3

4.1 INTRODUCTION

Metal overexposures, ranging from nonsymptomatic, elevated body levels to life threatening acute or chronic poisonings, should in general be treated by eliminating the exposure source, by various decontamination procedures, and by supportive treatment. However, in a quite extensive number of cases, various chelation treatment schedules offer an efficient way of handling the adverse effects of overexposure to metals, either by reducing the toxicity of the metal by forming a less toxic complex, by changing the toxicodynamics of the metal thereby reducing the interaction of the metal with a vulnerable target, and/or by changing the toxicokinetics of the metal thereby reducing its uptake and/or enhancing its excretion.

The present chapter offers a systematic review of the present state-of-the-art for chelation treatment of metal overexposures. Such exposures can be due to occupational, environmental, dietary, or life style factors, or iatrogenic procedures.

During recent decades a number of new chelating agents have been developed and tested in animal experimental models, some of these compounds are highly efficient compared to the classical, clinical chelators. Due to generally accepted ethical principles in pharmacology and medicine, experimental chelating agents proven efficient in animal experiments cannot be used in humans except in special cases, where the benefit clearly outweighs the potential toxicity of the agent. Because the economy is preventive for developing a new chelating agent for a situation with very few patients needing the compound, these drugs are considered "orphan drugs for orphan diseases." For diseases with a large number of users as some genetic diseases, especially the thalassemias, new drugs can be developed more easily. Due to extensive experimental work by dedicated scientists establishing safety profiles, also some of the new compounds are on their way into clinical practice.

Examples of chelating agents that have already been licensed for various metal poisonings are dimercaptosuccinic acid (DMSA) and dimercaptopropane sulfonate (DMPS) decades ago, and more recently deferiprone (L1) and deferasirox for iron.

A basic principle in chelation therapy, discussed in the chapter: General Chemistry of Metal Toxicity and Basis for Metal Complexation, is that metal (Lewis acid) and chelator (Lewis base) should have high affinity (high stability constant), thus soft metals (eg, Pd^{+}, Ag^{+}, Au^{+}, Hg^{2+}, Cu^{+}, Cd^{2+}, Pt^{2+}, Pb^{++}) should be chelated by chelators with soft ligands (eg, DMSA and DMPS), and hard metals (eg, Cr^{3+}, Ti^{4+}, Fe^{3+}, Be^{2+}, Al^{3+}) with chelators with hard ligands (eg, the polyaminopolycarboxylic acids EDTA and DTPA). Intermediate metals (eg, Fe^{2+}, Co^{2+}, Ni^{2+}, Zn^{2+}) prefer, for example, N-containing ligands, but can be chelated by both hard and soft bases. However, the pharmacokinetics of the chelating agent is highly important also, especially whether the chelator and the metal-chelator complex formed are hydrophilic with enhanced renal excretion as result, or lipophilic with enhanced biliary excretion or brain deposition as a potential result.

Some important questions are: Can the chelator be administered orally, and will it enhance the systemic uptake of toxic metal remaining in the gastrointestinal tract or will it prevent metal uptake? Is the chelator metabolically stable to allow extended treatment with few doses?

Yokel (2002) summarized some properties characterizing an ideal Al chelator and the benefits obtained from these properties. Below is provided a modified version of his summary. It can be seen that most of these properties and benefits are in fact true for any chelator used for any metal. The chelator should:

- Be sufficiently lipophilic or small-molecular to permeate membranes by diffusion or by a membrane carrier and thus distribute to intracellular sites of metal storage.
- Be a hard base to complex with the hard acid Al^{3+}.
- Have high affinity and reasonable selectivity for Al (or in general the toxic metal in question) to minimize depletion of Fe and other essential metals.

- Have a stability constant with Al (or any toxic metal in question) that is greater than that of the metal with endogenous ligands to favor metal:chelator complex formation to remove it from endogenous ligands and sites.
- The free chelator should have a long endogenous half-life to provide sufficient time to chelate free toxic metal diffusing out of storage sites since the free metal concentration should be reduced by complexation.
- Form a chelate that completely shields the toxic metal ions and thus block its potential toxicity either via interactions with vulnerable targets or by inducing oxidative stress via Fenton like mechanisms.
- Form a water soluble complex to enhance renal metal clearance, alternatively biliary clearance.
- The metal:chelator complex should be resistant to hydrolytic breakdown at physiological pH-values, that is, 7.4 extracellularly and about 6.8 intracellularly, and resistant to metabolic degradation to promote metal decorporation rather than redistribution.
- To promote metal elimination, the metal–chelator complex should not be reabsorbed in kidneys or via enterohepatic circulation.
- Minimal toxicity of both the chelator and the metal chelate formed in vivo.
- Good oral bioavailability to allow easy off-clinic administration, broader acceptance of use ensuring better compliance. This safer route of drug administration provide potential application also in treatment of neurodegenerative disorders.

The present review of chelation in metal overexposures is ordered alphabetically from aluminum to zinc citing animal experimental studies and epidemiological and clinical studies for each metal, if available. The chapter deals with both nonessential and essential metals. Therefore, it is relevant to state that the term "toxic metal" should be used with care, and may be misleading, since any metal is toxic at the wrong dose, as discussed in chapter: General Chemistry of Metal Toxicity and Basis for Metal Complexation.

4.2 ALUMINUM

Aluminum (Al, element no 13 in group 13 of the periodic table of element, atomic weight 26.981536, density 2.70 g/cm) is considered a light metal. Due to its strong affinity to oxygen, elemental Al is almost never found. Instead Al occurs in oxides or silicates. Al is the most abundant metal (about 8.3% by mass) in the Earth's crust, found in more than 270 different minerals (Shakhashiri, 2008). Pure Al metal is produced in highly energy demanding processes mainly from bauxite ores containing different oxo and hydroxy compounds of Al. Accordingly, recycling of Al is becoming increasingly important since it requires less than 10% of the energy cost of primary production. Aluminum metal is highly resistant to corrosion due to a thin oxide layer rapidly formed upon contact with air. Al is used in different alloys in a wide range of products ranging from airplanes and vehicles via the production industry to kitchen utensils. Al compounds have medical uses both as adjuvants in vaccines (eg, [$KAl(SO_4)2 \cdot 12H_2O$], alum), as over-the-counter antacids and as phosphate binders (Krewski et al., 2007) and are further used as food additives and in cosmetics. Al salts are used in large quantities as flocculants for treating drinking water.

The primary exposure source of Al for occupationally nonexposed humans is food, with intakes around 3–9 mg/day for adults in the western countries (Yokel, 2012, Willhite et al., 2014). Occupational exposure to aluminum compounds occur during production and processing, for example, welding (Sjögren, Elinder, Lidums, & Chang, 1988). Studies of pulmonary Al absorption in various occupational and experimental settings indicate about 2% absorption (reviewed by Sjögren, Iregren, Montelius, & Yokel, 2014). While occupational and iatrogenic exposures have been demonstrated in epidemiological studies to induce lung, brain, and bone toxicities of various kinds, dietary exposures cannot be demonstrated to lead to adverse effects in Europe and USA (Sjögren et al., 2014).

In biological systems Al exists only as the Al^{3+} ion present in different chemical forms greatly influencing Al toxicokinetics and toxicodynamics. Al prefers the coordination number 6 forming octahedral complexes. In water, Al normally occurs as solvated hydrophilic Al^{3+} ions with very low ligand exchange rate. This leads to low reactivity and minimum membrane passage. Accordingly, the intestinal Al absorption is limited conferring very low toxicity to most Al compounds. This allows the use of Al in the aforementioned antacids and in kitchen utensils. Al absorption from orally administered water studied using the ^{26}Al isotope measured by atomic absorption spectroscopic methods was estimated to be around 0.3% in humans and experimental animals (Reviewed by Yokel & McNamara, 2001).

Calculated by comparing measured intake and urinary excretion, 0.1–0.3% of dietary Al is absorbed (Ganrot, 1986; Priest et al., 1998; Nieboer, Gibson, Oxman, & Kramer, 1995). Absorbed Al is distributed systemically via blood. Al in plasma is mainly bound to transferrin (about 90%) and citrate (Yokel & McNamara, 2001). Data from different groups of nonoccupationally exposed humans show high Al levels in bone, kidney, liver and muscles, and lower levels in brain. Due to size differences, bone is the largest and brain the smallest Al compartment among these organs (Priest, 2004; Yokel & McNamara, 2001; WHO/IPCS, 1997). Elevated brain levels of Al have been measured in dialysis encephalopathy patients (Alfrey & Froment, 1990). Whether brain Al levels are increased in Alzheimer disease (AD) patients remains debatable (Krewski et al., 2007), data on association between copper exposure and AD risk seem stronger (Brewer, 2012). Al enters the brain via the blood–brain barrier, likely by endocytosis of Al-transferrin complex (Roskams & Connor, 1990) or by aluminum citrate influx mediated by a cystine/glutamate transporter system (Nagasawa et al., 2005; Yokel, 2006). Carrier mediated Al efflux from brain via citrate binding was discussed by Yokel (2006).

The main Al excretion route is renal, accounting for more than 95% of Al elimination while biliary excretion accounts for less than 2%. Accordingly, reduced renal function strongly affects Al kinetics potentially resulting in bone, blood and brain toxicity.

The long-term kinetics of Al is determined by bone turnover. Internalized Al^{3+} ions mainly bind to bone surface, however, intracellular Al^{3+} ions bind to the high phosphate content of DNA in the nucleus, of importance for the sensitivity of the brain to Al toxicity. Due to the slow ligand exchange rate noted earlier, excretion of Al is slow resulting in a long half-life: After a single i.v. dose of ^{26}Al-transferrin complex (the dominant Al species in blood) to rats, Yokel, Rhineheimer, Sharma, Elmore, and McNamarqa (2001) observed transfer of Al to the brain consistent with previous data indicating very slow brain transfer. The brain half-life of this single Al dose was estimated to be around 150 days. In workers occupationally exposed to aluminum flake powders the half-life of Al in urine was calculated to be 5–6 weeks during vacation without Al exposure, however, in retired Al workers the urinary Al half-life increased with retirement period, being up to 8 years, indicating excretion from several compartments, some with very long half-life (Ljunggren, Lidums, & Sjögren, 1991). Due to the very slow decay of ^{26}Al ($t_{1/2}$ 7.17×10^5 years) salts of this isotope can be administered to humans resulting in very low internal radioactive doses allowing detailed kinetic studies in humans. The half-lives of ^{26}Al in blood, trabecular bone and cortical bone of humans after intravenous injection of Al as the citrate salt were about 1 h, 1.4 years, and 29 years, respectively, indication very long body retainment of Al (Priest, 2004).

In the past, systemic Al exposure of chronic renal failure hemodialysis patients and patients on total parenteral nutrition led to numerous cases of serious neurodegenerative, hematopoietic, or bone diseases (Alfrey, Mishell, & Burks, 1972; Alfrey, LeGendre, & Kaehny, 1976). Subsequent investigations led to extensively modified medical techniques, that is, use of reverse-osmosis treated water, discontinuation of Al-containing phosphate binders, and avoidance of citrate-treated blood products and Al-based antacids for renal patients (Arenas et al., 2008). Also, the production of total parenteral nutrition solutions and preterm infant nutrition formulas was extensively modified to avoid Al contamination. Initiated about 3 decades ago, these measures extensively reduced the frequency of new cases of iatrogenic Al toxicity. However, despite the reduced iatrogenic Al exposure described above, end-stage renal disease patients still may develop microcytic anemia, osteomalacia or adynamic bone disease due extensively reduced renal Al excretion.

In a few cases, the procedures to avoid Al exposure during renal dialysis failed due to inappropriate treatment of raw water. In one case described by Barata et al. (1996), extremely high use of aluminum sulfate for raw water treatment resulting in very high Al levels in municipal water led to blocking of cartridge filters and reverse osmosis membranes in a hemodialysis center. This resulted in rapid acute Al intoxication in 71 patients on dialysis, 11 died within 2 weeks, 14 critically ill patients were transferred to intensive care, and 41 acutely intoxicated patients not presenting severe encephalopathic symptoms were chelated with DFO, 5 mg/kg b.w. after changing the water source and installing new Al cleaning devices in the dialysis unit.

The daily intake of Al as antacids may be several grams, apparently without toxic effects; 0.1% or less of aluminum hydroxide is absorbed in the GI tract (Krewski et al., 2007). Citrate chelates the Al^{3+} ion in a complex that is rapidly and efficiently absorbed in duodenum and jejunum due to paracellular transport induced by citrate scavenging of Ca^{++} thereby opening cellular tight junctions (Froment, Molitoris, Buddington, Miller, & Alfrey, 1989). Several other studies found that citrate increased Al uptake (reviewed by Krewski et al., 2007). Concominent intake of an oral solution of citrate and aluminum hydroxide gel as phosphate binder in a group of female renal failure patients led to rapid development of encephalopathy and eventually death (Kirschbaum & Schoolwerth, 1989). Extensive, potentially toxic, systemic Al exposure may result from antacid consumption with juice or other citrate containing beverages in otherwise healthy individuals.

Al chelation is performed to reduce Al organ levels (especially in bone) and reduce toxicity of Al. This may benefit patients with end-stage renal disease or with neurodegenerative disorders as well as patients suffering from neurobehavioral toxicity due to prolonged occupational Al exposure. In chronic hemodialysis patients chelation therapy is indicated at serum Al concentration higher than 80 μg/L (Canteros-Piccotto, Fernandez-Martin, Cannata-Ortiz, & Cannata-Andia, 1996). Optimal chelation in these different patient groups may require different treatment schedules regarding choice of chelator and administration routes.

Previously, the only available chelator for treating Al overloaded patients was deferoxamine (DFO) originally developed for decorporation of iron in transfusional iron overload in thalassemia and sickle cell anemia patients (see later).

The hydrophilic chelator DFO is poorly absorbed in the gastrointestinal tract and must be administered parenterally, either subcutaneously (s.c.), intramuscularly (i.m.), or intravenously (i.v.). DFO is distributed mainly in the extracellular space and enhances the excretion to the urine of Al from vascular and well perfused extracellular sites. Despite DFO cannot access brain deposits of Al it can decrease brain and bone levels of Al in experimental animals (Dang, Rasmussen, & Levine, 1994; Huang et al., 1995; Gomez et al., 1998a; Yokel et al., 2001). In the study by Gomez et al. (1998a), DFO was superior to four 3-hydroxypyrid-ones (see later) in enhancing urinary Al excretion and in reducing bone, kidney and especially brain levels of Al. In this study, the now clinically established oral Fe chelator L1 (1,2-dimethyl-3-hydroxy-4-pyridone, deferiprone, trade name Ferriprox) was unable to reduce brain and bone levels of Al and only marginally increased urinary Al excretion. A study of the brain kinetics of a single i.v. ^{26}Al dose in rats by Yokel et al. (2001) demonstrated that repeated DFO chelation extensively decreased the half-life of brain Al. DFO chelates extracellular Al thereby reversing the flux of Al from blood and extracellular fluids to brain and bone to be from bone and brain to extracellular fluid and blood and further to excretion in urine. By changing the toxicokinetics of Al in this way DFO chelation as a net result decreases organ loads of Al. After prolonged repetitive chelation, also the brain Al level may decrease as demonstrated by Yokel et al. (2001).

In Al overloaded dialysis patients, advantage can be taken from the high serum Al levels due to chelation, allowing Al to be removed during dialysis: The standard chelation regimen is i.v. infusion of DFO during the last period of dialysis. The resulting elevated serum Al level will remain high until the next hemodialysis course, which will therefore remove a significant fraction of serum Al. An alternative chelation procedure involves extracorporal chelation with DFO immobilized in a device attached to the dialysis apparatus (Anthone et al., 1995).

DFO is not an ideal chelating agent due to the high frequency of side effects, the need for parenteral administration restricting off-clinic self-administration, and high price. However, despite the advent of alternative chelators for Al chelation, DFO still has an important role in treatment of Al intoxication (Kan et al., 2010). Alternative Al chelators have been developed during recent decades, mainly in parallel to development of new iron chelators. Two series of derivatives of hydroxypyridinones have been developed, the 3-hydroxypyridin-2-ones and the 3,4-hydroxypyridinones. These compounds are orally administrable, somewhat less toxic, and much cheaper than DFO (Yokel, 2002). They are bidentate and form 3:1 closed complexes that shield Al, thereby preventing or reducing toxicity due to Fenton like generation of oxidative stress by reaction with H_2O_2 which could occur during formation of less than hexacoordinated Al complexes.

An extensive body of evidence from in vitro and experimental animal studies demonstrates the potential of hydroxypyridinone derivatives from both series to reduce Al toxicity and promote Al decorporation. These studies were reviewed by Yokel (2002). Some of these compounds enhanced the excretion of Al in animal studies (Gomez et al., 1998a, 1998b; Yokel, Meurer, Skinner, & Fredenburg, 1996b), however, toxicity prevented clinical use of several of these compounds. The most promising compound among the hydroxypyridinones for iron chelation after extensive animal experimentation, 1,2-dimethyl-3-hydroxy-4-pyridone (deferiprone, L1) went into clinical trial initially for iron decorporation and is licenced in USA and Europe for treatment of iron overload in thalassemia major. However, L1 was also shown to efficiently enhance Al excretion after oral administration to renal dialysis patients suffering from Al overload (Kontoghiorghes, Barr, & Baillod, 1994; Kontoghiorges, 1995).

Like L1, Deferasirox was developed as an orally administrable chelator for treating transfusional iron overload in thalassemias and other anemias, and is licenced in USA and Europe for treatment of transfusional iron overload.

Since Al^{3+} has a high affinity for the phosphate groups in nucleic acids, intracellular Al is to a high degree bound inside the nucleus. Several different research groups have experimented with combined chelation with two (or more) chelating agents, one with access to the nucleus due to lipophilic characteristics, and one remaining in the extracellular space due to hydrophilic characteristics. If the stability constants for the participating Al complexes are $K_{Al:DNA} < K_{Al:Chel(lip)} < K_{Al:Chel(hydr)}$ the combined complexation processes should mobilize nuclear Al to extracellular Al which should then be decorporated. This principle was first suggested for lead decorporation combining BAL (dimercaprol) and EDTA by Chisholm (1968).

4.2.1 Selected Representative Animal Studies

Giordano et al. (1989) loaded rats with a total Al dose of 128 mg per rat by i.p. injections of aluminum lactate for 109 days and measured organ Al levels before starting Al decorporation by DFO administration, 270 mg over 6 week or 675 mg over 15 weeks. DFO chelation reduced bone Al levels with only minor effect in other organs.

Gomez et al. (1994) compared the Al mobilizing effects of various chelators in Al-loaded uremic rats. DFO, L1, citric acid and succinic acid were administered s.c. at doses equal to 1/8 of LD_{50} for 5 days after daily i.p. doses of of 45 mg/kg aluminum nitrate nonahydrate for 3 weeks. L1 was also administered orally, 200 mg/kg. DFO enhanced urinary Al excretion while citric acid and succinic acid had very little effect. L1 effectively enhanced urinary Al excretion, however the mortality in animals given both Al and L1 was very high. None of the chelators significantly changed Al levels in bone, kidney, and brain, and oral or s.c. L1 and citric acid reduced liver Al levels. Since Al or L1 alone did not cause mortality, the mortality may be caused by the Al–L1 complex.

Xi, Ping, W, Shue, and Benjie (1997) studied effects on urinary Al excretion and Al tissues and serum levels in rabbits of oral administration of 750 μmol/kg per day L1 for 7 days starting two days after s.c. injection of 600 μmol Al/kg per day for 2 weeks. L1 mobilized aluminum from tissues to blood and increased urinary aluminum excretion, and reduced bone and kidney Al levels but not brain Al levels, compared to levels in Al-only controls.

Gomez et al. (1998a) studied the effects of several chelating agents on the urinary excretion and tissue distribution of Al in rats given a single i.p. Al dose, 0.24 mmol/kg. Ten minutes after Al injection, chelators were administered orally by gavage at 1.79 mmol/kg. Positive and negative control groups received a sc injection of DFO, 1.79 mmol/kg or distilled water. These experimental conditions are far from the situation in patients suffering from chronic Al overload, but still offer relevant toxicokinetic data: Measurement of urine and brain, bone, liver, kidney, and spleen Al levels demonstrated that several of the tested chelators enhanced the urinary Al excretion but also increased Al deposition in bone. Several compounds reduced the brain deposition of Al, most efficiently

1-benzyl-(4-carboxyl acid)-3-hydroxy-2-methyl-4-oxopyridine (Molenda et al., 1994) and 1-(p-methoxybenzyl)-2-methyl-3-hydroxypyrid-4-one (Jones et al., 1996) which both almost completely prevented brain deposition of Al.

In a study using a more relevant exposure scenario (Gomez et al., 1998b), different groups of rats loaded with 16 mmol/kg Al per day for 2 months received 0.89 mmol/kg per day of a chelator for 5 consecutive days. Four 3-hydroxypyrid-4-ones including L1 and 1-(p-methoxybenzyl)-2-methyl-3-hydroxypyrid-4-one were given orally by gavage and DFO was given by s.c. injection. All chelators enhanced the urinary Al excretion, however, DFO was at least twice as efficient as L1, enhancing the urinary Al excretion, on an average by a factor of 4. DFO, 1-(p-methoxybenzyl)-2-methyl-3-hydroxypyrid-4-one and 1-(p-methylbezyl)-2-ethyl-3-hydroxypyrid-4-one reduced the brain deposition of Al. DFO was the most efficient chelator.

Esparza, Gómez, Domingo, del Castillo, and Hernández (2000) studied the effects of DFO and L1 alone or in combination on Al excretion in uraemic rats after Al loading with 45 mg/kg per day $Al(NO_3)_3{\cdot}9H_2O$ i.p. for 5 weeks. Young and adult rats were given 0.90 mmol/kg per day sc DFO, 90 mmol/kg per day of oral L1, or 0.45 mmol/kg per day of DFO plus 0.45 mmol/kg per day L1. DFO and L1 increased the urinary Al excretion during 5 consecutive days, DFO plus L1 were less effective than either chelator given alone. However, DFO plus L1 reduced the Al level in liver of young rats, not seen in adult rats. The results of the current study show that a combined therapy with deferoxamine and deferiprone (at half-doses of each drug) can also be effective in mobilizing Al from the body of Al-loaded uremic rats.

Blanusa et al. (2000) chelated rats with L1 orally or DFO i.p. or both in combination, administered at 100 or 200 mg/kg b.w. 30 min after i.p. injection of 6 mg/kg Al as $AlCl_3 \times 6H_2O$. As noted for Gomez et al. (1998a), this experimental model is far from the situation in chronic Al overload patients. At the high chelator level, L1 increased the 24 h urinary Al excretion by a factor of 4 compared the unchelated control ($p < 0.05$), DFO increased the excretion by a factor of 6 ($p < 0.05$) while the combination increased the excretion by a factor of 7, marginally better than DFO alone.

Kruck, Cui, Percy, and Lukiw (2004) investigated the potential of Al chelators, including ascorbate (AS), DFO, and Feralex-G (FG) alone or in combination, for to removing Al from intact human brain cell nuclei. Nuclear bound Al was highly refractory to mobilization, however, combined chelation with AS and FG effectively mobilized Al from the nuclear matrix. The data indicate that chelators with *cis*-hydroxy ketone groups such as FG have potential for mobilizing Al from complex biological systems. The authors propose that AS chelates Al and deliver to FG, calling this proposed mechanism molecular shuttle chelation.

Liu et al. (2005) studied Al mobilizing effects of L1 in rabbits after giving injections of 600 μmol Al/kg 5 days per week for 3 weeks. One week after the last Al injection 750 μmol/kg per day L1 was given intragastrically for 2 weeks.

Compared to rabbits given the same Al dosage with out chelation, L1 effectively mobilized Al from tissues without affecting tissue levels of copper, zinc, and manganese.

Chaves et al. (2009) investigated the potential of combined chelation with tetradentate 3-hydroxy-4-pyridinones (3,4-HP) and bidentate *N*-glycosyl mono-(3,4-HP) for Al-chelation. Combined chelation with the tetradentate and the most promising bidentate ligand resulted in formation of ternary complexes with high thermodynamic stability at physiological pH. A ^{67}Ga in vivo model for Al kinetics demonstrated that combined administration of a mono- and a bis-(3,4-HP) chelator rapidly eliminated metal from organs and whole body.

Saljooghi (2012) studied the Al mobilizing effects of L1 and deferasirox, alone or in combination, using an experimental setup similar to that used by Gomez et al. (1998a) (Al 6 mg/kg i.p., chelators 100 or 200 mg/kg oral 30 min after Al). The high doses of L1 and deferasirox and the combination of both chelators increased the 24 h urinary Al excretion by factors of 4, 7, and less than 8, respectively, demonstrating only a marginal effect of combined chelation.

4.2.2 Selected Representative Clinical Studies

The use of DFO as an Al chelator in dialysis encephalopathy was initiated in a patient in1979 by Ackrill, Ralston, Day, and Hodge (1980). This treatment resulted in striking improvement of the status of the patient. Several other studies confirmed the efficiency. Rather large and varying doses were used in different clinical studies.

Malluche, Smith, Abreo, and Faugere (1984) administered DFO to renal-failure patients with muscle or bone pain affecting physical activity. DFO was given i.v. 14.25 mg/kg b.w. during the first 2 h of dialysis 3 times per week to patients undergoing long-term maintenance dialysis. Serum Al levels increased initially after treatment. Within 2–4 weeks of chelation the patients' symptoms in the patients improved with reduced pain and increased physical activity.

McCauley and Sorkin (1989) reported dramatic deteriorations of neurological symptoms in two hemodialysis patients with aluminum encephalopathy after initiation of chelation with large DFO doses, 1 g and 2 g per treatment. One patient developed paranoid delusions, visual hallucinations, seizures, and speech deterioration after each dialysis session with DFO chelation. The second patient became confused with reduced short-term memory and speech deterioration. The neurological symptoms regressed in both patients after decreasing or discontinuing DFO chelation. This report demonstrates the dangers of using high doses of DFO.

Canavese et al. (1989) administered DFO during the first hour of hemofiltration (superior to conventional dialysis for DFO chelation), 20–100 mg/kg per week for several years, to 3 Al overloaded uremic patients. Despite the Al mobilization was very low, not exceeding 100 mg/year, and the ratio (DFO used/Al removed) was only about 25 mg Al/150 g DFO after two years, the neurological symptoms improved. The effect of DFO chelation apparently decreased after about 2 years.

McCarthy, Milliner, and Johnson (1990) performed a diagnostic DFO infusion test (dose 36.9 ± 11.2 mg/kg) in 50 dialysis patients undergoing diagnostic bone biopsy. The serum-Al (s-Al) levels increased on an average 373 ± 250.4 ng/mL after infusion in 30 patients whose bones stained positively for aluminum, while the increase was 231 ± 179.2 ng/mL ($p < 0.05$) in aluminum-negative patients. The dialysis patients with aluminum toxicity were chelated with DFO once weekly for 11.0 ± 4.3 months. After chelation treatment for 5–7 months s-Al levels had decreased from 401 ± 262 ng/mL to 245 ± 217 ng/mL ($p < 0.01$). Fractures decreased from 1.7 to 0.1 fractures/patient per year.

Vogelsang (1994) studied the effect of two months DFO chelation on Al clearance in ten patients with increased serum aluminum. DFO induced a dose-dependent mobilization of tissue aluminum and plasma aluminum levels increased distinctly. "Low doses" of 10 mg/kg b.w. DFO per week were recommended for some cases.

Kontoghiorghes et al. (1994) administered L1 orally to renal dialysis patients to mobilize aluminum during dialysis. Plasma Al levels almost doubled during the first hour after administration of 40–60 mg/kg L1, then gradually decreased. L1 showed potential as Al chelator in Al overloaded patients.

With the approval of the US Food and Drug Administration, Anthone et al. (1995) developed a cartridge with immobilized DFO for extracorporeal chelation of blood aluminum, that is, without the chelator entering the body. This "Aluminum DFO-HP" was placed in the extracorporeal circuit in series with the dialyzer to study its efficiency and safety for removing aluminum during dialysis sessions in end stage renal disease patients with aluminum overload. Hematologic or clinical laboratory changes other than those associated with dialysis, or side effects and toxic reactions, did not occur during use of the device. Average aluminum clearance with the DFO-HP device was 25.3 mL/min, aluminum clearance with a F-60 polysulfone high-flux dialyzer was 8.4 mL/min. A 2-h treatment with the DFO-HP removed from 94 to 628 μg of Al, corresponding to 1/3 to 2 X the aluminum in the circulation before treatment, accordingly, aluminum was released from tissues into the circulation during the treatment. Up till the early 1990s DFO chelation during dialysis employed doses of 30–80 mg/kg often resulting in severe side effects (Verpooten et al., 1992).

Despite the advent of the new chelators L1 and deferasirox for treatment of iron and potentially aluminum overload, DFO still has an important role to play in treatment of Al overload in (fortunately much more seldom) cases of Al overload in renal patients (Kan et al., 2010). Barata et al. (1996) following recommendations of The Consensus Conference on Diagnosis and Treatment of Aluminum Overload in End-Stage Renal Failure Patients, Paris, 1992 (No authors listed, 1993), used the proposed low-dose DFO treatment for the first time in 41 acutely aluminum-intoxicated patients after high Al levels in municipal water blocked cartridge filters and reverse osmosis membranes in a hemodialysis center as described earlier. Nine patients with post-DFO serum Al>300 μg/L and two patients below this level in the diagnostic test of Al overload by D'Haese et al. (1995): single administration of 5 mg/kg DFO in the last hour of a dialysis session), had DFO-related neurological/ophthalmological toxicity. These symptoms disappeared after introduction of a DFO chelation schedule with administration of 5 mg/kg DFO 5 h prior to the start of a hemodialysis session. In 14 patients chelated with this low DFO dose schedule for extended time periods, serum Al levels and post-DFO chelation serum Al increment decreased significantly during the first 6 months. Similar results were observed in 27 patients receiving conventional DFO chelation. These results demonstrate that 5 mg/kg DFO chelation is as efficient as conventional high dose chelation.

Kan et al. (2010) used even lower DFO doses. Hemodialysis patients with aluminum overload diagnosed by predialysis serum Al > 20 μg/L and serum Al increment > 50 μg/L after 5 mg/kg DFOA challenge received either the new standard DFO chelation of 5 mg/kg per week (21 patients) or an even lower dose of 2.5 mg/kg per week (21 patients). Successful treatment was defined as a serum aluminum increase of <50 μg/L by DFO test. Response rates were similar, standard-dose: 12/21 versus low-dose: 13/21. Low-dose DFO may offer similar therapeutic effects as standard-dose DFO therapy.

4.2.3 Conclusions

Different forms of chronic Al exposure still cause severe human toxicity, and DFO is the presently used chelator in Al overload. L1 and deferasirox have been used with good results in animal experiments. Due to the toxicity of the most efficient Al chelators, an ideal chelation treatment is presently not available. Accordingly, studies to improve the possibility of Al chelation are needed in the future.

4.3 ANTIMONY

Antimony (Sb from latin: Stibium, element no. 51, metalloid in group 15 of the periodic table of the elements together with arsenic and bismuth, atomic weight 121.76, density 6.697 g/cm^3). Geologically, Sb occurs as sulfides and oxides, more rarely as the free metal. Sb is mined mainly from Stibnite (Sb_2S_3) or mixed sulfide ores with other metals. Low grade ores are burned to produce the gas Sb_2O_3 which polymerases and solidifies upon cooling. Free Sb metal is then formed by heating with coal forming CO_2. Alternatively Sb_2S_3 is transformed into Sb(0) by reaction with Fe(0) forming FeS (Anderson, 2012). Sb mainly occurs as Sb(III and Sb(VI) forming both inorganic and organic compounds, other oxidation steps occur as well. Sb and its compounds are used in various alloys, pigments, flame retardants, pesticides, and drugs. Since ancient times antimony compounds have been used as cosmetics and for medicinal purposes. Antimony(III) sulfide, Sb_2S_3, was used as an eye cosmetic (kohl) in predynastic Egypt as early as about 3100 BC (Shortland, 2006).

Antimony(III) sulfide also exist in a red form used as rouge for lips in Ancient Egypt and Rome (McCallum, 1977). Kohl is still a widely used traditional cosmetic worn around the eyes in Africa, Asia and the Middle East, where Kohl specimens may contain a variety of metals including substantial amounts of lead (Alhazzaa & Krahn, 1995).

Antimony compounds have been used as emetic and diaphoretic, also up through the Middle Ages: Wine stored in beakers of antimony metal was taken to induce sweating and vomiting, believed to help cure various diseases (McCallum, 1977, 2001). Most likely, tartaric acid in the wine reacted with Sb forming a highly toxic salt with a composition close to the classical drug "tartar emetic," antimony potassium tartrate.

This compound later followed by other Sb compounds was introduced as a drug to treat the tropical diseases trypanosomiasis, leischmaniasis, and schistosomiasis during the first decades of the 20th century (Low, 1916; Christopherson, 1918). Due to its extensive gastrointestinal toxicity, antimony potassium tartrate had to be administered by i.v. infusion. In 1954, Friedheim, DaSilva, and Martins (1954) introduced the far less toxic antimony(II)-DMSA complex as antischistosomiasis drug. Sb based drugs were completely phased out by the anthelmintic Praziquantel (Biltricide) in the 1970s (Hagan, 2009, Bentham Science, 1996).

In the US, tartar emetic was used as a patent medicine for alcohol intoxication. It was first ruled as ineffective in a court trial raised by the newly established FDA against manufacturer and sellers in 1941(United States vs 111/4 DOZEN PACKAGES, ETC., 40 F. Supp. 208 - Dist. Court, WD New York 1941). http://law.justia.com/cases/federal/district-courts/FSupp/40/208/2340292/. Likely, many deaths attributed to alcohol induced liver damage were caused by the use of tartar emetic.

The gastrointestinal absorption of the trivalent antimony salts tartrate and trichloride was estimated to 2–15% in various animal experiments (Felicetti, Thomas, & McClellan, 1974; Gerber, Maes, & Eykens, 1982). Soluble antimony salts absorbed from the gastrointestinal tract undergo extensive enterohepatic circulation [Bailly, Lauwerys, Buchet, Mahieu, and Konings (1991), and the main excretion route is via urine. The effects of antimony compounds in humans vary extensively, depending on the compound. Most antimony compounds exhibit rather low toxicity, tartar emetic is a notorious exception. Pulmonary exposure to various poorly soluble Sb(III) compounds is considered harmful and probably carcinogenic by indirect mechanisms (lung overload, inflammation and eventually tumor formation) Tylenda, Sullivan, and Fowler (2014)]. Skin exposure to antimony dust may cause dermatitis, and antimony chloride is corrosive to the skin. An extensive review of environmental and occupational fate and effects of antimony compounds was recently published by Tylenda et al. (2014).

4.3.1 Animal Experiments

Braun, Lusky, and Calvery (1946) investigated BAL as antidote in acute intoxications in rabbits with antimony tartrate, the Schistosomiasis drug Fuadin (sodium antimony-bis-catechol-2,4- disulfonate) and neostam (nitrogen glucoside of sodium p-aminophenylstibonate) administered in increasing doses to estimate LD_{50}. BAL was given as 4 doses of total 75 mg/kg over 48 h starting 1 h after antimony administration. For all compounds, BAL chelation almost doubled the LD_{50}.

Eagle, Germuth, Magnuson, and Fleischman (1947) studied effects of BAL chelation in rabbits after single i.v. injections of LD_{95} of the Sb compounds Fuadin, tartar emetic, Anthiomaline (antimony lithium thiomalate) and p-methylphenylstibonic acid. BAL exerted some protection against lethal doses of the 4 antimonials, 4 injections of BAL at 10–15 mg/kg BAL 4 times at 4-h intervals saved approximately half the animals.

DMSA was first recognized as a potent antidote for many metals including antimony in China where both oral and i.v. formulations of DMSA were used in experimental and clinical studies before 1960, well before the introduction of DMSA in USA. Ding and Liang (1991) reviewed experimental animal chelation studies with various antimony compounds. Consistently, DMSA had higher efficiency than BAL in reducing mortality. In several studies BAL had no antidotal effect at all.

In a study in mice of 16 different potential chelating antidotes for potassium antimonyl tartrate poisoning (i.p. administered at $>2 \times LD_{50}$) only few had antidotal effects; DMSA and DMPS were most effective while BAL and $CaNa_2EDTA$ had no antidotal effect (Basinger & Jones, 1981a).

Ruprecht (2008) summarized effects of DMPS on acute toxicity of various Sb compound including stibine and antischistomiasis drugs in experimental leichmaniasis. In essence, DMPS reduced toxic signs including histopathological changes, reduced organ levels of Sb and enhanced the excretion of Sb. In one study (Chin, 1958) the LD_{50} of potassium tartrate after s.c. administration was increased by a factor of 8.

4.3.2 Clinical Cases

Human poisonings are rare. Two patients given a high i.v. dose of tartar emetic by mistake instead of sucrose were chelated with DMSA and survived (Zhang & Ye, 1962).

Blanc et al. (1980) described a case of possible pentavalent antimony poisoning. A 70-year-old 60 kg French lady with cutaneous mediterranian leischmaniasis attracted during a holiday in Spain was treated with i.m. injections of glucamtine (meglumine antimonite) up to 4 ampoules of 425 mg Sb per day, total 50–52 ampoules over 2 weeks, slightly more than the recommended dose of 20 mg/kg per day for 2 weeks. She did not tolerate the treatment well and developed lipothymies at injection sites, asthenia, dyspnea, jaundice, and fever and was hospitalized 3 days after the last injection. She was transferred to respirator in the intensive care unit with acute dyspnea but died 5 day after admission due to severe irreversible circulatory collapse. Chelation treatment was not administered. In Europe, i.v. DMPS is an option for treatment of systemic intoxications with metals including antimony. Despite other antischistosomiasis drugs have been developed, pentavalent Sb based drugs are still the preferred treatment of cutaneous forms of leishmaniasis http://www.cdc.gov/parasites/leishmaniasis/treatment.html 2014).

In one severe acute oral poisoning, a three-year-old girl drank nearly 50 mL of a sweet tasting liquid against ants containing 2.3 g tartar emetic, several times the lethal dose for children. She presented heavily vomiting with a massive diarrhea, soon becoming apatic and cyanotic, so i.v. fluids were given. Both blood and urine Sb levels were high and DMPS chelation was initiated, 65 mg i.v. followed by oral 100 mg DMPS 3 times per day for 10 days followed by 3 times 50 mg per day for another 10 days. Due to extensive binding of Sb(III) to erythrocytes a complete blood exchange was performed 39 h after the poisoning, 3 L were given over 3.5 h. This late intervention was due to the blood type of the child, A_1B rhe pos. Her gastrointestinal conditions normalized over about 2 weeks. She was discharged without internal or neurological adverse symptoms. (Iffland & Bösche, 1987).

Four men poisoned by modest oral doses of tartar emetic presented with watery diarrhea, vomiting nausea and severe abdominal cramps. During baking a cake after an old recipe tatar cream was by mistake exchanged with tatar emetic, about 6 g were used. Gastric lavage and activated charcoal, rehydration, oxygen by face mask were rapidly instituted, and all 4 patients were chelated with BAL, 200 mg i.m. as soon as the poisoning agent was identiofied. Furosemide was given due to low urine flow. BAL chelation continued for 10 days with decreasing doses from 600 mg/day to 200 mg/day. Three patients were discharged on day 12 in good health and had normal clinical results and no adverse indications at 1 month follow-up. An elderly patient with a history of chronic heart disease had cardiac-respiratory failure and received mechanical ventilation and i.v. dopamine. Despite massive transfusion the patient died from multiorgan failure on day 3 (Lauwers, Roelants, Rosseel, Heyndrickx, & Baute, 1990).

Konstantopoulos, Ewald, and Pratt (2012) described a case of acute antimony tartrate poisoning. A 34-year-old Central American male presented in the emergency department of Massachusetts General Hospital with diarrhea, vomiting and abdominal pain. He had been drinking in the night. When he arrived home his wife gave him a glass of lemonade in which she had dissolved a powder she believed would prevent him from drinking alcohol. The patient received close monitoring and supportive treatment, i.v. fluid, and sodium polystyrene sulfonate was administered. At the emergency department his wife was carefully questioned and informed that unless she told what she had given him, he might die. She produced a package labeled "tartaro emetico." Contact with the regional poison center disclosed that the content could be antimony potassium tartrate, and that the dose he had consumed was in fact potentially lethal. He was given activated charcoal and chelated with BAL, 3 mg/kg i.m. every

4–6 h. He tolerated BAL very badly and instead DMSA chelation was started 23 h after admission. The article does not report any adverse late sequelae. Registered drugs for alcohol aversive therapy in the US and Europe are Antabuse (disulfiram), naltrexone and Campral (acamprosate). In certain countries tartar emetic is still sold for this purpose with potentially severe life threatening poisonings as result.

4.3.3 Conclusion

In animal experiments, DMPS increased the survival rates after acute poisoning with various antimony compounds and was a considerably more efficacious antidote than BAL, which had only moderate antidotal effect. The limited clinical experience indicates that DMSA and alternatively DMPS are drugs of choice to be preferred over BAL.

4.4 ARSENIC

Arsenic (As, atomic number 33 in group 15 of the periodic system, atomic weight 74.9216) is a widely distributed metalloid in the Earth's crust, occurring in many minerals, often together with other metals in sulfide ores.

The most common arsenic containing mineral is arsenopyrite. Arsenic is mainly produced as arsenic trioxide. During smelting ores of lead, copper, and gold, the As content gasses off and is collected as a dust by electrostatic precipitation. Roasting produces arsenic trioxide, which is used as starting material for production of the majority of commercial arsenic compounds. Arsenic is used in alloys, mainly with lead or copper, in semiconductors, in pigments, in glass and enamels. The widespread uses of As based pesticides—insecticides (eg, lead arsenate, calcium arsenate, and sodium arsenite), herbicides (eg, monosodium arsenate and cacodylic acid), wood preservatives (eg, copper chromium arsenate), and cotton dessicants (eg, arsenic acid), have caused and still cause numerous acute poisonings, mainly in the developing countries.

The use of inorganic arsenic compounds as medicines is known to begin at least 4000 years ago (Frost, 1967), and inorganic As based drugs were widely used until a few decades ago, and still may be used in a few places in developing countries. Fowler's solution containing 1% potassium arsenite ($KAsO_2$) was first used in England in 1786. From 1845 it was used for leukemia treatment (Jolliffe, 1993), later for chronic bronchial asthma and psoriasis. The prescription of Fowler's solution for several diseases including pellagra, syphilis, malaria, and the dyskinesia chorea continued in the USA until the late 1950s.

Organic arsenic compounds, for example, arsenobenzene were used to treat pellagra and protozoal and spirochetal infections. Arsphenamine (salvarsan) became the drug to treat syphilis from 1911 until less toxic derivatives neosalvarsan and mapharsen were developed (Jolliffe, 1993). Most organic arsenic-based drugs are now almost totally phased out in the Western countries.

The main reason for the discontinuation of As based drugs is their toxicity, since As compounds have side effects as liver cirrhosis, portal hypertention, and skin, lung, and urinary bladder cancer. Medical interest in As compounds has resumed since an arsenic trioxide based drug used to treat acute promyelocytic leukemia was approved in 2001 by the US FDA (Chen et al., 2011). However, already in 1931 Forkner and Scott introduced Fowler's solution combined with irradiation for treatment of chronic myeloid leukemia—the treatment of choice until busulphan came into use in 1953 (Sears, 1988).

BAL and DPA were originally used as antidotes in human poisonings with various inorganic or organic arsenic compounds. Experimental animal studies in mice, rats, and rabbits by several research groups have, however, clearly demonstrated that DMSA and DMPS are much more efficient antidotes, DPA being virtually without antidotal effect, and BAL having only marginal effect, being more than 10 times less efficient than DMPS and DMSA (see later).

A major arsenic related environmental problem is pollution of household water from As containing soil. Some regions in developing countries including Bangladesh, China, India, Mexico, and Vietnam have highly elevated As levels in drinking water. More than 50 millions of inhabitants in West Bengal and Bangladesh depend on drinking arsenic-contaminated water potentially resulting in health problems with arsenicosis, including severe skin lesions ("black foot disease"), neuropathy, or skin, bladder, kidney or lung cancer (http://www.who.int/water_sanitation_health/diseases/arsenicosis/en/, IARC, 2012). Tens of millions could be at risk by living in areas where the As content in water has not been measured. (Wyatt, Fimbres, Romo, Méndez, & Grijalva, 1998a; Wyatt, Lopez Quiroga, Olivas Acosta, & Olivia Méndez, 1998b; Berg et al., 2001; Tondel et al., 1999). The present treatment of arsenicosis is prevention of deterioration and attempt to relieving symptoms by securing clean drinking water, a gigantic task, combined with conservative supportive care. Chelation as an option for treating chronic arsenic toxicity by reducing arsenic stores in the body, thereby relieving clinical symptoms and reducing subsequent cancer risk, has been investigated only scarcely in chronic arsenicosis patients or in other chronically As exposed patients. (Guha Mazumder et al., 1998, 2001).

Arsenic is probably the element responsible for most acute and chronic human poisonings, mainly via pesticides and contaminated drinking water. Below are representative animal experiments briefly reviewed followed by a chronologic series of clinical studies and case reports of As poisonings. In several of the cases patients survived despite the intake of several times the lethal dose of arsenic, in some cases more than 10 times.

4.4.1 Selected Animal Experiments

A very large database on effects of chelators on the toxicity of different As compounds exist, a representative selection is briefly reviewed later.

Graziano et al. (1978a) treated inorganic arsenic (As_2O_3) poisoned rats with DMSA or BAL, 30 mg/kg per /day for 4 days. The arsenic content of brain, liver, kidney, and spleen and the arsenic elimination did not differ between DMSA and BAL treated rats. Both drugs reduced the tissue arsenic content to approximately 40% of that of unchelated controls. The LD_{50} of DMSA was more than 3 g/kg in rats and mice, about 30 times that of BAL.

Aposhian, Tadlock, and Moon (1981) studied effects of i.p. administered DMSA and DMPS on the acute toxicity of inorganic As. The LD_{50} of $NaAsO_2$ was found to be 0.129 mmol/kg in mice exposed only to As. The i.p. administration of 0.80 mmol/kg DMPS or DMSA immediately after and 90 min after $NaAsO_2$ increased the LD_{50} of $NaAsO_2$ about 4.2- and 4.4-fold, respectively. D-penicillamine or *N*-acetyl-DL-penicillamine administration did not reduce the acute toxicity of $NaAsO_2$ under the same conditions. The i.p. LD_{50} of DMPS or DMSA was found to be 5.22 or 13.58 mmol/kg. The ED_{50} was 0.066 mmol/kg for DMPS and 0.065 mmol/kg for DMSA for chelating mice 10 min after 0.15 mmol/kg $NaAsO_2$ corresponding to LD_{100}. The therapeutic index of DMSA at this dose was 209, 2.6 times larger than that of DMPS, which is more toxic than DMSA. Monomercaptosuccinic acid, mercaptopropionylglycine, diethyldithiocarbamate (DDC), α-DL-*N*-acetylhomocysteine thiolactone and a series of polymercapto compounds did not increase the LD_{50} of $NaAsO_2$.

Aposhian et al. (1984) compared the water soluble BAL analogs DMSA, DMPS, and *N*-(2,3-dimercaptopropyl)-phthalamidic acid (DMPA) to BAL as antidotes for acute inorganic As toxicity. The therapeutic indexes at LD_{99} of sodium arsenite were found to be 42:14:4:1. The relative efficiency accordingly is DMSA > DMPS > DMPA > BAL. Since DMPS, DMPA, or DMSA mobilize tissue arsenic and BAL increases the brain arsenic content these results indicate that BAL should not be used as chelating antidote for systemic arsenic poisoning, except may be for systemic lewisite poisoning (see later).

Inns, Rice, Bright, and Marrs (1990) evaluated the antidotal efficacy of the dimercapto chelating agents BAL, DMPS, and DMSA for systemic organic arsenic poisoning by i.v. administration of 0.05 mL/kg dichloro-(2-chlorovinyl)-arsine (lewisite) to rabbits. The chelators were administered i.m. at equimolar doses (40 μmol/kg) based upon realistic doses for the most toxic agent, BAL. They were all efficient antidotes against the lethal systemic effects of lewisite with similar therapeutic efficacy. Mortality was due to pulmonary damage after i.v. lewisite in chelated and unchelated rabbits.

BAL (2,3-dimercaptoethanol) was originally developed as a war fare gas antidote ("British Anti Lewisite") for Lewisite (Peters, Stocken, & Thompson, 1945), however, in animal experiments both DMSA and DMPS were more efficacious antidotes than BAL for treating the systemic toxicity of Lewisite after percutaneous administration (Inns & Rice, 1993). A drawback for BAL as a chelating agent is high toxicity (low LD_{50}), the need for painful parenteral administration and severe side effects. Further, BAL has a tendency to redistribute metal compounds including arsenicals to the brain (Andersen, 1999). While oral administration of DMSA or DMPS could mobilize As from organs of mice after injection of AsO_3 without leading to increased brain deposition, oral administration of BAL resulted in an extensive increase in the brain deposition of As (Schäfer, Kreppel, Reichl, Fichtl, & Forth, 1991): While DMSA and DMPS are suited for both oral and parenteral administration, BAL is normally administered by i.m. injection only. However, Schäfer et al. (1991) compared these 3 drugs after oral administration for mobilizing As from organs of mice. At 30 min after s.c. injection of 8.4 mg/kg of As_2O_3, 0.7 mmol/kg of the chelators were administered via gastric tube in saline, BAL also in peanut oil. All chelators including BAL in saline reduced the body burden of As almost equally, however, BAL in peanut oil was only marginally efficient. DMSA and DMPS did not increase the As level in brain, however both preparations of BAL extensively increased the brain deposition of As.

Kreppel et al. (1993) compared the therapeutic efficacy of 6 DMSA analogs (diesters with varying lipophilicity and some with shielded SH-groups—prodrugs) with that of DMSA in mice s.c. injected with inorganic arsenic (65 μmol/kg As_2O_3–LD_{80}). Chelators (0.7mmol/kg) were given i.p. or by gastric tube 30 min after As. The DMSA analogs had some antidotal effects, but DMSA was superior. All DMSA analogs lowered the As content of various organs except the brain.

Flora, Seth, Prakash, and Mathur (1995) studied the efficacies of DMSA and DMPS in chronic arsenic intoxication in rats. Both chelators effectively promoted urinary arsenic excretion and counteracted As induced inhibition of blood 6-aminolevulinic acid dehydratase activity and low hepatic glutathione (GSH) level. Both chelators significantly reduced As levels in blood, liver and kidneys. As induced histopathological lesions were effectively reduced by both chelators, more by DMSA than by DMPS. DMSA and DMPS are both effective antidotes for chronic arsenic toxicity in experimental animals.

Flora and Kumar (1996) studied the As mobilizing capacity of the BAL analogs DMSA and DMPS in gallium arsenide (GaAs) loaded rats. Gallium arsenide exposure significantly inhibited blood δ-aminolevulinic acid dehydratase (ALAD) activity, increased urinary ALA excretion and blood zinc protoporphyrin level and reduced blood GSH levels and renal alkaline phosphatase activity. Further, GaAs exposure affected relative thymus and spleen weight, spleen cellularity, antibody forming cell (AFC) response to sheep RBC and delayed type of hypersensitivity (DTH), indicating that chronic GaAs exposure adversely affect hematopoietic, renal and immune systems, while serum transminase activity and hepatic GSH levels were unaffected. DMPS was more effective than DMSA in reversing affected immunological variables and reducing arsenic concentration of spleen, liver, kidney, and blood. Except for a significant effect of DMSA on recovering blood ALAD activity, DMPS was more efficient than DMSA in restoring biochemical variables.

Flora, Pant, Tripathi, Kannan, and Jaiswal (1997) studied four diester derivatives of DMSA as antidotes in subchronic arsenic intoxication in rats. Dimethyl

DMSA (DMDMSA), diethyl DMSA (DEDMSA), diisopropyl DMSA (DiPDMSA) and diisoamyl DMSA (DiADMSA) were administered for two 5 day courses to rats preexposed to 100 ppm arsenic for 8 weeks. The diesters decreased blood and soft tissue arsenic levels but were only moderately effective in reversing biochemical indicators of arsenic toxicity. Although the diesters were effective arsenic chelators they were inferior to DMSA in reversing subchronic arsenic toxicity.

Muckter et al. (1997) investigated the As mobilizing effect of BAL, DMPS, and DMSA in different cell- and tissue in vitro/ex vivo models The results indicate that hydrophilic DMPS and DMSA less efficiently than BAL mobilized As that has escaped from the extracellular space across tight epithelial barriers. The authors conclude that DMPS and DMSA may replace BAL in situations where intervention time is not critical. The question which one is preferable for optimal therapy of arsenic poisoning is still open to discussion. Major drawbacks of BAL include (1) its low therapeutic index, (2) its tendency to redistribute arsenic to brain and testes, for example, (3) the need for (painful) intramuscular injection and (4) its unpleasant odor.

Flora et al. (2002a) investigated effects of DMSA and monoisoamyl DMSA (MiADMSA) on gallium arsenide (GaAs) induced hepatic damage. Rats were exposed to 10 mg/kg GaAs, orally, once daily, 5 days a week for 24 weeks followed by single oral daily dose of 0.3 mmol/kg DMSA or MiADMSA for two 5 days treatment courses. After sacrifice a series of biochemical analyses was performed and hepatic histopathological lesions assessed by light microscopy. MiADMSA treatment more efficiently than DMSA treatment mobilized arsenic and induced recovery of several biochemical indicators.

Flora, Kannan, Pant, and Jaiswal (2002b) investigated effects of DMSA or its analog, MiADMSA administered alone or combined with oxalic acid in rats exposed to 10 mg/kg GaAs orally, 5 days a week for 8 weeks. Rats were then given 0.5 mmol/kg i.p. DMSA or MiADMSA, oxalic acid or their combinations once daily for 5 consecutive days. GaAs reduced blood δ-aminolevulinic acid dehydratase (ALAD) activity and blood GSH levels and increased urinary delta-aminolevulinic acid (ALA) excretion and increased erythrocyte malondialdehyde (MDA) levels. Hepatic glutathione (GSH) levels decreased, whereas GSSG and MDA levels increased indicating involvement of oxidative stress in GaAs-induced hematological and hepatic damage. DMSA and MiADMSA administration reversed changes in most biochemical variables. Combined administration of DMSA and oxalic acid was more effective in removal of both gallium and arsenic from body organs, MiADMSA administration induced losses of essential metals copper and zinc. Oxalic acid is reported to be an effective gallium chelator.

Flora et al. (2004) studied dose-response relations in alleviating effects of DMSA, monoisoamyl and monomethyl esters of DMSA administered i.p. at 0.1, 0.3, or 0.5 mmol/kg once daily for 5 days on biochemical, immunological, oxidative stress, and DNA damage indicators in rats exposed to 10 mg/kg GaAs, orally once daily for 12 weeks. Also, the mobilizations of gallium and arsenic were examined. MiADMSA most effectively reversed the inhibited blood ALAD activity and zinc protoporphyrin level. All three chelators reduced urinary ALA excretion, compared to controls exposed to GaAs. Particularly at 0.3 mmol/kg, MiADMSA corrected the inhibited hepatic transaminase activities. All chelators significantly restored the altered immunological variables while oxidative stress parameters responded less to chelation therapy. MiADMSA was however relatively more effective than the other two chelators. The chelation treatment had moderate but significant effect in reducing GaAs induced DNA damage in liver and kidneys. MiADMSA was most effective in reducing arsenic concentrations in blood and other soft tissues while chelation therapy did not change gallium levels. MiADMSA administration induced a significant loss of copper.

Bhatt and Flora (2009) investigated effects of α-lipoic acid, quercetin and captopril on gallium arsenide induced inhibition of blood ALAD activity, liver, kidney, and brain reduced GSH levels, and elevation of oxidized glutathione (GSSG). Administration of GaAs with α-lipoic acid was most effective in reverting GaAs induced changes while captopril effectively reduced thiobarbituric acid reactive substance and quercetin reduced levels of reactive oxygen species in liver and kidney. The results indicate beneficial effects of α-lipoic acid administration during GaAs compared to captopril or quercetin. The potential clinical use in GaAs intoxication must await further studies.

Flora, Bhatt, Dwivedi, Pachauri, and Kushwah (2011) investigated effects of monoesters of DMSA administered individually or combined on As levels in organs of animals after oral exposure to 0.0014 mol/kg GaAs for 8 weeks. MiADMSA, monocyclohexyl DMSA (MchDMSA) or monomethyl DMSA (MmDMSA) were administered orally either individually at 0.3 mmol/kg or combined at 0.15 mmol/kg each for five consecutive days. GaAs exposure inhibited blood ALAD and increased reactive oxygen species levels and lipid peroxidation in blood, liver and kidney and disturbed glutathione metabolism, decreased hepatic and renal catalase activity and marginally increased hepatic and renal superoxide dismutase and serum transaminases activity. Administration of MiADMSA combined with MchDMSA had better therapeutic effect, including reduction of arsenic level, compared to the other combination or individual treatments.

MiADMSA has emerged as a lipophilic chelating agent for arsenic. Flora, Bhadauria, Pachauri, and Yadav (2012) explored the optimum dose and route of administration for maximum elimination of arsenic with minimal side effects and the pharmacokinetics of the compound for supporting arsenic chelation. Rats exposed to 25 ppm arsenic as sodium arsenite in drinking water for 6 months received 50 or 100 mg/kg MiADMSA orally or i.p. for 5 days. Arsenic levels in soft organs, liver and kidney histopathology, oxidative stress parameters, and liver function test were investigated. Arsenic exposure induced hepatotoxicity and oxidative stress; 50 mg/kg MiADMSA reduced body arsenic burden and oxidative stress after oral and i.p. administration, oral administration more efficiently than i.p. administration. Pharmacokinetic analysis indicated that oral administration gave longer availability of MiAMMSA indicating that MiADMSA was more effective after oral than after i.p. administration.

4.4.2 Clinical Studies

Lentz et al. (1981) described a man who ingested 2 g As_2O_3 in a suicide attempt. After admission, gastric lavage and administration of charcoal was initiated. His condition deteriorated rapidly and chelation therapy with DMSA was started, about 21 h after the ingestion of As_2O_3. 4 × 300 mg of DMSA were administered orally per day for 3 days. The cumulative elimination of As during the 3 days of chelation was 27.03 mg, and the urinary As (u-As) level decreased extensively after cessation of DMSA chelation. The patient had clinical signs of polyneuropathy, but survived.

A 21-year-old man was admitted to hospital in shock after oral intake 2 g of arsenic trioxide. Intensive treatment including hemodialysis and i.m. BAL chelation was unable to prevent death within 37 h. Clinical data indicated multisystem toxicities of arsenic (Levin-Scherz, Patrick, Weber, & Garabedian, 1987).

In Argentina, addition of sodium arsenite to meat by vandals resulted in a mass poisoning, where 718 individuals were affected. Urine samples were obtained from 307 individuals. Increasing symptomatology reflected urine arsenic levels with increasing diarrhea, vomiting, and systemic symptoms at urine arsenic > 0.75 g/L. Since supplies of BAL were very low, patients with u-As up to 0.75 g/L were not chelated, 49 patients with u-As 0.76-5 mg/L received 2 mg/kg BAL i.m. for 10 days, 12 patients with u-As > 5 mg/L received 3 × 2 mg BAL for 2 days, 2 × 2 mg for 2 days and 2 mg the following 6 days. No patients, chelated and nonchelated, reported arsenic toxicity related symptoms at 1 month and 2 years after the poisoning (Roses et al., 1991).

A 28-year old man died after ingesting 75 g of arsenic trioxide. He presented with profuse vomiting and watery diarrhea. X-ray showed radioopacities in the stomach. His bowel was purged with extensive amounts of saline and charcoal was administered. DMSA capsules were administered orally but were vomited, so i.m. BAL was administered. The patient died 16 h after the ingestion (Jolliffe, Budd, & Gwilt, 1991).

A 30-year-old male ingested about 10 g of sodium arsenate. This suicide attempt resulted in anuria, cardiovascular collapse, and hepatic damage. After hospital admission, the patient was immediately given gastric lavage and oral activated charcoal, and supportive measures and hemodialysis were instituted. On the next day, he was chelated with 250 mg BAL i.m. and hemodialysis was repeated. BAL chelation did not increase the hemodialytic As excretion. After 15 days the patient was discharged. (Mathieu et al., 1992).

A 39-year-old 28 weeks pregnant woman and a 30-year-old man were both poisoned by eating arsenic trioxide containing chocolate. They both developed multiple organ failure around 8–10 days after poisoning with life-threatening adult respiratory distress syndrome. Treatment in both patients was intubation and mechanical ventilation with positive end expiratory pressure. The poisoning resulted in intrauterine fetal death (Bolliger, van Zijl, & Louw, 1992).

After a contamination of food with As_2O_3, 117 individuals presented with abdominal pain, vomiting, nausea, and diarrhea. They were treated for 6 weeks with oral or parenteral DMSA due to gastrointestinal symptoms typical of acute As intoxication. All patients recovered, despite liver or cardiac toxicity symptoms or neuritis were observed in several patients (Dong, Wang, & Ma, 1993).

Two men (19 and 21 years) presented with gastroenteritis, one with acute renal failure. They had ingested approximately 1 and 4 g, respectively, of As_2O_3 believing that it was a substance of abuse. They were chelated with i.v. DMPS, 5 mg/kg every 4 h. Both recovered without renal or neurological symptoms (Moore et al., 1994).

A 20-year-old male cocaine addict drank about 500 mL of a 16% monosodium methanearsenate solution to commit suicide. He was hospitalized in a state of shock after extensive vomiting with early liver and renal involvement and transferred to intensive care. He was chelated with 30 mg/kg per day DMSA, for 4 periods of 5 days over 30 days. In this period the s-As declined from more than 2.8 mg/L down to 6 μg/L and the u-As from almost 80 mg/L to 20 μg/L. While kidney function was normalized, elevated s-transaminases indicated liver damage, most likely due to a subsequently diagnosed chronic hepatitis. The DMSA therapy was without side effects (Shum, Whitehead, Vaughn, Shum, & Hale, 1995).

A 22-month-old girl ingested about 0.65 g of sodium arsenate. She immediately developed diarrhea and vomiting. After presentation to an emergency department she had a gastric lavage followed by a single i.m. BAL administration, 3 mg/kg before transfer to an emergency unit. After 12 h oral D-penicillamine (DPA) was administered, 9 doses of 17 mg/kg every 6 h. After discharge on day 6 she returned with high U-As levels and a diffuse erythemous rash. The patient was discharged with DMSA, 10 mg/kg (Cullen, Wolf, & St. Clair, 1995).

A 33-year-old woman rapidly developed gastroenteritis and oral mucosal burns upon ingestion of about 1.8 g of As_2O_3 in a dental paste, more than a lethal dose. She was treated with hemodialysis and chelated with DMPS and recovered without complications or side effects of chelation (Kruszewska, Wiese, Kołaciński, & Mielczarska, 1996).

Three workers developed mild symptoms of As intoxication after exposure to Vinyzene, 10,10'-oxydephenarsine, in a chemical factory. After a few days BAL chelation they were discharged without symptoms. Urine analysis did not show increased arsenic excretion (Johansen, Abildtrup, Ebbehøj, Kristensen, & Eshøj, 1996).

DMPS chelation of subjects with recent, long-term ingestion of As in drinking water was associated with a rapid increase in urinary As excretion, several fold above prechelation levels (Aposhian et al., 1997). In 13 subjects consuming As in drinking water (528 μg/L) until one day prior to the administration of a single oral 300 mg dose of DMPS, total urine As increased from a baseline of 605 ± 81 μg/g creatinine (Cr) to a peak of 2325 ± 258 μg/g Cr in the first 2 h postchelation. In 11 control subjects chronically consuming water containing As at a concentration of 21 μg/L, DMPS resulted in baseline urine As concentration of 91 ± 17 μg/g Cr transiently increasing to 305 ± 79 μg/g Cr. The data are consistent with chelation accelerating the decorporation of As in chronically exposed humans. However, animal experiments suggest that compared to cessation of exposure alone, DMPS chelation may predominantly affect the rate of As excretion, rather than long-term net excretion (Maiorino & Aposhian, 1985).

A 23-year-old male ingested about 1 g of As_2O_3. Gastrointestinal symptoms did not start until after 7 h. During the next 5 h, he drank 5 L of water. As the major symptoms had subsided when he was admitted to the hospital 20 h later, the only treatment instituted was BAL chelation (Kamijo, Soma, Asari, & Ohwada, 1998).

A study evaluating the efficacy of DMSA chelation in chronic arsenicosis patients did not show lower clinical scores for arsenicosis than seen in the placebo control group (Guha Mazumder et al., 1998).

Chelation of 5 West Bengal chronic arsenicosis patients with 250 mg DPA × 3 daily for 15 days did not alleviate symptoms compared to control patients (Guha Mazumder et al., 1998). In contrast, Bansal, Haldar, Dhang, and Chopra (1991) reported significant clinical improvement in a patient with acute arsenic neuropathy with asymmetric bilateral phrenic nerve involvement after DPA chelation, 750 mg/day. DPA was found to be ineffective in acute As poisoning in mice (Kreppel, Reichl, Forth, & Fichtl, 1989).

In a single blinded trial study using DMPS as chelating agent, a significant reduction in clinical scores was observed among chelated cases compared to controls. Twenty-one consecutive patients were given As free water and randomized into groups receiving either 100 mg DMPS capsules, 4/day for 1 week, repeated in the 3rd, 5th, and 7th week (11 patients) or placebo capsules (10 patients). Clinical scores of chronic arsenicosis symptoms were reduced in the placebo group, however, much more in the DMPS treated group. u-As excretion was increased in the DMPS group but not in the placebo group (Guha Mazumder et al., 2001). Accordingly, DMPS (but not DMSA or DPA) is a potentially effective chelator in chronic arsenicosis.

A 33-year-old female with a history of multisystem disease was diagnosed with arsenic poisoning. She was initially chelated with DMSA. After she developed neuropathy requiring ventilator dependence, intravenous chelation with DMPS was started, resulting in marked neuropathic improvement allowing extubation. After 1 year, remaining neuropathy was mild distal lower extremity weakness and sensory loss (Wax & Thornton, 2000).

A 41-year-old woman ingested about 5 g of a trivalent arsenic powder to commit suicide. Abdominal X-ray showed multiple gastric opacities persisting despite repeated gastric lavage with saline, supportive therapy and BAL chelation, and a gastroscopy showed nonremovable agglomerates. A continuous gastric alkaline irrigation was performed. After 3 days abdominal X-ray was normal but gastroscopy still showed agglomerates. After further 3 days of alkaline irrigation gastroscopy showed total disappearance of agglomerates. Total 46.2 mg of inorganic arsenic, less than 1% the ingested dose, had been extracted from the stomach. The patient was discharged after 20 days without sequelae (Michaux et al., 2000).

Chou, Tsai, Tsai, Lee, and Lin (2002) studied 17 patients in the Poison Control Center of Kaohsiung Medical University Hospital in the period 1996–2001 (23–64 years old, 5 females, and 12 males) suffering acute organic arsenic intoxication for attempted suicide. The main symptoms were abdominal pain and vomiting. The clinical outcomes were similar for patients treated with and those treated without chelating agents.

A 22-month-old boy developed acute hemodynamic compromise with gastrointestinal symptoms, poor urine output, hypertention, and tachycardia after ingestion of As_2O_3 containing ant bait (approximately twice the estimated lethal dose). He received sodium bicarbonate by i.v. drop and i.m. BAL, 5 mg/kg every 6 h for 3 days, then DMSA three times a day for 5 days and thereafter twice daily until the urine u-As was below 50 µg/L. He was discharged symptom free (Stephanopoulos, Willman, Shevlin, Pinter, & Gummin, 2002).

A 26-year-old man with a heavy drug misuse for about 2 weeks was hospitalized with severe toxic hepatitis and pancreatitis. He developed acute renal failure, cardiovascular disturbances and respiratory distress besides neurological disorders. He had taken an oral dose of As_2O_3, likely about 10 g. Besides general supportive therapy, the patient was treated with extrarenal elimination techniques and chelation with BAL and DMSA for 2 days, then with DMSA only. DMSA was given intravenously and intraperitoneally, 20 mg/kg per day for five days, then 10 mg/kg per day for 6 days). Despite continuous chelation, venovenous hemofiltration, hemodialysis, and peritoneal dialysis, the combined As elimination was only around 60 mg during 11 days treatment, a negligible amount compared to the probable dose. The patient died after 26 days due to multiple organ failure, subarachnoid hemorrhage and a *Aspergillus fumigatus* systemic infection (Hantson, Haufroid, Buchet, & Mahieu, 2003).

Pélissier-Alicot, Salério, Marquet, Panteix, and Léonetti (2003) reported an unusual case of acute As poisoning by i.v. administration. A 38-year-old man injected a solution of sodium arsenite to commit suicide. He was admitted to an emergency unit with aqueous diarrhea, hypotension, and abnormal electrocardiogram. BAL chelation was immediately started but discontinued after 48 h later due to acute renal failure. The patient survived. The symptomatology of this acute intravenous As poisoning was similar to that of oral As poisoning.

Isbister, Dawson, and Whyte (2004) reported two cases of acute poisoning with an unwettable formulation of arsenic trioxide. Both patients presented with gastrointestinal toxicity and were given whole bowel irrigation. DMSA chelation was started within 24 h and continued for at least 2 weeks. Neither patient had any adverse outcome despite high urine and blood levels of arsenic.

Vantroyen et al. (2004) described a case of a massive arsenic trioxide overdose that was treated by continuous gastric irrigation with sodium bicarbonate, forced diuresis, and chelation with BAL and DMSA. A 27-year-old woman had ingested 9 g As_2O_3. She presented with vomiting, gastrointestinal cramps, diarrhea, ECG abnormalities, and abnormal liver function. As absorbtion was reduced by gastric irrigation with highly concentrated $NaHCO_3$ and intestinal cleansing with NaHCO3 and polyethyleneglycol. Forced diuresis, BAL, and DMSA chelation as well as forced As methylation therapy were initiated to reduce As toxicity and enhance As excretion. The patient survived with only polyneuropathy one year later despite the massive As dose, many times a lethal dose.

Two siblings, a 4-month-old boy and a 2-year-old girl, both ingested an inorganic arsenic containing pesticide solution stored in a spring water bottle. The 4-month-old boy died despite attempts to remove arsenic by extracorporeal membrane oxygenation, exchange transfusion, and hemodialysis. BAL was given i.m., 5 mg/kg every 4 h. The 2-year-old girl survived with conventional therapy including i.m. BAL, 5 mg/kg every 4 h. On day 4 she continued chelation by oral DMSA (Lai, Boyer, Kleinman, Rodig, & Ewald, 2005).

Magdalan, Smolarek, Porebska, Zawadzki, and Dyś (2007) described two acute suicidal arsenic trioxide intoxications. A 38-year-old alcohol abuser ingested 2.2–2.7 g arsenic trioxide in 4–5 g dental paste. He developed gastritis with vomiting and abdominal pain. Diarrhea, renal failure or cardiovascular collapse were not observed. Central nervous system symptoms were observed (minor left paresis). Transient hepatic impairment recovered after few days. The patient was discharged on 2 day. A 57-year-old man ingested a few grams of pure arsenic. He developed vomiting, severe diarrhea, and abdominal pain. Myocardial dysfunction, vasodilatation, and cardiovascular collapse due to intravascular volume depletion were observed, resulting in the death of the patient on day 1 of hospitalization. Both patients were treated with gastric lavage, hemodialysis and supportive measures, and BAL chelation.

Stenehjem et al., 2007 described a severe arsenic poisonoing in a 39-year-old woman, who presented with nausea, vomiting and diarrhea, and general weakness. Her condition severely worsened and multiple organ failure developed. Measurement of arsenic in serum and urine (290 μg/kg and 2 mg/L, respectively) indicated severe arsenic poisoning. Chelation with DMSA, 600 mg $\times$ 3 for a period of 45 days, resulted in increased urinary As elimination and modestly decreased blood As concentrations. Clinical signs of arsenic poisoning disappeared slowly, and 5 years later the patient still suffered from peripheral neuropathy. The authors reasoned that the DMSA treatment probably had no significant effect on the total body burden of As in their patient.

Yarris et al. (2008) described the clinical course in 6 preschool children, 8 months to 4-years-old, who had unintentionally ingested various amounts of arsenic trioxide (0.46%) containing ant bait gel bars. The children all vomited shortly after exposure. All children were chelated with DMSA.The prechelation u-As ranged from 1.858 to 13.981 mg/L and fell to normal levels 14–35 days after chelation. Further As related toxicity was not observed.

A cross-sectional survey by Joshi and Bhandari (2008) involving 7683 individuals of all ages living in an arsenic-affected region in the Indo-Nepal Border area was conducted between Apr. 2006 and Mar. 2007. Water containing As below or above 0.05 mg/L was consumed by 3467 and 4216 people. The prevalence of all arsenicosis related symptoms (eg, pigmentation, keratosis, hepatomegaly, weakness, nausea, lung disease, and neuropathy) was significantly higher in the group exposed to water As > 0.05 mg/L compared to the group exposed to water As < 0.05 mg/L. DMSA chelation was not superior to placebo treatment, while DMPS chelation significantly reduced clinical scores of arsenicosis.

An 18-year-old male ingested an extensive dose of arsenic trioxide in a termiticide for suicidal purpose. He received intensive support for multisystem organ failure and was chelated with DMSA replaced by BAL on Days 2–5. He recovered slowly. Nine weeks after the ingestion slowly improving mild peripheral neuropathy persisted (Kim & Abel, 2009).

A 77-year old male dentist with a history of major depression presented at hospital with nausea and vomiting 5 h after attempting suicide by ingesting 4 g of arsenic trioxide. Abdominal radiograph showed opaque material in the stomach and small intestine. Nasogastric lavage and activated charcoal were used to remove arsenic. He was stabilized with i.v. fluid and chelated with i.m. BAL, 3 mg/kg every 3 h for 2 days, every 6 h on day 3 and every 12 h on the following days. On day 3, endoscopy indicated gastritis and superficial ulcers. On day 7 significant anemia without hemolysis was diagnosed. The patient gradually recovered during 5 months and did not suffer any chronic toxic effects (Yilmaz et al., 2009).

4.4.3 Discussion and Conclusion

The case reports reviewed earlier describe several survivals, apparently without sequelae, despite ingestion of extensive doses of organic or inorganic arsenic compounds, several times the lethal doses, sometimes more than $10 \times LD_{100}$. Due to the delay and low intensity of the chelation treatment in some of the cases, survival is likely to be due to supportive treatment. Also, in several cases, the arsenic compound ingested had low solubility so intensive support and GI cleaning were effective in improving the clinical outcome.

The low toxicities and high therapeutic indexes of DMPS and DMSA and the possibility of both oral and intravenous administration due to high water solubility make them candidates for replacing BAL in treatment of acute and chronic inorganic arsenic poisoning. They may be less effective in acute intoxication with lipophilic organoarsenicals due to reduced intracellular availability. Despite clear evidence of the superior efficiacy of DMSA and DMPS, BAL and DPA are however still used in clinical treatment of acute As poisoning.

Based on the earlier review, the recommended therapy in acute oral As poisoning is oral and/or parenteral chelation with DMPS, instituted as fast as clinically possible. If DMPS is not available, DMSA should be employed as the second choice. In severe poisonings by organic arsenicals, BAL may still have a role as As antidote. Chelation should be initiated in symptomatic As-poisoned patients and in patients with urine arsenic levels exceeding 200 μg/L. If renal failure occurs, hemodialysis combined with DMPS chelation should be initiated. Treatment of arsine gas exposure differs in that chelating agents appear to be ineffective. Exchange blood transfusions may be necessary in arsine poisonings to overcome the hemolytic response, and hemodialysis may be needed for arsine induced renal failure.

4.5 BERYLLIUM

Beryllium (Be, atomic number 4, in group 2 of the periodic table of the elements, atomic weight 9.0122, density 1.848 g/cm^3) is among the lightest metallic elements. Be metal has a very high hardness with melting point 1278°C. Due to a beryllium oxide film rapidly formed on surfaces on exposure of Be to air it is highly resistance to corrosion. Be confers resistance to vibration fatigue and shock in alloys with other metals. Be easily forms compounds with covalent bonds. Beryllium is mainly produced from silicate ores, beryl ($Al_2Be_3Si_6O_{18}$) and bertrandite ($Be_4(OH)_2Si_2$). Beryllium compounds are important materials in the electronic, automotive, aerospace, nuclear, and defense industries despite their relatively high cost. Despite limited geological resources of Be, its uses are increasing. Three forms of beryllium are important: pure beryllium metal, copperberyllium alloy, and beryllium oxide ceramics. Beryllium is produced from beryl by smelting, fritting, and grinding producing water soluble sulfate. Bertrandite is crushed with water to a slurry and heated with sulfuric acid. The sulfates formed are transformed via several steps into beryllium hydroxide used for producing beryllium metal, copper–beryllium alloy, and beryllium oxide ceramics (Kolanz, 2001). Copper–beryllium master alloy is produced by arc furnace reduction of beryllium oxide by carbon at 1800–2000°C in the presence of molten copper to form a master alloy with 4.0–4.25% beryllium by weight. Other beryllium alloys are produced by melting this master alloy with copper or other metals including Ni, Fe, and Al (Jakubke & Jeschkeit, 1994).

Due to the high toxicities of various beryllium compounds, control of occupational exposures is an important health issue. Accordingly environmental standards have been set at increasingly lower exposure levels, present time weighted average (TWA) concentrations are around 0.01–1 $\mu g/m^3$. Be compounds are poorly absorbed after oral exposure while inhalation may results in long-term storage in lung tissues including pulmonary lymph nodes and eventually in the skeleton, an important Be depot during chronic exposure (Jakubowskij & Palczynski, 2014).

Be salts are strong immunotoxins inducing various pathological changes based on delayed allergic hypersensitivity. Acute inhalation may cause acute pneumoconiosis while chronic inhalation may cause berylliosis [chronic beryllium disease (CBD), a chronic pulmonary granulomatosis], that may be misdiagnosed as sarcoidosis (Newman & Kreiss, 1992). Thus, the increased incidence of sarcoidosis reported in fire-fighters, for example, after the World Trade Center disaster in 2001, may in part be related to Be-containing dust. (Izbicki et al., 2007).

Berylliosis is a T cell-mediated disorder induced by Be acting as a hapten which interacts with pulmonary antigen-presenting cells. Skin exposures to soluble Be salts have caused erythematous, edematous, and papulovesicular dermatitis while insoluble beryllium salts may cause granulomatous necrotic changes and ulcerations due to skin penetration. An increased incidence of lung cancer has been observed among beryllium exposed workers. The International Agency for Research on Cancer (IARC, 2012) has classified beryllium as a group 1 substance (ie, sufficient evidence for carcinogenicity in humans).

Clinical studies of berylliosis patients indicate that systemic glucocorticosteroid (GCS) treatment improve pulmonary function and alleviate symptoms. Patients not responding to GCS or developing severe side effects from GCS may be treated with other immunosuppressants, for example, azathioprine, cyclosporine or methotrexate (Mroz, Balkisson, & Newman, 2001, Salvator et al., 2013). Other treatment options involve immunization against respiratory pathogens, bronchodilators, and oxygen (Maier & Newman, 1998).

4.5.1 Experimental Chelation Studies

The knowledge about potential beneficial effects of chelation treatment of beryllium poisoning is scarce. Basinger, Johnson, Burka, and Jones (1982) studied 11 water soluble chelating agents as antidotes for acute beryllium sulfate intoxication in mice. The most effective of these was sodium 4,5-dihydroxy-1,3-benzenedisulfonate (Tiron).

Mathur, Flora, Mathur, and Gupta (1993) studied 3 polyaminopolycarboxylic acids as antidotes for experimental beryllium intoxication in male rats. *N*-(2-hydroxyethyl) ethylene diamine triacetic acid (HEDTA) was more effective than $CaNa_2EDTA$ in reducing both histopathological lesions in the liver and spleen, beryllium-induced inhibition of hepatic alkaline phosphatase activity, and blood, kidneys and spleen levels of beryllium. Calcium trisodium diethylene triaminepentaacetic acid ($CaNa_3DTPA$) induced severe liver and systemic toxicity. This study indicates that HEDTA is a potential chelator for beryllium poisoning.

In a following study of effects of DMSA and DMPS on biochemical indicators of toxic effects and on body beryllium burden in rats, Mathur, Flora, Mathur, Kannan, and Gupta (1994) found DMPS to be a more efficient chelator for acute Be poisoning than DMSA. Chelators, 50 mg/kg once a day for 3 days, were injected i.p. starting immediately after one i.p. injection of 2.5 mg/kg Be as the nitrate. DMSA and DMPS both alleviated most Be-induced changes in alkaline and acid phosphatase, glutathione, hepatic lipid peroxidation, and porphyrin metabolism. Histopathological lesions in liver and kidneys and tissue Be levels and were significantly reduced by DMPS, less so by DMSA.

An experimental study by Flora, Mathur, and Mathur (1995c) demonstrated that in male rats repeatedly dosed with $Be(NO_3)_2$ (0.5 mg/kg, orally, daily 5 days/week for 21 days) both DMPS and DMSA chelation (50 mg/kg, twice daily for 5 days) decreased organ Be concentration and enhanced fecal Be excretion. DMPS was more efficient than DMSA in enhancing Be mobilization and decreasing biochemical and histological indications of tissue damage induced by Be. The authors conclude that DMPS chelation likely is beneficial in beryllium poisoning.

Sharma, Johri, and Shukla (2000) studied Tiron (disodium 4,5-dihydroxy-1,3- benzenedisulfonate) and $CaNa_2EDTA$ as chelating antidotes in rats given one i.m. injection of 50 mg/kg beryllium nitrate. EDTA and Tiron were injected i.p., 111 mg/kg and 471 mg/kg respectively, for 3 consecutive days. Tiron was more efficient than EDTA both in correcting biochemical indicators of Be toxicity and in reducing beryllium levels in liver, kidney and lungs.

Johri, Shukla, and Sharma (2002) and Johri, Shrivastava, Sharma, and Shukla (2004) studied alleviating effects of 0.3 mmol/kg GSH i.p. or DMPS 0.3 mmol/kg p.o. combined with 0.5 mg/kg sodium selenite s.c. or 0.3 mmol/kg DPA with 0.5 mg/kg sodium selenite, on Be toxicity in rats given a single i.m. dose of 50 mg/kg beryllium nitrate. Therapy was performed for 3 consecutive days and all treatments reduced biochemical indicators of poisoning and organ Be levels compared to the Be treated control group, most effectively by DPA + Se followed by DMPS + Se and GSH.

Nirala, Bhadauria, Mathur, and Mathur (2007) investigated tiron as antidote for subchronic beryllium poisoning in rats i.p. injected with 1 mg/kg beryllium nitrate daily for 28 days followed by chelation for 5 consecutive days. Exposure to beryllium increased Be levels in liver, kidney, and serum and changed serum bilirubin, creatinine and urea levels and the activities of an extensive suite of biochemical indicators of acute poisoning, as well as induced severe histopathological damage in liver and kidneys. Tiron (300 mg/kg, i.p.) alone or combined with α-tocopherol (25 mg/kg, p.o.) or piperine (10 mg/kg, p.o.) alleviated Be toxicity seen as reversed alterations of indicators toward control levels. Tiron combined with α-tocopherol was more efficient than tiron alone, however, the combination of tiron with piperidine offered the best therapeutic potential.

Nirala et al. (2008) in the same experimental model studied the effect of propolis (honey beehive product; 200 mg/kg, p.o.) combined with tiron (300 mg/kg, i.p.) after exposure of rats to beryllium nitrate (1 mg/kg, i.p.) daily for 28 days. Tiron combined with propolis more effectively than either compound alone alleviated Be toxicity seen as reversed alterations of indicators toward control levels their individual treatment.

4.5.2 Clinical Experience

Only one small study has been identified: Cash, Shapiro, Levy, and Hopkins (1959) investigated EDTA salts as chelating agents in 2 patients suffering from occupationally induced beryllium pneumoconiosis with pulmonary insufficience. In a short-time clinical study, Na_3HEDTA administration by i.v. infusion (total 2.8 g to one patient, and 3 g to the other patient over 3 days) extensively increased the daily urinary Be elimination (5–7 times in case one, much more in case 2). Case 2 was chelated with 3 g Ca_2EDTA on day 4, also increasing Be elimination extensively. There are no comments on clinical effects of this chelation, which would not be expected, but potentially chelation could be alleviating symptoms in acute pulmonary and dermal Be disease.

4.5.3 Conclusion

The available animal experimental evidence indicates than among generally available chelators for use in humans, DMPS, DMSA, EDTA, and DPA are potential antidotes. Since a direct comparison between these chelators has not been done in animals, a conclusion on which is the optimal choice must await further experimental generated information. Early studies (Schubert & Lindenbaum, 1954) indicated that the chelator aurintricarboxylic acid through its oxygen donor groups had high affinity for beryllium, that is a "hard" calcium-resembling metal. In accord with these observations, $CaNa_2EDTA$ might turn out to be a first choice in the clinical treatment of acute cases, whereas corticosteroids should be added in chronic cases.

4.6 BISMUTH

Bismuth (Bi, atomic number 83, in group 15 of the periodic system of the elements together with antimony and arsenic, atomic weight 208.98, density, 9.7 g/cm^3) is a crystalline metal with a white slightly pink color. Geologically, bismuth occurs as bismuthinite (Bi_2S_3) and bismite (BiO_3) together with tin dioxide and lead and copper sulfide ores. Metallic bismuth is produced in relation to copper and lead refining. Bismuth occurs in inorganic and organic compounds in oxidation states +3 and +5.

Bismuth is mainly used in low-melting alloys and metallurgical additives and in electronic industry. Other uses are in various industrial chemicals, catalysts, cosmetics, and pharmaceuticals; bismuth salts have been used medically for centuries, and the previous therapeutic uses of a wide range of bismuth compounds were an important exposure source. Bismuth compounds alone or in combination with organic arsenic compounds were previously used to treat syphilis, treatments now replaced by penicillin and other antibiotics (Slikkerveer & de Wolff, 1989). Cosmetic uses of various bismuth compounds are still common.

Large doses (occasionally several grams of bismuth salts per day) were earlier used to treat a variety of gastrointestinal diseases with over-the-counter drugs. This led to severe epidemics of nephropathies and especially encephalopathies in the mid-1970s in France affecting about 1000 people and with fatal outcomes in 70 cases (Martin-Bouyer, 1976; Slikkerveer & de Wolff, 1989). Dresow et al. (1991) calculated the gastrointestinal absorption of ^{205}Bi in rats to 0.26–0.33% for oral bismuth citrates (basic bismuth citrate, colloidal bismuth subcitrate) and 0.04–0.11% for oral basic bismuth nitrate, salicylate, gallate, and bismuth aluminate based on ^{205}Bi whole body retention and accumulated ^{205}Bi urinary excretion. Retained bismuth mainly accumulated in the kidney, followed by bone, red blood cells and the lung. The whole body retention, fecal and urinary excretions of ^{205}Bi followed a three-compartment model with half-lives of 10, 36, and 295 h. This low absorption would not lead to extensive renal and neurological toxicity.

The present standard treatment of patients with peptic ulcers due to *Helicobacter pylori* infection is one-week combined therapy with the antibiotics clarithromycin and amoxicillin combined with a proton pump inhibitor, for example, omeprazole (Malfertheiner et al., 2012). Variations of this therapy are used in patients allergic to one of the drugs or harboring antibiotic-resistant bacteria. These patients are treated with alternative drugs often including a bismuth compound such as colloid bismuth subsalicylate or colloidal bismuth subcitrate, CBS (DeNol, tripotassium dicitratobismuthate) (Kung et al., 1997; Laine et al., 2003; Graham, Opekun, Belson, El-Zimaity, & Carlson, 2005; Kuo et al., 2012). The intestinal absorption of CBS and of basic bismuth salicylate is about 0.35 and 0.08% in rats, respectively (Dresow et al., 1991). Also, patients receiving CBS had higher p-Bi than those receiving basic bismuth salicylate (Raedsch, Walter-Sack, Weber, & Blessing, 1990). This therapy is therefore expected to be strictly local, however high-level oral exposures have caused kidney and liver damage (proximal renal tubule epithelial necrosis potentially leading to tubule degeneration and renal failure and hepatic fatty changes and necrosis) as well as neurological dysfunction including severe lethal encephalopathy. Even though the uses of bismuth based drugs have been extensively reduced after previous frequent intoxications, cases of CBS induced systemic toxicity (renal failure, encephalopathy) are still seen due to continued use for extended time periods or accidental or deliberate overdose.

4.6.1 Animal Chelation Studies

Basinger, Jones, and Mc. Croskey (1983) tested the antidotal efficacy of nine chelating agents in acute bismuth poisoning. After a single parenteral administration of a lethal dose of $Bi(NO_3)_3H_2O$ to mice, DMSA and DMPS effectively protected against mortality and DMSA reduced bismuth deposition in liver and kidneys, so effective chelators should have vicinal thiol groups combined with adjacent hydroxyl groups. DPA had some antidotal effect.

Allain, Krari, Chaleil, Lagier, and Jouglard (1991) studied concentrations of Bi in tissues of rats given 400 mg/kg per day of a suspension of bismuth nitrate Basic Recaptur (Prolabo) by intubation for one month. Different experimental groups received 10 mmol/L of one of the chelators $CaNa_2EDTA$, nitrilotriacetic acid (Na_3NTA), tripolyphosphate (TPP), cysteine or DDC. Cysteine and DDC most effectively increased Bi levels in tissues but with a wide dispersion of levels. EDTA increased Bi levels in kidney, brain and bone and NTA increased kidney levels. Even the rats with the highest Bi levels showed no signs of behavioral problems or obvious sign of toxicity. The study did not succeed in reproducing in rats the Bi toxicity observed in patients in the mid-seventies in France.

Slikkerveer, Jong, Helmich, and De Wolff, 1992 compared the ability of several chelators to mobilize Bi in rats loaded with a sublethal CBS dose (50 μmol/kg i.p. per day for 14 days). Groups were chelated by i.p. doses of 250 μmol/kg per day for 3 consecutive days of either BAL, DMPS, DMSA, DFO, $CaNa_2EDTA$, or DPA. The dithiol compounds (DMPS, DMSA, and BAL) effectively reduced Bi levels in most organs (especially in kidney and liver) and DMPS and BAL increased urinary Bi elimination. The only chelator lowering brain bismuth levels was BAL, while EDTA increased brain bismuth levels. DPA and DFO were without effects. DMSA and DMPS may be clinically useful while BAL should only be used in very severe cases of poisoning due its own toxicity.

Tubafard and Fatemi (2008) studied effects of DFO and L1 on bismuth toxicity after oral administration of bismuth as bismuth nitrate to rats at doses of 20 μg/L drinking water or 40 mg/kg food for 55 days. L1 and DFO (110 mg/kg b.w.) were given orally (L1) or intraperitoneally (DFO) for 1 week as single or combined chelation. Combined DFO and L1 chelation extensively increased bismuth excretion. DFO more effectively than L1 reduced Bi tissues levels. The efficiency of DFO + L1 is higher than those of DFO or L1 in removing bismuth from organs.

4.6.2 Clinical Chelation Studies

Only few cases of chelation treatment of humans exposed to bismuth are reported. BAL, DPA, DMPS, and DMSA have been used.

Molina, Calandre, and Bermejo (1989) reported two cases of Bi induced encephalopathy chelated with BAL. A 68-year-old man with a 20 years lasting occasional use of bismuth subgallate for abdominal complaints developed tremor and confusion. He was hospitalized due to rapid deterioration and after clinical assessment chelated with i.m. BAL, 600 mg/kg every 8 h for 3 days, then 150 mg/12 h until day 13. The patient rapidly recovered. Only mild tremor remained after 1 month. A 32-year-old woman was admitted with seizures, speech impairment and episodes of memory loss after intake of 2–3 g bismuth subgallate per day for 4 weeks for constipation. After medical evaluation i.m. BAL chelation was started, 300 mg/kg per 4 h day 1, per 6 h day 2, per 8 h day 3–4, per 12 h day 5–10. The neurological symptoms disappeared during the period of chelation. The patient was asymptomatic 2 weeks after initiation of chelation.

Playford et al. (1990) described a 68-year-old patient with chronic renal failure who by mistake took twice the recommended dose of DeNol liquid to treat gastrointestinal bleeding, totally 864 mg bismuth per day for 2 months. He developed encephalopathy with hallucinations, ataxia, and an abnormal EEG. DeNol treatment was suspended and the patient was chelated with oral DMPS for 10 days resulting in about 10 times increased Bi clearance compared to the clearance before and after chelation. The patient completely recovered his mental function.

Stevens, Moore, House, Volans, and Rainford (1995) reported a suicidal case of acute Bi poisoning. A 21-year-old man had taken 50–60 DeNol tablets corresponding to about 7 g of bismuth. He was hospitalized 48 h after in an anuric state. After initial oral activated charcoal and polyethylene glycol and i.m. chelation with BAL he was dialyzed daily for 6 days simultaneously with repeated i.v. infusions of DMPS (250 mg/kg per 4 h for 2 days, 250 mg/kg per 6 h for 2 days, followed by 2 × 250 mg/kg daily for the next 14 days. BAL failed to mobilize bismuth to dialysate despite a blood level of 590 μg/L Bi, but i.v. DMPS combined with dialysis mobilized extensive amounts of Bi into the dialysate and reduced blood Bi to below 50 μg/L.

Slikkerveer et al. (1998) compared the mobilization of Bi by DMPS and DMSA in 24 human volunteers treated with CBS for *Helicobacter pylori*-associated gastritis. Twelve patients received a single oral dose of 30 mg/kg DMSA or DMPS in a randomized single blinded design. The blood Bi levels were extensively increased during the first 4 h after DMSA intake, only marginal increases were seen for DMPS. Both chelators increased the urinary bismuth excretion 50-fold. Both treatments were well tolerated.

Hruz, Mayr, Löw, Drewe, and Huber (2002) described an acute suicidal CBS poisoning. After ingesting of 5.4 g colloidal bismuth subcitrate in a suicide attempt a 22-year-old woman presented with Fanconi's syndrome and acute renal failure progressing to anuria on day 3. Accordingly i.v. DMPS chelation combined with hemodialysis was started 60 h after intoxication. During 6 days serum bismuth decreased from 640 μg/L to 15 μ/L. Renal function improved and hemodialysis was discontinued on day 14. Her renal damage appeared completely reversible.

Cengiz, Uslu, Gök, and Anarat (2005) reported another suicidal case where a 16-year-old girl presented with nausea, vomiting, and facial paresthesia ten days after intake of 60 tablets of DeNol corresponding to 18 g of colloidal bismuth subcitrate. Clinical tests indicated minimal fluid overload but no signs of encephalopathy and a serum bismuth level of 495 μg/L. The patient received fluid therapy and and was chelated with DPA. Due to acute renal failure hemodialysis was instituted. Renal function gradually returned to normal over 9 weeks.

Ovaska et al. (2008) described a patient with neurological complications after packing a wound with bismuth iodoform paraffin paste (BIPP). After a 67-year-old man had a pelvic tumor surgically resected a severe postoperative infection requested intensive cleaning and BIPP packing was performed for surgical wound breakdown. Five days after he developed clinical signs of bismuth toxicity (confusion, tremor, gastrointestinal discomfort, and nausea). His condition deteriorated over the next 5 days, blood and urine Bi levels were 340 μg/L and 2800 μg/L, respectively. The BIPP packing was removed and i.v. DMPS chelation initiated (5 mg/kg × 4 per day for 5 days, 5 mg/kg × 3/day for 5 days, 5 mg/kg × 2/day for 17 days) followed by oral DMPS (200 mg × 3/day for 10 days, 200 mg × 2 for 14 days). This resulted in rapid improvement of his symptoms. There were no adverse effects during chelation.

Reynolds, Abalos, Hopp, and Williams (2012) described a case of progressing neurologic dysfunction in a 56-year-old woman who had taken toxic doses of bismuth salicylate to treat diarrhea. This medication was held, and her condition rapidly improved over 2 days, and further during a stay in a rehabilitation clinic without any chelation treatment. Follow-up several months later showed normal mental status.

In a case described by Erden et al. (2013) acute Bi poisoning in a 21-year-old woman after suicidal ingestion of 20 tablets of CBS corresponding to 2.4 g Bi metal resulted in chronic renal damage requiring hemodialysis one year after the incidence. In this case chelation was not instituted.

4.6.3 Conclusion

Taken together, the limited available data indicate that DMPS is an efficient antidote in even very severe acute Bi poisoning, with DMSA being an alternative drug. Further studies of DFO and L1 as chelators in chronic Bi intoxication are needed.

4.7 CADMIUM

Cadmium (Cd, atomic number 48, in group12 of the periodic table of the elements, atomic weight 112.414, density 8.65 g/mL^3) is a soft bluish-white metal with a low-melting point preferring oxidation state 2. The γ-emitting isotope ^{109}Cd ($t_{½}$ 462.6 d) is very well suited for studies of Cd kinetics (Andersen, 1989b). Cadmium is produced as a by-product of metal production from sulfide ores, mainly of zinc. It has been used in pigments, plastic stabilizers, corrosion-resistant electroplating on steel, alloys, nickel–cadmium batteries, and the nuclear industry (IPCS, 1992). These use are decreasing due to environmental and human toxicity and Cadmium is listed in the European Union Restriction of Hazardous Substances Directive 2002/95/EC (Eu-lex.europa.eu, 2003). Especially its use in batteries is replaced by lithium ion and nickel-metal- hydride batteries. Cadmium is increasingly used in solar panels as cadmium telluride.

Acute human cadmium poisonings are very rare and mainly due to suicidal oral intake of cadmium compounds, accidental cadmium contamination of food items, or accidental inhalation of cadmium oxide fumes during welding or flame cutting cadmium-coated metal. Beton, Andrews, Davies, Howells, and Smith (1966) described accidental poisoning of five workers by cadmium oxide fume during dismantling a frame of girders in a confined space by cutting bolts unaware that the bolts were cadmium plated. 4 survived severe pulmonary chemical pneumonia while one died from alveolar metaplasia of the lung and bilateral cortical necrosis of the kidneys. His lungs contained 2.5 mg cadmium oxide per gram wet tissue.

The frequencies of industrial and environmental chronic low-level cadmium exposure have been reduced, yet still exist in some areas resulting in renal and bone toxicities (Nordberg, Nogawa, & Nordberg, 2014). Accordingly, there is a clinical need for chelation therapy of aged cadmium deposits in liver and kidney. The literature on animal experiments to optimize treatment of acute cadmium poisoning and to develop chelation strategies to prevent or alleviate chronic cadmium toxicity by mobilizing aged cadmium depots is extensive.

Effective long-term chelation of deposited cadmium is challenged by the special toxicokinetics of cadmium. After systemic entrance, cadmium is rapidly localized intracellularly, mainly in the liver, and bound to metallothionein (MT). Liver Cd-MT complex is subsequently slowly transferred via blood to be renally deposited in proximal tubular cells. This may lead to tubular cell necrosis resulting in urinary loss of filtrable proteins, calcium, and other small molecules (Fanconi like syndrome) thereby initiating the chronic toxicity of cadmium, development of osteomalacia (Nordberg et al., 2014). This special toxicokinetics lead to rapid decline in efficacy of hydrophilic chelators for treatment of acute cadmium poisoning demonstrated by Eybl, Sykora, and Mertl (1965) and confirmed several years later by Bakka and Aaseth (1979) and Cantilena and Klaassen (1982).

4.7.1 Animal Chelation Experiments

An extensive number of chelating agents from several groups of chemical compounds have been studied as antidotes in acute cadmium poisoning experiments in animals, in most cases cadmium and chelator were administered parenterally by various injection routes, reducing the relevance in relation to acute human poisonings. Already in 1955, Dalhamn and Friberg (1955) demonstrated that BAL potentiated the toxicity of Cd in rabbits, increasing cadmium-induced proteinuria, weight loss and anemia. In general, hydrophilic polyaminopolycarboxylic acids and dithiol compounds effectively reduced mortality and enhanced cadmium excretion in injection studies, if the chelator was administered rapidly after cadmium (Bakka & Aaseth, 1979; Ding & Liang, 1991; Cantilena & Klaassen, 1981; Eybl et al., 1984; Jones, Weaver, & Weller, 1978; Basinger et al., 1981a). These studies demonstrate that DMSA but especially DTPA are efficient antidotes in the experimental condition of injecting both metal and chelator; BAL is contraindicated in Cd poisoning (Dalhamn & Friberg, 1955).

Andersen et al. (Andersen, 1989a, 1989b; Andersen, Nielsen, & Svendsen, 1988c) developed an experimental model relevant for acute human oral metal poisoning and demonstrated that oral administration of chelating agents after oral administration of a highly toxic cadmium dose reduced intestinal cadmium absorption, histological tissue damage, and mortality (Andersen, 1989a; Andersen, Nielsen, & Svendsen, 1988b). Parenteral administration of chelating agents reduced the toxicity of orally administered cadmium (Andersen, 1989a). Oral administration of DMSA efficiently reduced intestinal uptake and toxicity of highly toxic oral doses of cadmium, while i.p. administration of DMSA only marginally protected against Cd toxicity. DMPS was also an efficient oral antidote. Oral administration of disodium DTPA extensively reduced intestinal absorption of orally administered cadmium and reduced mortality, and i.p. injection of CaDTPA efficiently reduced the toxicity of orally administered cadmium. Also, triethylenetetraminehexaacetic acid (TTHA) effectively protected against oral cadmium toxicity (Andersen, 1989a). Based on these animal experiments the optimum treatment of acute oral human cadmium poisoning by chelating agents that are in clinical use would be oral administration of DMSA and parenteral administration of CaDTPA.

The development of chelating agents capable of mobilizing aged cadmium depots was previously reviewed by Jones (1991) and Jones and Cherian (1990). This work was based on the mobilizing effects on aged body depots of cadmium exerted by the lipophilic chelators BAL (Shaik & Lucis, 1972; Cherian, 1980) and DDC (Gale, Atkins, & Walker, 1982), presumably by chelating intracellular and MT-bound cadmium. However, Andersen, Nielsen, and Svendsen (1988a) and Andersen and Nielsen (1989) demonstrated that both after oral and parenteral administration, DDC increased the acute toxicity of orally administered cadmium, increased the intestinal uptake and enhanced the brain deposition of cadmium. The DDC dimer tetraethylthiuram disulfide (TTD, disulfiram, Antabuse) had similar effects on oral cadmium toxicity (Andersen & Grandjean, 1989). In conclusion, neither DDC nor BAL have any antidotal roles in acute oral cadmium poisoning.

Based on these initial cadmium mobilization studies, Jones and Singh and their coworkers developed compounds capable of efficiently mobilizing aged cadmium depots from liver and kidneys during prolonged parenteral administration without enhancing cadmium toxicity or increasing cadmium deposition in the brain. Only few of a large number of studies are cited below. Based on the molecular structures of BAL and DDC series of compounds have been synthesized and tested for cadmium mobilizing efficiency: Monoalkylesters or monoalkylamides of *meso*-2,3-dimercaptosuccinic acid (Jones, Singh, Gale, Smith, & Atkins, 1992, Jones et al., 1994a, Singh et al., 1996) and amphipathic carbodithioates as, for example, *N*-(4-methoxybenzyl)-D-glucamine carbodithioate (Jones, Cherian, Singh, Basinger, & Jones, 1991a) and *N*-(4-methoxybenzyl)-4-0-(β-D-galactopyranosyl)-D-glucamine carbodithioate (Jones et al., 1991b) were effective mobilizers, monoisoamyl-DMSA was effective after oral administration (Jones et al., 1992). *N*-aryl-4-O-(β-D-galactopyranosyl)-D-glucamine-*N*-carbodithioates were effective mobilizers of aged cadmium deposits, with the aryl groups benzyl (Eybl et al., 1998) or 4-methylbenzyl (Blaha et al., 1995; Eybl, Kotyzova, Koutensky, Jones, & Singh, 1995). The supposedly intracellular action of DMSA esters is conceivably mediated by active transport, as inhibitors of organic ion transporters reduced the mobilization of Cd by these compounds (Jones et al., 1994; Tasende, Gale, Smith, Jones, & Singh, 1992).

These compounds have presently been used only in experimental animals and their toxicities preclude clinical use. The most promising compounds could however be further developed into clinically useful chelating agents. Persons eligible for cadmium chelation mobilization by such compounds due to large hepatic and renal cadmium depots will most often have marginal renal damage (reduced proximal tubular reabsorption capacity leading to increased urinary calcium loss). In itself, this condition is not serious but can eventually develop to more severe renal disease and osteomalacia. The potential usefulness of mobilization of aged cadmium depots by chelation must be weighed against the reversibility of slight tubular damage. To be ethically acceptable, such chelation treatment must be very safe and without adverse effects.

Saric et al. (2004) studied the mobilizing effect of oral DMSA and i.p. CaDTPA and their combination on orally administered cadmium in female albino rats. The efficiency of Cd removal from the body (kidneys and liver) decreased with time. DMSA was more efficient than CaDTPA in mobilizing Cd, and combined chelation was most efficient.

Saljooghi and Fatemi (2010) studied the mobilizing effect of deferasirox in weanling rats on cadmium administered in drinking water or food. After 45 days Cd exposure deferasirox chelation for 1 week significantly reduced Cd blood levels compared to unchelated controls and blood iron levels returned to the level in untreated animals.

Fatemi, Saljooghi, Balooch, Iranmanesh, and Golbafan (2011) studied effects of oral administration of deferasirox (140 mg/kg b.w.) or L1 (300 mg/kg b.w. for one week or both deferasirox (70 mg/kg b.w.) and L1 (150 mg/kg b.w.) in rats after 60 days exposure to cadmium in drinking water. Both chelators reduced the Cd levels in liver, heart, kidney, and intestines compared to levels in unchelated controls, combined chelation was more effective than chelation with one of the compounds.

Ivanovaa et al. (2012) investigated the effect of chelation with the tetraethylammonium salt of monensic acid in Cd-intoxicated mice. Compared to controls the monensic acid salt reduced the kidneys liver, heart, lungs, spleen, and testes levels of cadmium by 50% in the kidneys and by 90% in the hearts. Cd was not redistributed to the brain, and the endogenous levels of copper and zinc were not adversely changed. The chelation treatment significantly ameliorated

Cd-induced iron depletion in liver and spleen and corrected transferrin-bound Fe levels and total iron binding capacity in plasma. The authors consider the tetraethylammonium salt of monensic acid an efficient antidote for Cd-poisoning.

4.7.2 Clinical Chelation Studies

Very few human cadmium intoxication cases have been treated with chelating agents. Gil et al. (2011) measured the renal excretion of cadmium and β2-microglobulin, proteinuria, and hematuria after intravenous administration of 50 mg/kg glutathione and 500 mg Ca-EDTA in 1 L saline over 24 h to a 54-year old patient with chronic cadmium intoxication. Basal levels with only saline administration were determined during 3 days. During the next 3 days, Ca-EDTA was administered, then Ca-EDTA and GSH were administered for 3 days, and then GSH was administered for 3 days. The protocol was repeated after one month. Infusion of EDTA with GSH increased the blood cadmium level (7.44 + 0.73 mg/L, $p < 0.01$) compared to the basal level (4.6 + 0.44 mg/L) and increased the renal cadmium excretion significantly than in the basal treatment (23.4 + 15.81 mg/g creatinine vs 89.23 + 58.52 mg/g creatinine, $p < 0.01$). The protein/creatinine and β2-microglobulin/creatinine ratio in the urine ($p > 0.05$) did not differ among the treatments. Furthermore, microhematuria and proteinuria did not develop over an observation period of 6 months. These results suggest that GSH administration with EDTA might be a potential treatment of patients with cadmium intoxication.

Cao, Chen, Bottai, Caldwell, and Rogan (2013) analyzed the lead and cadmium blood levels in children from a randomized trial of DMSA for lead poisoning and found that DMSA did not lower blood cadmium in children with background exposure.

4.7.3 Conclusion

Acute human cadmium poisonings are rare, and a clinical chelation scheme is not established. However, animal experiments clearly demonstrate that oral EDTA, DTPA, DMSA, and DMPS are efficient antidote in *oral* cadmium poisoning while DDC as well as BAL are contraindicated. Various derivatives of BAL, or DDC, and DMSA including several esters have been developed as potential chelators for mobilization of aged cadmium deposits. To be clinically acceptable, such compounds must have very low toxicity. Further studies of deferasirox as chelator in chronic Cd intoxication are needed.

4.8 CHROMIUM

Chromium (Cr, atomic number 24, first element in group 6, atomic weight 52, density 7.2 g/cm^3) is a lustrous, steel-gray metal, very hard but brittle, named after the Greek word chroma, (color) because many chromium compounds have intensive colors. Chromium metal was used in weapon production in the Chinese Quin dynasty more than 2000 years ago. Chromium metal is highly corrosion resistant due to formation of an ultrathin oxide layer upon contact with oxygen allowing its use to produce stainless steel. Chromium metal and ferrochromium alloy as well as chromium pigments are produced from chromite (iron chromium oxide, $FeCr_2O_4$) with Cr in the trivalent Cr(III) form. Stainless steel (an alloy of steel and 13% or more carbon free chromium), chrome electroplating and pigments are dominating used of chromium, which also has a wide range of other minor applications (Langård & Costa, 2014).

Chromium compounds exist in oxidation steps from 0 to +6 and Cr also forms organic compounds, none of those have toxicological importance. Cr(VI) and Cr(III) compounds dominate chromium chemistry, Cr(III) being 500–1000 × less toxic than Cr(VI). Also, Cr(VI) is rapidly absorbed in lungs and gastrointestinal tract while the uptake of Cr(III) is very low, 0.4–2.5%, fecal excretion amounting to about 98% (ATSDR, 2012). Cr(VI) compounds are strong oxidizers and are rapidly reduced to Cr(III) in biological material (Langård & Costa, 2014) and excretion of Cr(III) is primarily via urine, in humans about 60% of gastrointestinally absorbed Cr(VI) is excreted as Cr(III) in urine within 8 h while about 10% is excreted in bile. Smaller amounts are excreted in sweat, hair, and nails (Kiilunen, Kivisto, Ala-Laurila, Tossavainen, & Aitio, 1983; Langård & Costa, 2014).

The toxicity of Cr(VI) is dominated by the corrosive action of its compounds inducing skin ulcers (Maloof, 1955) and ulceration and perforation of the nasal septum in chromate workers (Kleinfeld & Rosso, 1965). Also, Cr(VI) is a lung carcinogen upon inhalation, mainly in chromate workers. Certain Cr(VI) compounds are highly potent carcinogens, partially via mechanisms exerted by the reduction product Cr(III). Further, Cr(VI) compounds are strong skin allergens (Langård & Costa, 2014). Liu and Shi (2001) presented data suggesting that Cr(VI) toxicity is mediated via redox mechanisms by Cr(V).

In acute systemic Cr(VI) poisoning supportive treatment stabilizing the patient is indicated, while hemodialysis and charcoal hemoperfusion is not indicated if renal function is normal (Ellis et al., 1982). In renal failure, hemodialysis is necessary for management of the renal failure itself (Geller, 2001). CaEDTA chelation does not seem to have any clinical benefit (Geller, 2001). If skin and eyes are exposed, extensive flush with water should be done. Topical ascorbic acid has been used in management of chromium dermatitis. Its efficacy is not established in controlled clinical trials (Bradberry & Vale, 1999a). Chromate ulcers often heal spontaneously without specific treatment. Wet ascorbic acid dress or 10% EDTA ointment have been used to treat chromate scabs (Geller, 2001; Lewis, 2004). In most cases of chronic low-dose chromate exposure, no specific treatment is needed.

4.8.1 Animal Experimental Studies

Nowak-Wiaderek (1975) investigated effects of various chelating agents on elimination of ^{51}Cr(III) injected i.m. in rats. Intraperitoneal administration of

$CaNa_2EDTA$ did not increase total Cr(III) elimination while sc administration of α-lipoic acid slightly decreased elimination. Oral administration of diphenylcarbazid, sc administration of DPA, or i.m. administration of BAL reduced the elimination rate significantly. Accordingly, these compounds are of no use for Cr(III) elimination after Cr(VI) OR Cr(III) exposure.

Tandon and Gaur (1977) investigated the chromium mobilizing effect from liver, brain and testes of various chelators in chromium intoxicated animals and from subcellular organ fractions and erythrocytes of poisoned animals. EDTA and DTPA were efficient mobilizers in vivo while 3,4-dihydroxy-L-phenyl alanine and ascorbic acid were effective in vitro. A relationship between structure or molecular weight of the chelating agents used and chromium mobilizing efficiency could not be established.

Behari and Tandon (1980) examined the Cr mobilizing effect of polyaminocarboxylic acids from certain organs, subcellular fractions, and blood cells of rats poisoned by K_2CrO_4. Ethylene diamine di(O-hydroxylphenyl acetic acid) (EDDHA), triethylene tetramine hexaacetic acid (TTHA), and hexamethylene 1,6-diamino tetraacetic acid (TDTA) had some mobilizing capacity and potential for reducing chromate toxicity. A relationship between chromium-removing capacity and structure of the chelating agents could not be established.

Banner et al. (1986) studied the antidotal effect of *N*-acetylcysteine (NAC), CaEDTA, and/or DMSA in rats poisoned by potassium dichromate, lead tetraacetate, or boric acid. NAC was most effective in increasing urinary excretion of chromium and boron and in reversing toxin induced oliguria.

Wang et al. (2010) investigated the effect of NAC on the rate of chromium sensitization development, severity of skin reaction by intradermal and epicutaneous elicitation tests and the formation of reactive oxygen species (ROS, H_2O_2, and MDA in the skin and the oxygen radical absorbance capacity (ORAC) in plasma) during chromium hypersensitivity development in a coadjuvant chromium-sensitized guinea pig model. The sensitization rate and the skin reaction in intradermal and epicutaneous elicitation tests and the H_2O_2 and MDA levels in the skin were all significantly reduced and the ORAC in plasma was significantly increased by a dose of 1200 mg/kg NAC per day indicating that NAC could have potential in preventing the progression of chromium hypersensitivity.

Molina-Jijón et al. (2012) evaluated DFO as antidote in dichromate induced nephrotoxicity and oxidative stress. Single i.p. injections of 100, 200 or 400 mg/kg of DFO 30 min before a single s.c. injection of 15 mg/kg $K_2Cr_2O_7$ reduced chromate induced renal damage and biochemical indicators of Cr(VI) toxicity (proteinuria, blood urea nitrogen, serum creatinine and creatinine clearance, plasma glutathione peroxidase activity, urinary excretion of *N*-acetyl-β-d-glucosaminidase) and Cr(VI) induced renal oxidative stress seen as decreased activities of catalase, superoxide dismutase, glutathione peroxidase, glutathione reductase, glutathione-S-transferase. Also, 400 mg/kg DFO reduced the renal Cr level. Another experiment demonstrated that DFO posttreatment did not alleviate Cr(VI) induced nephrotoxicity and oxidative stress and was unable to enhance urinary Cr excretion.

Iranmanesh et al. (2013a) studied the potential efficiency of deferasirox and deferiprone given alone or in combination for 1 week after 60 days administration of 15 or 30 mg/kg b.w. of $K_2Cr_2O_7$ to rats. Combined chelation therapy was able to remove chromium from various tissues while iron concentration returned to normal levels and poisoning symptoms also decreased.

4.8.2 Clinical Cases

Schiffle, Weidmann, Weiss, and Massry (1982) reported a case of a chromium poisoned 19-year-old man with third-degree burns after accidental contact of both legs with chromium acid. Initial serum chromium levels were 2,2 μg/mL, a usually lethal level. The patient had hepatic damage, anuria and progressive anemia. Aggressive peritoneal dialysis for 252 h between the 4th and 22nd day decreased serum chromium levels. The patient had complete recovery after 35 days. The chromium removing efficacy of peritoneal dialysis was compared to hemodialysis in 5 acute renal failure peritoneal dialysis patients and 6 end-stage renal failure hemodialysis patients. After i.v. administration of 500 μCi $^{51}CrCl_3$ chromium clearance after peritoneal dialysis was 0.8 + /− 0.3 mL/min ($n = 50$) and after hemodialysis 2.5 + /− 0.8 mL/min ($n = 24$), respectively. The authors conclude that hemodialysis per unit of time about 3 more effective in removing chromium than is peritoneal dialysis. Since uninterrupted peritoneal dialysis can be performed for several days it is considered at least equivalent to hemodialysis in the initial stage of poisoning. It should be noted that removal of Cr in this case likely is Cr(III) only.

Ellis et al. (1982) reported a fatal case of chromate poisoning: A 22-month-old boy died after drinking sodium dichromate that his father had brought from work. He was treated with folic acid and chelated with BAL (that would not chelate hexavalent Cr and was shown to reduce Cr(III) elimination), hemodialysis, and exchange transfusion. To evaluate this treatment, four dogs were hemodialyzed after receiving intravenous sodium dichromate: their renal Cr clearance during dialysis was similar to their undialyzed renal chromium clearance and BAL administration did not significantly change chromium clearance.

Wallpole et al. (1985) reported a case of acute chromium poisoning in a 2-year-old boy accidentally drinking 50 mL or less of a 10% solution of sodium dichromate. The boy immediately vomited profusely and became pale, drowsy, and lethargic and he was brought to an emergency ward. When the type of poisoning was realized, aggressive therapy was initiated with gastric lavage, activated charcoal, and repeated gastric sodiumbicarbonate addition. Generous i.v. fluids were given and diuresis promoted. Nasogastric tube was left and used for further supportive treatment including ascorbic acid. Peritoneal dialysis started at 5 h postingestion. BAL chelation was administered during 72 h, 4 mg/kg every 4 h but was inefficient in enhancing Cr excretion, in agreement with published animal experiments. The patient was discharged after 6 days. Later radiological investigation indicated no structural anomalies.

Anderson, Bryden, and Waters (1999) reported that NaEDTA chelation therapy in cardiovascular disease patients did not increase urinary Cr excretion, independent on previous chelation history. Urinary Cr losses were strongly influenced by Cr supplementation.

Kolacinski, Kostrzewski, Kruszewska, Razniewska, and Mielczarska (1999) reported a suicidal case: A 48-year-old man was admitted 7 h after drinking 22.5 g of potassium dichromate in aqueous solution. He immediately received hemodialysis. The total chromium elimination via hemodialysis and urine was estimated to 36.7 mg, only 0.16% of the dose. CaEDTA administration significant increased the Cr elimination rate in the dialysate but did not influence urine, serum, or erythrocyte Cr levels. The patient was discharged after 21 days, and esophageal radiography 3 month after the incidence did not show disturbed motility or constriction.

Hantson, Van Caenegem, Decordier, Haufroid, and Lison (2005) described a suicidal case of ingestion of a lethal dose of potassium dichromate, 2–3 g, with a drink by a 17-year-old girl during a chemistry lesson at school. She developed epigastric pain and vomiting. About 1 h after the intake she received gastrointestinal decontamination with activated charcoal. Also, she immediately received i.v. infusion of 3 g ascorbic acid and 150 mg/kg *N*-acetylcysteine. Liver parameters were normal. Her increased urinary levels of β2-microglobulin and retinol binding protein but normal glomerular filtration and creatinine clearance rates indicated mild proximal tubular damage. She developed a minor ulceration in the gastric fundus but no further complications. After 48 h she was transferred to a psychiatric ward.

Baresic et al. (2009) described a 55-year-old man accidentally poisoned from a sip of 20% chromic acid (estimated intake: 2.3 g Cr). Renal and liver failure developed in the course of disease. Hemodialysis was initiated, chelation or other methods for enhancing Cr elimination were not performed. Liver and renal function improved slowly. The patient was discharged 45 days after the incidence without need for dialysis. His renal function remained stable but depressed during eight months follow-up.

Lin et al. (2009) reported a case of a chemical burn of 15% of the body surface due to accidental chromate skin exposure. Short time after the exposure severe chromium poisoning with multiple organ failure resulted due to transdermal Cr(VI) uptake. Besides mechanical ventilation, continuous venovenous hemofiltration and plasmapheresis, the patient received intravenous administration of DMPS, NAC, and ascorbic acid. After 33 days, the patient was discharged without long-term sequelae.

Illner, Gerth, Pfeiffer, Bruns, and Wolf (2009) describe a 22-year-old man who ingested a lethal dichromate dose in a suicidal attempt. He presented with liver and renal toxicity and very high serum Cr levels. Occupational toxicology literature states that hemodialysis and hemoperfusion are not efficient in removing chromium, so the patient was submitted to five plasmapheresis sessions resulting in significantly lowered serum and urinary Cr levels. Chelation therapy was not used. The patient survived without organ damage. Plasmapheresis is suggested as therapeutic option to reduce chromium concentrations.

Pazzaglia et al. (2011) described a patient with a total hip replacement who developed acoustic, peripheral, and optic neuropathy, due to metal intoxication from wear products from the prosthesis, most likely due to cobalt toxicity (see later). The patient was chelated with EDTA at regular intervals from diagnosis until removal of the prosthesis (74 days) and for a further 33 days. EDTA chelation only marginally reduced blood Cr levels.

4.8.3 Conclusion

Most established clinical chelators have been used in experimental studies and (rather few) clinical chromate poisoning cases. Due to the rapid metabolism of chromate, both Cr^{6+} and Cr^{3+} should be chelated. BAL and DPA are without beneficial effects and even reduced the Cr^{3+} elimination, and EDTA gave contradictory results. At present, the knowledge of the chromium-antidotal effects of DFO, L1, and deferasirox is limited.

4.9 COBALT

Cobalt (Co, atomic number 27, in group 9 of the periodic table of the elements, atomic mass 58.9, density 8.9 g/cm^3) is a shiny gray, hard, ductile, and brittle metal with magnetic properties. Cobalt prefer oxidation states (II) or (III), the former is most stable. Cobalt carbonyl $Co_2(CO)_8$ is white in the pure state but often presents as an orange-brown solid. Cobalt is an essential element and is a constituent of vitamin B12. The γ-emitting isotopes ^{57}Co, ^{58}Co, and ^{60}Co with half-lives of 272 days, 71 days and 5.271 years are discussed in chapter: Decorporation of Radionuclides. Cobalt often occurs in ores with iron, lead, nickel, copper, and silver and is mainly mined from erythrite, [$Co_3(AsO_4)2.8H_2O$], cobaltite (CoAsS), and smaltite ($CoAs_2$). Cobalt consumption is increasing due to its use in Ni-Cd and Li-ion rechargeable batteries and in aircraft engines (Lison, 2014). Cobalt compounds were used in the manufacture of blue Egyptian faience about 4000 years ago (Nicholson, 2009).

Cobalt is mainly used in rechargeable batteries and in steel and more than 2000 other alloys. Superalloys of cobalt, chromium, and other metals are employed for very hard cutting tools and for surfaces in turbines and space vehicles. Hard metals are composite materials produced by powder techniques from cobalt metal particles (up to 10%) and tungsten carbide (about 90%). Hard metals have extreme hardness (close to that of diamond). Cobalt alloys including Vittalium (CoCrMo) are used in hip and knee prostheses. Alloys of 90% tungsten with 5% nickel and 5% cobalt are used for munitions as an alternative to depleted uranium. Other uses are in pigments. Cobalt carbonyl is used for preparation of ultra-pure cobalt and as catalyst in organic chemistry (Lison, 2014).

The gastrointestinal Co absorption in animal studies varies from less than 0.5% of cobalt oxide CoO of very low solubility (Wehner & Craig, 1972) to about 30% of highly soluble $CoCl_2$ (Comar & Davis, 1947; Taylor, 1962). Human studies indicate gastrointestinal cobalt uptake rates from 5 to 45% in different individuals. After oral or parenteral administration cobalt is mainly distributed to liver, kidneys, spleen, adrenals, and thyroid with largest concentrations in liver and kidney (Comar & Davis, 1947; Taylor & Marks, 1978; Domingo, 1989). The free Co(II) concentration in vivo is low because Co(II) precipitates at physiological phosphate concentrations and binds to proteins, as, for example, albumin. This mechanism enhances the solubilization of Co from nanoparticles from corrosion and wear of prosthetic materials by offering a sink for free Co (II) ions in biological fluids (Lison, 2014).

Cobalt-containing prosthetic materials release Co ions and nanoparticles from corrosion and wear, stress, and fatigue giving elevated serum and tissue Co levels (Bradberry, Wilkinson, & Ferner, 2014; Polyzois, Nikolopoulos, Michos, Patsouris, & Theocharis, 2012). Polyzois et al. (2012) estimated that a Metal on Metal (MoM) prosthesis releases between 10^{13} and 10^{15} metal particles per year. Blood cobalt levels in patients receiving MoM prostheses slowly raise and stabilize after about 1 year at 5–10 × higher levels than presurgery levels (Polyzois et al., 2012; Sampson & Hart, 2012). These elevated levels are common in patients with MoM hip prostheses. Neurotoxicity, including anxiety and headache, peripheral neuropathy with hand tremor, diminished coordination capacity, reduced cognition and memory, tinnitus, optical and auditory nerve atrophy, and convulsions have been reported in cases with very high cobalt levels in urine, blood, plasma or serum. Surgical prosthesis revision often alleviates or removes these signs and symptoms (reviewed by Catalani, Rizzetti, Padovani, & Apostoli, 2012 and Keegan, Learmonth, & Case, 2007). Even cardiomyopathy and/or hypothyroidism have been observed in some orthopedic patients (Oldenburg, Wegner, & Baur, 2009). Similar toxicity has been observed in anemic patients after high doses of cobalt chloride (Schirrmacher, 1967; Licht, Oliver, & Rachmilewitz, 1972). Evidence of neurotoxicity due to occupational Co exposure is very limited (Lison, 2014), however, cobalt allergy occurs over a wide range of branches besides the cobalt and hard metal industries. It generally manifests as an erythematous and/or papular dermatitis (Lison, 2014). Endemic outbreaks of cardiomyopathy with heart failure, polycythemia, and thyroid lesions resulting in high mortality rates have previously occurred in heavy beer drinkers consuming beer in which the froth was stabilized with cobalt chloride in Quebec, Canada; Minneapolis, USA; and in Belgium (Morin & Daniel, 1967; Kesteloot, Roelandt, Willems, Claes, & Joossens, 1968; Alexander, 1972). Cobalt compounds are mutagenic and carcinogenic after certain exposures (Reviewed by Lison, 2014).

4.9.1 Chelation, Animal Experiments

Domingo, Llobet, and Corbella (1983) investigated the effect of EDTA on acute cobalt toxicity in rats. Oral or i.p. administration of $CoCl_2$-EDTA chelate did not induce mortality even at the LD_{100} dose of $CoCl_2$. However, intraperitoneally administered EDTA was not an efficient antidote for orally administered $CoCl_2$.

Domingo and Llobet (1984) investigated the antidotal effect of L-methionine in rats after an oral dose of 2.73 mmol/kg $CoCl_2$ or an intraperitoneal dose of 0.21 mmol/kg. Both doses are higher than LD_{50} for $CoCl_2$ at these administration routes. L-methionine was administered i.p. at a dose of 0.63 mmol/kg, and orally at 8.19 mmol/kg. L-methionine did not have any appreciable antidotal effect. Oral or intraperitoneal administration of the preformed L-methionine-Co^{2+} chelate resulted in 10% or 30% mortality. In contrast, cysteine-Co^{2+} and *N*-acetylcysteine-Co^{2+} chelates did not induce mortality.

Eybl et al. (1985) injected 22 μmol/kg DTPA, DMSA, or DMPS into mice immediately after i.v. administration of a lethal dose of $CoCl_2$, 2.2 μmol/kg. All mice receiving DTPA or DMPS survived, while mortality was reduced in mice receiving DMSA. DTPA reduced the total body levels of cobalt slightly.

Domingo, Llobet, and Tomas (1985) administered 2.28 mmol/kg $CoCl_2$ chelated by 6.84 mmol/kg NAC to rats and observed reduced toxicity compared to $CoCl_2$ alone. Oral administration of 6.84 mmol/kg NAC immediately after an oral dose of 2.28 mmol/kg $CoCl_2$ or i.p. administration of 0.537 mmol/kg NAC 5 min after oral administration of $CoCl_2$ marginally reduced mortality.

Llobet, Domingo, and Corbella (1985) compared 14 chelating agents as antidotes in acute Cobalt chloride poisoning, 0.70 mmol/kg injected i.p. in mice. The chelating agents were injected i.p. at 2:1 or 5:1 molar ratio to cobalt. DMSA, DTPA, EDTA, L-cysteine, NAC, GSH, DPA, and L-histidine had significant antidotal effects. At the $CoCl_2$ dose level 1.18 mmol/kg i.p., injection of DMSA, DTPA, EDTA, L-cysteine, NAC, and GSH significantly enhanced the survival rate. EDTA and DTPA were the most effective antidotes.

Llobet, Domingo, and Corbella (1986) investigated effects of BAL, EDTA, DTPA, L-cysteine (CYS), DMSA, NAC, GSH, and DPA administered at doses equalling one-fourth of their respective LD_{50} values on the toxicity, distribution and excretion of various doses of $CoCl_2$ (0.60–1.80 mmol/kg) injected intraperitoneally into mice. BAL enhanced $CoCl_2$ toxicity by increasing the mortality over that in controls given only $CoCl_2$ while DPA was without antidotal effect. EDTA was most effective in preventing mortality, leading to almost 100% survival at a $CoCl_2$ dose beyond LD_{100}. Next in efficiency followed DTPA, NAC, CYS, DMSA and GSH. EDTA, DTPA, CYS, NAC, and GSH were most effective in increasing the urinary cobalt excretion and reducing tissue levels of cobalt.

Llobet, Domingo, and Corbella (1988a) investigated effects of daily i.p. administration of EDTA, DTPA, DMSA, NAC, and GSH on the distribution and excretion of cobalt in groups of rats injected i.p. with 0.06 mmol CoCl2/kg/day 3 × per week for four weeks. Chelation started 24 h after the last Co injection and lasted 5 days. Glutathione, EDTA, NAC and DMSA effectively increased fecal cobalt elimination while NAC and DTPA significantly increased urinary cobalt excretion. The only chelators decreasing cobalt tissue levels were NAC (liver and spleen), and GSH (spleen).

4.9.2 Chelation, Clinical Studies

Only few clinical studies describe chelation treatment of cobalt intoxication despite several cobalt poisonings due to release of cobalt ions from wear products from prosthetic materials have been described. Bradberry et al. (2014) reviewed this subject and identified 18 cases where systemic toxicity had developed months or several years after placement of a metal-containing prosthesis. The symptoms seen in these cases have previously been associated with cobalt poisoning: cardiotoxicity (11 patients); thyroid toxicity (9 patients); peripheral neuropathy (8 cases); sensorineural hearing loss (7); neuroocular toxicity (14 patients), ocular toxicity presented as visual impairment (6). Cognitive decline (5 patients) has not previously been associated with Co toxicity.

Henretig and Shannon (1988) described an 11-year-old boy who developed vomiting, weakness, weight loss, and a neckmass following ingestion of several magnets. He was chelated with EDTA which increased his urinary cobalt excretion 4× and resulted in clinical improvement.

Waters, Bryden, Patterson, Veillon, and Anderson (2001) measured urinary Co excretion in 16 individuals receiving EDTA chelation therapy. The infusion contained a mix of vitamins including hydroxycobalamin and between 1.2 and 3 g EDTA. The postchelation urinary Co elimination was equal to the amount of cobalt in the infusion making interpretation of effect of chelation on cobalt excretion impossible.

Pazzaglia et al. (2011) described a patient with a total hip replacement who developed acoustic, optic, and peripheral neuropathy due to release of metal ions from wear products released from the prosthesis. The patient was chelated with EDTA at regular intervals from diagnosis until removal of the prosthesis (74 days) and for a further 33 days. Each chelation session resulted in reduced blood and plasma cobalt levels and increased urine cobalt levels, but blood and plasma cobalt levels rebounded after few days. The blood Co level was slowly reduced from 400–500 μg/L to 100–150 μg/L during the first chelation period and further to below 100 μg/L during the second chelation period after removal of the prosthesis.

Pelclova, Sklensky, Janicek, and Lach (2012) described a 56-year-old male patient who had a ceramics-on-ceramics implant replaced by a metal implant containing cobalt, chromium, and titanium. He developed weight loss, neurologic toxicity with severe hearing loss, heart, and thyroid toxicity symptoms. He was chelated with DMPS, which increased his cobalt excretion. Apart from deafness his clinical symptoms gradually resolved.

4.9.3 Conclusion

The clinical experience with Co chelation is limited but indicates that CaEDTA or DMPS chelation enhance Co excretion, DMPS being the first drug of choice. However, animal experiments offer additional information: Both EDTA, DTPA and DMSA were efficient antidotes and mobilizers of Co while BAL enhanced mortality and tissue retention of Co and is strongly contraindicated.

4.10 COPPER

Copper (Cu, atomic number 29, in group 11 of the periodic table of elements, atomic weight 63.54, density 8.94 g/cm^3) is a reddish-brown metal and a good conductor of heat and electricity. Copper occurs in oxidation states 0, +1, +2, and +3. Cu(I) is easily oxidized to Cu(II), the most stable form, while Cu(III) is highly unstable with little biological significance (Ellingsen, Møller, & Aaseth, 2014).

Copper has been used for at least 10,000 years, and its discovery is estimated to be around 9000 BC in the Middle East. A copper pendant found in Northern Iraq dates to 8700 BC when Neolithic humans apparently first used lumps of native metallic copper. Copper was used for the earliest known artifacts made from smelted metal, and slags from the smelting of copper found in excavations at the first Neolithic settlement in Southern Anatolia date to as early as 7,000 BC (http://dragonseedcave.com/copperhistory.htm) Accessed 19/8-2015.

Copper is mainly mined from sulfide ores, chalcocite (Cu_2S) and chalcopyrite ($CuFeS_2$) but also from oxidic ores, cuprite (Cu_2O), malachite ($Cu_2(OH)_2CO_3$) and azurite [$Cu_3(OH)_2(CO_3)_2$] (Barceloux, 1999). Copper is used in wires and electric cables, in the electronic industry, water pipes and tubes, roofing and facing materials in buildings, in vessels and containers, and in alloys as brass (copper-zinc), bronze (copper-tin) and cupronickels as coinage material (Ellingsen et al., 2014). Copper nanowires are becoming important in small integrated cirquits (Yang, He, & Yang, 2014). Other uses are in wood preservatives, fungicides, pigments and antifouling agents in paints. Minor uses include intrauterine contraceptives and copper-based alloys in dentistry (Barceloux, 1999).

Copper is an essential element of high toxicity, so homeostatic mechanisms regulate its uptake, distribution, and excretion. Copper is important in many biological processes as catalytic cofactor in enzymes involved in, for example, cellular respiration, connective tissue formation, antioxidative defense, peptide hormone maturation, neurotransmitter biosynthesis, keratinization, and pigmentation.

Dietary copper is absorbed in the small intestines facilitated by the apical high-affinity copper transporter CTR1, which is endocytosed at high dietary copper levels, offering a potential mechanism reducing copper uptake (Petris, Smith, Lee, & Thiele, 2003). In the enterocyte the free copper level is extremely low due to complexation by scavengers as metallothionein, glutathione, and metallochaperones as well as small molecules (Rae, Schmidt, Pufahl, Culotta, & O'Halloran, 1999; Huffman & O'Halloran, 2001).

Copper efflux from enterocytes to the portal circulation is mediated by the ATP7A transporter (Menkes protein) (Tapiero, Townsend, & Tew, 2003; van den Berghe & Klomp, 2009). Copper in portal blood is bound to ceruloplasmin which contains 60–95% of the copper in human serum, to transcuprein, to albumin and to low molecular weight components (Linder & Hazegh-Azam, 1996; Linder et al., 1998; Hyun & Filippich, 2004). ATP7B mediates copper export out of hepatocytes and also mediates holoceruloplasmin synthesis by supplying copper to apoceruloplasmin in hepatocytes. Metallothioneins bind excess copper in hepatocytes (Wijmenga & Klomp, 2004). High copper levels indirectly induce metallothionein synthesis by competing zinc out of metallothionein so zinc can bind to and activate the metallothionein transcription factor MTF-1 (Zhang et al., 2003). In healthy individuals about 98% of copper excreted is via bile and 2% via urine (Wijmenga & Klomp, 2004). Intracellular copper levels are regulated tightly by transmembrane transporters and metallochaperones to protect against Cu(I) and Cu(II) catalyzed oxidation and reduction reactions, which could lead to production of hydroxyl radicals (Gaetke & Chow, 2003). The biological half-time of orally administered Cu in healthy human subjects was estimated to 13–33 days (Johnson, Milne, & Lykken, 1992).

Menkes disease is characterized by progressive neurological impairment, connective tissue disturbances, and "kinky" hair. The disease results from mutations in the *ATP7A* gene. Because of the presence of the ATP7A transporter in many tissues and its role in export of copper from enterocytes to the bloodstream, Menkes disease is a copper deficiency disease affecting many organs (Kim et al., 2010). The copper transport across the blood–brain barrier is affected, resulting in copper deficiency in the brain (Horn, Tonnesen, & Tumer, 1992). Menkes disease infants most often die before 3 years of age.

Wilson disease (hepatolenticular degeneration) is the major cause of chronic copper intoxication. It is an autosomal recessive disease of copper transport caused by mutations in the *ATP7B* gene resulting in defective biliary copper excretion and hepatic copper accumulation subsequently leading to copper accumulation in other organs, including the brain and kidneys, causing copper induced neurological and/or hepatic symptoms. Copper deposition in the cornea results in formation of the Kayser-Fleischer ring used as a diagnostic tool aside with high urinary copper levels and low blood ceruloplasmin levels (Llanos & Mercer, 2002; Moller, Ott, Lund, & Horn, 2005). DPA was originally used for chelation treatment of Wilson's disease, but triethylene tetramine hydrochloride (TETA) has been the recommended first drug in the western world for decades (Walshe, 1956, 1973, 1982). In China, oral DMSA has been used to treat hundreds of Wilson's disease patients over the last 40 years, resulting in increased urinary Cu excretion and clinical improvement, even in the later stages of this disease Wang et al. (2003). Continuous lifelong chelation with a copper-chelating agent is necessary to prevent disease progression. This requires frequent clinical and laboratory analyses to detect possible side effects of the treatment. DPA treatment has several side effects, including proteinuria, thrombocytopenia and leukocytopenia (Roberts & Schilsky, 2003). Apparently, TETA is better tolerated than DPA (Andersen, 1999; Roberts & Schilsky, 2003; Flora & Pachauri, 2010). Oral zinc administration inducing metallothionein synthesis in enterocytes is used to reduce intestinal copper uptake along with diets low in copper (Barceloux, 1999; Roberts & Schilsky, 2003; Brewer, 2009). The final option is liver transplantation (Roberts & Schilsky, 2003).

The clinical signs in acute oral copper poisoning are dominated by gastrointestinal symptoms and in severe cases hemolysis, renal symptoms as anuria or oliguria and eventually multiorgan damage. Naha, Saravu, and Shastry (2012) reported that among 35 adult patients with acute copper sulfate poisoning, 69% of patients were diagnosed with hemolysis. In 48 patients suffering acute copper sulfate poisoning 13 patients developed anuria or oliguria (Chuttani, Gupta, Gulati, & Gupta, 1965).

4.10.1 Animal Chelation Studies

Koutenský et al. (1971) found that DDC reduced the acute LD_{50} of $CuCl_2$ in mice by almost a factor of 4, an extensive increase in Cu toxicity, and also extensively increased the retention of Cu in various organs, most notably in the brain, where Cu deposition was increased by a factor of 3.

Jasim, Danielsson, Tjälve, and Dencker (1985) investigated effects of DDC on $^{64}CuCl_2$ administered intravenously to male mice and to pregnant female mice at various stages of gestation. Administration of DDC before or after $^{64}CuCl_2$ injection extensively increased ^{64}Cu levels in most tissues of adult mice and increased fetal Cu uptake. The brain deposition was increased by a factor of 20–35. Both studies indicate that DDC is strongly contraindicated in Cu poisoning.

In acute parenteral copper poisoning in mice, DPA, TETA, DMSA, and DMPS were all efficient antidotes with DMPS being most efficient (Ding & Liang, 1991, Jones, Weaver, & Basinger, 1981). Also, copper-induced hemolysis of human red blood cells in vitro was reduced by these chelating agents, although high concentrations of DMPS could promote hemolysis (Aaseth, 1983). Increased urinary Cu excretion after administration of TETA or DPA to normal or cupper loaded animals has been demonstrated in several species. Further, the urinary copper excretion in rats injected with copper was increased by oral administration of DMSA (Yan et al., 1993).

4.10.2 Human Clinical Chelation Studies

Few clinical cases of chelation treatment in acute human Cu intoxications are reported: Jantsch, Kulig, and Rumack (1985) described a suicide attempt in a 42-year-old male ingesting about 250 g of crystalline $CuSO_4$. Upon admission he was vomiting but fully alert. Intramuscular BAL chelation was immediately started. Vomiting subsided after 10 h. Activated charcoal and magnesium sulfate were administered and then DPA chelation was initiated. After 3 days acute liver damage was indicated by blood levels of liver enzymes. The patient recovered completely.

Hantson, Lievens, and Mahieu (1996) described an acute poisoning in an 86-year-old woman who accidentally drank a solution of copper and zinc sulfate, 3 g of each. This tonic "Eau de Dalibour" is used in diluted form to treat skin ulcers. She arrived at hospital vomiting and soon after delivered a watery diarrhea. Endoscopy showed that her gastric mucosa was erythematous with areas of bleeding, the peak plasma concentration was 19.8 mg/L for zinc and 2.09 mg/L for copper, suggesting preferential absorption of zinc After initial gastric lavage and intravenous fluid she was chelated with i.m. BAL and with DPA by nasogastric tube for 48 h, apparently with little benefits in addition to supportive therapy. The patient became hypotensive on the next day. Inflammation and ulceration in the bronchial tree was revealed on day 3 by fiber-optic bronchoscopy. Mechanical ventilation was instituted due to deteriorating respiratory function. Renal function deteriorated during the following days. Starting from day 11 the patient made a complete recovery.

Takeda, Yukioka, and Shimazaki (2000) reported a case of suicidal ingestion of approximately 8 g of cupric sulfate by a 18-year-old man. He was brought to the hospital 1 h after lethargic and vomiting spontaneously. Blue staining of the oral mucosa and vomitus on his clothes were noticed. Radiographs of chest and abdomen were unremarkable. He was intubated and received gastric lavage and was then chelated with BAL 1.8 g/day, and DPA 0.9 g/day. The next day, hemolysis and rhabdomyolysis were diagnosed, and acute tubular necrosis was suspected. He was hydrated to maintain urine output. The patient was treated with 4 sessions of direct hemoperfusion with activated charcoal for 4 h and 5 sessions of hemodiafiltration for 4 h without volume depletion using a polysulfone hollow fiber dialyzer during 6 days to remove copper, hemoglobin, myoglobin and other debris from injured tissue. The patient was discharged after 15 days, and treatment with DPA was continued for 4 weeks until hemolytic anemia was resolved. No complications were noticed during a 8-weeks follow-up period.

Bhowmik et al. (2001) described a 21-year-old man admitted after injecting copper sulfate into the left antecubital vein in a suicidal attempt. He developed acute renal failure and intravascular hemolysis, metabolic acidosis, and septicemia. Intensive hemodialysis with blood transfusions and antibiotics were started, chelation treatment was not instituted. He remained anuric for 4 weeks, then urine output gradually started and he became dialysis independent after six weeks, however, his renal function only partially recovered. Renal biopsy 8 weeks after the poisoning demonstrated chronic tubulo-interstitial nephritis, not reported before after acute copper sulfate intoxication.

Faure, Mathon, Poupelin, Allaouchiche, and Chassard (2003) described a case of acute copper sulfate intoxication after a very high dose in a 38-years-old patient with a minor mental deficit. After he had ingested half a glass of copper sulfate he presented with nausea and vomiting, then developed intravascular hemolysis during treatment in the intensive care unit. He received DPA as a copper chelator and packed red cell transfusion besides general intensive care. He left the intensive care unit after 9 days.

Franchitto et al. (2008) described a case of suicidal copper sulfate poisoning in a patient presenting with vomiting, diarrhea, and fever. Intravenous $CaNa_2EDTA$ chelation, 1 g/12 h, was given for 3 days followed by by oral BAL, 3 mg/kg X 4 for 5 days. Intravascular hemolysis occurred on day 3 after poisoning. The patient developed hematuria, oliguria, and tachycardia, without other signs of hypovolaemic shock. Endoscopy revealed a perforating ulcer in the pyloric antrum with signs of recent hemorrhage and duodenal mucosal bleeding. Four packed red cell transfusions were given for anemia. Hemodialysis was not required as diuresis was well maintained. After 9 days in the intensive care unit the patient was transferred to a psychiatric department.

Sinkovic, Strdin, and Svensek (2008) described acute poisoning of a 33-year-old woman attempting suicide by ingesting an unknown amount of copper sulfate pentahydrate. She presented with symptoms of dehydration, renal dysfunction, severe hemorrhagic gastroenteritis, and methemoglobinaemia with normal serum copper level. She had immediate gastric lavage and antiemetic drugs, fluid replacement, vasoactive drugs, furosemide, and DMPS. The patient developed intravascular hemolysis, acute hepatic and renal failure, and adrenal insufficiency. Prolonged intensive treatment with hemodialysis and i.v. hydrocortisone allowed the patient to be discharged with mild liver and renal damage.

Hassan, Shaikh, Ali, and Riaz (2010) describe a case of accidental ingestion of copper sulfate leading to severe acute toxicity. Intensive supportive care was successful in managing this patient. BAL chelation was used, the effect cannot be evaluated.

4.10.3 Conclusions

Oral copper sulfate poisoning should as soon as possible be treated with gastric lavage and then instillation of potassium ferrocyanide or activated charcoal to minimize absorption. Delayed gastric lavage or charcoal may be dangerous due to potential copper sulfate induced mucosal damage and perforation. Hemoglobinuria due to intravascular hemolysis may induce acute renal failure, requiring hemodialysis (Oldenquist & Salem, 1999). Due to their side effects the classic chelators EDTA and BAL are obsolete as chelators in acute copper poisoning (Andersen & Aaseth, 2002). Based on results from animal experiments, DDC is strongly contraindicated in copper poisoning, and BAL and EDTA are contraindicated as well. Again based on animal experiments, DPA, TETA, DMSA, and DMPS are all potential antidotes for use in acute human copper poisoning. The clinical experience is related to treatment of Wilson's disease patients and indicates TETA as a first drug of choice for low level copper poisoning. The clinical experience with chelation in acute copper poisoning is very small and does not offer clues for chelation treatment.

4.11 GALLIUM

Gallium (Ga, atomic number 31, group 13 of the periodic table of the elements, atomic weight 69.735, specific gravity 5.904 at 29.6°C) is a soft, silvery brittle metal solid at low temperatures (melting point, 29.78°C) with minor highly specific uses, mirrored by a world production of less than 200 metric tons.

Elemental gallium in free form does not occur in nature, common valence states are +2 and +3. Gallium(III) compounds occur in trace amounts in bauxite and in zinc ores. The gallium compounds Gallium arsenide (GaAs) and gallium nitride (GaN) are used in the semiconductor industry in silicon computer chips, in semiconductors, solar cells, photodetectors, light-emitting diodes and lasers (Fowler & Sexton, 2014). Gallium compounds have several diagnostic and medical uses. The intestinal uptake of gallium salts is normally low requiring parenteral exposure during pharmacologic use of the metal; gallium maltotate has however high oral gallium bioavailability and is absorbed rapidly (Bernstein, Tanner, Godfrey, & Noll, 2000) offering development of oral gallium based drugs. Gallium in the circulation binds to transferrin. Major depots are liver, kidneys, spleen and bone, and bone marrow with urinary and fecal excretion routes (Collery, Domingo, & Keppler, 1996; Rosner & Carter, 1987; Yamauchi, Takahashi, & Yamamura, 1986). Gallium isotopes, eg ^{67}Ga are used as diagnostic tools for various oncological (Wirth et al., 2002; Ng et al., 2005; Shah Syed, Younis, Usmani, & Zafar, 2004; Tuli et al., 2004) and non oncological diseases (Sosabowsky, Melendez-Alfort, & Mather, 2003; Love & Palestro, 2004; Nakazawa et al., 2004). The medical uses of gallium compounds including the antitumerigenic use of gallium nitrate for bladder and lymphatic tumors were recently reviewed by Chitambar (2010).

4.11.1 Experimental Animal Chelation Studies

Domingo, Llobet, and Corbella (1987) compared the efficacy (prevention of mortality) of 12 chelating agents administered i.p. to mice after a single i.p. administration of gallium nitrate. Effective chelators were DFO, citric acid, succinic acid, malic acid, and oxalic acid. EDTA, DTPA, DMSA, Tiron, DDC, L-cysteine, and sodium salicylate did not possess antidotal effects.

Santos et al. (2002) investigated three *N*-carboxyalkyl 3-hydroxy-4-pyridinones as bidentate chelators for Fe(III), Al(III), and Ga(III) offering potential oral administration. The effects of the compounds on ^{67}Ga biokinetics in ^{67}Ga-citrate loaded rats were investigated. A *N*-carboxyethyl derivative possessed the highest affinity for all 3 metals, and could even compete with transferrin. All the ligands enhanced the excretion of Ga.

Graziano et al. (2009) developed and studied two new chelators based on trishydroxypyridinone, KEMPPr(3,4-HP)$_3$ and KEMPBu(3,4-HP)$_3$ as strong sequestering agents for iron and group III metal ions with the aim of application in chelation therapy. Their structures are based on the KEMP acid scaffold to which three 3-hydroxy-4-pyridinone chelating moieties are attached via two different size spacers. After characterization of the compound's chemical properties and metal binding affinity and lipophilicity the in vivo metal sequestering capacity of KEMPPr(3,4-HP)$_3$ was investigated in ^{67}Ga overloaded animals. The in vivo results indicated that the compounds have higher metal chelating efficacy than DFO, indicating the compounds to be potential candidates for chelating therapy.

4.11.2 Clinical Chelation

Baker and Manno (1988) described a 23-year-old black male with homozygous sickle cell anemia and transfusional iron overload evaluated for response to i.v. DFO therapy. The patient developed an intraventricular hemorrhage and then after hospitalization developed a persistent fever of undetermined origin. A ^{67}Ga scan was performed as part of the diagnostic evaluation of his fever, but gave no result due to DFO chelation of Ga. After discontinuation of DFO a repeat scan showed a lesion above the left kidney. To avoid in vivo interaction of DFO with ^{67}Ga citrate, DFO chelation should be discontinued before use of ^{67}Ga scanning.

4.11.3 Conclusions

Based on limited experimental animal and clinical knowledge, among clinically available chelating agents, only DFO is a potential choice in acute human gallium poisoning.

4.12 GOLD

Gold (Au, atomic number 79 in group 11 of the periodic table with copper and silver, atomic mass 196.97, density 19.3 g/cm^3) occurs in nature as a single stable isotope, there are 14 radioactive isotopes, all with short half-times. Gold can occur in oxidation states +1, +2, +3, +4, +5, and +7, but only +1 (aurous) and +3 (auric) are common. Au(0) is chemically very stable, inert to most chemicals and does not oxidize. Gold is unstable in most compounds and easily reduced to Au(0), so free Au ions hardly exist in aqueous solutions, however, coordination complexes as gold cyanide $[Au(CN)_2]^-$, gold sulfite $[Au(SO_3)_2]_{3-}$, and gold thiosulfate $[Au(S_2O_3)_2]^{3-}$ are highly stable (Butterman & Amey, 2005). Due to its chemical characteristics gold is mainly mined as the free metal, with an estimated world production of 2560 tons/year in 2010. Leading gold producing-countries are China, Australia, the United States, Russia, South Africa, Peru, Indonesia, and Canada, (Aitio, Kiilunen, Santonen, & Nordberg, 2014).

By far the majority of gold is used in jewelry production, investment and bullions. Minor uses of metallic gold are in electronics, dentistry, imitation coins, medals, and various commemorative objects. Very small amounts of gold have other uses, for example, in various medical uses including the traditional Ayurvedic medicines in India and Sri Lanka and in gold thiolates used in the therapy of rheumatoid arthritis (Butterman & Amey, 2005). Gold nanoparticles find increasing uses in electronics and as catalysts, and for biomedical diagnostics and analytics as, for example, in computed tomography and medical applications of Raman spectroscopy and photoacoustic imaging (Thakor, Jokerst, Zavaleta, Massoud, & Gambhir, 2011).

The environmental, occupational, medical, and toxicological properties of gold were recently reviewed by Aitio et al. (2014). Various therapeutic uses of gold nanoparticles are being developed, for example, for photothermal heating of tumors killing their cells (Pitsillides, Joe, Wei, Anderson, & Lin, 2003) and for the targeted delivery of anticancer drugs to tumor cells (Kumar, Zhang, & Liang, 2013) and as direct therapeutic agents in cancer and rheumatoid arthritis (Bhattacharya & Mukherjee, 2008; Tsai et al., 2007). Gold compounds have been used for treatment of rheumatoid arthritis since 1928. The advent of other treatment options as methotrexate and biological drugs has reduced this use of gold compounds (Cohen, 1988; Kean & Kean, 2008). The most used gold compounds are auranofin which can be administered orally, aurothioglucose, aurothiosulfate, and aurothiomalates which are administered intramuscularly. Intramuscular administration of aurathiolates was therapeutically more effective than oral auranofin but induced more unwanted side effects (Felson, Anderson, & Meenan, 1990). Despite a high incidence of toxic side effects including dermatitis, sometimes exfoliative as erythroderma, colitis, nephropathy, or hepatic damage, in some cases with a fatal outcome, gold treatment is still important in the management of rheumatoid arthritis. The high frequency of side effects may be related to patients with rheumatoid arthritis could be an unusually sensitive population subgroup (Aaseth, Haugen, & Førre, 1998).

The absorption of a single oral dose of ^{195}Au auranofin in humans was 15-33% with peak plasma levels after 1–2 h. After i.m. administration of aurothiomalate, peak levels occurred after 2−6 h (Blocka et al., 1982; Tozman & Gottlieb, 1987). In rats orally loaded with ^{195}Au-auranofin for 29 days, blood Au and kidney Au levels were increased approximately 5-fold and 20-fold compared to levels after a single dose, and Au also accumulated in spleen and lungs (Intoccia et al., 1982). In humans 92−98% and about 82% of gold in plasma was bound to albumin after aurothiosulfate and auranofin administration (Eberl & Altmann, 1970). After i.m. administration of aurothiomalate to humans 70% of gold was excreted in urine, while after oral administration of auranofin approximately 85% of gold was excreted in feces and 15% in the urine (Blocka et al., 1982; Tozman & Gottlieb, 1987).

4.12.1 Animal Experimental Studies

Rubin, Sliwinski, Photias, Feldman, and Zvaifler (1967) used thermal neutron activation to study effects of BAL, DPA, and thiomalic acid on gold kinetics in rats injected with gold thioglucose, gold mercaptoethyliminodiacetic acid and gold 1.8-diamino-3,6-dimercaptooctane-*N*,*N*-tetraacetic acid. DPA was most effective and increased urinary gold excretion and decreased gold levels in spleen and lungs but increased gold deposition in liver and kidneys.

Aaseth, Jellum, and Munthe (1980) administered 35 μmol/kg ^{195}Au-thiomalate intramuscularly to mice. Daily administration of 1 mmol/kg DMSA increased the urinary ^{195}Au excretion. Administration of 1 mmol/kg of penicillamine or DMSA for 7 days reduced the blood and kidney gold levels by 30–50% compared to controls. Oral administration of 1−10 mmol/kg penicillamine increased the urinary excretion of ^{195}Au on the first day after ^{195}Au-thiomalate injection, on subsequent days the gold excretion was unaffected by chelation. Daily administration of 300 μmol/kg DPA gave insignificant increased urinary gold excretion, accordingly, DPA is an inefficient chelator of gold at low clinical doses. Also, Dvorac and Ehrig (1970) and Brown and Smith (1977). demonstrated DPA to be inefficient as antidote for gold and for mobilizing gold.

Gabard (1980) studied DMPS as chelator for removing gold in rats after i.v. injection of 2 mg Au/kg as Auro-Detoxin. Oral administration of DMPS reduced gold levels and increased urinary gold excretion in Auro-Detoxin treated rats. In a long-term experiment, DMPS significantly decreased kidney gold levels. DMPS is suggested as a potential chelation antidote to replace BAL.

Mason (1983) investigated effects of DMSA on gold levels and protein binding in kidneys in rats exposed to 10 mg Au/kg as sodium aurothiomalate (AuTM). The renal gold level increased for 4 days and then slowly declined. Gold accumulated in metallothionein-like, low molecular weight proteins. Daily i.p. injection of 50 mg/kg DMSA for 2 weeks to AuTM treated rats reduced the gold concentration in high and low molecular weight proteins of the soluble fraction and in the nonsoluble fraction of renal homogenate.

Basinger, Gibbs, Forti, Mitchell, and Jones (1985) investigated 8 compounds for efficacy as antidotes in acute gold intoxication after i.p. injection of 200 mg/kg of $Na_3[Au(S_2O_3)_2]2H_2O$. DMSA was the most effective antidote while DPA resulted in faster death of animals than in unchelated control animals. Administration of 140 mg/kg $Na_3[Au(S_2O_3)_2]2H_2O$ DMSA reduced gold levels in kidneys by a factor of about 5 and gold levels in liver by a factor of approximately 2.

Kojima, Takahashi, Kiyozumi, and Tagawa (1991) investigated effects of chelating agents on renal damage induced by AuTM in rats. Urinary excretion of protein, aspartate aminotransferase (AST), and glucose was increased after i.v. administration of AuTM. Urinary gold excretion was high on the first day after AuTM injection and then gradually decreased. Intraperitoneal administration of 1.2 mmol/kg DPA, DMSA, DMPS, or *N*-(2-mercapto-2-methylpropanoyl)-L-cysteine (bucillamine) after i.v. administration of 26 μmol/kg, AuTM reduced the urinary excretion of protein, AST, and glucose and the BUN level. DPA, DMSA, and DMPS enhanced urinary gold excretion while bucillamine enhanced fecal gold excretion. The chelating agents reduced the kidney and liver gold levels.

Takahashi, Funakoshi, Shimada, and Kojima (1994) studied effects of the chelating agents EDTA, L-cysteine (L-Cys), D-cysteine (D-Cys), NAC, dithiocarbamate (BGD), and (2S)-1-(3-mercaptopropionyl)-L-proline (captopril), *N*-(2-mercaptopropionyl)-glycine (tipronin), on organ levels, excretion, and renal toxicity of AuTM in rats injected i.p. with the chelating agents (1.2 mmol/kg each) immediately after i.v. injection of AuTM (0.026 mmol/kg). Captopril or tiopronin reduced the increases in the urinary levels of protein, aspartate aminotransferae (AST), and glucose and blood urea nitrogen (BUN), while L-NAC and D-Cys reduced the increases in urinary levels of protein, AST, and glucose after AuTM injection. BGD, EDTA, or L-Cys did not prevent AuTM-induced increases in urinary levels of protein, AST, and glucose and BUN level. Tiopronin increased urinary gold excretion. Captopril slightly increased both urinary and fecal gold excretion, increasing total gold excretion. Tiopronin and captopril decreased gold levels in kidneys and liver. L-Cys, D-Cys, L-NAC, BGD, and EDTA had no significant effect on excretion or organ levels of gold at 7 days after AuTM injection. In a study of effects of DMPS, bucillamine, captopril, and tiopronin at 1.2, 0.4 or 0.2 mmol/kg on the distribution and renal toxicity of gold, DMPS was effective in reducing renal gold levels and in protecting against renal toxicity after AuTM injection even at 0.2 mmol/kg DMPS. Bucillamine and tiopronin protected against the renal toxicity of gold at dose levels of 0.4 and 1.2 mmol/kg and captopril ameliorated the gold toxicity only at higher dose level (1.2 mmol/kg).

Takahashi, Funakoshi, Shimada, and Kojima (1995) investigated effects of DMPS and bucillamine on gold sodium thiomalate (AuTM) induced renal damage in adjuvant-arthritic rats (induced by adjuvant using Mycobacterium butyricum). Rats received an intraperitoneal injection of 0.6 mmol/kg of a chelating agent immediately after intramuscular injection of 66 µmmol/kg of AuTM every other day for 21 days. DMPS and bucillamine chelation protected against increased urinary protein excretion of protein, and increased aspartate aminotransferase, and glucose and blood urea nitrogen level due to AuTM exposure. AuTM reduced hindfeet volumes in both adjuvant-treated and untreated rats. These effects of AuTM were not affected by DMPS or bucillamine. Both chelators reduced gold levels in kidney and liver after AuTM injection without affecting copper, zinc, iron, and calcium levels in liver and zinc, iron, and calcium levels in kidneys, indication that DMPS and bucillamine are useful chelating antidotes in gold intoxication.

4.12.2 Clinical Studies

Bureau, Barriere, Nicolas, and Leroux (1962) described two cases of erythroderma induced by gold treatment of rheumatoid arthritis. In the first case, a pruritus starting some time after initiation of gold therapy in a 53-year-old man rapidly developed into erythroderma on hands, trunc, and face after administration of total 0.9 g gold over 2 months. A 10 days i.v. EDTA chelation course, total 5 g EDTA, mobilized extensive amounts of gold into urine paralleled by rapid healing of the skin lesions. The second case, a 76-year-old female, had a rapid, serious and painful aggravation of her rheumatoid arthritis. She then received 6 injections of 0.2 g Aurotioprol ("allochrysine") followed 3 months later by weekly injections of 0.1 g Aurotioprol. After 5 injections in the second course she rapidly developed a generalized pruritus worsening to a vesiculobullous edematous erythroderma over most of the body, requiring hospitalization. She received 2 daily i.v. EDTA infusion of 0.5 g EDTA for 5 days, then 1 infusion per day for 6 days. She experienced rapid healing of her erytherma paralleled with extensive mobilization of gold in urine.

Davis and Barraclough (1977) monitored serum and urinary gold levels during chelation with DPA in 18 patients treated with gold salts for rheumatoid arthritis. DPA did not increase urinary gold excretion statistically significantly. Serum gold levels in chelated and unchelated patients fell at similar rates. Analysis of protein binding of gold salts in vitro indicated high affinity between gold and albumin and low levels of unbound gold even at very high gold levels suggesting that only small amounts of gold are available for chelation by DPA, which is considered an unreliable chelator of gold in vivo and its use in gold poisoning remains speculative.

Thompson, Pegelow, Singsen, Powars, and Hanson (1978) described development of severe neutropenia in five children receiving gold injections for treatment of systemic onset juvenile rheumatoid arthritis within eight weeks after starting therapy in four patients, and 24 weeks after start in the fifth. In two children leukopenia preceded neutropenia. One child died from septicemia. In the four surviving children neutropenia resolved within 1–2 weeks. BAL chelation in one child did not appear to influence the recovery.

Perry and Jacobsen (1984) described a patient treated with therapeutic doses of gold for presumed rheumatoid arthritis. The patients developed encephalopathy, generalized muscle fasciculations, and peripheral neuropathy. BAL chelation resulted in remission of the symptoms.

Dubowitz, Hughes, Lane, and Wade (1991) described a case of gold induced neuroencephalopathy in a 56 y old man starting 5 months after starting AuTM therapy (50 mg injection weekly) for rheumatoid arthritis. The patient presented anorectic after loosing 20 kg, with painful paraesthesia in hands and feet, muscle waisting and fasciculations. He was confuse and disoriented and these conditions rapidly worsened. Gold induced polyneuropathy and neuroencephathy was diagnosed and gold therapy was discontinued. The patient was chelated with BAL, 150 mg $\times$ 2 daily for 2 days, 150 mg daily for 6 days. His condition improved and he was discharged after 10 days, alert and with appetite.

4.12.3 Conclusions

Animal studies indicate that DMSA and DMPS are efficient antidotes in acute gold poisoning and efficiently reduce the toxicity of sodium bis(thiosulfato)-gold(I) after i.p. administration. Unfortunately, the cited studies did not compare DMSA and DMPS with the two chelators previously used in human gold intoxication, BAL and DPA. The conclusion based on available data that DMPS and DMSA are more efficient antidotes and mobilizing agents than BAL and DPA in gold poisoning is therefore preliminary. Literature search has not disclosed any examples of DMSA or DMPS chelation in human gold intoxication. Limited experience with EDTA chelation disagree between animal and clinical data. The old studies in humans are from 1935 and forwards, and apparently high doses were used, today other gold compounds in lower doses are used and the frequency of poisonings has decreased (renal damage or bone marrow suppression), still 35% of gold treated rheumatoid arthritis patients discontinue due to these and other side effects. Today many other medications are used, often as a 3 drug therapy where the combined effect is more effective than each drug alone. Still a good chelation treatment of gold poisoning is needed, but this would require further experimental and clinical studies.

4.13 IRON

Iron (Fe, atomic number 26, in group 8 of the periodic table of the elements, atomic weight, 55.8, density 7.9 g/cm^3) occur with major valences +2 and +3 and exist in a large number of inorganic compounds, for example, magnetite, carbonate, sulfur, chloride, and carbonyl compounds. Soluble Fe (II) compounds readily oxidize and precipitate as $Fe(OH)_3$. Because of malleability and ductility of iron in the hot state and the hardness in the cold state iron has widespread technological uses ranging from structural elements in buildings, various vehicles, and machineries. Other uses are iron-based pigments and pharmaceuticals. Mined magnetite, hematite, and taconite iron ores are cleaned and smelted to metallic iron. Large producers are the United States, South Africa, China, Australia, Japan, Russia, Brazil, and India. The worldwide iron production in 2010 came from about 2.6 billion metric tons of mined ore. Raw iron is an important alloying metal for, for example, stainless steel and numerous other alloys (Ponka, Tenenbeim, & Eaton, 2014). Steel typically contains small amounts of carbon (<2%).

Iron-containing medications with iron alone or in combination with vitamins are highly toxic and have been and still are the causes of the most frequent childhood poisonings, often fatal (Litovitz & Manoguerra, 1992; Morris, 2000; Singhi & Baranwal, 2003; Tenenbein, 2005). Deliberate overdoses for suicidal purpose also occur in both adolescents and adults resulting in a high frequency of mortality (Watson et al., 2004). During 1983–1994, 6744 cases of DFO treatment of acute iron poisonings were reported, likely an underestimation (Bowden & Krenzelok, 1997).

According to Bronstein et al. (2010), almost 16,000 iron exposures are reported annually in the United States in children below six years of age. The vast majority of these resulted in no or minimal toxicity. Serious exposures involved adult pure iron preparations containing ferrous sulfate tablets with more elemental iron per tablet (60–65 mg) than the content in other iron preparations. Children's chewable vitamins with iron are unlikely to cause serious toxicity, no fatalities were reported among 195,780 exposures to chewable children's vitamins with iron between 1983 and 1998 (Bronstein et al., 2010) as compared to 60 deaths among 147,079 ingestions of adult iron containing preparations during the same time period. Fortunately the frequency of iron tablet induced fatalities has decreased considerably during the latest decades (Morris, 2000; Tenenbein, 2005).

Despite more efficient methods of supportive care and chelation with DFO have improved the possibility for treating severe iron poisoning, the frequency of such poisonings and the number of fatalities due to ingestion of concentrated iron supplements have been substantial (Mills & Curry, 1994). Iron used to be the most common cause of overdose mortality in children under 6 years of age (Cheney, Gumbiner, Benson, & Tenenbein, 1995). The symptoms include gastrointestinal injury due to corrosive effects of iron salts, hypotension, metabolic acidosis, coagulopathies, and multiorgan failure.

4.13.1 Selected Animal Studies

Pfister, Catsch, and Nigrović (1967) compared DFO, DTPA, and Prussion Blue (PB) as orally administered antidotes toward the toxicity of orally administered ferrosulfate in mice. The most efficient antidote was PB, increasing LD_{50} of oral ferrosulfate from 4.5 to 15.4 mmol/kg, DFO and DTPA were less efficient, with LD_{50} 7.7 and 12.3, respectively, all with administration immediately after ferrosulfate. The chelation efficacy was reduced by delayed administration and increased by repeated administration. After testing various mixed chelation courses the authors found that oral PB followed by repeated oral DTPA most effectively reduced acute mortality. This study is of interest, since oral PB clearly was more efficacious than oral DFO, and since i.p. DTPA was a more efficient antidote than i.p. DFO for oral ferrosulfate.

Dean, Oehme, Krenzelok, and Hines (1988) used a pig model to closely simulate iron poisoning in a 2 year child. Fasted male pigs orally dosed with 300 mg/kg FeSO4 (60 mg Fe/kg) received either 50 mL 5% sodium bicarbonate, 50 ml 5% sodium dihydrogen phosphate, DFO (10 g) or 50 mL water (control). Bicarbonate or phosphate did not reduce intestinal Fe uptake compared to controls while DFO reduced iron absorption. This study indicates that digestive tract complexation of iron with bicarbonate or phosphate is of no value.

To avoid the severe complication of high dose i.v. DFO induced hypotension additive to that caused by iron poisoning, Mahoney, Hallaway, Hedlund, and Eaton (1989) covalently attached DFO to high molecular weight dextran or hydroxyethyl starch. Even very large i.v. doses of these macromolecular DFO conjugates did not decrease the blood pressure in mice. Polymer attached DFO persisted in blood much longer than free DFO. The DFO-polymers were highly efficient antidotes in acute oral iron poisoning, more than 90% survival at 30 h after i.p. injection of a dose of ferrous sulfate corresponding to LD_{90} in mice compared to 0% survival in unchelated controls and 10% in mice given free DFO.

Bentur et al. (1990) investigated the effect of orally active iron chelator L1 on iron handling in experimental acute iron intoxication. The results indicate that L1-iron complex is not absorbed from the gi tract.

Fassos et al. (1996) investigated the efficacy of L1 in rats after an oral dose of 612 mg/kg elemental iron followed by an i.p. loading dose of 400 mg/kg L1 and additional intraperitoneal injections of 200, 100, and 100 mg/kg L1 at 1 h intervals. The mortality was 15% compared to 58% in controls given only iron

($p = 0.013$). L1 induced urinary iron excretion which did not occur with iron alone. Iron levels were reduced in liver and gastrointestinal tract.

Dean, Oehme, Krenzelok, Griffith, and Hines (1996) used a pig model to study wether gastrointestinal DFO will inhibit or enhance Fe uptake in acute oral poisoning. Fasted pigs weighing an average of 10 kg received an oral dose of 60 mg/kg iron followed by either 50 mL water or 10 g DFO (1 g/kg). There was no mortality in either group. In the DFO group characteristic urine discoloration occurred at 4 h. Despite statistical differences in serum iron levels occurred at 6 and 8 h, DFO did not diminish the total iron uptake.

Barr et al. (1999) investigated whether enteral L1 reduces or enhances intestinal iron uptake. Rats given an oral dose of 20 mg/kg ferrous sulfate solution + 1 mEq sodium bicarbonate per kg received an oral dose of 150 mg/kg L1 immediately or after 15 min. Within 20 min of oral iron dosing, s-Fe levels rapidly increased to > 3.50 mg/L. L1 given immediately after iron decreased s-Fe levels and increased fecal iron excretion twofold. Effectiveness was reduced when L1 was given 15 min after the iron dosing.

Berkovitch et al. (2000) administered 612 mg/kg elemental iron orally to rats followed by 800 mg/kg oral L1, another group received another dose of 800 mg/kg 2 h later. L1 administration decreased mortality from 30 to 6.6% after 2 h, from 40 to 16.6% after 12 h, and from 53.3 to 20% after 24 h. Two doses of 800 mg/kg L1 reduced mortality to 0, 9, and 18% at 2, 12, and 24 h after L1 administration. Histologically, there was a dose-dependent decrease in iron accumulation in the gastrointestinal tract. Oral L1 is potentially an effective chelator in treatment of acute iron poisonings in humans.

Eybl, Kotyzova, Kolek, Koutensky, and Nielsen (2002) used an iron feeding, iron-overload model in mice to study effects of DFO and L1 on tissue iron, lipid peroxidation (LP), and oxidative status. The hepatic Fe level reached 600% of the control level. Administration of 7 i.p. doses of DFO or 0.72 mmol/kg L1 orally every 48 h during the 9th and 10th week reduced hepatic, renal, and heart iron levels in both iron-loaded and control mice. DFO and L1 treatment also equally reduced LP and increased hepatic GSH levels in iron loaded mice. The glutathione peroxidase and catalase activities were not affected by iron loading, however, both DFO and L1 decreased GSH-Px activity.

4.13.2 Clinical Chelation Cases

Peck, Rogers, and Rivenbark (1982) described a 19-year-old female patient who ingested an estimated 50–60 ferrous sulfate tablets, 9.8–11.7 g of iron. She presented with a s-Fe level of 9.15 mg/L (164 μmol/L) and a saturated total iron binding capacity. She received i.v. DFO, 15 mg/kg per h via continuous infusion. Her total dose over 52 h was 37.1 g, halted when her urine no longer showed evidence of DFO-Fe chelation. This case report indicates safety and efficacy of slow i.v. infusion of DFO in an adult patient, using a regimen recommended for pediatric patients.

Jackson, Ling, and Washington (1995) studied the effects of orally administered DFO on the intestinal absorption of orally administered iron. Seven informed adult human volunteers received an oral dose of 5 mg/kg iron in a control phase and again in an experimental phase followed by an equimolar oral dose of DFO. There was no significant difference in peak s-Fe levels, time to peak s-Fe level or area-under-the-curve between the two groups. Equimolar oral doses of DFO do not appear to reduce the intestinal absorption of low oral iron doses in humans.

Cheney et al. (1995) described a 22-month-old boy brought to the emergency department after ingesting estimated 50 ferrous sulfate tablets with 60 mg iron/tablet. Despite spontaneous emesis and gastric lavage his condition deteriorated and his serum iron increased to 2992 μmol/L, 167 g/L. He developed coma, metabolic acidosis, hypovolemic and cardiogenic shock, liver failure, coagulopathy and adult respiratory distress syndrome over the following 4 days. He received a DFO dosage of 25 mg/kg per h 12 h/day for 3 day, mechanical ventilation, dopamine/nitroprusside therapy, blood products, bicarbonate, electrolyte, and volume replacement. Despite his hospital course was complicated by gastric outlet obstruction, he was dismissed on full oral feedings, gaining weight, and neurologically intact. Swan-Ganz catheter monitoring had been used to guide the management of his shock, iron-induced cardiac failure, and deferoxamine mesylate induced adult respiratory distress syndrome. This case describes the highest reported s-Fe level allowing survival after massive iron overdose.

The use of high i.v. doses of DFO in acute iron poisoning is complicated by toxicity, mainly hypotension, and short plasma half-life. Dragsten et al. (2000) administered a DFO-hydroxyethyl starch high-molecular-weight iron chelator (HES-DFO) to healthy male subjects by i.v. infusion during 4 h. The drug was well tolerated, and signs of acute DFO toxicity were not observed. The maximum plasma chelator levels were around 3 mmol/L with the HES-DFO, more than an order of magnitude higher than with DFO administration. Plasma residence time was increased, initial half-life 22–33 h. Urinary Fe excretion was 7.1+/−2.2 mg during 48 h in the highest dose group, and 0.06+/−0.15 mg in controls who received saline infusions. Intravenous infusion of HES-DFO was well tolerated, with prolonged plasma chelator levels, and increased urinary iron excretion.

Daram and Hayashi (2005) reported a case of severe hepatic injury in an adult after a suicidal overdose of iron tablets. Although peak serum iron level (3.4 mg/L) was significantly lower than that reported to cause hepatotoxicity (>17 mg/L), rapid and significant elevations in aminotransferases, total bilirubin, and prothrombin time occurred within 48 h. DFO chelation was rapidly followed by empiric NAC. The patient was minimally symptomatic and had a full recovery.

Matteuchi et al. (2006) investigated the effect of orally administrated EDTA with or without activated charcoal (AC) on iron absorption after a mild iron ingestion in healthy human volunteers. Subjects ingested 5 mg/kg of elemental iron as ferrous sulfate. 1 h postingestion, subjects were randomized to receive 35 mg/kg EDTA, EDTA plus 50 g of AC, or water. Serial serum iron levels were obtained at baseline and every hour for the first 6 h, then at 8, 12, and 24 h. A 2-week washout was used between study arms. Baseline serum iron levels did not differ among treatment groups. AUCs were not different among groups at 24 h. Peak serum iron levels did not differ among groups. Orally administered EDTA administered 1 h after iron did not significantly reduce iron absorption.

Skoczynska, Kwiecinska, Kielbinski, and Lukaszewski (2007) described a 27-year-old female who were treated with high oral and parenteral iron doses for anemia. Within 20 days she received total doses of 4 g Fe^{2+} orally and 700 mg Fe^{2+} i.v. A final 100 mg i.m. dose resulted in development of clinical manifestations characteristic of acute iron poisoning starting the next day. Gastrointestinal symptoms and hypotension were followed by high leucocytosis, shock, multi-organ failure and disseminated intravascular coagulation. The patient received intensive liquid support, i.v. saline, electrolytes, colloids, and albumin, then i.v. heparin and plasma infusion. Chelation was initiated on day 3 after renal function restarted on day 2, total 2 g DFO were administered i.m. to avoid hypotension by i.v. DFO. About 5 days after the iron exposure respiratory failure necessitated ventilatory support. She started to slowly recover at day 9. This case of iatrogenic iron poisoning demonstrates full recovery with minimum chelation.

Haider, De Carli, Dhanani, and Sweeney (2009) described the use of laparoscopic-assisted gastrotomy in the treatment of a suicidal iron overdose in a 14-year-old girl with a calculated potentially lethal dose of 70 mg/kg iron. Due to her level of consciousness, emesis was not induced, and gastric lavage was not performed, but she was started on i.v. DFO chelation therapy. A gastric iron bezoar was seen on plain radiograph. Upper endoscopy confirmed the presence of iron tablets and showed dense adherence to the gastric mucosa. It was therefore decided to surgically remove the iron tablets via an incision at the umbilicus allowing insertion of a 5-mm laparoscope and instruments for digital disimpaction of the bezoar and removal parallel with plenty of saline irrigation. After a rapid recovery the patient underwent psychiatric treatment. This case describes the usefulness of laparoscopic-assisted physical removal of solid material by gastrotomy.

Milne and Petros (2010) described a toddler who was admitted to the regional pediatric intensive care unit after ingestion of a large amount of ferrous sulfate. He had a high serum iron level of 700 μmol/L. After gastric lavage, bowel irrigation, and intravenous DFO he received continuous veno-venous hemofiltration. Serum Fe levels quickly returned to normal. After a good recovery he had no permanent sequelae from the ingestion.

Griffith, Fallgatter, Tantama, Tanen, and Matteucci (2011) performed a double-blinded, placebo-controlled, randomized, crossover study of effects of deferasirox on intestinal iron absorption in 8 healthy human volunteers ingesting 5 mg/kg of iron as ferrous sulfate. 1 h after iron ingestion, subjects received 20 mg/kg deferasirox or placebo. After a 2-week washout the other study arm took place. Baseline s-Fe levels were similar in the 2 groups. Oral deferasirox reduced s-Fe AUC curves compared to placebo. The study indicates that deferasirox may be a potential chelator in acute iron poisoning.

Sankar, Shukla, Khurana, and Dubey (2013) described a 10 months old girl presenting after ingestion of almost 130 mg/kg of iron with signs of serious poisoning in the form of hypotension, metabolic acidosis, and irritability. Her s-Fe level was 3.60 g/L. She immediately received oxygen, fluid therapy for severe dehydration, and i.v. antiemetics and antacids for gastric irritation, within 30 min of her arrival she had whole bowel irrigation with polyethylene glycol, 30 mL/kg per h until she passed clear stools after about 3 h. Intravenous DFO, 15 mg/kg/h, started within about 2 h of admission. Although the ingested iron dose was lethal and she had evidence of serious toxicity, conservative therapy with DFO and supportive care was chosen with exchange transfusion as an option in case of worsening. After 6 h of therapy, the child had become normovolaemic. Despite her extensive s-Fe level, she had an uneventful recovery.

Simonse, Valk-Swinkels, van't Veer, Ermens, and Veldkamp (2013) describe a suicidal intentional iron overdose in a 16-year-old girl. She was brought comatose to an emergency department. She had hyperglycaemia and mild metabolic acidosis. A computed tomography scan showed no signs of intracerebral haemorrhage or elevated intracerebral pressure. She woke up and confessed having ingested Fero-Gradumet(®). Her s-Fe 7 h after ingestion was 62 μmol/L corresponding to a moderate iron poisoning. After whole bowel irrigation with 2 L polyethyleneglycol solution she received 8 h intravenous chelation with DFO 20 mg/kg. She was discharged in a good clinical condition after three days.

Gumber et al. (2013) described an 18-year-old girl who ingested 50 tablets of ferrous sulfate (100 mg of elemental iron per 335 mg tablet corresponding to about 100 mg/kg body weight of elemental iron. She developed acute gastrointestinal and neurologic signs of poisoning and severe anion gap metabolic acidosis. The patient received gastrointestinal decontamination, DFO infusion, and hemodialysis resulting in reduction of serum iron from 21.50 to 1.60 g/L at 24-h postingestion and improved mental status.

4.13.3 Clinical Reviews

Unintentional (accidental) iron overdose cases has been and still is a leading cause of poisoning-related injury in young children in USA and other countries.

Morris (2000) analyzed the nature, trend, and hazard patterns of national data on pediatric iron ingestion-related injuries and deaths in the United States from 1980 to 1996 using data from the US Census Bureau, the US Consumer Product Safety Commission, the American Association of Poison Control

Centers, and the National Center for Health Statistics. Annual pediatric reported and diagnosed iron poisonings were stable until 1986 where the incidence increased 150% from an annual average of 1200 from 1980 through 1985 to 3000 from 1986 through 1996. Most children were below 6 years, 1/3 below 2. The number of iron-related pediatric fatalities increased in 1986, peaked at 10 in 1991, and then declined to 2 by 1995. Unit-dose packaging of hig-dose iron supplements was mentioned to be expected to reduce the frequency of severe pediatric iron overdose incidents.

Singhi and Baranwal (2003) studied the incidence of acute iron intoxication in children attending Pediatric Emergency service of a teaching hospital in a retrospective study during a 5 years' period. Among 27125 patient visits to Pediatric Emergency, 337 (1.2%) were for accidental poisoning, 21 patients had iron poisoning; 18 were transferred to PICU. The most common signs in Fe poisoned children were vomiting (83%), diarrhea (72%), malena (44%), and hemetemesis (33%) generally within 6 h of ingestion. Nine children developed shock and/or impaired consciousness, 7 of these patients responded to saline (33 + /−15 mL/kg) and dopamine (10 + /−4 μg/kg per min) within 4–24 h. The remaining two with acute liver failure died from shock or acute liver failure with coagulopathy and/or severe acidosis. The amounts of ingested iron and clinical signs were more useful to evaluate poisoning severeness and guide to treatment decisions than was se-Fe levels. Gastric lavage removed fragments of iron tablets in 10 patients. DFO infusion and supportive care was instituted in all patients. Vin rose-colored urine was not seen in 31% of patients despite high se-Fe levels.

Tenenbein (2005) described the effects of the US FDA proclaimed regulation for unit-dose packaging of iron supplements in 1997 as a preventive measure against unintentional iron poisoning death in young children in a preintervention-postintervention study comparing 10 years prior to the intervention with 5 years after based on iron ingestion and iron poisoning deaths incidences for children younger than 6 years from the annual reports of the American Association of Poison Control Centers (Washington, DC). The average number of calls to poison control centers related to iron ingestion decreased from 2.99 per 1000 to 1.91 per 1000 ($P < 0.001$). The number of deaths decreased from 29 to 1 ($P = 0.03$). These data are the first to show decreases in the incidence of nonintentional ingestion by young children and in poisoning mortality for a specific drug after introduction of unit-dose packaging.

4.13.4 Conclusions

Supportive care is highly important in acute oral iron poisoning. Treatment may include mechanical removal of remains of tablets, GI decontamination, careful management of body fluid volume, and chelation with DFO. Clinical experience indicates that i.v. infusion of DFO is an efficient route of chelation treatment in acute iron poisoning. There is some animal experimental evidence, that rapid enteral chelation may be effective in reducing oral iron toxicity. Oral PB was more efficacious than oral DTPA which was more efficacious than oral DFO in oral ferrosulfate poisoning in an animal study. Trial of enteral DFO have not demonstrated adverse effects. Oral PB, DTPA, L1 or deferasirox are potentially effective chelators in treatment of acute iron poisonings but further animal studies are needed to pave the way for clinical studies.

4.14 LEAD

Lead (Pb, atomic number 82, member of group 14 of the periodic table of the elements, atomic weight 207.19, density 11.3 g/cm^3, melting point 327.5°C) is a soft, malleable and heavy posttransition metal. The most common oxidation step in inorganic lead compounds is +2, but +4 also occurs. Since all stable lead isotopes but ^{204}Pb are end products of radioactive decay (^{206}Pb from the uranium series, ^{207}Pb from the actinium series, ^{208}Pb from the thorium series), the isotopic composition of lead depends on its geological origin. Metallic lead is rarely found in nature, lead often occurs in ores with copper, zinc, and silver. The main lead ore is gallena (PbS), other important ores are cerussite ($PbCO_3$) and anglesite ($PbSO_4$) (Holleman, Wiberg, & Wiberg, 1985). The annual world primary lead production is about 5.4 million tons, recycling of lead scrap contributes a similar amount to cover the world annual use of around 10 million tons. The largest producers are China, Australia, USA, Peru, and Mexico (USGS, 2014). The present main use of lead is in automobile and industrial batteries and electric backup systems. Present and past minor uses of lead are in ammunition, cable sheathing, solders, various alloys, water piping and in the fitting of water pipes, and importantly, in pigments for corrosion protection of steel constructions and in house paint as ($2PbCO_3 \cdot Pb(OH)_2$) (International Lead and Zinc Study Group, 2012).

The past large-scale use of organic lead compounds as antiknocking agent in gasoline annually consumed about 400,000 tons mainly emitted to the environment (Nriagu, 1996). This use has decreased extensively since the 1970s, due to outphasing of tetramethyllead (Me_4Pb) and tetraethyllead (Et_4Pb) as antiknock additives (IARC, 2006). This has significantly reduced environmental lead levels. Because of lead's comparatively low melting point and high vapor pressure, industrial uses of inorganic lead have also caused extensive local environmental pollution. Organolead poisonings, sometimes fatal, have occurred from gasoline sniffing and in production and distribution of organoleads.

The earliest identified use of lead was found in the El Miron cave in Spain, where lead sulfide was used in an almost 16,000 years old burial stained by red ochre (Strauss et al., 2011). Galena bead production dates back to about 6500 BC in Turkey and Iraq; the production of lead together with silver started around 3500 BC. In the Roman Empire, lead produced as a by-product of silver production had increasing uses in aquaducts and in kitchen utensils and for wine sweetening (Nriagu, 1998).

Lead is absorbed from the lungs, to some degree from the skin, and from the gastrointestinal tract. In humans the absorption after oral lead exposure varied from an average of 60% in fasting subjects to an average of 8% for soluble lead salts taken with a meal (James, Hilburn, & Blair, 1985; Rabinowitz, Kopple, & Wetherill, 1980). In small children the gastrointestinal lead absorption could be much larger (Scheuplein, Charnley, & Dourson, 2002). Lead in blood is associated with erythrocytes due to binding to δ-aminolevulinic acid dehydratase (ALAD) generally with less than 1% of the total blood lead (b-Pb) in plasma. At high b-Pb ≥ 4–5 μmol/L plasma lead (p-Pb) increases over 1% of total b-Pb. (Bergdahl, Schutz, & Grubb, 1996; Bergdahl, Schutz, Gerhardsson, & Skerfving, 1997; Bergdahl et al., 1998). Liver and kidneys have the highest lead levels among soft tissues, and lead can pass the blood–brain barrier and also accumulate in peripheral nerve tissue (Barry, 1975; Skerfving et al., 1985). The skeleton is the main lead depot, containing > 90% of body lead, in lead workers even more (Barry, 1975). Due to slow turnover, bone lead indicated both long-term lead and total body lead burden. Bone lead is slowly released to blood due to bone remodeling and then redistributed and excreted, mainly via urine and feces (Bergdahl et al., 1997; Rabinowitz et al., 1980). U-Pb excretion after administration of a chelating agent (EDTA or DMSA) has been used as an index of total body burden and risk (Sakai, Ushio, & Ikeya, 1998; Lee, Schwartz, Stewart, & Ahn, 1995). Chelatable lead is however not an accurate measure of body burden, reflecting mainly blood and soft tissues lead levels (Gerhardsson et al., 1998) and may be trabecular bone (Tell et al., 1992). Since EDTA may redistribute lead to the brain (see later), EDTA diagnostic challenge is potentially dangerous and should not be used.

Inorganic lead exposure may cause a wide range of toxic effects depending on exposure route and dose. At lower exposures, effects on the central and peripheral nervous system may develop, higher exposures lead to gastrointestinal symptoms ("lead colic") and very high acute exposures may cause lead encephalopathy most often seen in children, potentially lethal if not swiftly treated by chelation. The condition is partly reversible. High level lead exposure may cause anemia, renal dysfunction (partly reversible glomerular and tubulointerstitial nephritis) leading to elevated blood pressure and increased risk of cardiovascular disease and stroke and eventually to chronic renal failure (Skerfving & Bergdahl, 2014). The CNS effects due to acute or chronic lead exposure vary from mild depression of mental development and function in children via concentration problems, irritability, fatigue, anxiety, hostility, depressed mood, tension, and interpersonal problems seen in lead workers to acute encephalopathy (Goodman et al., 2002; Seeber, Meyer-Baron, & Schaper, 2002).

Childhood lead poisoning has been and still is a serious health problem in less affluent population groups living in low-standard housing and in polluted environments in developing countries. Environmental lead poisoning in young children represents the most common preventable childhood disease in the United States. In the US and elsewhere, indoor lead paint in old houses is still an important source of childhood lead exposure despite extensive renovation programs. Despite most exposed children have no clinical signs of lead intoxication discernible on an individual basis, they are at risk for developing irreversible neuropsycologic dysfunction. The issue whether abatement of lead pollution should be combined with chelation treatment has been a matter of debate for decades (Shannon, Graef, & Lovejoy, 1988; Graziano et al., 1992; Liebelt, Shannon, & Graef, 1994; Besunder, Anderson, & Super, 1995; Yeoh et al., 2014). Epidemiological studies from all over the world have been published on effects of lead exposures on mental development in children http://ntpsearch.niehs.nih.gov/texis/search/?query=lead+epidemiology&pr=ntp_web_entire_site_all&mu=Entire+NTP+Site, (WHO/IPCS, 2000; EFSA, 2010; JECFA, 2011; USNTP, 2012. The combined epidemiology on low level lead exposure in children indicates a supralinear relationship between blood lead and reduced IQ which could mean that a threshold does not exist (Lanphear et al., 2005; USNTP, 2012; Pawlas et al., 2012; Lucchini et al., 2012; Skerfving & Bergdahl, 2014).

4.14.1 Animal Chelation Studies

An extensive body of evidence from experimental animal studies clearly indicates that DPA, BAL, and EDTA are less efficient chelating antidotes in acute lead poisoning than DMSA, while DMSA and EDTA are efficient in mobilizing lead in chronic lead exposure, DMSA from soft tissues and EDTA from bone:

DMSA more efficiently than DPA reduced tissue levels and increased urinary lead excretion and corrected disturbances in porphyrin metabolism in rats, mice, and rabbits. DMSA reduced lead levels in bone, spleen, liver, and kidneys, and most importantly, the brain (Friedheim, Corvi, & Wakker, 1976; Graziano et al., 1978b; Okonishnikova, Rozenberg, & Rezina, 1976).

Sharma, Kachru, Singh, and Tandon (1986) studied effects of some alpha-mercapto-beta-aryl acrylic acids as antidotes in lead poisoning in rats. Alpha-mercapto-beta-(3,4-dimethoxyphenyl)acrylic acid (MDA) was most effective. Other substituted acrylic acid had similar effects but less so than MDA in reducing tissue Pb levels and enhancing renal Pb excretion. MDA was the only chelator reducing Pb levels in brain. Also MFA more effectively than structurally related compounds reduced the body burden of lead and enhanced fecal and urinary Pb excretion. All compounds counteracted lead induced inhibition of blood delta-aminolevulinic acid dehydratase (delta-ALA-D) activity and increased urinary delta-aminolevulinic acid excretion.

Sharma, Khandelwal, Kachru, Singh, and Tandon (1987) compared the ability of β-1,2-Phenylene di-a-mercaptoacrylic acid (1,2-PDMA), 3-1,4-phenylene di-a-mercaptoacrylic acid (1,4-PDMA) and a-mercapto-Q-(2-hydroxyphenyl) acrylic acid (MHA) to counteract toxic effects of lead in rats with that of DMPS. DMPS and 1,2-PDMA effectively reduced Pb body levels and enhanced Pb excretion, and restored most biochemical alterations induced by

Pb. MHA reduced Pb tissue levels and enhanced urinary Pb excretion. The results indicate the efficiency of vicinal thio groups and participation of the hydroxy group on the benzene nucleus besides the SH group of the MHA molecule, in chelation of Pb.

Parenteral administration of EDTA to rats exposed for several months to lead temporarily increased the lead level in brain, up to 2 × the prechelation level; The brain lead level was not reduced by 5 days treatment, however, blood, kidney, and bone lead levels were reduced compared to levels in unchelated rats (Cory-Slechta, Weiss, & Cox, 1987).

After long-term exposure of rats to lead in drinking water, repeated DMSA injections extensively reduced blood, brain, liver, and kidney lead levels, but bone lead levels were not reduced. Four months after cessation of chelation, lead levels in blood and soft tissue had increased due to redistribution of lead from bone. This experimental setup is realistic in relation to occupational or environmental lead poisoning (Cory-Slechta, 1988).

Xu and Jones (1988) compared a series of chelating agents injected i.p. as antidotes for acute and chronic poisoning from i.p. injected lead in mice. DMSA and cyclohexanediaminetetraacetic acid (CDTA) were most efficient among 16 chelators. EDTA, DMPS, and DPA did not protect against mortality, data for BAL are not given. DMPS more efficiently than DMSA and other chelators including EDTA removed lead from kidneys and brain. DPA increased the brain lead level. In a small experiment, chelation with BAL reduced bone lead. Oral administration of DMSA significantly reduced kidney, liver, brain, and bone lead levels while oral DPA and EDTA were marginally efficient.

Kapoor, Wielopolski, Graziano, and LoIacono (1989) administered a single oral dose of $^{203}Pb^{2+}$ to rats. Whole-body γ-counting, and γ-counting of total urine showed that parenteral administration of EDTA, DMSA, DPA, or BAL immediately after lead administration increased the intestinal absorption of lead estimated as the whole-body retention plus the cumulative urinary lead output at 144 h after dosage. Chelation did not affect the net retention of lead estimated from the whole-body retention, except for a slightly increased retention in BAL-treated animals. Oral administration of chelating agents immediately after oral administration of lead did not increase the intestinal uptake of lead, and the whole-body retention of lead was reduced extensively in rats given EDTA or DMSA orally but not in rats given BAL or DPA orally. The results indicate that DMSA treatment of childhood lead poisoning on an outpatient basis does not pose a risk for increased Pb absorption.

Pappas, Nuttall, Ahlquist, Allen, and Banner (1995) investigated effects of oral administration of DMSA on urinary lead and δ-aminolevulinic acid excretion, blood zinc protoporphyrin levels and organ lead levels in rats exposed for 35 days to lead in drinking water, both after cessation of lead exposure and during continued lead exposure. DMSA reversed hematologic effects of lead, increased urinary lead excretion, and decreased blood, liver, kidney, brain, and bone lead levels in rats, even during continued lead exposure.

Llobet, Domingo, Paternain, and Corbella (1990) investigated the efficacy of EDTA, DTPA, EGTA, CDTA, NAC, BAL, ascorbic acid, DDC, DMSA and DMPS as mobilizing agents and antidotes for acute lead intoxication in mice. Chelators were given i.p. at doses approximately equal to one-fourth of their respective LD_{50} values 15 min after s.c. administration of 37.8 mmol/kg lead acetate. CDTA, ascorbic acid, DMSA, and DMPS increased survival. CDTA (2.33) and EDTA (1.73) had the highest therapeutic effectiveness. EDTA, DTPA and CDTA most effectively increased the urinary lead excretion, while DTPA, CDTA, and DMSA increased the fecal lead excretion. EDTA, DDC, and CDTA most effectively reduced tissue lead levels.

Tandon, Hashmi, and Kachru (1990) studied the lead mobilizing effectiveness of substituted dithiocarbamates in rats given 10 mg Pb/kg per day orally for 8 weeks and then chelated with 400 μmol/kg i.p. daily for 5 days of DMSA, DDC, tetraammonium ethylenediamine diacetic acid dithiocarbamate (EDDTC), morpholine dithiocarbamate, ammonium diethanolamine dithiocarbamate (ADDTC), or *N*-benzyl-D-glucamine dithiocarbamate (NBGDTC). All chelaters reduced renal and hepatic Pb levels. ADDTC, EDDTC, and NBGDTC also reduced bone Pb levels. The reduction of Pb levels did not correlate with ameliorating effects on Pb-induced hematopoietic alterations. The relatively low lipophilicity of substituted dithiocarbamates due to hydrophilic groups seems to be advantageous in preventing transport of lead chelate into the brain. The substituted dithiocarbamates did not induce excessive excretion of Cu and Zn. ADDTC and EDDTC appear to be potential antidotes in Pb poisoning.

Jones et al. (1994b) gave 10 or 20 i.p. injections of lead acetate to mice during 12 or 26 days. Parenteral administration for 4 or 8 days of DTPA, EDTA, or DMSA consistently reduced lead levels in brain and kidneys. Lead in bone was mobilized after some EDTA or DMSA chelation treatments, however, less effectively than soft organ lead levels. In a summary of data on effects of EDTA and DMSA on brain lead levels the authors conclude that DMSA reduces lead levels in brain under all chelation conditions examined.

Flora et al. (1995a, 1995b) investigated the lead mobilizing effects of DMSA or EDTA after acute parenteral lead intoxication in rats. Injected EDTA and orally administered DMSA equally efficiently increased erythrocyte δ-aminolevulinic acid dehydrase activity and decreased urinary δ-aminolevulinic acid levels toward normal levels. The chelators were even more effective with combined administration. Oral DMSA more effectively than injected EDTA lowered blood, kidney, liver, and brain lead levels, while EDTA slightly increased the brain lead level. The urinary lead excretion was similar for the chelators. Combined administration of both chelators more effectively enhanced urinary lead excretion and reduced organ lead levels, except in brain. However, the kidney lead levels remained high after combined treatment, indicating a potential extra renal lead burden. Also, the combined treatment resulted in elevated creatinine level and serum transaminase activity and reduced blood zinc levels.

In a neurobehavioral investigation in mice using a forced swim model, 7 weeks DMSA chelation alongside lead exposure in drinking water enhanced the behavioral anomaly induced by lead (Stewart et al., 1995). Cory-Slechta and Weiss (1989) previously found similar adverse effects of EDTA chelation during lead intoxication potentially explained by EDTA induced transiently increased brain deposition of lead, an explanation not available for the effect of DMSA chelation.

Intraperitoneal injection of 1–4 doses of DMPS daily to rats starting 4 days after exposure to lead acetate in drinking water for 86 days did not increase the lead level in brain (Aposhian, Maiorino, Xu, & Aposhian, 1996).

In an experimental study of lead-induced hyperactivity in mice, administration of DMSA starting 6 weeks after cessation of lead exposure corrected lead-induced behavioral anomaly and reduced blood lead levels in both sexes, most effectively in males (Stewart, Blaine, Cohen, Burright, & Donovick, 1996).

In a habituation study of lead-induced hyperactivity in rats, DMSA chelation after cessation of lead exposure reduced lead induced neurological anomalies and toxicity (Gong & Evans, 1997).

Tandon, Singh, Prasad, and Mathur (1998) obtained similar results in a dose-response experiment with the same experimental model as used by Flora et al. (1995a, 1995b). An important result of this study was extensive and consistent reduction of lead levels in brain and bone in groups treated with combinations of EDTA and DMSA or with one of these chelators at a high dose.

Smith, Bayer, and Strupp (1998) exposed rats to lead in the drinking water for 30 or 40 days to study relationships between blood and brain lead levels during oral administration of DMSA. One week of chelation reduced the blood lead level much more than the brain lead level. Chelation for 21 days decreased the lead level in brain compared to unchelated controls but did not reduce blood lead levels further.

Smith et al. (2000) studied effects of DMSA on the urinary excretion of essential elements in infant rhesus monkeys (Macaca mulatta) as a primate model of childhood Pb exposure. Monkeys exposed to Pb from birth to 1 y of age with resulting b-Pb levels around 400–500 μg/L were chelated with DMSA, 30 mg/kg per day $\times$ 5 days then 20 mg/kg per day $\times$ 14 days. Urine samples were analyzed for Ca, Co, Cu, Fe, Pb, Mg, Mn, Ni, and Zn. DMSA chelation reduced b-Pb levels compared to controls and increased total urinary Pb excretion >fourfold. DMSA chelation increased the urinary excretion of essential elements, but only when total cumulative excretion day 1–5 for all elements were considered. DMSA does contribute to increased urinary excretion of essential elements, although not significantly for any single element. Pb-exposed children may have suboptimal trace element status due to nutritional deficiencies.

Ambrus et al. (2001) developed a "Lead-Hemopurifier" (L-HP) with an immobilized chelator, an amerlite IRC 718 resin with high affinity for lead. The L-HP device reduced lead concentrations in lead solutions in vitro. Also, the L-HP removed lead from the blood of lead poisoned dogs. Increased B-Pb mobilized from bone was removed until the skeleton was cleared from lead. The L-HP offers a safe alternative to EDTA chelation of lead poisoned children. The device should however be compared with DMSA for efficiency.

Bradberrry and Vale (2009a,b) reviewed experimental studies of lead chelation by equimolar and clinically relevant doses of DMSA and $Na_2CaEDTA$. These chelators had similar effects on urine lead excretion and/or blood lead concentrations, though direct comparison between the antidotes was not performed. DMSA reduced kidney lead levels more effectively than EDTA while EDTA more effectively than DMSA reduced bone lead levels. The experimental studies did not demonstrate consistent effects of chelation on brain lead levels.

Jin et al. (2011) investigated the therapeutic efficiency of DMSA administered with ascorbic acid and calcium in mild lead poisoning in mice exposed to lead in drinking water. DMSA, 50 or 100 mg/kg b.w. or 50 mg/kg b.w. succimer with calcium and ascorbic acid was administered by gavage. DMSA alone reduced blood and bone lead levels and improved blood ALAD activities. However, DMSA administered with ascorbic acid and calcium more efficiently mobilized bone lead.

Sangvanich et al. (2014) developed a thiol containing nanoporous silica material called SH-SAMMS to be used as oral therapy for metal poisoning. SH-SAMMS had higher affinity for methyl mercury and inorganic mercury, lead, and cadmium in artificial gastrointestinal fluids and in biologically digested fish tissue than carboxylic acid or phosphonic acid containing SAMMS or commercial metal chelating sorbents. SH-SAMMS added to a diet with lead offered to rats reduced b-Pb significantly compared to levels in rats given only the metal containing diet. SH-SAMMS was non toxic to common intestinal bacteria (Escherichia coli) and to an in vitro intestinal epithelium model (Caco-2 cells) and seems to offer a potential oral chelator for metal poisoning.

The studies reviewed above together indicate that oral DMSA alone or combined with parenteral EDTA may be the most efficient chelation treatment for lead intoxication, and that the EDTA provocation test for diagnostic estimation of the lead body burden is dangerous for the patient. The combined animal data together with human data reviewed below indicate that DMSA chelation mobilizes soft tissue lead and recently deposited bone lead, however, DMSA can only indirectly mobilize aged bone lead deposits during prolonged chelation by depleting soft tissues of lead, thereby promoting flow of lead from bones. EDTA less efficiently than DMSA mobilizes soft tissue lead deposits, however, EDTA can mobilize aged bone lead deposits. An important question in chelation treatment of lead intoxication is the enhancing or inhibiting effect of chelating agents on intestinal lead uptake. The results of animal studies indicate that EDTA should only be used after cessation of lead exposure while results with DMSA are not entirely clear.

4.14.2 Clinical Studies

Several cohort studies and case studies of chelation of lead-poisoned humans are published: Friedheim, Graziano, Popovac, Dragovic, and Kaul (1978) chelated five lead-poisoned lead smelter workers with oral DMSA in doses increasing from start doses of 8.4–12.7 mg/kg b.w. and up to 28.1–42.2 mg/kg b.w. on day 6). Chelation reduced blood lead levels to about 50% of prechelation levels.

Bentur, Brook, Behar, and Taitelman (1987) diagnosed a chronic lead poisoning due to use of a primitive flour mill for home production of bread. $CaNa_2EDTA$ provocation followed by oral DMSA challenge increased the urinary lead excretion by a factor of 11. Five days DMSA chelation alleviated clinical symptoms of lead poisoning symptoms, decreased b-Pb and increased urinary lead excretion. Clinical symptoms of lead poisoning did not reappear during follow-up for several months. This case indicates that oral DMSA challenge could be a diagnostic test for lead poisoning less dangerous than the EDTA provocation test.

Fournier et al. (1988) treated nine lead-poisoned workers with DMSA chelation. Seven workers received 30 mg/kg per day DMSA for 5 days, two workers were started with lower doses, one was chelated for 15 days due high initial blood lead level, and one had a history of atopy. Chelation on an average increased the urinary lead excretion by 1 order of magnitude and reduced b-Pb levels by 35–81%. At three weeks after chelation treatment, clinical indices of lead poisoning had stabilized or improved in all patients.

Shannon et al. (1988) reviewed clinical experience with DPA as chelating agent in low level lead poisoning (b-Pb levels 250–400 μg/L). 84 subjects treated with a mean daily dose of 27.5 mg/kg DPA were compared to 37 unchelated control subjects. After a mean period of 76 days of DPA chelation b-Pb levels in chelated patients were reduced by 33%. In 64 patients (76%), b-PB was reduced to "acceptable levels", less than or equal to 250 μg/L). There were eight treatment failures (10%). The mean b-Pb level did not change significantly in the control group during 119 days of observation. Fourteen control subjects were chelated with $CaNa_2EDTA$, and 17 were lost to follow-up. DPA chelation induced adverse reactions in 28 cases (33%); rash in 7, transient platelet count depression in 7, transient leukopenia in 8, enuresis in three, and abdominal pain in two. Chelation was terminated in eight cases (10%) due to an adverse reaction.

A challenge to be met during chelation treatment of chronic lead poisoning is a rebound of the blood lead level occurring soon after cessation of a chelation course. This rebound is observed with all chelating agents that have been used in lead intoxication and is likely due to the continued slow mobilization of lead in bones, and in many cases it necessitates repeated chelation schedules.

Another challenge in chelation treatment of lead poisoning with BAL or EDTA is management of iron deficiency induced by lead, as both BAL and EDTA form toxic iron complexes (Singh, Khodr, Tayler, & Hider, 1995; Tilbrook & Hider, 1998) precluding iron therapy. Haust, Inwood, Spence, Poon, and Peter (1989) treated a worker with a severe occupational lead poisoning with extensive oral doses of DMSA for several years simultaneously with i.m. iron administration which normalized serum-ferritin levels without toxic effect.

Before initiation of DMSA chelation, combined chelation therapy with BAL and $CaNa_2EDTA$ followed by $CaNa_2EDTA$ chelation during 3 years reaching a total of 64.5 g did not alleviate the patient's clinical symptoms and at four years after cessation of lead exposure the patient suffered from insomnia, colic, anorexia and various neuropsychiatric symptoms and the b-Pb level was 900 µg/L. At the time of reporting this case 189 g of DMSA had been administered in 6 chelation courses totaling 141 days of treatment during 2 years. This had mobilized about 375 mg of lead. The urinary lead excretion increased about 7 times and the b-Pb level was reduced to about 1/5 of pretreatment levels during chelation courses but gradually rebounded to pretreatment levels after each treatment. Subjective and clinical symptoms of lead poisoning were alleviated but gradually reappeared parallel to increased b-Pb level after the chelation courses. The patient's body-burden of lead was still very high despite this intensive chelation treatment, so he is most likely bound for repeated chelation for his entire lifetime.

Grandjean, Jacobsen, and Jørgensen (1991) reported a similar however less severe lead poisoning case. DMSA chelation initially reduced the b-Pb level by a factor of about 10. After cessation of chelation the b-Pb gradually rebounded. Chelation was discontinued after three courses since the patient developed DMSA hypersensitivity. The 3 chelation courses apparently had a long-lasting effect on the patient's mental capacity and on blood lead levels.

Tell et al. (1992) observed close correlation ($r = 0.86$, $P < 0.001$) between prechelation b-Pb levels and 24 h urinary Pb excretion after i.v. infusion of 1 g $CaNa_2EDTA$ in 20 lead workers. Also, significant correlations were found between Pb levels in bones measured by in vivo X-ray fluorescence (tibia/calcaneus, $r = 0.93$, $P < 0.001$; tibia/phalanx, $r = 0.67$, $P < 0.002$; calcaneus/phalanx $r = 0.80$, $P < 0.001$). In currently exposed workers chelated lead and bone lead correlated (eg, for calcaneus, $r = 0.62$).

Graziano (1993) and Graziano et al. (1992) chelated lead-exposed children and workers with DMSA. DMSA increased urinary lead excretion and reduced b-Pb levels. Biochemical indicators of lead poisoning were corrected. DMSA chelation was more effective than $CaNa_2EDTA$ chelation in restoring function of the heme pathway and was tolerated in nine patients receiving iron supplementation and two homozygous for glucose-6-phosphate dehydrogenase deficiency. The cumulative lead excretion via urine was much larger than the calculated reduction in the blood lead store indicating that DMSA chelation mobilized lead from other tissues. Administration of 700 mg/m^2 DMSA per day on an outpatient basis delayed the typical rebound in b-Pb values and reduced the need for repeated hospitalizations. Studies of Liebelt et al. (1994) and Besunder et al. (1995) also indicated high efficacy of DMSA chelation in lead poisoning.

Smith, Markowitz, Crick, Rosen, and Flegal (1994) used the stable isotope ^{204}Pb to study oral lead kinetics in adult humans. Oral DMSA administration immediately after oral intake of 200 µg lead labeled by ^{204}Pb increased the urinary and decreased the fecal lead output. The fraction of the dose recovered in urine and feces after the experimental period was reduced by DMSA exposure, indicating that DMSA enhanced the intestinal lead absorption, at variance with results of animal studies reviewed above. The experiment involved only four individuals in each of two DMSA groups and four controls. The differences did not reach statistical significance, however, this study pinpoint the importance of removal from lead exposure before chelation with DMSA is initiated. Oral administration of DMPS or DMSA after oral administration of inorganic mercury or cadmium salts to mice reduced the intestinal Cd and Hg metal uptake (Andersen et al., 1988b; Andersen, 1989a; Nielsen & Andersen, 1991a).

Lee et al. (1995) performed a provocative chelation test with DMSA and an EDTA provocation test in the same subjects to compare lead excretion after these two chelating agents. Oral DMSA enhances excretion of lead from storage sites in the body relevant for health effects of lead. Thirty-four male Korean lead workers received a single oral dose of 10 mg/kg DMSA. Urine volume and urinary lead level were determined at 0, 2, 4, 6, 8, and 24 h. 17 of these workers also received 1 g i.v. EDTA with similar urine collection 2 weeks before or two weeks after DMSA. U-Pb levels peaked 2 h after DMSA and 4 h after EDTA. Lead excretion after DMSA was less than after EDTA. Multiple linear regression demonstrated that b-Pb was a predictor of EDTA-chelatable lead and urinary aminolevulinic acid was associated with lead chelatable by DMSA. When EDTA was given before DMSA, excretion after DMSA was greatly increased indicating EDTA induced lead transfer from bone to soft tissues.

Besunder et al. (1995) investigated the short-term efficacy of DMSA chelation in mild to moderate pediatric lead poisoning by retrospective review of medical records of pediatric patients receiving 19 days of DMSA between June 1991 and May 1993 with prechelation bPb levels 1.21–2.36 μmol/L (250–490 μg/L). Homes were abated of major lead hazards before chelation therapy. Approximately 10 mg/kg DMSA was given every 8 h for 5 days, followed by 10 mg/kg every 12 h for 14 days. 18 out of 46 children chelated with DMSA were excluded from analysis. The percent reduction in b-Pb compared with baseline was 43% ± 20.8%, 26% ± 16.9%, and 31% ± 20.2% on days 18, 30, and 80. Eighty percent of patients had 20% or more reduction in their pretreatment BPb and/or ZnP after completion of DMSA chelation. No significant adverse effects were observed except for neutropenia in one patient. This study demonstrates short-term efficacy of DMSA chelation in mild to moderate lead poisoning.

Gordon, Roberts, Amin, Williams, and Paloucek (1998) reported a case of a 3-year-old girl with pica behavior presenting almost unconscious with severe lead encephalopathy and a very high bPb level, 26.4 μmol/L (5.5 mg/L) due to exposure to lead paint in a home not well maintained. She was treated with extensive gut decontamination by whole bowel irrigation and i.m. BAL chelation, i.v. EDTA chelation and oral DMSA chelation. The treatment was well tolerated and effective in promoting lead excretion and inducing an extensive reduction in bPb levels. During oral DMSA chelation alone lead blood levels increased so

EDTA chelation was reinstituted combined with oral zinc sulfate. She was discharged from the hospital with oral DMSA, zinc sulfate, and iron sulfate to be cared for by her mother and grandmother in a location approved by the Illinois Department of Public Health.

Chisholm (2000) reported a study on the safety and efficacy of DMSA for chelation of children with lead toxicity. 59 children 12–65-months old, with pretreatment b-Pb of 250-660 μ/L received 116, 26–28 day courses of oral DMSA either in the Pediatric Clinical Research Unit of the Johns Hopkins Hospital or in lead-safe housing as outpatients. Children completing the study had sharp decreases in b-Pb levels during chelation, but 2–3 weeks after completion of chelation, b-Pb levels rebounded to an average of 58% of their average pretreatment b-Pb levels. No adverse reactions were caused by DMSA. Two patients reexposed to defective lead paint had sharp increases in b-Pb levels during therapy. For one child, the b-Pb level raised from 200 to 900 μg/L in 1 week. DMSA appears safe for mobilizing lead into the urine. The study does not allow conclusions on long-term beneficial effects.

Torres-Alanis et al. (2002) performed a pilot experiment in Mexico where DMSA at that time was not approved, to evaluate this chelating agent in workers with occupational lead exposure and b-Pb levels >0.5 mg/L. Ten men without clinical symptoms of lead poisoning received 600 mg oral DMSA per day for five days. DMSA chelation therapy did not influence hepatic, renal or hematologic functions and effectively decreased blood lead levels without inducing adverse drug reactions.

Mikler, Banovcin, Jesenak, Hamzikova, and Statelova (2009) described a severe acute lead poisoning in a 17-year-old girl admitted to emergency department after suicidal ingestion of 20 g of lead nitrate, more than 10 × a lethal lead dose. Her very high lead blood level of 4.227 mg/L (20.4 μmol/L) at 90 min after ingestion was treated by gastric lavage with one dose of charcoal, 1 g/kg and continuous infusion of 1500 mg/m^2 per day of $CaNa_2$ EDTA as single chelating agent. Blood levels above 0.7 mg/L (3.37 μmol/L) persisted for approximately 24 h. Gastrointestinal toxicity disappeared during 2 days and organ dysfunction or anemia were not observed. Chelation continued for 5 days without inducing signs of $CaNa_2$ EDTA toxicity and with normal renal function tests. Follow-up of the patient showed no clinical or subclinical signs of neurological deficiency or psychiatric pathology.

Bradberry, Sheehan, and Vale (2009) administered DMSA to 17 consecutive patients $\geq$ 16 years who presented with lead poisoning regardless of the source (occupational or intake of lead-containing traditional remedies) and with blood lead levels $\geq$ 0.5 mg/L. The patients received 35 oral chelation courses, each of 30 mg/kg per day. B-Pb levels were significantly reduced and urine lead excretion was significantly increased by a median increase in daily urine lead excretion 12-fold over the prechelation level with wide individual variation. Clinical and subjective signs of lead poisoning rapidly improved or resolved during the first 2 days of treatment in more than 50% of the patients. DMSA was well tolerated, however, one patient developed a severe mucocutaneous reaction and treatment was discontinued. Transient increases in alanine aminotransferase activity occurred in 14% of patients. DMSA increased urine copper and zinc excretion significantly. This study indicates that oral DMSA at the dose of 30 mg/kg per day is effective as chelating antidote in lead intoxication despite wide inter- and intra-individual variation in the response.

Only two clinical studies are available comparing urine lead excretion after equimolar or similar doses of EDTA and DMSA; they did not find significant differences between the antidotes, and EDTA and DMSA had similar blood lead lowering capacity at similar molar chelator doses: Bradberrry and Vale (2009a) calculated the relative lead mobilizing effects in the study by Wang, Ting, and Wu (1965), the first clinical study comparing DMSA and EDTA. Fourteen patients suffering from chronic occupational lead poisoning were chelated with i.v. $CaNa_2EDTA$ 1–2 g daily or i.v. DMSA 1–2 g on alternate days (14.3–28.6 mg/kg per day for each antidote). Compared to each patient's prechelation urine lead excretion the lead excretion increased 6.5 ± 6.2 (range 2.1–10.9)-fold after one 2 g i.v. $CaNa_2EDTA$ dose and 8.0 ± 2.9 (range 6.2–11.3)-fold after 1 g DMSA. The difference is not significant. The size of the patient group is small, however, these data are the only human data comparing equimolar doses of EDTA and DMSA both administered i.v. Bradberrry and Vale (2009b) compared the effects of DMSA chelation, 30 mg/kg/day with effects of i.v. $CaNa_2EDTA$ chelation, 75 mg/kg/day (molar ratio for DMSA: $CaNa_2EDTA$ 1.0:1.25) in lead poisoned patients (data from Bradberry, 2009 and Bradberry et al., 2009). The median prechelation blood lead levels did not differ significantly and the lead excretion over 4 days did not differ significantly between the two groups.

Jin et al. (2011) investigated the therapeutic efficiency of DMSA combined with calcium and ascorbic acid for treatment of mild lead poisoning in 72 preschool children aged 48–72 months. The children were randomly assigned to two groups: 40 subjects received combined treatment with 10 mg/kg per day DMSA every second day, and 1250 mg calcium carbonate and 200 mg ascorbic acid every day for four weeks; 32 subjects were assigned into a nutritional intervention group, and given 1250 mg calcium carbonate and 200 mg ascorbic acid every day for 4 weeks. The reduction in b-Pb levels during chelation in the combined treatment group was significantly larger than the reduction in the nutritional intervention group. The fraction of children with b-Pb levels below 0.1 mg/L at the end of therapy and at 8 weeks later was significantly higher in the combined treatment group than in the nutritional intervention group. Since both groups received 1250 mg calcium carbonate and 200 mg ascorbic only the effect of DMSA compared to nutritional intervention can be evaluated in this study.

Rehani and Wissman (2011) described an unusual lead poisoning from a gunshot wound in a 30-year-old male who presented with right knee pain due to intrarticular invasion of bullet fragments from a gunshot several years ago. He had microcytic anemia and high b-Pb levels. He was chelated with DMSA and surgical removal of bullet fragments.

Carrier et al. (2012) described a 21-year-old man presenting with colicky abdominal pain. Abdominal radiograph showed several intracolonic metal bodies. The diagnosis of lead poisoning was confirmed from elevated serum levels of lead and zinc protoporphyrin. The patient reported to chew fishing lead sinker and sometimes might swallow them during preparation of a fishing rod. Colonic emptying by polyethylene glycol was combined with chelation therapy with 20 mg/kg DMSA per 8 h and 75 mg/kg EDTA per day until the blood lead level was below 1 mg/L followed by 20 mg/kg DMSA per 12 h alone until the blood lead levels was below 400 μg/L. Total colonoscopy was performed to remove residues of lead. The clinical development was very satisfactory.

Wu, Deng, Lin, and Tsai (2013) described a case of cutaneous lead poisoning. A 75-year-old man presented with nausea, vomiting, constipation, headache, dizziness, anorexia, weight loss, weakness, and anemia after 3-month treatment of a chronic leg ulcer with a herbal patch which was found to contain 517 mg lead per gram. His blood lead level was 2260 μg/L. Chelation with EDTA and DMSA was followed by clinical recovery.

Breeher, Gerr, and Fuortes (2013) described a case of adult lead poisoning following use of Ayurvedic herbal medication. These medications may be intentionally combined with metals, for example, lead, since users believe that the toxic properties of the metals are reduced or eliminated during preparation and processing. A 69 year old Caucasian male with a prior history of stroke presented with constipation, anorexia, weight loss, depression, fatigue and generalized weakness. The patient was previously diagnosed at another hospital to have a severe anemia for which no etiology was found. The b-Pb level was 940 μg/L. The Ayurvedic "Bhasma" medication was found to contain 19.4 g/kg lead and 1.43 g/kg arsenic. The patient was chelated with 5 mg/kg BAL i.m. each 4 h for 3 days, and with 1500 mg/m^2 per day $CaNa_2EDTA$ i.v. for 5 days. The patient was discharged from the hospital after 6 days with b-Pb 255 μg/L. The patient was instructed to take 10 mg/kg × 3 oral DMSA daily for 5 days, then 10 mg/kg × 2 daily for 14 days. His symptoms improved during and after chelation and he could discontinue antidepressant medication.

Petracca, Scafa, Boeri, Flachi, and Candura (2013) described four male Italian patients who had worked in Chinese battery recycling plants for 7–13 months. They suffered from recurrent abdominal pain and on return to Italy, three had normocytic, normochromic anaemia. They had high blood and urine lead levels. Chelation with EDTA increased the urinary lead excretion and improved the clinical picture.

Yeoh et al. (2014) performed a metaanalysis of studies of effectiveness of household interventions in preventing or reducing lead exposure as measured by reductions in blood lead levels and/or improvements in cognitive development. Studies were identified through various electronic databases. Fourteen studies involving 2656 children were selected as randomized and quasirandomized controlled trials of household educational or environmental interventions to prevent lead exposure in children where at least one standardized outcome measure was reported. All studies reported blood lead level outcomes and none reported on cognitive or neurobehavioral outcomes. The studies were subgrouped according to intervention types and a metaanalysis of data for subgroups was performed where appropriate. Educational interventions did not reduce blood lead levels. Analysis of the dust control subgroup presented no evidence of effectiveness. Soil removal and replacement and combination intervention studies could not be metaanalyzed due to major differences between studies.

Greig et al. (2014) described investigations by Medecins Sans Frontieres (MSF) of reports of high mortality in young children in Zamfara State, Nigeria. The cause was identified to be widespread acute severe lead poisoning. Blood lead levels were analyzed to identify thresholds and risk factors for encephalopathy in children aged $\leq$ 5 years with recorded neurological status and with b-Pb $\geq$ 450 μg/L before chelation. Increasing b-Pb and age 1–3 years were strongly associated with neurological signs.

Thurtle et al. (2014) described a medical treatment program including oral chelation with DMSA in a cohort of 1,156 children $\leq$ 5 years of age with severe lead poisoning with b-Pb $\geq$ 450 μg/L who received between one and 15 chelation courses of 19 or 28 days duration. The effect of chelation was estimated from end-course b-pb as a percentage of precourse b-Pb. No clinically severe adverse drug effects were observed, and no laboratory findings required discontinuation of treatment. The results demonstrate that oral DMSA chelation was effective for treatment of severe childhood lead poisoning in a resource-limited setting.

A randomized trial of the efficacy of oral DMSA chelation treatment of children with moderately elevated b-Pb supported by the US NIEHS and NIH was initiated with enrollment of 780 children between 1994 and 1996 to be allocated to placebo or DMSA chelation, 77% were black, 5% were hispanic. The baseline data on this study have been published (Rogan, Bornschein, & Chisholm, 1998). The results were published by the TLC trial group (2000). The trial consisted of up to 3 26-day DMSA chelation courses in 12–33 month old children with b-Pb levels of 200-440 μg/L (1.0–2.1 μM) living in deteriorating inner city housing. Results showed that placebo-treated children had a gradual decrease in b-Pb levels. DMSA treated children had a sharp fall in b-Pb level, followed by rebound. The mean b-Pb level of DMSA chelated children during 6 months after initiation of the trial was 45 μg/L (0.22 μM) lower than that of placebo-treated children. DMSA-treated children had more scalp rashes and an unanticipated excess of trauma, but few other side effects. Further results on the neuropsychological development of this cohort were published by Rogan et al. (2001) who tested cognitive, motor, behavioral, and neuropsychological function in the cohort. At 36 months of follow-up, the mean IQ score of DMSA chelated children was 1 point lower than that of placebo exposed controls, and the behavior of DMSA chelated children was slightly worse by parent rating. However, DMSA chelated children scored slightly better on the Developmental neuropsychological Assessment test battery designed to measure neuropsychological deficits believed to interfere with learning. All differences were small and statistically nonsignificant. The results of this large epidemiological trial indicate that chelation therapy is not indicated for children with low blood lead levels.

Organic lead poisoning used to be a problem due to gasoline sniffing, this problem has transformed into one of organic solvent induced brain damage due to the discontinuation of the use of organolead gasoline additives. Tenenbaum (1997) summarized this addiction to be worldwide but especially frequent in northern Canada, southwestern USA and the Australian Outback, with high prevalence in certain ethnic groups such as American and Canadian Indians living in isolated areas (Fortenberry, 1985). Organolead poisoining is today a limited problem except in very few developing countries. Chronic, heavy "sniffing" of gasoline results in cerebellar and corticospinal symptoms and signs, dementia, behavioral alterations, and organic psychosis, mainly due to gasoline hydrocarbons. Tetraethyl lead is responsible for altered mental status and persistent psychosis. There is no effective chelation treatment (with, eg, BAL, EDTA, DMSA, DPA) of alkyllead poisoning.

4.14.3 Summary and Conclusions

The traditionally used chelators in acute and chronic lead poisoning have been BAL DPA and CaEDTA. The advent of DMSA several decades ago have led to extensive reduction in the use of BAL and DPA and to some degree CaEDTA. Due to BAL's high toxicity and unpleasant side effects, the need for painful parenteral administration, and the increased brain levels of several toxic metals after BAL chelation seen in the light of the very high efficiency and low toxicity of DMSA, BAL should not any longer be used as a chelation agent for lead.

Comparison of intervention studies of childhood low-level lead exposure cohorts, unchelated or chelated (Markowitz et al., 1993a,b; Besunder et al., 1995; Besunder, Super, & Anderson, 1997) indicate that lead abatement alone marginally reduces b-Pb and biochemical indicators of lead toxicity. Chelation by EDTA, BAL + EDTA, DMSA, or EDTA + DMSA results in significantly reduced b-Pb. Conclusively, DMSA appears to be the least toxic and best tolerated chelating agent, as well as having the option of oral or i.v. administration. This chelator is now the first choice in low to moderate lead poisoning. The frequency of side effects is high in groups chelated by DPA. Because of its toxicity and its tendency to increase lead absorption from the gastrointestinal tract, DPA should not be used for lead chelation.

Acute lead encephalopathy previously occurred frequently, most often due to extensive oral intake of lead-based paint chips in infants, and led to very high mortality and chronic morbidity. This poisoning which is fortunately rare today, requires immediate chelation treatment. Different chelation schedules have been advocated in clinical toxicology texts (Henretig, 1998; Klaassen, 2006), for example, intravenous CaEDTA infusion combined with intravenous administration of BAL. This combined EDTA and BAL treatment was advocated and previously extensively used based on Chisholm (1968) finding that this combined chelation lowered b-Pb more effectively than either agent alone. The reason for the recommendation of combined BAL-EDTA chelation is that the soft tissue mobilizing effect of BAL should counteract the increasing effect of EDTA on brain lead levels, however, animal experimental or clinical data supporting this hypothesis does not exist. In fact, the arguments for combined EDTA-BAL chelation have been invalid for decades, since DMSA, p.o. and/or i.v., which does not increase brain lead, is available as an alternative with much lower toxicity. Unfortunately, animal studies comparing the effect of DMSA chelation with combined BAL-EDTA chelation in severe experimental lead intoxication are, to the author's knowledge, not available. Such studies would show whether DMSA is the superior antidote in all kinds of lead intoxication.

4.15 MANGANESE

Manganese (Mn, atomic number 25 in group 7 of the periodic table of the elements, atomic weight 54, density 7.43 g/cm^3) is the 12th most abundant element in the earth's crust. Mn does not occur as a free element. It is present in many minerals, often with iron. Mn has one stable isotope, ^{55}Mn, the moste stable radioactive isotopes are ^{53}Mn ($t_{1/2}$ 3.7 million years, ^{52}Mn ($t_{1/2}$ 5.591 days) and ^{54}Mn ($t_{1/2}$ 312.3 days). Another 14 isotopes have very short half-lives. Oxidation states from −3 to +7 are known, the most common are +2, +3, +4, +6, +7. The +7 (permanganate state) is strongly oxidizing as are compounds with oxidation states +6, +5 and +4 which can disproportionate. The most stable oxidation state is +2. Manganese is mainly produced from pyrolusite, MnO_2. The largest producer is South Africa, possessing about 80% of known resources. The main uses of Mn are in alloys, mainly with iron. Ferromanganese (30–80% Mn) is produced by reducing mixed ores of iron and manganese in a blast furnace or in an electric arc furnace. Other important uses of manganese are in aluminum alloys with 0.8–1.5% Mn improving corrosion resistance and as manganese phosphating to prevent rust and corrosion on steel, as the gasoline octane booster and antiknocking agent methylcyclopentadienyl manganese tricarbonyl, as pigment in paint and as catalyst in organic industry. MnO_2 is used as the cathode in alkaline and zinc–carbon batteries.

Mn is an essential trace mineral for all living organisms as cofactors for many enzymes with diverse functions, particularly in detoxification of superoxide radicals from oxygen metabolism. Overexposures, mainly by inhalation in occupational settings can cause neurological damage (manganism) developing to dementia. The mechanism is not known but seems to involve the nigrostriatal functioning, mainly affecting striatum and globus pallidus with disturbed chatechol metabolism and oxidative stress generation. The cortex may also be affected. Manganism is sometimes irreversible, and sometimes resembles Parkinson's disease. However, manganism does not induce the characteristic total symptom picture of Parkinson's disease including i.a. loss of smell (Lu, Huang, Chu, & Calne, 1994), and their response to antiparkinson drugs such as L-dopa is only partial. High pulmonary burden of MnO or MnO_2 in ferromanganese welders may cause chemical pneumonitis and impaired resistance to lung infections. Mn is not considered carcinogenic.

Historically, manganese was named for it occurence in black minerals, for example, pyrolusite in the region Magnesia in Greece which also named the iron ore magnetite and the essential element magnesium. Many manganese oxides are abundant in nature and have been used as pigments since prehistoric times. The 30,000–24,000 years old cave paintings in Gargas, Haute-Garonne were made with manganese pigments (Chalmin et al., 2006). Manganese was used in glass making in Egypt and this use was continued by Roman glassmakers (Sayre & Smith, 1961) and through Venetian 14th-century glass (Mccray, 1998) until modern times.

4.15.1 Animal Experimental Chelation Studies

Animal studies on antidotal and decorporating effects of chelators in manganese poisoning are scarce. Eybl, Sykora, and Mertl (1969) compared effects of various polyaminopolycarboxylic acids on the toxicokinetics of $MnCl_2$ in the rat after injection of both chelator and Mn. The chelators all reduced the hepatic and renal Mn deposition and increased the urinary Mn excretion. EDTA and DTPA were effective, DTPA more than EDTA.

Tandon, Chandra, Singh, Husain, and Seth (1975) investigated structurally different chelating agents for ability to mobilize Mn from liver and testis of rats given i.p. injection of manganese sulfate for 25 days. Most chelators significantly reduced Mn levels, most efficient were NTA, CDTA, DTPA, DDTA, and ascorbic acid.

Tandon (1978) investigated the Mn mobilizing effects of CDTA and p-aminosalicylic acid (PAS) individually and in combination in rabbits given MnO_2. Both increased fecal excretion more than urinary excretion. CDTA enhanced both urinary and fecal Mn excretion while PAS only enhanced fecal elimination. Combined chelation was not more effective than the individual compounds.

Khandelwal, Kachru, and Tandon (1980) investigated effects of 2 polyamino-polycarboxylic acids HEDTA and DTPA and 2 thiol containing chelators DDC and DMSA on decorporation of i.p. injected Mn into rabbits to study the efficacy of N, O and S containing chelators for Mn. HEDTA and DTPA effectively enhanced urinary and fecal Mn excretion, while DDC and DMSA were ineffective indicating greater affinity of Mn with chelators having N and O, than with those having S as electron donors.

Tandon and Khandewal (1982a) studied effects of selected polyaminocarboxylic acids and thiol containing chelators on tissue distribution and urinary and fecal excretion of ^{54}Mn in rats. HEDTA, CDTA, DTPA and TTHA very efficiently reduced tissue levels and enhanced excretion of ^{54}Mn. The thiol containing chelators DPA, NAPA and DMSA did not influence tissue distribution and excretion of ^{54}Mn again suggesting low affinity of SH groups for Mn.

In a parallel study, Tandon and Khandewal (1982b) studied effects of structurally different metal chelating agents on mortality at much higher Mn doses in mice. Polyaminocarboxylic acids with oxygen and nitrogen as ligands more effectively than sulfhydryl chelating agents prevented mortality after a lethal manganese chloride dose.

Wieczorek and Oberdörster (1989) gave seven daily i.p. injections of CDTA or DTPA to rats starting immediately after inhalation exposure to a $MnCl_2$ aerosol for 1 h. Both chelators enhanced the urinary excretion of Mn extensively while the excretion was almost nil in the control group and in a group exposed to DMPS. Postponing the chelation treatment for 7 days resulted in even more effective decorporation of Mn by CDTA or DTPA.

Zheng et al. (2009) studied effects of PAS on Mn levels in body fluids and tissues in rats after daily i.p. injections of 6 mg Mn/kg as $MnCl_2$, 5 days/week for 4 weeks, which increased Mn levels in brain and soft tissues, plasma, red blood cells, and cerebrospinal fluid. Daily s.c. injection of 200 mg/kg PAS for 2, 3, or 6 weeks after Mn exposure reduced Mn levels in liver, spleen, heart, and pancreas by 25–33%. After 6 weeks, Mn levels in frontal cortex, hippocampus, thalamus, striatum, and choroid plexus were reduced by 16–29%. Three weeks of 100 mg/kg PAS injection had no effect.

4.15.2 Clinical Chelation Studies

In clinical studies chelation by EDTA in patients with chronic Mn poisoning, CaEDTA efficiently increased urinary Mn excretion. DMSA was without effect. Neither EDTA nor DMSA had alleviating effects on clinical symptoms (Whitlock, Amuso, & Bittenbender, 1966; Cook, Fahn, & Brait, 1974; Smyth, Ruhf, Whitman, & Dugan, 1973).

Jiang et al. (2006) described a female patient exposed to airborne Mn for 21 years. She had severe neuropathy with hand tremor, hypermyotonia, palpitations, and lower limb myalgia. She received 15 courses with the FDA-approved anti-tuberculosis drug PAS, 6 g i.v. per day for 4 days, and 3 days rest before the next course. Her symptoms were significantly alleviated, and her handwriting improved. At follow-up in 2004, 17 years after the treatment, she had normal clinical and neurologic status and a normal brain magnetic resonance imaging. This case indicates that PAS is a potentially effective drug for treatment of manganism.

4.15.3 Conclusion

Based on the limited information available, chelating agents with O- and N-ligands seem to be effective in acute Mn poisoning. A chelation schedule in chronic manganese poisoning (manganism) is not established, but DTPA, EDTA, and PAS are available as potential chelators. PAS appears to be the most promising agent, although clinical experience is limited, and animal experiments indicate that i.v. administration of relatively high doses are required in acute cases. The Mn-PAS chelate is supposed to be dialyzable. PAS may also exert an antiinflammatory action, as its molecular congeners, aspirin and salazopyrin.

4.16 MERCURY

Mercury (Hg from greek *hydrargyros* ὑδράργυροζ, or quicksilver, atomic number 80 in group 12 of the periodic table of the elements, atomic weight 200.6, density, 13.6 g/cm^3, oxidation states, +1, +2) is named after the Roman god Mercury who also named the planet Mercury. Hg is the only metal liquid at room temperature. Hg(0) is highly volatile and to some degree soluble in water and lipids, and many inorganic and organic Hg salts have high vapor pressure. In presence of oxygen, Hg(0) is rapidly oxidized. Most mercury salts and also $MeHg^+$ and $EthylHg^+$ are water soluble, the organic Hg compounds also in lipids. Organic Hg compounds have high affinity for HS-groups in proteins.

Historically, Hg had medicinal uses in China and Tibet believing it to give good health, heal fractures, and prolong life. Mercury has been found in Egyptian and Mexican tombs dating from 1500 BC. In ancient Egypt, Greece, and Rome Hg was used in ointments and cosmetics.

Mercury was produced in Almaden (Spain), Monte Amiata (Italy), and Idria (Slovenia) starting 500 years BC (Eisler, 2006).

Mercury occurs at very low levels in the Earth's crust, averaging only 0.08 ppm (Ehrlich & Newman, 2008). However, mercury ores can be very concentrated, up to 2.5% Hg. Geologically, Hg occurs as the native metal or as cinnabar (HgS, the most common ore), corderoite ($Hg_3S_2Cl_2$), livingstonite ($HgSb_4S_8$) and other ores (Rytuba, 2003). Mercury is produced from cinnabar by heating in a current of air and condensing Hg(0) vapor: $HgS + O_2 \rightarrow Hg + SO_2$.

The world production has fallen extensively over the last decades and many mines have been closed. The world production in 2003 was less than 2000 tons (USGS, 2015). Mercury is released to the environment by combustion of fossil fuels, waste disposal and industrial activities, together amounting to more than 7000 tons per year during the 1970s, however, these emissions have decreased during recent decades except in Asia (Berlin, Rudolfs, Zalups, & Fowler, 2014). Degassing from oceans and the Earth's crust is the largest contribution to environmental mercury cycling, estimated at 30,000–150,000 tons per year (Korringa & Hagel, 1974). The major anthropogenic contributions to global atmospheric Hg emissions are artisanal gold mining, burning of coal, production of nonferrous metals and cement production (Bjerregaard, Andersen, & Andersen, 2014).

Mercury is used in various instruments (thermometers, manometers, barometers) and fluorescent lamps, mercury switches and relays, float valves and many other devices. Hg toxicity and environmental spread have resulted in out phasing of many uses of Hg in favor of alternatives using newer electronic technologies. Mercury is still used in amalgam for dental restoration, in scientific research and in fluorescent lamps. The organic mercury compound thiomersal (Ethyl(2-mercaptobenzoato-(2−)-O,S) mercurate(1−) sodium) is used as preservative in vaccines, skin test antigens, antivenins, immunoglobulin preparations, ophthalmic and nasal products, mascara, and tattoo inks.

Due to the wide use of elementary mercury in industrial and scientific operations and dentistry, exposure to Hg vapor has been an important occupational health problem. Also, uses of inorganic Hg salts in the chemical industry and of organic mercury compounds in paper industry and in seed dressing has led to human exposures and extensive environmental pollution.

Occupational mercury exposure is dominated by exposure to mercury vapor, for example, in gold and mercury mining, chloralkali factories, production of instruments and fluorescent lamps and in physics and medical laboratories. Spillage of elemental Hg or (mainly organic) mercury compounds is an important exposure source. Gold miners have been extensively exposed to Hg vapor from heating mercury-gold amalgams resulting in neurological and renal effects (Aitio et al., 2014).

The mercury release from ingested metallic mercury is very low and without toxicological importance. The skin uptake of mercury vapor is also low, approximately 1% of the uptake from inhalation. Mercury vapor is lipophilic and is efficiently absorbed (about 80%) through the alveolar membrane. Erythrocytes or hemoglobin transport Hg(0) in blood, and during exposure to Hg vapor, some Hg(0) is oxidized to Hg^{2+} and excreted in the urine. Due to its lipophilicity a fraction of Hg(0) in blood is deposited in the brain and other organs with subsequent oxidation to Hg^{2+}. Since Hg^{2+} does not pass cell membranes easily, this mechanism captures Hg in the central nervous system. Mercury vapor also penetrates the placental barrier and accumulate as Hg^{2+} in the fetus when the mother is exposed to mercury vapor. At high acute exposure, mercury vapors induce extensive alveolar necrosis, often rapidly fatal. The brain is the critical organ during Hg vapor exposure.

Inorganic mercury salts are poorly absorbed in the intestinal tract, about 10% in the mouse (Nielsen & Andersen, 1989) and deposited mainly in the kidney, which is a target organ for Hg^{2+}.

Absorbed mercury vapor and salts are mainly excreted in urine and feces. Small amounts of mercury vapor are exhaled before oxidation has taken place and due to reduction of Hg^{++} in tissues. The majority of Hg in humans is excreted with a halftime of about 60 days while Hg accumulated in the brain has a half-time of several years. (Hursh, Cherian, Clarkson, Vostal, & Mallie, 1976; Kosta, Vyrne, & Zelenko, 1975; Rossi, Clemente, & Santaroni, 1976).

The mercury retention in different organs varies extensively with half-times from few days to months. The brain, kidneys, and testicles have the longest retention times and accumulate mercury during prolonged exposure and dominate organ distribution at steady state (Berlin et al., 2014).

Organic Hg compounds as, for example, CH_3Hg^+ are highly lipophilic and completely absorbed after oral exposure (Nielsen and Andersen, 1991b) and deposited in the brain or in the fetus after passing the placenta barrier making neurotoxicity and fetotoxicity important toxic effects of these compounds.

Treatment of mercury poisonings is complicated due to the large differences in the toxicokinetics and target organs of inorganic salts, Hg(0) vapor, and organic mercury compounds. Human poisonings by various mercury compounds have been treated by chelation with BAL, DPA, NAPA, DMSA, or DMPS. The traditional treatment was i.m. BAL followed by oral DPA. Since BAL increases the brain deposition of CH_3Hg^+ (Berlin & Ullberg, 1963) this chelator is contraindicated in organic mercury poisoning.

As described later, DMSA and DMPS are the antidotes of choice in various types of Hg poisoning, due to their low toxicity and high efficacy. Even though CH_3Hg^+ does not form chelates, bonds formed between CH_3Hg^+ and deprotonated thio groups in various thio compounds have a high degree of covalent character. Thus, chelators with HS-groups influence the toxicokinetics of CH_3Hg^+ by forming stable complexes.

4.16.1 Experimental Animal Studies

Several experimental animal studies investigated chelating antidotes against acute poisoning by inorganic or organic mercury compounds. DMSA is an efficient antidote and Hg mobilizing agent in acute systemic $HgCl_2$ or CH_3HgCl poisonings, increasing the urinary excretion of Hg and reducing Hg levels in various organs (Friedheim & Corvi, 1975; Magos, 1976). In the study by Magos (1976) on kinetics of $MeHg^+$ injected in mice chelation by DMSA increased the urinary Hg excretion more than 10 times and administration of DMSA in drinking water reduced whole-body, kidney, liver and brain levels of injected $MeHg^+$ in mice by 50–70%.

Gabard (1976) tested 15 chelating agents including DTPA, BAL, NAPA, and DPA for inorganic Hg mobilizing potential. DMPS was superior in enhancing the urinary Hg excretion and lowering Hg levels in all organs.

In the studies of Aaseth and Friedheim (1978) 8 days oral administration of DMSA after injection of CH_3Hg^+ reduced the brain Hg level by 75%, while DPA, NAPA, and DMPS were less effective.

Jones et al. (1980) compared the antidotal efficacy of BAL, DPA, NAPA DMSA and DMPS injected 20 min after injection of a $HgCl_2$ dose > LD_{98} and found BAL to be the least effective chelator. In a subsequent study, Basinger et al. (1981b) used the same $HgCl_2$ dose and administration route and found that DMPS, DPA and NAPA more efficiently than BAL and DMSA reduced mortality.

Kostyniak (1983) dosed dogs with 2.5 mg Hg/kg of ^{203}Hg labeled CH_3Hg^+ followed by continuous i.v. DMSA infusion resulting in similar DMSA plasma levels as those observed during DMSA chelation hemodialysis, to study effects on CH_3Hg^+ kinetics. DMSA infusion resulted in a shift in ^{203}Hg binding in blood from the erythrocytes to plasma consistent with association of DMSA with the plasma fraction, and increase in urinary clearance of ^{203}Hg. In four dogs 5-h DMSA infusion removed an average of 6.5 μg of Hg via urine, compared to 0.007 μg in saline-infused dogs. DMSA chelation hemodialysis removed an additional 5 μg Hg being significantly more effective than infusion. ^{203}Hg tissue concentration after DMSA infusion was 6.5-fold decreased in liver and threefold decreased in kidneys compared to controls.

In several studies DMSA and DMPS effectively enhanced Hg excretion estimated from increased urinary Hg excretion or reduced kidney levels or body burden of Hg after injection of mercury salts in mice or rats, DMPS being more efficient than DMSA (Planas-Boehne, 1981; Aaseth, 1983; Eybl et al., 1985). Repeated injections of either of these chelators eventually mobilized the same amounts of Hg from kidneys (Buchet & Lauwerys, 1989).

Most studies of effects of chelating agents on inorganic mercury toxicity used parenteral administration of both of Hg and chelators. In relation to acute human Hg poisoning two studies are of special interest by using relevant exposure routes: Buchet and Lauwerys (1989) reported that DMSA enhanced the urinary Hg excretion in rats after pulmonary exposure to different levels of Hg vapor and mobilized Hg accumulated in kidneys and to a lesser extent in liver. DMSA could, however, not mobilize Hg accumulated in the brain after Hg vapor exposure.

Oral administration of $^{203}HgCl_2$ to mice induced dose-related mortality in the study by Nielsen and Andersen (1991). Parenteral or oral administration of DMSA or DMPS 15 min after $HgCl_2$ reduced mortality and intestinal stasis induced by $HgCl_2$ more efficiently than did BAL and NAPA. Oral administration of DMSA or DMPS also reduced the whole body retention and the brain deposition of orally administered Hg more efficiently than after parenteral administration.

Sc injection of DMSA immediately after oral administration of a teratogenic CH_3Hg^+ dose to mice on day 10 of gestation reduced the frequency of cleft palate, skeletal anomalies and embryo lethality in a dose-dependent manner (Sanchez, Gomez, Llobet, & Domingo, 1993). A subsequent study compared effects of BAL and DMPS on the acute maternal toxicity and embryotoxicity of CH_3Hg^+ in mice. BAL did not protect against maternal and fetal mortality or structural malformations while DMPS reduced maternal and fetal toxicity and teratogenicity of CH_3Hg^+ in a dose-dependent manner (Gomez et al., 1994).

Gale, Smith, Jones, and Singh (1993) evaluated monoalkylesters of DMSA as mobilizing agents for mercury in Hg-loaded mice. Parenteral administration of several esters more effectively than DMSA and DMPS increased the urinary Hg excretion and reduced the whole-body retention, the monoisoamyl ester of DMSA (Mi-ADMS) being most effective. Also in rats, monoalkyl esters of DMSA more effectively than DMSA mobilized Hg (Kostial, Blanusa, Simonovic, Jones, & Singh, 1993). Also at protracted time after administration of Hg^{2+}.

Mi-ADMS more effectively than DMSA decreased whole-body and organ levels of Hg, except in the brain. Both chelators were equally effective in this organ (Kostial et al., 1994).

Bellés et al. (1996) studied effects of Mi-ADMS on CH_3Hg^+ induced maternal and developmental toxicity in mice. Mi-ADMS was injected sc at 0.25, 6, 24, and 48 h after oral administration of 25 mg/kg of CH_3Hg^+ on day 10 of gestation. Mi-ADMS was administered at 23.8, 47.6 and 95 mg/kg. CH_3Hg^+ administration increased the number of resorptions, decreased fetal weight, and increased the incidence of cleft palate, micrognathia, and skeletal variations. Mi-ADMS at 23.8, 47.6, and 95 mg/kg significantly reduced CH_3Hg^+ induced fetotoxicity compared to non chelated controls.

de la Torre, Belles, Llobet, Mayayo, and Domingo (1998) compared effects of parenterally administered BAL and DMSA on the nephrotoxicity of parenterally administered Hg in the rat. At the lowest dose applied BAL decreased the urinary Hg excretion. At the highest dose applied, BAL exacerbated proteinuria induced by Hg. DMSA offered a dose related increase in urinary Hg excretion and significantly decreased renal Hg levels.

Joshi et al. (2010) administered 1.5 mg/kg dimethylmercury per day orally to rats for 21 days followed by chelation for 5 days with 2 mmol/kg i.p. NAC combined with 2 mM/kg zinc p.o as $(CH_3COO)_2$ Zn H_2O and 0.5 mg/kg selenium p.o. as Na_2SeO_4. Dimethylmercury exposure increased serum bilirubin, γ-GT, cholesterol, triglycerides, urea, creatinine, uric acid levels and decreased albumin levels. These indicators of hepatic and renal damange were partially reversed by the combined NAC-Zn-Se treatment, which also reduced Hg levels in brain, liver and kidney and counteracted reduced acetylcholinesterase levels in fore brain, mid brain and hind brain induced by dimethylmercury exposure.

Clarke, Buchanan, Gupta, and Haley (2012) speculated that inorganic mercury toxicity occurs mainly at the intracellular level due to binding of Hg^{2+} to HS-groups in proteins and induction of oxidative stress, and therefore chelation treatment of Hg poisoning would potentially be efficacious by using a chelator with antioxidant properties able to cross the blood brain barrier and cell membranes, and forming nontoxic Hg chelates. They initially made a toxicity profile of the chelator, N,N′-bis(2-mercaptoethyl)isophthalamide (NBMI) including mutagenicity test, metabolic profiling, and pharmacokinetics. Further, the effect of sc injected NBMI on the toxicity, organ distribution and excretion of sc injected HgCl2 was studied in rats. NBMI chelation resulted in extensively increased survival time and reduced mortality after increasing doses of $HgCl_2$ and reduced Hg levels in liver and kidneys but increased Hg deposition in the brain. Both urinary and fecal Hg excretion was statistically nonsignificantly reduced by chelation with NBMI.

Iranmanesh et al. (2013b) investigated the antidotal effects of orally administered deferasirox and deferiprone in male rats after exposure to mercury vapor for 2 weeks. Chelation reduced symptoms of mercury toxicity. Analysis of mercury in heart, liver, kidneys, intestine, spleen, and testicles showed that combined chelation therapy enhanced mercury excretion besides decreasing toxicity symptoms.

Joshi, Mittal, Shukla, Srivastav, and Srivastav (2014) investigated the effects of NNAC, 0.6 mg /kg, i.p. for 5 days), dithiothreitol (DTT, 15.4mg/kg i.p. for five days), and selenium (Se, 0.5 mg/kg oral for 5 days) given alone or in combination on CH_3Hg^+ induced oxidative stress and biochemical alterations in rats orally exposed to 1.5mg/kg CH_3Hg^+ daily for 21 days. CH_3Hg^+ administration increased serum levels of alkaline phosphatases, transaminases, and lactate dehydrogenases as well as lipid peroxidation levels in liver, kidney, and brain with concomitant decreased GSH levels and decreased hepatic aniline hydroxylase and amidopyrine *N*-demethylase activities of CYP2E1. Histological alterations were also observed in kidney, liver, and brain. Chelation treatment induced recovery of methylmercury induced alterations, but combined treatments with DTT and Se or NAC and Se were more effective than treatments with single agents. All data including Hg levels in liver, kidneys and brain indicate that NAC + Se is superior to DTT +Se.

4.16.2 Clinical Studies

Several case and cohort studies on chelation treatment of Hg poisonings are published. Kanluen and Gottlieb (1991) described four men exposed to Hg vapor during smelting of dental amalgam in a private home to obtain silver. They were admitted to hospital with severe pulmonary incapacitation 24 h later. They received chelation treatment with BAL, and all four died from severe pulmonary damage 9–23 days after the exposure.

Rowens, Guerrero-Betancourt, Gottlieb, Boyes, and Eichenhorn (1991) described a similar case where 4 members of a family died from respiratory failure after an attempt to extract silver from dental amalgam. They received BAL chelation treatment.

Florentine and Sanfilippo (1991) described three siblings poisoned by inhalation of elemental mercury after a brother had spilled 15–30 mL elemental mercury in the house. A 4-year-old girl was admitted with fever, fatigue, increasing irritability, malaise, headache, insomnia, anorexia, and ataxia but discharged after 2 days with a diagnosis of acute cerebellar ataxia. Her condition worsened over the following 18 days and she was hospitalized again. Her 11-year-old sister was hospitalized due to fatigue, lower back pain, weakness and ataxia. The older girl's b-Hg level was 55 µg/L. In both children Hg poisoning was confirmed from 24 h urine Hg screening. The two girls had two courses of BAL chelation therapy. Since symptoms persisted in all three children, they received five 10-day NAPA chelation therapy courses. The youngest girl had a third BAL chelation course. All three children continued to receive NAPA chelation therapy until the results of repeated urine mercury concentration determinations were normal.

An oral provocation dose of DMSA or DMPS has been used as a diagnostic tool to estimate Hg vapor exposure and body stores of Hg. Roels, Boeckx, Ceulemans, and Lauwerys (1991) studied three groups of workers, one group presently exposed to high Hg vapor levels, another group with reduced Hg exposure and a group removed from Hg exposure. One oral dose of 2 g DMSA increased the average 24 h urinary Hg excretion to around 20 μg Hg in workers removed from exposure and to 600 μg in workers presently exposed to high Hg vapor levels. The excretion was 4 μg in an unexposed control group. The ratios between the average 24 h u-Hg excretions after and before DMSA administration varied between 2.5 and 4, with the highest ratios in those workers who had the highest and most recent Hg vapor exposure. This study indicates that DMSA-induced urinary Hg excretion could be an indicator of renal Hg deposits in individuals without recent Hg exposure. The results suggest that DMSA mobilizes Hg in more shallow depots and that the extent of mobilization could indicate the intensity of recent exposure.

Bluhm et al. (1992) described a group of 53 workers exposed to Hg vapor during repair work in a chloralkali factory. Flame cutting of mercury pipes resulted in spreading of boiling Hg over the workers and high Hg vapor levels. Several workers became ill. Elevated urinary Hg levels several days after the exposure indicated Hg poisoning. Totally 26 workers were hospitalized 19 days or later after the incidence. A 2 week DMSA or NAPA chelation treatment was started at 26 days after the exposure. A group of 12 patients with elevated u-Hg levels 73 days after the exposure received a 4 days chelation treatment with DMSA or NAPA. DMSA chelation increased the u-Hg excretion 3.5–5-fold while the excretion was increased only 2–2.5-fold by chelation with NAPA.

Atta, Faintuch, do Nascimento, R, and Ados (1992) described a gold prospector who presented with headache, fever, and tachypnea. Chelation with BAL and DPA and intensive supportive care were instituted. The patient died from acute respiratory distress.

Aposhian et al. (1992) used the DMPS mobilization test to study Hg exposure and systemic Hg load in populations without occupational Hg exposure. In a group of volunteers a statistically significant correlation was observed between the "amalgam score" (number and size of dental amalgam fillings) and the DMPS-provoked urinary excretion of Hg.

In similar studies Zander, Ewers, Frier, and Brockhaus (1992) and Herrmann and Schweinsberg (1993) found 6–7-fold and 9-fold increases in the average urinary Hg excretion in DMPS mobilization tests. In both studies the urinary Hg excretion was larger in individuals with amalgam fillings than in those without amalgam fillings, both before and after DMPS provocation. Herrmann and Schweinsberg (1993) observed a significant correlation between the "amalgam filling index" and Hg excretion.

Houeto, Sandouk, Baud, and Levillain (1994) described two jewelers who inhaled Hg vapors during melting a Hg containing block of gold. They were admitted to hospital on the next day, short of breath with fatigue, nausea, and pain at various sites and normal renal function. They received chelation treatment first with i.m. BAL for 5 days, then with oral DMSA chelation for another 5 days. Urine and blood Hg levels rapidly fell from high initial values. The urinary Hg elimination increased after change from BAL to DMSA treatment. Blood Hg remained at the same levels.

Singer, Mofenson, Carracio, and Ilasi (1994) described a patient who ingested a stool fixative containing 675 mg $HgCl_2$. The patient was given extensive hydration and rapidly chelated with BAL. The patient did not show systemic signs of mercury poisoning.

Toet, van Dijk, Savelkoul, and Meulenbelt (1994) described a 38-year-old man who in a suicide attempt drank 100 mL of a $HgCl_2$ solution of unknown concentration. He presented with consistent vomiting and bloody diarrhea. He was treated with gastric lavage and activated charcoal and received i.m. BAL chelation. He rapidly deteriorated and developed renal failure. After about 10 h hemodialysis together with plasma expander due to hypovolumic chock and i.v. DMPS chelation was initiated. Despite very high blood Hg levels (>2 mg/L), his kidney function recovered after 10 days. DMPS chelation was reduced from 1.5 to 0.75 g/day and continued for 4 weeks, followed by oral DMSA chelation, 0.9 g/day for another 3 weeks. The patient recovered completely.

Sallsten, Barregard, and Schutz (1994) administered a single oral dose of 0.3 g DMPS to groups of industrial workers and dentists exposed to mercury vapor, a control group with amalgam fillings, and a control group without amalgam fillings. DMPS significantly increased the urinary mercury output in all groups. The increased Hg excretion was larger than in the study by Roels et al. (1991), 3–12 X increase compared to 2.5–4 X increase despite a much lower cherlator dose (0.3 g DMPS vs 2 g DMSA). The Hg excretions during 6 and 24 h after DMPS administration correlated strongly, accordingly a long period of urine collection period is not necessary.

Gonzales-Ramirez et al. (1995) used the DMPS mobilization test to investigate Hg exposure in dentists and dental technicians. The urinary Hg excretion after DMPS provocation was extensively higher than in non-Hg-exposed controls, highest in dentists. The post-DMPS and pre-DMPS Hg excretions correlated strongly. The amount of mercury mobilized by DMPS and scores in neurobehavioral tests showed a significant inverse relationship. This indicates a potential value of the test in diagnosis of adverse Hg exposure.

Koriakov and Gol'dfarb (1995) described symptoms and treatment of 56 patients suffering from Hg poisoning due to use of Hg_2Cl_2-containing creams. The patients had gastrointestinal, hepatic, renal, or dermal disorders. The highest blood Hg level recorded was 800 μg/L. The patients were chelated with DMPS, the most serious poisoning cases were treated with hemoperfusion.

Torres-Alanis, Garza-Ocanas, and Pineyro-Lopez (1995) administered a single oral dose of 300 mg DMPS intended as a Hg mobilization test to 7 men 3 years after long-term mercury vapor exposure had ended. The average 24 h urinary Hg excretion was increased by a factor of 7.6. Further, 10 mercury-exposed workers with high basal urinary Hg levels (50 μg Hg/g creatinin or higher) were given 300 mg DMPS as chelation treatment for 5 days. This increased the urinary Hg excretion significantly during the 5 days of DMPS chelation.

Pfab, Müchter, Roider, and Zilker (1996) described a 44-year-old man who drank a solution of about 5 g of thiomersal (sodium 2-(ethylmercurio)-thiobezoic acid) for suicidal purpose. He presented at the hospital with nausea and vomiting and hemorrhagic gastritis. He received gastric lavage followed by oral DMPS chelation as a solution via nasogastric tube. Acute renal failure developed rapidly and persisted till day 40. He was chelated with i.v. administrations of DMPS alternating with administration via the nasogastric tube. From day 17–29, alternating chelation courses with DMSA and DMPS were given. From day 33 till day 70, he was chelated with oral DMSA. During the early stages he developed fever and delirium and became comatose for a few days. Further he developed various cutaneous lesions and polyneuropathy. After 148 days, his neuropathy had completely resolved except for sensory defects in two toes.

In most uses of the DMPS mobilization test exposure to Hg vapor has been assessed. The test is however also a diagnostic tool for exposure to other Hg compounds. Maiorino et al. (1996) applied the test to 11 workers producing a skin lotion with Hg_2Cl_2, 8 individuals using the lotion and to 9 controls with no apparent exposure to Hg. In the exposed individuals the urinary Hg excretion over 6 h was increased between 1 and 2 orders of magnitude with average Hg excretions more than 5 mg in workers and 1.4 mg in users.

Eight of the workers participated in a second trial and also received DMPS chelation treatment 18 months after the first DMPS mobilization test. The average urinary Hg excretion during 6 h after DMPS administration was almost 7 mg in this mobilization test. All participants had normal kidney function. 3 oral DMPS chelation courses of 400 mg per day lasting 8, 7, and 6 days were administered to the workers. This mobilized more than 24 mg of Hg on average, including the mobilization test (Gonzales-Ramirez et al., 1998).

Hohage et al. (1997) described a case where a man injected 40 mL of metallic mercury intravenously in a suicide attempt. After 3 years apparently without symptoms of Hg poisoning he presented at hospital with sweating, intermittent pain, mild neuropsychiatric symptoms, and mild peripheral neuropathy. An X-ray showed a deposit of mercury in the right ventricle of the heart and multiple fine mercury granules in the entire pulmonary circulation. The patient received oral DMPS chelation for 6 months without any side effects. The chelation treatment reduced the blood Hg level only from about 100 to about 90 μg/L, however, the urinary Hg excretion increased from about 600 μg in 24 h before chelation to more than 2000 μg.

In another intravenous self-administration of elementary Hg described by Torres-Alanis, Garza-Ocanas, and Pineyro-Lopez (1997) the patient received long-term DMPS chelation. Despite very high urinary Hg excretion, the blood Hg level continued to be high. After 5 years Hg deposits were still present in the body. The patient had normal lung, liver and kidney function but suffered from lower extremity weakness and tremor.

Yoshida et al. (1997) described a young woman who ingested approximately 1 g of $HgCl_2$ in a suicide attempt. She developed acute renal failure and was treated with plasma exchange, hemodialysis, peritoneal dialysis and i.m. BAL chelation. She was anuric for 14 days. At follow up after 4 months renal function was normal.

Garza-Orcanas, Torres-Alanis, and Pineyro-Lopez (1997) described 12 patients who for 2–10 years had been using a facial cream containing Hg_2Cl_2. They had all high urinary Hg excretion. Chelation treatment with DMPS further increased the urinary Hg excretion.

Torres-Alanis, Garza-Ocanas, Bernal, and Pineyro-Lopez (2000) administered 3 mg/kg DMPS intravenously to 11 subjects concerned about mercury release from dental amalgam fillings. Urinary Hg excretion was significantly increased (3- to 107-fold) 1 h after DMPS administration, copper excretion was increased 2- to 119-fold, selenium 3- to 43.8-fold; zinc 1.6- to 44-fold, and magnesium 1.75- to 42.7-fold while manganese, chromium, cobalt, aluminum, and molybdenum excretions were unchanged.

Dargan et al. (2003) described a 40-year-old man presenting with hematemesis after suicidal ingestion of 1 g mercuric sulfate. His initial b-Hg level was 15.58 mg/L. DMPS chelation treatment was initiated 4.5 h after the ingestion. The patient rapidly deteriorated and required intubation and ventilation and developed acute renal failure, so continuous veno-venous hemodiafiltration for renal support were initiated and continued for 14 days. A total of 127 mg mercury (12.7% of the ingested dose) was recovered in the ultrafiltrate. The patient did not develop neurological features. He was discharged from hospital on day 50 and 5 months later he was asymptomatic, with normal creatinine clearance.

Eyer, Felgenhauer, Pfab, Drasch, and Zilker (2006) described a case of intravenous injection of metallic mercury in a 27-year-old man. Within 12 h after intravenous injection of 1.5 mL of elemental Hg he became febrile, tachycardic, and dyspneic. X-rays showed radiodense deposits scattered in the heart, lung, liver and kidney, and intestinal wall. The initial serum Hg level was 172 μg/L increasing to a peak level of 274 μg/L on day 6. A five day oral chelation treatment with DMPS mobilized 8 mg Hg, and a five day oral chelation treatment with DMSA mobilized 3 mg Hg.

Wang, Mahajan, Wills, and Leikin (2007) described a case of suicidal ingestion of mercuric chloride purchased through the internet. A 22-year-old male with a history of depression presented within 1 h after drinking a solution of 37 g mercuric chloride in water. Within minutes later he developed metallic taste and streaks of hematemesis but no other symptoms. Physical examination and abdominal X-ray were unremarkable except for tachycardia. His urine and blood mercury levels were 1.29 mg/g creatinine and 152 μg/L. Within 2 h of ingestion, i.m. chelation with 3 mg/kg BAL/4 h was started. On day 5 he developed a rash suspected to be due to allergy to peanut oil used as vehicle for BAL. The rash resolved after 5 days oral treatment with 60 mg prednisone/day. At this time he received DMSA chelation, 10 mg/kg X 3 daily for 5 days followed by 2 daily doses for 2 additional weeks. Ten days after ingestion, blood and 24-h urine and Hg levels were 26 μg/L and 160 μg/gram creatinine. Esophagogastroduodenoscopy showed mild fundal gastric erythema. His recovery was uneventful.

Vallant, Deutsch, Muntean, and Goessler (2008) described a case of probable consecutive i.v. administrations of metallic mercury. A 34-year-old man presented at the hospital with pleuritic chest pain. X-ray showed radio dense punctate material in both lung fields and around both elbows. The blood (140 μg/L) and urine (320 μg/L) Hg levels were highly elevated. The renal Hg excretion and blood Hg level were monitored during 5 months of DMPS chelation therapy, and the time-course of Hg in scalp hair was determined.

Van der Linde, Pillen, Gerrits, and Bouwes Bavinck (2008) described a case of Stevens-Johnson syndrome in an 11-year old boy with chronic exposure to mercury vapor. His 24-h u-Hg level was 37 μg/L. After cessation of exposure to Hg vapor he received oral DMPS chelation treatment. After 2 weeks of DMPS chelation the boy developed a disseminated cutaneous eruption of pruritic macules which over three days spread over his entire body with maculae becoming confluent. He developed crusts and erosions on the lips and blisters in the mouth. Stevens-Johnson syndrome was diagnosed and DMPS chelation was stopped. The symptoms gradually resolved.

Campbell, Leitch, Lewington, Dargan, and Baker (2009) described a 25-year-old man presenting with severe hypertension and nephrotic syndrome. He had worked at a fluorescent light factory with occupational exposure to mercury vapor. Minimal-change disease was diagnosed from a renal biopsy analyzed by light microscopy, immunofluorescence and electron microscopy. His blood and urinary mercury levels were elevated. He was chelated with DMPS and received steroids for minimal-change disease. Within 6 weeks his nephrotic syndrome had fully resolved. He remained well with normal blood pressure, renal function, and urine and blood mercury levels.

Ellis, Mullins, Galvin, Anthony, and Scalzo (2009) described a case involving a 19-year-old male. He presented with his father, who requested evaluation of a specimen surgically removed per request of the father from a "lump" under the skin of the son's lower abdomen. Gross inspection revealed that the specimen contained minor metallic droplets. The son denied injection of metallic mercury, despite a urine heavy-metal screen 10 weeks after removal of the "lump" revealed a high Hg level, 87.6 μg/g creatinine, falling to 11.9 g/g one month later. Analysis of the specimen by gross and microscopic examination, electron microscopy, and energy dispersive X-ray analysis of tissue small metal spherules demonstrated mercury to be present. Due to persistent elevated Hg levels potentially inducing mercury poisoning and the father's insistence, the young man received chelation therapy with DMSA. The urine Hg-creatinine ratio 2 days after initiation of chelation was 61.7 µg/g. The following month, 11 days after completion of chelation therapy, the urine Hg-creatinine ratio had decreased to 20.4 µg/g. Follow-up showed that the patient remained healthy without demonstrable signs of mercury poisoning.

Corsello, Fulgenzi, Vietti, and Ferrero (2009) described a 67-year-old Italian man presenting with periodical neurological symptoms such as shiver, pallor, asthenia. In 1984, the patient developed convulsions. In 2000 he developed headache, tremors, vertigo, memory loss, anxiety, depression, insomnia, muscular cramps, tachycardia. Despite several clinical examinations by internists and neurologists over 40 years his symptoms were never attributed to mercury poisoning. In 2003 he was examined by a physician with experience in chelation therapy who performed a "mercury challenge test" by slow infusion of 2 g disodium EDTA in 500 mL physiological saline followed by 12 h urine collection. The mercury level was 10 µg/g creatinine compared to <4 µg/g creatinine before chelation. The patient now remembered that he had received treatment for syphilis 40 years ago by weekly i.v. injections of a mercurial solution for 4 months. The patient was chelated with intravenous EDTA, 2 g in 500 mL saline once a week for two years. The neurological symptoms began to decrease 6 months after starting chelation therapy and had completely disappeared after 2 years of chelation. At the end of the chelation therapy, 12-h urine mercury levels after EDTA challenge was < 4 µg/g creatinine.

Sarikaya et al. (2010) described a case of elemental mercury poisoning in a 36-year-old woman who presented with diarrhea, abdominal pain and fever. One week before her daughter had brought liquid mercury from the school and placed it on a heating stove. The next day the14-month old breast fed sister got fever and passed away before hospital admission. Autopsy disclosed a suspected mercury poisoning potentially resulting in cardiorespiratory collapse. Chelation with NAC of the mother was instituted. After 7 days she was discharged without any sequelae. The Hg level in a blood sample taken on the discharge day was 300 µg/L. NAC chelation continued for 14 days.

Tezer et al. (2011) described three members of a family exposed to mercury vapor from metallic mercury brought home from school. The initial presentation and clinical picture lead to a misdiagnosis of an infectious disease, since symptoms occurred at different times in the family members and the exposure to mercury was not known. After identification of the cause mercury poisoning was diagnosed DMSA chelation therapy was initiated.

Malkani, Weinstein, Kumar, Victor, and Bernstein (2011) described a case of neurological dysfunction including diplopia, nystagmus, dysarthria, gait and limb ataxia, and vomiting in a 35-year-old Latin American man 1 year after sc injection of metallic mercury. He had an indurated plaque at the injection site on his right shoulder. His blood and 24-h urine mercury levels were high. Despite the mercury reservoir was excised and he was chelated with DMSA he showed only mild improvement after 1 year.

Cao et al. (2011) examined whether DMSA chelation would reduce blood mercury levels in low-level mercury exposed children. They analyzed total Hg and organic Hg (80–95% of blood Hg is methyl mercury in USA) in samples from a randomized trial of DMSA chelation in lead-exposed children aged 12–33 months, participating in the Treatment of Lead-exposed Children trial conducted between Sep. 1994 and Jun. 2003. Prechelation Hg levels were measured in blood samples from 767 children, in blood samples drawn 1 week after start of chelation (N = 768) and in a random sample of children receiving a maximum of 3 chelation courses (N = 67), and in a nonchelated placebo group. The mean organic Hg level in the DMSA chelated group fell from 99% at baseline to 82% after three courses of treatment relative to the placebo group. This result could be explained by prevention of age-related increase in the chelated group, so in conclusion, DMSA chelation had limited efficacy in low level organic mercury exposure in children

Mercer, Bercovitch, and Muglia (2012) described a case of acrodynia, also known as "pink disease," erythredema polyneuropathy, as a toxic reaction to metallic mercury exposure. Acrodynia occurred frequently in the early 20th century in babies due to use of diaper rinse with mercury chloride, but the disease is almost eradicated today. A 3-year-old girl presented with acrodynia due to exposure in the home to Hg vapor from spillage of metallic mercury on a carpet. She suffered from profuse sweats, redness, chills, edema of hands and feet, poor food intake, and periumbilical pain. Her blood pressure was 158/100. After extensive diagnostic evaluation mercury toxicity was suspected and confirmed by a urine Hg excretion of 178 μg/24 h. Her hypertension was treated with labetalol and amlodipine, and DMSA chelation therapy was initiated. After 5 weeks of DMSA chelation therapy, all symptoms had resolved.

Sasan et al. (2012) described accidental Hg poisoning initially diagnosed and treated as brucellosis in 2 brothers, 7 and 14 years old, presenting with salivation, sweating, pain in the lower extremities, anorexia and weight loss, and mood changes. Careful questioning revealed that they had played with metallic mercury brought home from a shool laboratory 3 months before admission. Urinary Hg levels in the younger and older brother were 125.9 and 54.2 9 μg/L. Both received chelation treatment with BAL, 3 mg/kg per day for 10 days. They were discharged after 24 days in good condition.

Brannan, Su, and Alverson (2012) reported a case of mercury poisoning in a 3-year-old girl without a known history of mercury exposure. She presented with acrodynia and hypertension after 3 weeks of intermittent abdominal pain, diaphoresis, and tachycardia. Her irritability and elevated catecholamine levels without a tumor together with acrodynia indicated possible Hg poisoning. Oral chelation with DMSA, 16 mg/kg per day, resulted in strongly increased urinary Hg excretion. Chelation continued for 2½ month. Her pain associated with acrodynia was treated until symptoms resolved. She received antihypertensive treatment for 2 months. Investigation of the home disclosed extremely high Hg vapor levels. A previous tenant had practiced rituals involving liquid mercury.

Alhamad et al. (2012) reported a case of metallic mercury poisoning via multiple exposure routes. A 36-year old Latin American man presented with rash, fever, sore throat and cough, chills, and diarrhea after chronic mercury vapor exposure and likely intravenous injection. The patient had been employed in thermometer recycling for 1 year, where he cut thermometers apart vaporizing mercury in the process. He had unusually heavy exposure prior to admission. He denied mercury injection, but radio-opaque deposits were observed in kidneys, bladder, and bowel wall. A concentrated mass of material was not observed. He was chelated with DMSA and DMPS, but deteriorated during development of renal failure and he passed away after 18 days.

Akyildiz, Kondolot, Kurtoğlu, and Konuşkan (2012) presented the largest pediatric series of metallic mercury poisonings in Turkey involving 26 cases. The poisonings were caused by skin contact and/or inhalation from a broken thermometer in a school laboratory. Of the patients, 21 inhaled, 3 inhaled and touched mercury, and 2 took mercury home. The children were observed for clinical symptoms, physical findings, and urine and blood mercury levels measured for 3 months. Sixteen children had poisoning symptoms and high b-Hg levels at admission. The 2 children who had taken mercury home had the highest blood mercury levels. Symptoms among the children were headache, abdominal pain, rashes, itching and fever. Twenty-one children with symptoms of mercury poisoning and high blood or urine Hg levels were chelated with DPA (25–50 mg/kg per day) and *N*-acetylcysteine (15 mg/kg per day). No adverse effects were observed during chelation therapy. Chelation was terminated after 1 or 2 weeks, based reductions in blood and urine Hg levels.

Mostafazadeh, Kiani, Mohamadi, Shaki, and Shirazi (2013) determined blood and urine mercury levels in 16 gold miners with neuropsychiatric symptoms. The patients received chelation treatment with BAL and DPA. The mean serum Hg levels before and after chelation therapy were 208.14 and 10.50 μg/L, respectively. The mean urinary mercury levels before and after chelation therapy were 134.70 and 17.23 μg/L, respectively. There were no significant differences in biochemistry parameters of patients before and after treatment. The study indicated exposure to high levels of mercury vapors in gold miners from the northwest of Iran.

Tang et al. (2013) described 4 female cases presenting with nephrotic syndrome and extensive proteinuria, 8.35–20.69 g/day after 2–6 months use of mercury-containing skin lightening creams with very high mercury levels, 7,420–30,000 ppm, for. Urine mercury excretions were 316–2,521 nmol/day and blood mercury levels were 26–129 nmol/L. Minimal change disease (MCD) was diagnosed in all patients by renal biopsy. The patients were chelated with DPA and their use of the skin lightening cream was stopped. Two patients also received steroids. Blood mercury levels normalized after 1–7 months, while urine mercury levels normalized after 9–16 months. Complete remission of proteinuria occurred after 1–9 months. Minimal change disease should be included as a pathological entity caused by mercury exposure or intoxication.

Mamdani and Vettese (2013) described a 40-year-old man presenting with dry cough, headache, and dyspnea for 3 days. He had labile mood, intention tremor, and tender subcutaneous nodules on the left forearm. Chest radiograph showed numerous small, high-density opacities distributed in both lungs. His urine Hg level was 1249 μg/L and his serum Hg was higher than 160 μg/L. The patient reported mercury exposure from his recently deceased father's old gun box; liquid mercury can be used to clean gun barrels and chambers from lead. A radiograph of the left wrist and forearm showed opacities corresponding to the subcutaneous nodules observed and following the course of veins indicating both subcutaneous and intravenous self-injection of mercury. The patient was chelated with DMPS. On day 5, his state of labile mood had decreased and his tremor had resolved. The urine Hg level had decreased to 692 μg/L. The patient was transferred to an inpatient psychiatric unit.

Beasley et al. (2014) described a suicidal case of mercuric chloride ingestion in a 19-year-old female. She presented with abdominal discomfort and nausea, diarrhea and vomiting of blood-stained fluid after ingestion of 2–4 g of mercuric chloride powder. Radiograph indicated opaque material in the gastric antrum. At 3 h postingestion the blood mercury level was 3.58 mg/L. The patient was transferred to intensive care unit and BAL chelation was initiated. Clinical signs included mild hemodynamic instability, fever, acidosis, leukocytosis, and hypokalemia. The symptoms improved after 2 days and completely resolved within a week.

Kobidze, Urushadze, Afandiyev, Nemsadze, and Loladze (2014) described a case of intentional self-injection of metallic mercury. A 22-year-old male with a medical history of suicidal poisoning with ethylene glycol presented with fatigue, pain and tremor in limbs, and skin rash 4 months after i.v. injection into his antecubital vein of metallic mercury from several thermometers. CT scan of the thorax and the abdomen showed numerous small, high density opacities in liver, both lungs, and right kidney. He had no clinical pulmonary malfunction or hepatic or renal biochemical abnormalities despite minor symptoms of tremor, erethism, knee joints arthralgia and lower extremities weakness. He was chelated with 20 mg/kg per day i.m. DMPS. After a month of chelation, blood mercury levels had decreased from 134 to 105 μg/L. The case demonstrated only mild acute toxicity after i.v. administration of an unknown amount of metallic mercury. The patient was recommended long-term DMPS treatments with repeated measurements of blood Hg levels.

Cicek-Senturk et al. (2014) described a 52-year-old woman admitted to hospital with high fever, a rash over the entire body, sore throat, nausea, itching, and muscle pain. Autoimmune diseases, infectious pathologies, and malignancy were excluded by diagnostic evaluation. Several organs of the patient were involved and fever persisted for 4 weeks. Repeated questioning about potential causes elicited that her son had taken liquid mercury from the school and put it on a heating stove, so the family had been exposed to mercury vapor for an extended time period. She was diagnosed with mercury poisoning and chelated with 300 mg DPA every 6 h for 7 days. Her clinical and laboratory data partially normalized during chelation treatment. DPA chelation had no side effects. The patient's son and husband had similar symptoms and were given the same chelation treatment.

Gencpınar et al. (2015) described a case where a 12 year old boy chronically exposed to mercury vapor presented after severe fatigue and weakness, and generalized muscle pain had been present for one month. He had decreased motor strength, painful extremities, and lack of deep tendon reflexes in lower extremities. Electromyography indicated mixed type polyneuropathy. Whole blood and 24-h urinary mercury levels were 23.2 μg/L and 175 μg/L, respectively. Family questioning revealed that the elder son had brought home circa 130 mL liquid mercury. Both boys had played intermittently with mercury during 6 months. On the 4th day of admission chelation therapy with DMSA was initiated. On day 7 the boy developed nausea and headache. Physical examination revealed bilateral papilledema and intracranial hypertension. He was treated with acetazolamide and after 1 month fundi examination was normal. The patient was discharged after 35 days with acetazolamide, gabapentin, and vitamin B6. Follow-up showed improved clinical findings. The authors conclude that the mercury poisoning caused the intracranial hypertension.

4.16.3 Conclusions

The data summarized above indicate that DMPS and DMSA are both effective chelating antidotes in acute inorganic and organic mercury intoxication in animal experiments, DMPS being most efficacious in inorganic poisoning while in poisonings with organic Hg compounds DMSA is more efficacious than DMPS. In chronic Hg exposure DMSA monoalkylesters, particularly the isoamyl ester, more efficiently than DMPS and DMSA mobilize Hg from body stores. Due to the possibility of oral as well as i.v. administration and repeated chelation courses for extended time periods with DMSA or DMPS and a low rate of adverse side effects, DMSA or DMPS are superior to DPA, NAPA and BAL in mercury poisoning. A growing number of human case and cohort data together indicate that the optimum Hg chelation antidote is DMPS, both in acute and chronic poisonings with inorganic Hg compounds, including Hg vapor. Experimental animal studies quantifying and comparing the antidotal efficacy of DMSA and DMPS with those of BAL, DPA and NAPA in both organic and inorganic mercury poisoning are available, although it would be useful to further verify in experimental animals that BAL should be dismissed in treatment of mercury poisoning and that DPA and NAPA are inferior to DMSA and DMPS.

4.17 NICKEL

Nickel (Ni, atomic number 28 in group 10 of the periodic table of the elements, atomic weight 58.71, density 8.908 g/cm^3) is a ferromagnetic transition metal. Naturally occurring nickel contains five stable isotopes: ^{58}Ni (most abundant), ^{60}Ni, ^{61}Ni, ^{62}Ni, and ^{64}Ni. Nickel often occurs in iron alloys as major component of iron meteorites. The use of such natural meteoritic iron–nickel alloy dates back to 3500 BC. Ni metal is silver-white, hard, ductile and malleable, and highly corrosion resistant. Nickel exist in the oxidation states −1, +1, +2, +3, and +4, the most common is +2. Nickel compounds can be described as falling into the distinct categories: soluble nickel, sulfidic nickel, oxidic nickel, and metallic nickel (Muñoz & Costa, 2012). The most important nickel compounds are nickel sulfate, nickel chloride, nickel oxide, nickel hydroxide, nickel subsulfide, and nickel tetracarbonyl, $Ni(CO)_4$, a colorless, volatile liquid.

Nickel is a relatively abundant element occurring mainly as oxide ores with other metals and as sulfide ores with metals as, for example, arsenic, iron and copper: Laterite Ni ores formed by tropical weathering of metal rich soils are either of the Limonite type - oxides with a very high iron content - or of the Silicate type formed beneath the Limonite zone. Laterite Ni ores represent the largest resources and are to take over as most important for Ni production. Sulfides as Millerite (NiS), nickeline (NiAs), and especially Pentlandite ($[Fe,Ni]_9S_8$), have been the most important ores, often occurring with a low content of Cu. Major nickel resources occur in Australia, New Caledonia, Canada, and Russia. The world nickel production was almost 1.6 million tons in 2011, matching the global demand for nickel, which increased about fivefold compared to the demand at the turn of the century (http://www.insg.org/prodnickel.aspx). Major industrial uses of nickel include steel and other alloys, stainless steel being the dominating product. Nickel alloys are used in ships, armaments, turbines, tools and a wide range of utensils. Electroplating, nickel–cadmium batteries, electronic components, and chemical catalysis are other important uses of nickel. Other uses include coins, jewelry, orthopedic and orthodontic implants (Klein & Costa, 2014).

While nickel is an essential cofactor in several bacterial enzymes (Hiron et al., 2010), there is still no clear prove that nickel should be essential to animals despite low nickel diet reduced animal growth (Anke, Groppel, & Kronemann, 1984).

The intestinal uptake of nickel from food is about 1% in humans but much higher from water (Sunderman et al., 1989). In mice given $NiCl_2$ orally, the intestinal uptake was less than 1% (Nielsen, Andersen, & Jensen, 1993). Absorbed nickel is efficiently excreted so tissue levels are low. Kidneys lungs, brain and pancreas retain some nickel upon exposure. Nickel and several other metals bind to transferrin (Quarles, Marcus, & Brumaghim, 2011) and to divalent metal transporter 1 (DMT-1) (Chen, Davidson, Singleton, Garrick, & Costa, 2005). Thereby iron and nickel transport interact on each other (Tallkvist, Bowlus, &

Lonnerdal, 2003). Nickel excretion is primarily via urine while feces, salivation and sweat are minor excretion routes (Klein & Costa, 2014). The half-time for nickel excretion in mice is very short (Nielsen et al., 1993) and plasma and urinary half-times of nickel in humans were found by Tossavainen, Nurminen, Mutanen, and Tola (1980) to be about 20–34 and 17–39 h, respectively. The excretion of pulmonarily deposited soluble nickel salts is also fast, while the lung clearance of deposited insoluble or low-solubility nickel dust, for example, welding fumes, is much slower (Antonini, Roberts, & Stone, 2011).

Skin absorption of nickel is an important exposure route, leading to nickel allergy and dermatitis, the Ni^{++} ion acting as a hapten. Nickel is the most frequent contact allergen in skin and patch tests (Lu, Warshaw, & Dunnick, 2009; Schmidt & Goebeler, 2011). The incidence of nickel sensitivity is higher in females than in males and has increased to reach about 30% in tested populations, mainly due to the use of nickel in jewelry (Brydl, Hindsberger, Kyvik, Agner, & Menné, 2004). Due to EU legislation on the use of nickel in jewelry and other items the incidence has recently been falling in certain European countries, especially after the full implementation in 2001 (Garg et al., 2013). Oral nickel intake from food items high in nickel and leaching from nickel-containing kitchen utensils may exacerbate nickel dermatitis. Treatment of severe nickel contact dermatitis should therefore include avoidance of nickel-containing items in the household and a diet low in nickel.

Acute intoxication by soluble nickel compounds or nickel carbonyl may manifest as vomiting and nausea, headache, vertigo, chemical pneumonia, and renal effects developing into pulmonary fibrosis (Klein & Costa, 2014). In nickel exposed workers, chronic pulmonary exposures are reported to induce liver damage, hypertrophic rhinitis, sinusitis, nasal polyps, asthma and nasal septum perforation, reduced olfactory function, and nasal mucosa epithelial dysplasia. As a transition metal, nickel can mediate toxic effects via induction of oxidative stress (Andersen & Andersen, 1989). Nickel induced hepatotoxicity can be alleviated by zinc administration (Sidhu et al., 2004). Inhaled $Ni(C0)_4$ rapidly decomposes into CO and Ni thereby inducing severe, often lethal, poisoning, initially manifesting as respiratory symptoms, worsening to dyspnoe, pneumonia, and acute respiratory distress.

Certain insoluble crystalline nickel compounds are carcinogenic in animals and humans inducing nasal and pulmonary cancers, and various nickel compounds have been demonstrated to induce a spectrum of epigenetic and genotoxic effects (Klein & Costa, 2014). Sufficient animal experimental and human epidemiological data have led to classification of Nickel subsulfide as an IARC Class 1 carcinogen (IARC, 1990).

4.17.1 Experimental Chelation Studies

Tandon and Mathur (1976) investigated the ability of six chelating agents for mobilizing nickel from organs in nickel loaded rats. CDTA effectively reduced nickel levels in the heart, brain, kidney and liver. DDC effectively reduced nickel levels in the heart, liver, kidney and brain.

Baselt, Sunderman, Mitchell, and Horak (1977) investigated the effectiveness in preventing mortality in rats of i.m. injection of 0.6 times their respective LD50 values of DDC, DPA, or TETA 10 min before or after 15 min inhalation exposure to 1.4 or 4.2 mg $Ni(CO)_4$ per liter of air. DDC was most effective. When chelators were administered 6 hr after exposure to nickel carbonyl, DPA was most effective. DDC and DPA were significantly more effective than TETA.

Basinger, Jones, and Tarka (1980) studied the efficacy of 14 chelating agents in acute nickel acetate poisoning in mice. After an i.p. dose of 62 mg/kg nickel acetate corresponding to LD_{90} or greater, $Na_2CaEDTA$ and DPA were the most effective antidotes. Several other chelating agents were almost as effective. Acetylation of the amino group in DPA to *N*-acetyl-D,L-penicillamine effectively abolished the antidotal potential indicating that coordination to the nitrogen is essential to the antidotal effect of DPA.

Oskarsson and Tjälve (1980) investigated effects of DDC and DPA on the toxicokinetics of $^{63}Ni^{2+}Cl_2$ injected into mice. Whole body autoradiography and liquid scintillation counting demonstrated that DDC caused tissue retention and -redistribution of $^{63}Ni^{2+}$. DPA reduced $^{63}Ni^{2+}$ tissue levels. The lipophilicity of the Ni-DDC complex and the hydrophilicity of the Ni-DPA complex may explain the different effects on $^{63}Ni^{2+}$ toxicokinetics.

Baselt and Hanson (1982) investigated the oral efficacy of the chelating agents disulfiram, DDC and DPA in preventing mortality after acute $Ni(CO)_4$ inhalation exposure. DDC and to some degree DPA were effective antidotes. Orally administered DDC gave moderately high prolonged plasma levels of DDC while disulfiram gave transient very high levels. The tissue distribution of inhaled ^{63}Ni-labeled $Ni(CO)_4$ at 24 h after exposure indicated that all three chelating agents reduced nickel levels in heart and lung, and DPA also reduced Ni levels in kidneys and blood. Disulfiram was the only chelator increasing the brain level of nickel. The results indicate caution in using oral disulfiram in human nickel carbonyl poisoning.

Tjälve, Jasim, and Oskarsson (1984) studied effects of DDC on toxicokinetics of ^{63}Ni labeled $Ni(CO)_4$ in mice after inhalation or intraperitoneal administration using whole-body autoradiography and liquid scintillation counting. DDC extensively changed the organ distribution of ^{63}Ni due to formation of lipophilic chelates redistributing among tissues. The lung levels were decreased by this possibly explaining the beneficial effect of DDC in nickel carbonyl poisoning—the lung is target tissue for $Ni(CO)_4$. The brain levels of ^{63}Ni were very high in mice after inhalation exposure to $^{63}Ni(CO)_4$, and DDC chelation reduced the brain levels. After i.p. injections of $^{63}Ni(CO)_4$ the brain Ni levels were low and DDC increased brain Ni levels likely due to affinity of lipophilic Ni-DDC complex for lipid-rich brain tissue.

Dwivedi, Athar, Hasan, and Srivastava (1986) investigated nickel mobilizing effects of chelating agents in nickel poisoned sham-operated or partially hepatectomized rats. The chelators effectively reduced nickel levels in both experimental groups. EDTA was more effective in reducing hepatic Ni levels while HEDTA and CDTA more effectively reduced renal Ni levels. The Ni levels in lung and heart were reduced to variable degrees by the chelators. The efficacy of the chelating agents was found to be in the order: EDTA > CDTA > HEDTA > TTHA > DTPA.

Sharma et al. (1986) studied effects of α-mercapto-β-aryl acrylic acids as antidotes in nickel poisoning in rats. α-mercapto-β-(3,4-dimethoxyphenyl)acrylic acid (MDA) was most effective. Other substituted acrylic acid had similar effects but less so than MDA in reducing tissue Ni levels and enhancing renal Ni excretion. MDA was the only chelator reducing Ni levels in brain. Also α-mercapto-β-(2-furyl) acrylic acid more effectively than structurally related compounds reduced the body burden of Ni and enhanced fecal and urinary Ni excretion. All compounds counteracted Ni induced inhibition of blood δ-aminolevulinic acid dehydratase activity and increased urinary δ-aminolevulinic acid excretion.

Sharma et al. (1987) compared the ability of β-1,2-Phenylene di-α-mercaptoacrylic acid (1,2-PDMA), 3-1,4-phenylene di-α-mercaptoacrylic acid (1,4-PDMA) and α-mercapto-Q-(2-hydroxyphenyl) acrylic acid (MHA) to counteract toxic effects of nickel in rats with that of DMPS. DMPS and 1,2-PDMA effectively reduced Ni body levels and enhanced Ni excretion, and restored most biochemical alterations induced by Ni toxicity. MHA reduced Ni tissue levels and enhanced urinary excretion. The results indicate the efficiency of vicinal thio groups and participation of the hydroxy group on the benzene nucleus besides the SH group of the MHA molecule, in chelation of Ni.

Athar, Misra, and Srivastava (1987) investigated effects of the macrocyclic chelators 1,4,8,11-tetraazacyclotetradecane (Cyclam) and 5,7,7′,12,14,14′-hexamethyl-1,4,8, 11-tetraazacyclotetradecane (Cyclam s) on organ distribution, excretion, and toxicity of nickel in rats compared with TETA and GSH. Cyclam and Cyclam s reduced nickel induced mortality even at low chelator doses, and enhanced biliary and urinary nickel excretion and restored altered levels of trace metals (viz., Cu, Zn, Fe, Mn) more effectively than TETA and GSH.

Oral or parenteral administration of DDC or tetraethylthiuram disulfide (disulfiram, Antabuse, TTD) dramatically changed the kinetics of orally administered $^{57}Ni^{++}$ in mice, since in some cases, the intestinal uptake of orally administered nickel increased about 10 times and the brain deposition of nickel was increased by a factor of about 700 (Nielsen & Andersen, 1994).

Tjälve and Borg-Neczak (1994) studied effects of a series of chelating agents forming lipophilic Ni^{2+} complexes (pyridinethiones, xanthates, dithiocarbamates, thiuram sulphides, and halogenated 8-hydroxyquinolines) on nickel kinetics in mice, rats and fish (brown trout) exposed to $^{63}NiCl2$ and chelators. Some of the chelators extensively increased tissue Ni levels. After inhalation exposure of mice to $^{63}Ni(CO)_4$ DDC decreased Ni levels in target tissues in nickel carbonyl poisoning, brain, lung, and heart. The antidotal ability of DDC may be limited to nickel carbonyl seen in the light of results of Nielsen and Andersen (1994).

Effects of several chelating agents as potential antidotes in acute nickel poisoning in mice were investigated by Xie, Funakoshi, Shimada, and Kojima (1994); Xie, Funakoshi, Shimada, and Kojima (1995); Xie, Funakoshi, Shimada, and Kojima (1996). Intraperitioneal injection of DMSA consistently protected to some degree against the acute toxicity of injected $NiCl_2$ estimated from hepatic, renal, pulmonary, or testicular lipid peroxidation, increased urinary and fecal Ni excretion, and decreased nickel levels in various organs.

Xie et al. (1995) found that DMSA and NBG-DTC effectively decreased testicular nickel levels and protected against Ni-induced testicular damage in mice.

Tandon, Singh, Jain, and Prasad (1996) studied nickel mobilizing effects of different chelating agents (DMSA, DMPS, DDC), α-mercapto-β-(2-furyl) acrylic acid (MFA), α-mercapto-β-(2-thienyl) acrylic acid (MTA), and *N*-benzyl-D-glucamine dithiocarbamate (NBG-DTC) and effects on nickel-induced biochemical alterations in rats after i.p. injection of nickel sulfate. MFA, DMSA, and NBG-DTC more effectively than their corresponding homologs, MTA, DMPS and DDC, respectively, decreased tissue nickel levels and enhanced fecal and urinary nickel excretion in rats exposed to nickel.

Ahmed, Rahman, Saleem, Athar, and Sultana (1999) studied effects of ellagic acid on biochemical alterations in serum, liver and kidney in nickel poisoned rats. Administration of 250 mmol Ni/kg body increased GSH levels and GST and GR activities in kidney and liver. Ellagic acid administration ameliorated Ni induced toxicity seen as reduced GSH level and reduced GST and GR and GPx activities in liver and kidney. Ellagic acid administration 30 min after nickel administration offered maximum protection against nickel induced biochemical alterations.

4.17.2 Clinical Studies

Creams containing low molecular weight chelators or ion-exchange resins to reduce skin uptake of nickel and to block the antigenic activity of nickel have been evaluated for potential to alleviate nickel contact dermatitis. Chelating agents in creams and ointments affect the in vitro skin penetration of Ni^{2+} quite differently. EDTA, DDC or dimethylglyoxim in creams decreased patch testing responses to solutions of nickel salts or nickel coins in nickel allergic patients (Allenby & Goodwin, 1983; Memon, Molokhia, & Friedman, 1994; Samitz & Pomerantz, 1958). Clioquinol appeared to be most effective (Memon et al., 1994), however, a range of different toxic effects prevents the use of this chelator as a preventive agent in Ni dermatitis (Gawkrodger, Healy, & Howe, 1995). A cation-exchange resin in a cream elicited some protective effect (Jarich et al., 1975). The available data indicates that besides reducing the skin penetration of Ni, chelation may reduce the antigenic potency of Ni^{++}, as suggested by Kurtin and Orentreich (1954).

Sunderman (1979, 1981, 1990) reported that DDC was an efficient chelating agent in $Ni(CO)_4$ poisoning, thus no deaths occurred among 375 DDC treated poisoned patients. Other chelating agents have much lower efficacy or may enhance nickel $Ni(CO)_4$ toxicity (NRC, 1975).

Several clinical studies reported healing of skin eruptions in nickel allergic patients by systemic chelation with oral TTD or DDC to reduce nickel stores in the body. The chelation treatment increased nickel excretion indicated by elevated nickel levels in urine and serum (Menne, Kaaber, & Tjell, 1980). The clinical improvement rate was, however, not high in most studies, and some patients developed hepatotoxicity (Menne and Kaaber, 1978; Spruit, Bongaarts, Jongh, 1978; Kaaber, Menne, Tjell, & Veien, 1979; Kaaber, Menne, Veien, & Hougaard, 1983; Kaaber et al., 1987; Christensen & Kristensen, 1982). The results of Nielsen and Andersen (1994) indicate that systemic chelation treatment of nickel allergic patients with DDC or TTD has the potential for increasing the brain deposition of nickel.

Kaaber et al. (1979) chelated a group of nickel-allergic patients with chronic, dyshidrotic hand eczema with TTD. The patients received 100 mg TTD 2–4 X per day for 4–10 weeks. Shortly after initiation of the treatment a flare of the dermatitis occurred in 9 of 11patients. The dermatitis cleared in 7 patients during the course of treatment, and improvement occurred in 2 patients. In 2 patients the dermatitis remained unchanged. In 6 patients a flare was seen upon discontinuation of chelation treatment. Side effects as dizziness, headache and fatigue occurred in 7 patients. Chelation of 4 patients was discontinued due to side effects. High serum and urine nickel levels were observed during the treatment.

Christensen (1982) administered oral TTD to three patients suffering from severe long-lasting nickel contact dermatitis. An initial dose of 50 mg/day was gradually increased to 100 mg or more twice a day. The eczema cleared in all 3 patients.

van Ketel and Bruynzeel (1982) investigated the blocking effect of locally applied DDC on patch test reactions to nickel. Patch test in nickel allergic patients with different nickel concentrations on skin treated with DDC were compared with control patch tests on areas pretreated with creambase only. There were no statistically significant differences between reactions on skin pretreated with DDC and skin treated with cream base indicating that a DDC-containing barrier cream is unlikely to help patients with dermatitis due to nickel allergy.

Shi (1986) described a series of 179 cases of $Ni(CO)_4$ poisoning due to various exposure causes including accidental spills or leaks, feeding raw material, repair processes, and fire fighting. Symptomatic treatment was offered to mild and moderate poisoning cases (rest in bed, bronchodilators and symptomatic drugs, oxygen, glucose, vitamin C, and corticosteroids according to needs). In 6 severe cases pulmonary edema or pneumonitis or both developed and 3 had toxic myocarditis. The severe cases were treated with a series of drugs and interventions, reduced water intake, oxygen administration, hibernation therapy, parenteral administration of corticosteroids, antibiotics, and other drugs combined with DDC chelation to treat pneumonia, pulmonary edema, and toxic myocarditis. All patients recovered without severe sequelae. About one third of the patients had weakness and neurasthenic syndrome after discharge, in some persisting for 3–6 months.

Kaaber, Mennem, Veien, and Baadsgaard (1987) reported a study of 3 men and 58 women with nickel allergy and hand eczema treated with 50–400 mg TTD per day for 4–56 weeks. Eleven patients developed biochemical evidence of hepatotoxicity, 5 patients developed evidence of hepatitis verified by liver biopsy in 4 patients. Patients showing hepatotoxity were older than those not having this side effect. The dermatitis healed in 29 patients, improvement was seen in 19, and 15 patients had no change. There was no difference in effects of TTD between maximum daily doses of 50, 200, or 400 mg. In 50% of the patients improving during TTD therapy the eczema recurred within a month after termination of therapy, in another 40% of the patients, recurrence was seen within 6 months.

Scott, Grier, Arnold, and Conrad (2002) described a case of acute $Ni(CO)_4$ poisoning with acute respiratory failure in a 39-year-old chemist exposed to of $Ni(CO)_4$ spilled in a laboratory. He presented with symptoms of cough and dyspnea. Diagnosed with pneumonia he was treated accordingly as outpatient. On day 2 after the spill he had respiratory distress and was given supplemental oxygen but later required endotrachial intubation and positive pressure mechanical ventilation after transfer to a medical intensive care unit. TTD chelation was initiated at 500 mg every 12 h via a nasogastric tube since DDC was unavailable. Over the next several hours, the patient had further deterioration in pulmonary function with increasing oxygen requirements. Therefor high-volume continuous venovenous hemofiltration was initiated. Chest radiograph continued to show interstitial infiltrates and the patient continued to require ventilatory support. However, after 16 days of mechanical ventilation, the patient improved with reduced oxygen requirements. The patient was extubated 24 days after the exposure and his pulmonary function gradually recovered.

4.17.3 Conclusions

In acute inorganic nickel poisoning, DDC is strongly contraindicated, since studies have demonstrated that oral or parenteral DDC administration extensively increased brain deposition of nickel after oral nickel exposure, while the effect of DDC on i.p. injected Ni is antidotal. EDTA, DPA, DMPS, and DMSA were all effective antidotes in animal studies. Clinical experience with chelation in nickel poisoning is limited; DDC has been demonstrated to be an effective antidote in acute nickel carbonyl poisoning, and both DDC and TTD have been used in many clinical trials to alleviate nickel dermatitis, apparently by promoting excretion of body levels of Ni.

4.18 PLATINUM

Platinum (Pt, atomic number, 78, member of group 10 in the periodic table of elements, atomic mass 195.078, density 21.41 g/cm^3) is lustrous, silver–gray, ductile and malleable, a precious noble metal together with gold and silver; the name platinum originates from Spanish *platina*, "little silver" (Encyclopædia Britannica and Online, 2012). Main oxidation states are +2 and +4, but +1, +5, and +6 also occur. Of 6 natural isotopes including ^{192}Pt, ^{194}Pt (32.9%), ^{195}Pt (33.8%), ^{196}Pt (25.2%), and ^{198}, one ^{190}Pt is radioactive with $t_{1/2}$ 6.9 × 1011 years. Several artificial radioactive isotopes are available for research. Platinum is the least reactive metal and it does not react with oxygen except at extremely high temperature, but it reacts with boiling aqua regia and with molten alkali cyanides. Important Pt compounds include halogenides. Tetravalent Pt compounds are water soluble, except for the oxide, which is soluble in strong acids and in potassium hydroxide solution. In aqueous solutions, hexacoordinate and tetracoordinate complexes dominate.

Platinum is a rare metal in the earth's crust (average 5 μg/kg). Platinum occurs as the pure native metal and as alloys with iron and other metals in alluvial deposits, for example, in Colombia and Russia (Lide, 2007). Platinum and other platinum-group metals are mainly obtained as by-products during nickel and copper mining and processing from mixed platinum containing sulfide and arsenide ores. Sperrylite (PtAs2) is mined in Canada, and braggite (Pt,Pd,Ni)S, cooperite ([Pt,Pd]S) and platinum chromites are mined in South Africa, which possesses the world's largest platinum resources (Seymour & O'Farrelly, 2001; Xiao & Laplante, 2004). The world platinum production was 184 tons in 2011(Kiilunen, Aitio, & Santonen, 2014).

The use of Pt in catalytic converters in cars previously consumed approximately 80% of total platinum use (Matthey, 2004). This use is decreasing due to development of palladium based catalytic converters (Kiilunen et al., 2014). The second largest use of platinum is as catalysts in chemical industry. Other important uses of platinum are in jewelry, glass, dental, and electronic industry, for example, as electrodes and contacts. Special uses are in neurological prostheses and in pacemakers. A number of platinum coordination complexes with various ligands are important cancer chemotherapeutic drugs, one of the most important being *cis*-diammoniumdichloroplatinum(II) ($Pt(NH_3)_2Cl_2$, cisplatin, *cis*-Pt), the *trans* isomer is inactive.

Exposure to platinum mainly occurs in occupational settings as inhalation in mining, production, and processing, for example, platinum refining and catalyst manufacture and during exposure to traffic dust (IPCS, 1991). Platinum is not essential for any known life form. Due to rapid complex formation with biological O-, N-, and S- containing ligands, free Pt ions are unlikely to exist in vivo.

The excretion of platinum after inhalation or intratracheal instillation of various radioactive platinum compounds in rats was biphasic with rapid fecal elimination of the majority of radioactivity followed by slow fecal and urinary excretion (Moore, Hysell, Hall, Campbell, & Stara, 1975a; Artelt, Kock, & Nachtigall, 1998). The gastrointestrinal absorption of platinum(IV) chloride is very limited (< %) in adult and suckling rats (Moore, Hysell, Crocker, & Stara, 1975b). The uptake of other orally administered Pt compounds including model particulates of car exhaust are also low (Lown, Morganti, Stineman, D'Agostino, & Massaro, 1980; Artelt, Creutzenberg, & Kock, 1999). The kidneys had the highest Pt levels after inhalation exposure, intratracheal instillation, oral administration to metallic Pt or intravenous administration of $PtCl_4$ in rats (Moore et al., 1975b,c; Artelt et al., 1998) and dietary administration of $Pt(SO_4)_2$ to mice (Lown et al., 1980).

Metallic platinum is rather nontoxic. Metallic Pt induced slight necrotic gastrointestinal epithelium changes and epithelial swelling in the convoluted renal tubules after oral administration to rats (IPCS, 1991). The toxicities of platinum salts after oral administration to rats increased in the order: $PtO_2 < PtCl_2 < Pt(SO_4)_2 \cdot 4H_2O < PtCl_4$ indicating that toxicity is positively related to solubility (Holbrook, Washington, Leake, & Brubaker, 1975). Orally administered chloride containing platinum coordination complexes are more toxic than platinum salts (IPCS, 1991). The kidney is the target organ for hexachloroplatinic acid, $H_2[PtCl_6]$ (Ward et al., 1976), and nephrotoxicity is a major side effect during use of *cis*-Pt in cancer chemotherapy (Bokemeyer et al., 1996; Ferrari et al., 2005; Markman, 2003; Taguchi, Nazneen Abid, & Razzaque, 2005). Neurotoxicity is another severe side effect (Sastry & Kellie, 2005).

Clinical effects of occupational exposure to platinum salts include hypersensitivity and allergic disorders. Platinum salts and complexes induce a high frequency of an asthma-like disease, "platinosis," with sneezing, wheezing, coughing, breathlessness, tightness of the chest, and watering of the eyes in exposed workers. Other effects are contact dermatitis and urticarial like skin lesions and mucous membrane inflammation (Hunter, Milton, & Perry, 1945; Roberts, 1951). Roberts (1951) observed 60–100% prevalences of platinosis among exposed while Niezborala and Garnier (1996) found >30% prevalence of platinum sensitivity developing within 3 years, indicating that platinum is a highly potent sensitizer. The induction of platinum hypersensitivity most likely follows a type 1 immunoglobulin E (IgE)-mediated mechanism, platinum acting as a hapten by combining with HS-groups in serum proteins, forming a complete antigen (Cromwell, Pepys, Parish, & Hughes, 1979; Merget, Reineke, Rückmann, & Bergmann, 1994; Schultze-Werninghaus, Roesch, Wilhelms, Gonsior, & Meir-Sydow, 1978).

Therapeutic uses of *cis*-Pt and other platinum-containing antineoplastic drugs as oxaliplatin, nedaplatin, and carboplatin (Wheate, Walker, Craig, & Oun, 2010) as highly efficient antitumor drugs may lead to serious side effects, primarily gastrointestinal symptoms, hematological disorders, neurotoxicity, ototoxicity, as well as nephrotoxicity which is dose-limiting (Loehrer & Einhorn, 1984). The toxic mechanism is believed to involve GSH depletion and induction of oxidative stress, and animal experimental and clinical studies have demonstrated that various nucleophilic thio compounds can protect against *cis*-Pt nephrotoxicity without affecting antitumor activity significantly (Basinger, Jones, Holscher, 1990; DeGregorio et al., 1989; Howell, Pfeifle, Wung, Olshen, 1983; Jones et al., 1991c). Some toxic effects are age-related, being less frequent in younger patients (POISINDEX, 2004).

4.18.1 Experimental Animal Studies

In animal experiments DDC and derivatives of DDC decreased renal and hepatic Pt levels, and increased especially the biliary excretion of Pt after *cis*-Pt administration, besides protecting against *cis*-Pt induced nephrotoxicity (Borch, Katz, Lieder, & Pleasants, 1980; Basinger et al., 1989; Jones & Basinger, 1989; Hidaka et al., 1994; Hidaka, Funakoshi, Shimada, Tsuruoka, & Kojima, 1995), conceivably by changing the preferentially renal excretion route to biliary excretion.

Subcutaneous administration of DMSA reduced mortality after i.p. administration of 50 mg/kg of H_2PtCl_6 to mice (Ding & Liang, 1991), and i.p. administration of DMSA after i.v. administration of *cis*-Pt reduced renal Pt levels in rats (Planas-Boehne et al., 1982). Both studies support studies by Graziano, Jones, and Pisciotto (1981), who found that repeated i.p. DMSA administration following i.v. injection of *cis*-Pt reduced hepatic and renal Pt levels and increased urinary Pt excretion in rats. The Pt mobilizing effect of DMSA was comparable to that of the effective dithiocarbamate derivatives, however, DMSA was unable to prevent *cis*-Pt-induced renal damage seen as weight loss, increased serum creatinine level, urinary *N*-acetyl-β-D-glucosaminidase excretion, and histological damage. Most likely, increased urinary Pt excretion induced by DMSA is responsible for the observed renal damage. In the same study, DFO reduced hepatic Pt levels more efficiently than did DMSA, however DFO potentiated *cis*-Pt induced toxicity, and BAL chelation increased organ levels of Pt (Graziano et al., 1981).

Appenroth, Winnefeld, Schröter, and Rost (1993) investigated effects of NAC on *cis*-Pt nephrotoxicity in rats. Sc administration of 1 g NAC/kg completely abolished the nephrotoxic effects of i.p. administration of 6 mg/kg *cis*-Pt. Also, the renal Pt level was reduced significantly by NAC due to enhanced urinary Pt excretion. Similar effect on *cis*-Pt nephrotoxicity was observed after injection of preformed *cis*-Pt-NAC complex, indicating that the protective effect of NAC on *cis*-Pt nephrotoxicity is due to chelation of platinum.

Delivery of *cis*-Pt directly into a tumor can be achieved if the tumor has a single, well defined artery; Ambrus et al. (2002) developed a device capable of removing *cis*-Pt in the venous drainage from a tumor before reaching systemic circulation, that is, performing extracorporeal removal of *cis*-Pt without the chelator entering the blood. A hollow fiber with an immobilized platinum chelator could remove 80% of *cis*-Pt from blood from melanoma patients. *Cis*-Pt was infused into the femoral vein of dogs at a dose of 100 mg/m^2 restricting the drug to the area to be treated. This device allows local application of high *cis*-Pt doses at the same time minimizing systemic side effects.

Kadikoylu et al. (2004) investigated effects of DFO on *cis*-Pt induced lipid peroxidation and activities of antioxidant enzymes in rat kidneys. Intraperitoneal injection of 250 mg/kg DFO 30 min before i.p. injection of 10 mg/kg *cis*-Pt reduced renal MDA levels at 72 h postdosage to control levels, partly restored SOD activity but could not restore catalase activity and H_2O_2 levels and glomerular filtration rate. In the same experiment i.p. injection of 100 mg/kg vitamin C or E more effectively restored antioxidant enzyme activities indicating a potential for combined administration to reduce renal *cis*-Pt toxicity.

Dickey et al. (2008) investigated effects of dosing and route of administration of NAC for protection against *cis*-Pt nephrotoxicity in rats after a single high i.p. dose of 10 mg/kg *cis*-Pt and after multiple low doses, 1 mg/kg i.p. twice a day for 4 days, 10 days rest, and then repeated. NAC (50-1, 200 mg/kg) was given by i.p., oral, i.v. or intraarterial (i.a.) routes. Renal toxicity occurred after both *cis*-Pt administration regimens. After single *cis*-Pt administration, i.p. or oral administration of 400 mg/kg NAC offered no renal protection as measured by BUN or CR compared to controls. After i.v. administration, NAC reduced nephrotoxicity, and 50 mg/kg NAC given i.a. offered even better protection. In the repeated-dose regimen 800 mg/kg NAC given i.v. but not i.p. prevented nephrotoxicity. Accordingly, protective effects of NAC depend both on dose and on route of administration.

4.18.2 Clinical Studies

Gandara et al. (1995) evaluated DDC as chelating agent in a randomized placebo-controlled trial in 221 patients receiving *cis*-Pt (100 mg/m^2) combined with cyclophosphamide or etoposide. DDC did not reduce the incidence of peripheral neurotoxicity, however, the incidences of nephrotoxicity and treatment withdrawal due to toxicity was higher in the DDC group than in the control group, at variance with results of animal experiment with DDC as antidote against *cis*-Pt toxicity.

Charlier, Kintz, Dubois, and Plomteux (2004) described a fatal *cis*-Pt overdosage due to an accidental administration of 750 mg instead of 170 m *cis*-Pt to a 63-year-old lymphoma patient. Postmortem heart, peripheral blood, urine, and bile platinum levels were 1515, 1253, 1038, and 501 pg/L, respectively. Renal dialysis was started immediately following *cis*-Pt perfusion. NAC was administered as adjuvant therapy followed by globule transfusion and erythropoietetin administration and repeated plasmapheresis. The patient deceased however on day 16 with renal and hepatic insufficiency, ototoxicity, and pancytopenia.

4.18.3 Conclusions

Presently there is no recommendation for chelation therapy in platinum exposure. Limited animal experimental and human clinical data indicate that DDC could be effective in alleviating side effects in patients receiving high-dose *cis*-Pt therapy, without significantly affecting *cis*-Pt antineoplastic effects, and that NAC could protect against renal damage by chelation and by acting as an antioxidant.

4.19 SILVER

Silver (Ag, greek άργυροζ, latin *argentum*, atomic number 47 in group 11 of the periodic table of the elements, atomic weight 107.868 g/mol, density 10.5 g/cm^3) is a soft, white, lustrous, ductile, and malleable transition metal with the highest reflectivity, and thermal and electrical conductivity of any metal. Silver occurs as free native silver in alloys with various metals including gold. Silver also occurs in argentite (Ag_2S) and in chlorargyrite (AgCl), but Ag is mainly obtained as a by-product during gold, lead, copper, and zinc refining. Silver occurs as 2 stable isotopes, ^{107}Ag and ^{109}Ag, with almost equal abundance, 28 radioactive isotopes (^{105}Ag, $t_{½}$ 41.29 days, ^{111}Ag, $t_{½}$ 7.45 days, 2 isotopes with $t_{½}$ of few hours, the rest with $t_{½}$ below 3 min) and several meta states (^{108m}Ag, $t_{1/2}$ 418 years), ^{110m}Ag, $t_{1/2}$ 249.79 days, ^{106m}Ag, $t_{1/2}$ 8.28 days).

Silver objects dating before 3000 BC have been found in the Sumerian city of Kish, in Anatolia in Turkey and in Greece (Ottaway and Roberts, 2008; Ozbal, 2001; Mesopotamia, 2003). Silver staining of glass was introduced in the 14th century using combinations of silver nitrate and silver sulfide to facilitate coloring in general and to obtain orange and yellow colors (Davison, 2003).

Holler, Fowler, and Nordberg (2014) recently published an extensive review of the chemistry and biology of silver. The 2011 world primary silver production was 23000 tons. Recycling and other sources than mining added 8400 tons (The Silver Institute, 2015). Silver is a precious metal more abundant than platinum and gold, and traditionally used in coinage, bullions and jewelry, mirrors, ornaments and tableware. Silver forms important alloys with copper and other metals. Silver compounds occur as Ag^+, for example, $AgNO_3$, Ag^{2+} (less common, eg, AgF_2), and (even less common) Ag^{3+} and Ag^{4+}, for example, $KAgF_4$ and K_2AgF_6 (Riedel & Kaupp, 2009). Important compounds include silver nitrate, silver lactate, silver picrate, silver acetate, silver chloride, silver bromide, and silver iodide (Riedel & Kaupp, 2009).

Industrial uses include a range of electric and electronic applications (computer keyboards use silver electrical contacts), amalgams in dentistry, chemical catalysts, disinfectants in a wide range of medical applications, water filtration (Ag prevents bacteria and algae from building up in filters), photographic and X-ray films, windows coatings, and photovoltaic solar panels and plasmonic solar cells. Almost 3000 tons of Ag are expected for these uses in 2015 (The Silver Institute, 2015). Thermal or infrared telescope mirrors are silver coated instead of the normal Al coating due to better infrared performance (Gemini Observatory, 2015).

The intestinal silver uptake was 10% or less in several experimental animal species, and more than 90% of silver was excreted via bile to feces after oral, pulmonary, i.p., or i.v. administration to experimental animals (Furchner, Richmond, & Drake, 1968), likely bound to GSH (Alexander & Aaseth, 1981). In a silver exposed human, the $t_{1/2}$ in lungs and liver were estimated to 1 day and 52 days, respectively (Newton & Holmes, 1966). Toxic effects of silver occur in hematopoietic, hepatic, and cardiovascular systems. Silver exposure of vitamin E-deficient rats induced hepatic ultrastructural lysosomal and mitochondrial changes and centrilobular necrosis (Grasso, Abrahan, & Hendy, 1970). Ventricular hypertrophy and cardiac enlargement were observed in turkeys fed 900 mg/kg silver nitrate in diet for 18 weeks (Jensen, Peterson, & Falen, 1974; Peterson, Jensen, & Harrison, 1973).

Silver compounds including silver nanoparticles are used as antimicrobials in creams and wound dressings, creams, and as coating on medical devices and in numerous industrial, healthcare and domestic applications due to the bactericidal action of Ag^+. Silver has low toxicity in humans conferring minimal risk from iatrogenic uses (Lansdown, 2006; Maillard & Hartemann, 2013).

Subchronic or chronic pulmonary or oral exposure to silver salts or colloidal silver may result in development of a bluish-gray discolorization of skin, argyria, mainly in skin exposed to light, due to dermis deposition of nanosize silver containing granules, mainly in sebaceous and sweat glands and around hair follicles (Schell & Hornstein, 1974; Nasemann, Rogge, & Schaeg, 1974). Based on a series of case studies, Drake and Hazelwood (2005) reported that soluble silver compounds caused argyria more often than less soluble or colloidal silver compounds. Silver deposition may cause functional impairment resulting in clinical symptoms in various organs. Aaseth, Olsen, Halse, and Hovig, 1981 demonstrated that silver deposited in renal basement membrane was in the form of silver selenide. Administration of selenite together with silver to rats enhanced silver retention in brain, kidneys, and blood, due to formation of insoluble silver-selenium complexes (Alexander & Aaseth, 1981). An effective treatment for argyria has not been developed, and the condition is more or less chronic even when silver exposure is discontinued. Chelation therapy is considered ineffective (Aaseth et al., 1981).

4.20 THALLIUM

Thallium (Tl, atomic number 81 in group 13 of the periodic table of the elements, atomic weight 204.4, density 11.85 g/cm^3 with indium, gallium, aluminum, and boron) is a blue-white metal with compounds in oxidation states +1, +3. Thallium metal is reactive and forms a brownish-black oxide on exposure to air. Thallium solubilizes in acids forming monovalent thallous and less stable trivalent thallic salts (Lee, 1971). Important compounds are thallous sulfate, thallous nitrate, thallous acetate, thallium(I) and thallium(III) oxides, thallous carbonate, and thallous sulfide. Thallium is widely distributed over the Earth but at low concentrations and does not exist as the free metal. Thallium is mainly obtained as a by-product from mining and refining of heavy metal sulfide minerals, for example, lorandite, $TlAsS_2$, and crookesite, one form is $(Cu,Tl,Ag)_2Se$. Tl is mined in the USA, Brazil, and China, and also produced from sulfuric acid production. The annual worldwide production of thallium is as low as approximately 15 tons and approximately 2000–5000 tons are mobilized by industrial processes (Kazantzis, 2000). Thallium has limited uses in alloys, but main uses are in electronics, photoelectric cells and lamps, and semiconductors, the remainder is used in alloys, pigments, glass coloring, imitation jewelry, and in the pharmaceutical industry (Blain & Kazantzis, 2014). Thallium has been used as catalysts in organic synthesis (Wade & Banister, 1973).

Formerly, thallium salts' large scale and widespread use as rodenticides led to many accidental, homicidal, and suicidal human poisonings. Thallium containing rodenticides were banned in several western countries in the 1970s, and anticoagulants and other biochemically acting but less toxic poisons became commonly used as rodenticides, but Tl salts were still readily available around the world. Due to development of warfarin resistance in rats, thallium salts are again increasingly used as rodenticide in some countries, so today, thallium poisonings still occur. Before introduction of ^{99m}technetium in nuclear medicine, the radioactive isotope ^{201}thallium ($t_{½}$ 73 h) was widely employed for nuclear cardiography. This thallium isotope is still used in stress tests in patients with coronary artery disease (Jain & Zaret, 2005).

Occupational inhalation exposures to thallium have occurred in flue dust and pyrite roasting processes, during extraction of the metal, production of thallium based rodenticides and thallium-containing lenses, and separation of industrial diamonds (Richeson, 1958), however, the main sources of poisoning in thallium workers are skin absorption and gastrointestinal absorption (Ewers, 1988).

Thallium salts are rapidly and extensively absorbed after inhalation or skin contact and are widely distributed in the body with highest levels in the kidneys (Lie, Thomas, & Scott, 1960). The gastrointestinal absorption and absorption after intratracheal instillation are close to 100% in the rat (Lie et al., 1960; Lund, 1956a). Also in chronic feeding experiments in the rat, the highest concentration occurs in kidneys, followed by bone, liver, lung, spleen, and brain (Downs, Scott, Steadman, & Maynard, 1960) In both animal and humans thallium is excreted in urine and feces with minor excretions into hair and milk and over the placental barrier (Blain & Kazantzis, 2014). In rats, $t_{½}$ was found to be around 3.3 days independent on the administration route (Lie et al., 1960).

The toxicity of the Tl^+ ion is partly due to similarity with the K^+ ion, leading to substitution of K^+ in biochemical processes, most importantly in Na^+/K^+ ATPases. Also, Tl binds to HS-groups in proteins thereby acting as enzyme inhibitor: Tl inhibits the sodium-potassium-adenosine triphosphatase and interferes with energy production at essential steps in glycolysis and the TCA cycle and in oxidative phosphorylation (Hoffman, 2003).

The similarity to K^+ results in extensive intestinal uptake and tubular reabsorption. Accordingly, i.v. K^+ administration to compete for biochemical sites and to increase renal clearance by competing for reabsorption is important as supportive treatment in Tl poisoning (Gehring & Hammond, 1966; Chamberlain, Stavinoha, Davis, Kniker, & Panos, 1958). The critical targets in acute thallium poisoning are the digestive, nervous and renal systems. In chronic poisoning, loss of hair is characteristic of thallium poisoning, most likely due to blocked cell proliferation in hair follicles (Cavanagh & Gregson, 1978).

Acute thallium poisoning rapidly induces gastroenteritis with abdominal pain, diarrhea, vomiting, and nausea. After few days nervous system toxicity develop with paresthesia, weakness, tender, painful extremities, convulsions, mental confusion or delirium, and respiratory and circulatory failure resulting in death. Gastric lavage and laxative treatment have been employed after acute oral poisoning, and forced diuresis offers a means to increase Tl excretion (Nogue et al., 1982). Also Hemodialysis and hemoperfusion are employed to reduce thallium blood levels. The clinically available chelators BAL, DPA, EDTA, and DTPA were unable to enhance Tl excretion (Heydlauf, 1969; van der Stock & de Schepper, 1978; Lund, 1956a, 1956b). DPA increased Tl induced mortality in rats and enhanced the brain deposition of Tl (Rios & Monroy-Noyola, 1992). As has been observed for most other metal cations, DDC enhanced the brain deposition of Tl, augmenting Tl neurotoxicity, however, the urinary Tl excretion was increased in rats (Schwetz, O'Neil, Voelker, & Jacobs, 1967; Rauws, ten Ham, & Kamerbeek, 1969; Kamerbeek et al., 1971a).

Kamerbeek, van Heijst, Rauws, and ten Ham (1970) reported that DDC chelation in humans resulted in clinical deterioration likely caused by thallium redistribution to the brain. None of the clinically used antidotes listed earlier are recommended in thallium poisoning, and DDC and DPA are contraindicated. The ion exchanger Prussian blue (PB) was originally proposed as a thallium chelating antidote by Heydlauf (1969), and PB turns out to be the most effective thallium antidote investigated so far (Yang et al., 2008). Up to 20 g of oral PB can be administered per day after initial gastric lavage (Malbrain et al., 1997).

If survival extends about 1 week various neurological symptoms dominate, with headache, tremor, paresthesias, ataxia, and muscular atrophy. At later poisoning stages involvement of the cranial nerve lead to ophthalmoplegia, ptosis, retrobulbar neuritis, or facial paralysis. In the subacute cases distal neuropathy begins with numbness and sensory loss in the fingers and toes spreading proximally progressing to motor weakness. Recovery may be full, but neurological defects as mental abnormalities, tremor and ataxia may remain for extended time periods (Bank, Pleasure, Suzuki, Nigro, & Katz, 1972; Gastel, 1978; Kalita & Misra, 2006; Lu et al., 2007; Pelclová et al., 2009).

The efficiency of PB is due the extensive enterohepatic circulation of Tl. The intestinal Tl absorption was reduced by 70% in rats given oral PB before oral Tl administration (Rauws, 1974). Thus, the protective mechanism of oral

PB in oral thallium poisoning is exchange of K^+ ions in PB with thallium ions thereby blocking enterohepatic Tl cycling and increasing fecal Tl elimination since neither PB nor its Tl complex are systemically absorbed. In chronic Tl poisoning long-term PB administration is an efficient decorporation procedure by prolonged intestinal trapping of Tl by PB, which is also used for decorporation of cesium. Various chemical forms of PB with different physical properties have been used clinically. Especially ammoniumferrichexacyanoferrat (AFCF) is widely used both in animal experimental cerium and thallium detoxification and in human clinical treatment of cerium and thallium poisoning. The synthesis and further preparation of the three main types of PB determine the Tl-binding capacity, especially are colloid solubility or insolubility and particle size, that is, specific surface area, and K^+ content main determining factors for Tl binding capacity (Dvorak, 1970, 1971; Kamerbeek et al., 1971a; Kamerbeek, Rauws, ten Ham, & van Heijst, 1971b).

4.20.1 Animal Studies

Leloux, Lich, and Claude (1990) evaluated various Tl mobilization treatments in acute oral Tl poisoning in the rat. Enhanced fecal elimination by oral PB administration and forced urinary excretion by K^+ administration were the most efficient treatments while furoseimid enhanced diuresis was ineffective by itself. Combined i.p. furoseimid and oral PB administration however resulted in extensive total urinary and fecal Tl excretion.

Kravzov, Rios, Altagracia, Monroy-Noyola, and López (1993) evaluated the potential of a commercially available PB product and a freshly prepared colloidal PB preparation for reducing blood and organ Tl levels administered orally 24 h after i.p. injection of Tl in mice. Both PB preparations efficiently reduced Tl levels in all investigated organs, however, freshly prepared PB was significantly more efficient, confirming previous studies cited earlier.

Three days chelation with oral PB combined with i.p. DPA starting 1 day after i.p. injection of thallium acetate in rats significantly reduced histological cerebellar damage compared to PB chelation alone, which only marginally protected against toxicity while DPA chelation alone potentiated brain damage. The mortality in the different treatment groups closely followed the degree of brain damage (Barroso-Moguel, Villeda-Hernandez, Mendez-Armanta, Rios, & Monroy-Noyola, 1994).

Meggs, Cahill-Morasco, Shih, Goldfrank, and Hoffman (1997) compared effects of PB and *N*-acetylcystein (NAC) administered singly or in combination on acute Tl poisoning in mice. NAC only marginally reduced mortality induced by a s.c. thallium acetate dose corresponding to LD_{90}. PB alone and PB and NAC combined were slightly more effective. PB alone was the only treatment offering some protection after a Tl dose >LD100.

Mulkey and Oehme (2000) evaluated the antidotal effects of PB and DMPS given alone or in combination after acute oral Tl poisoning in rats. Relative

Tl levels were kidney ≫ heart > liver approximately equal brain. While PB administration and combined PB + DMPS administration reduced TI levels in all tissues and increased fecal TI excretion, DMPS did not reduce Tl levels significantly except in whole blood and only marginally enhanced fecal Tl excretion. The combined treatment was not more efficient than PB alone. This study confirms and expands results of previous studies cited earlier that DMPS has no use in Tl poisoning.

Rusyniak et al. (2003) compared PB and DMSA as chelating antidotes in acute Tl poisoning in rats. Survival in PB chelated rats was higher than in DMSA chelated rats, which was higher than in unchelated controls. Brain Tl levels were elevated by DMSA (not significant) but extensively reduced by PB chelation.

Montes et al. (2011) compared the efficacies of oral PB and i.p. D,L-penicillamine (DL-P) as chelating antidotes in acute thallium poisoning in rats. DL-P was without effect on survival while PB and DL-P chelation increased survival compared to PB alone. Organ levels of Tl were marginally reduced by DL-P chelation, more so by PB chelation, but combined chelation most efficiently reduced organ Tl levels. Most importantly, the same effects were observed in the brain regions hypothalamus, striatum, mesencephalon, hippocampus, and cortex.

Wang, He, and Zhang (2012) chelated orally Tl poisoned mice with i.p. ZnDTPA, oral PB or both. Histologic damage in intestines, liver, and kidneys was reduced by chelation compared to the unchelated control group, most after combined chelation, and brain damage was slightly reduced. PB chelation and combined chelation reduced blood Tl levels and increased urine and feces Tl levels, most in the combined treatment group. Brain Tl levels were not reduced by the chelation treatments. This experiment indicates some increased efficiency of combined chelation compared to PB chelation alone.

4.20.2 Clinical Cases

In cases of acute oral thallium poisoning cases oral administration of PB led to clinical improvement and survival even after lethal doses, granted that PB chelation was instituted rapidly after thallium intake (Kamerbeek et al., 1971b; van der Merwe, 1972; Stevens, van Peteghem, Heyndrickx, & Barbier, 1974; Pelclová et al., 2009), in some cases combined with hemodialysis and forced diuresis (Pedersen et al., 1978). However, fatal outcome may occur despite early treatment with activated charcoal and PB. Thus, Riyaz, Pandalai, Schwartz, and Kazzi (2013) reported a fatal suicidal ingestion of an unknown amount of thallium sulfate by a 36-year-old man presenting 45 min after ingestion with abdominal pain and vomiting. He was initially treated with multidose activated charcoal (MDAC), and PB chelation was initiated 18 h postarrival. His condition rapidly deteriorated with tachycardia and hypertension and subsequently renal failure. Despite initiation of continuous renal replacement therapy on day 3 the patient died shortly after. His last blood and spot urine Tl levels were 5.369 mg/L and >2 mg/L.

Wainwright et al. (1988) described a severe thallium poisoning in a young man presenting with transient loss of consciousness and a b-Tl-level of 5.75 mg/L, He rapidly developed severe neuropathy and required temporary mechanical ventilation and nasogastric feeding. Different method were used to decorporate thallium during a long hospitalization. DDC increased b-TL and induced a clinical deterioration and its use should be abandoned in Tl poisoning, hemofiltration was ineffective while oral PB, forced diuresis and hemodialysis were most. The patient survived with severe chronic neurological damage.

Niehues et al. (1995) described a suicidal ingestion of Tl containing rat poison in 16-year-old girl. After various enteric detoxification procedures, forced dialysis, and then hemodialysis were instituted combined with PB chelation. She had no intoxication symptoms at any time. She was discharged after 10 days, but 5 days later she was again admitted in a state of agitation with vomiting and abdominal pain, and paraesthesias of the hands and feet, after again having ingested rat poison. Physical examination only revealed diffuse alopecia. She was treated with hemodialysis, forced diuresis, PB chelation, orthograde intestinal infusions, and potassium substitution. She was transferred to psychiatric care after 28 days.

Atsmon, Taliansky, Landau, and Neufeld (2000) reported the first registered case of Tl poisoning in Israel in almost 30 years. A 40-year-old man was apparently poisoned by unknowingly drinking Tl containing alcoholic beverages at several occasions served by a business associate. Due to recurrent thallium ingestion and delayed admission he presented with both acute and chronic symptoms. PB chelation and forced diuresis were employed. The patient survived, some neurologic sequelae remained.

Pau (2000) described a case of acute thallium poisoning in a 67-year-old Chinese woman presenting with pain in the chest, abdomen, and lower limbs. Diagnosis was delayed until alopecia developed after about 2 weeks, then PB chelation was initiated. The patient's motor function was recovered after about 1 year, but residual sensory neuropathy remained likely due to the delay in chelation treatment.

Sun et al. (2012) described a series of 14 patients treated after considerable delays, 9–19 days, for acute Tl poisoning via food. The patients presented with gastrointestinal symptoms, painful combined polyneuropathy, fatigue, skin pigmentation, and allopecia. The patients were hemodialysed and chelated with oral PB and DMPS. One patient diagnosed with pulmonary fibrosis died from respiratory failure. Liver damage, delirium, and coma occurred in the minority of patients. Symptoms slowly improved and blood or urine Tl levels normalized before discharge after several weeks. Follow-up after ½ year showed minor chronic peripheral neuropathy in 1 patient; 1 patient developed a deep venous thrombosis in the left lower limb, not necessarily related to the Tl poisoning. In another patient numbness in the lower limbs remained.

Huang et al. (2014) reported survival of a patient despite supralethal blood Tl levels, 3.764 mg/L. He presented with numbness and stabbing pains in arms and legs and a pricking sensation that started 2 days before examination. The symptoms worsened over the following 2 days. His girlfriend then admitted to have intentionally poisoned him by thallium nitrate in his supper. He was then chelated with oral PB, 250 mg/kg per day divided in 4 doses. He received several rounds of combined hemoperfusion (HP) and continuous veno-venous hemofiltration (CVVH). Both treatments extensively reduced blood thallium levels. This treatment combined with intramuscular injection of 250 mg DMPS per day and general supportive therapy resulted in survival of the patient without lasting neurological damage.

4.20.3 Conclusions

Development of an optimal treatment of acute and chronic Tl poisoning is limited by the lack of controlled clinical trials of treatments in thallium-poisoned patients combined with case reports with limited data, However, in most clinical cases (and in animal experiments) PB chelation induced high fecal thallium excretion and also urinary excretion. The literature on experimental animal studies is growing but still incomplete. The presently considered optimal strategy for treatment of thallium poisoning is based on such available information: a combination of the following elements according to need and severity of the poisoning: oral PB administration after gastric lavage alone or with single- or multiple-dose activated charcoal, K^+ infusion, forced diuresis with furosemide and mannitol, hemodialysis, hemoperfusion or charcoal hemoperfusion, continuous veno-venous hemofiltration or double-filtration plasmapheresis as needed. Forced potassium diuresis appears harmful. Since the safety profile of PB is superior to that of other proposed therapies, it is considered the chelating drug of choice in acute thallium poisoning (Stevens et al., 1974; IPCS, 1992; Wainwright et al., 1988; Hoffman, 2003).

4.21 TIN

Tin (Sn from Latin *stannum*, atomic number 50 in Group 14 of the Periodic Table of the Elements, atomic weight 118.71, density 7.265 g/cm^3) has 10 stable isotopes. Metallic tin is insoluble in water and resistant to oxygen and occurs in 3 allotropic forms, gray cubic α tin, white tetragonal β tin, and rhombic, brittle γ tin. Cooling white β tin below 13.2°C results in change to the gray α form, a process called "tin pest." Tin exist in four oxidation states: −2, 0, +2, and +4, in inorganic compounds the oxidation state +2 in stannous compounds readily oxidizes at high pH, and +4 in stannic compounds is more stable than stannous compounds. Both tend to hydrolyze in solution. Tin is a relatively rare element, with an abundance in the Earth's crust of about 2.2 parts per million. Tin does not occur as a free metal in nature. The major ore for tin mining is cassiterite

(SnO_2), ores of less importance are tin containing sulfide minerals as stannite (Cu_2S-FeS-SnS_2), teallite ($PbSnS_2$), cylindrite ($Pb_3Sn_4FeSb_2S_{14}$), and frankeite ($Fe(Pb,Sn)_6Sn_2Sb_2S_{14}$).

Global tin reserves are estimated to be 4.7 million tons, the total tin production was 240,000 tons in 2012 and 230,000 tons in 2013. Major tin producing countries are China (44%), Indonesia (21%), and Peru (14%) (USGS, 2015). Important inorganic tin compounds are the chlorides $SnCl_2$ and $SnCl_4$, and SnO, and SnF_2. Organic tin compounds exist as mono-, di-, tri-, and tetraorgano-tin compounds with covalently bound alkyl or aryl groups and coordinated ligands as halides, oxides, hydroxides, carboxylates, or mercaptides. Tetra- and triorganotin compounds have low water solubility but are soluble in organic solvents, dimethyltin dichloride is soluble in water, and monoorganotins are hygroscopic and hydrolyze in acidic water. Most environmental organic tin compounds are leached from, for example, man-made biocides and stabilizers, naturally occurring organotin compounds are produced by microbial methylation of inorganic tin in sewage and estuarine waters and in sediment (Quevauviller, Lavigne, Pinel, Astruc, 1989).

Decreased use of lead in plumbing has led to increased demands for inorganic tin as substitute. Rising tin prices have resulted in increased recycling, the largest producers are France and USA. A major use of inorganic tin is in solder, an alloy of 63% tin and lead, primarily used for electronic applications and accounting for more than 50% of tin use. Lead-free tin solders, containing up to 5% silver or antimony, are used at high temperatures. Other important uses of tin are in cans and containers, alloys, electrical applications, construction, electrolytes, dental implants, and intermediates in the manufacture of other compounds. Stannous chloride is the most commercially used inorganic tin compound in organic and inorganic synthesis and tin galvanizing.

Alkyltin compounds have been widely used in skin contact textiles, wall and floor coverings, soft PVC profiles, coated fabrics for outdoor use, outdoor pipes, roofing materials industry, as biocides in ship paint and in agriculture, and as catalysts. Restrictions on organotin uses in many of the above products have resulted in gradual decrease in organotin production.

Tin has no known natural biological role in living organisms, the intestinal uptake and tissue retention are very limited, and inorganic tin compounds have very low toxicity allowing the use of tin in kitchen utensils (Johnson and Greger, 1982; Krigman and Silverman, 1984; Winship, 1988). High levels of tin in drinks or solid foods have induced vomiting, diarrhea, fatigue, and headaches (WHO, 2001, 2006).

Organic tin compounds have very high toxicity, and various organic tin compounds induce bile duct damage and thymus atrophy. Major toxic manifestations are strong neurotoxity. Organotin compounds are metabolized by dealkylation reactions leading to potential systemic exposure to mixtures of mono- di- tri- and tetra alkyl/aryl tin compound, depending on the exposure compounds.

4.21.1 Animal Experimental and Clinical Studies

BAL chelation only marginally reduced dibutyltin-induced thymus and bile duct damage in mice, DMSA being more efficacious, but without reducing mortality. DMSA was however an antidote in rats: Merkord, Weber, Kröning, and Hennighausen (2000) investigated the antidotal effects of DMPS and DMSA on toxic effects of dibutyltin dichloride (DBTC) in rats. DMPS and DMSA reduced DBTC induced liver, bile duct, and pancreatic damage more than they reduced thymus atrophy. DMPS and DMSA reduced development of pancreatic fibrosis and hepatic cirrhosis several weeks after single administration of DBTC. The antidotal effects on serum parameters were observed after oral as well as i.p. administration. DMPS more effective than DMSA corrected DBTC induced deviations in serum parameters; decreased biliary DBTC excretion induced by DMPS and DMSA is likely the reason for the antidotal effects of DMPS and DMSA on bile duct, pancreas, and liver.

Kreyberg, Torvik, Bjørneboe, Wiik-Larsen, and Jacobsen (1992) described poisoning of two women by trimethyltin added to redwine by the spouse of one of the women. She presented with lightheadedness, aggression, tinnitus, and episodes of unresponsiveness. She gradually developed coma and died from multiorgan failure after 1 week despite intravenous DMSA chelation. Pathologic findings included neuronal chromatolysis in brain, spinal cord and spinal ganglia, and recent neuronal necrosis in fascia dentata of the hippocampus and spinal ganglia. The other woman recovered gradually from severe neuropsychiatric symptoms over several months after several weeks of oral DMSA chelation mentioned by the authors to apparently improve her clinical condition.

4.21.2 Conclusions

The toxicology of tin is dominated by organotin compounds, and examples of chelation in inorganic tin poisoning have not been identified. The experience with chelation treatment of organotin poisoning is very limited, and recommendation cannot be offered.

4.22 ZINC

Zinc (Zn, atomic number 30, first element of group 12 of the periodic table of the elements, atomic weight, 65.38, density 7.14 g/cm^3, most common oxidation states 0, +1 and +2) is a bluish-white transition metal with five stable isotopes, ^{64}Zn (49%), ^{66}Zn (28%), ^{67}Zn (4.1%), ^{68}Zn (19%), ^{70}Zn (0.62%), and 19 known radioactive isotopes, ^{65}Zn ($t_{1/2}$ 243.8 days, ε and γ decay) is suited for biokinetic studies. Paracelsus is believed to have taken the name for this element from the German word *Zinke*. The oldest documented production of pure zinc was in Zawar, Rajasthan, in the 9th century AD (Kharakwal & Gurjar, 2006). Brass, an alloy of copper and zinc, was used in Judea since the 10th century BC and in Ancient Greece since the 7th century BC (Craddock, 1978).

Metallic Zn reacts with O_2 to form ZnO, Cl_2 to form $ZnCl_2$, and with elemental S to form ZnS (Greenwood & Earnshaw, 2011). Zinc is stable in dry air, but in moist air it forms Zn oxide or basic carbonate on the surface. Zinc is the 24th most abundant element, 0.02% by weight of the Earth's crust. The most important ore is sphalerite [zincblende, (Zn,Fe)S with varying proportion of iron], major deposits are found in Australia, Asia, and USA. The world zinc production was 13.5 million tons in 2012 and in 2013 (USGS, 2015). Zinc is used as a protective coating for other metals, in the construction industry, and in noncorrosive alloys. Zinc oxide is the most common Zn compound used in industry and is used in pigment production ("zinc white") and in production of rubber. Inorganic Zn compounds are further used in automotive equipment, storage and dry cell batteries, and dental, medical, and household applications. Soldering flux solutions with zinc salts are highly corrosive. Skin ointments and creams contain zinc oxide at levels toxic upon oral intake. Organic Zn compounds are used as fungicides, lubricants, and topical antibiotics (Simon-Hettich, Wibbertmann, Wagner, Tomaska, & Malcolm, 2001).

Zinc is an essential element necessary for an extensive number of biological structures and processes (Maret, 2013). Zinc is redox neutral in biological systems (Maret, 2013) and readily binds to various amino acid motifs in numerous proteins. More than 3000 proteins with such motifs are known (Andreini, Banci, & Bertini, 2006). Zinc is especially important for pre-, peri-, and postnatal development. Severe deficiency leads to retarded growth and delayed development in infants. Subclinical biochemical and functional disturbances precede clinical symptoms as dementia and acrodermatitis (Kay, Tasman-Jones, Pybus, Whiting, & Black, 1976; Arakawa, Tamura, & Igarashi, 1976; Neldner, Hambidge, & Walravens, 1978). Intestinal zinc uptake is facilitated by the zinc transporter ZIP4 in the apical membrane of the enterocyte (Cousins, 2010) and takes place in the entire small intestine, the largest amounts are absorbed in the duodenum (Solomons, 1982), but zinc is also absorbed in the colon (Sandstrom, Cederblad, Kivisto, Stenquist, & Andersson, 1986). The main Zinc excretion routes are via pancreatic and intestinal secretions to feces (Sandstrom, 1997), with some reabsorbtion in the jejunum, ileum, and colon.

Exposures to Zn metal and Zn compounds occur in Zn mining and smelting, welding, and other industrial activities using zinc (Simon-Hettich et al., 2001). Inhalation of Zn oxide fumes formed at high temperature, for example, welding on zinc-plated items, can induce acute respiratory distress with flu-like symptoms as fever, chills, nausea, myalgia, fatigue, and shortness of breath, a form of metal fume fever known as zinc fever, brassfounder's ague, or Zn chills.

Dietary zinc poisoning seldomly occur but could result from intake of acidic juice stored in galvanized containers. Signs and symptoms include severe nausea, vomiting, abdominal cramps, diarrhea, and tenesmus (Brown, Thom, Orth, Cova, & Juare, 1964). Ingestion of Zn chloride can induce pancreatitis leading to exocrine insufficiency (McKinney, Brent, & Kulig, 1995).

4.22.1 Experimental and Clinical Chelation Studies

Eybl, Sykora, and Mertl (1970) compared the mobilizing effects of polyaminopolycarboxylic acids in zinc-loaded rats, DTPA, and TTHA most efficiently increased fecal and urinary zinc excretion and decreased organ zinc levels.

Aaseth, Søli, and Førre (1979) found that DDC enhanced the zinc deposition in the brain of mice.

Basinger and Jones (1981b) compared the antidotal efficacy of several chelating agents against acute parenteral zinc poisoning in mice and found that DMSA efficiently reduced acute mortality.

Llobet, Domingo, and Corbella (1988b) found that among 16 chelators DTPA, CDTA, EDTA with decreasing effectiveness were effective antidotes in acute zinc intoxication, both enhancing zinc excretion and preventing mortality. DMSA afforded some protection at a higher ratio between chelator and zinc dose, while DMPS and DPA had rather low antidotal effects.

Llobet, Colomina, Domingo, and Corbella (1989) studied the effect of time between zinc- and chelator administration in acute zinc poisoning in mice by measuring zinc excretion and organ zinc levels. DTPA and CDTA increased fecal and urinary zinc excretion with decreasing effectiveness at later times after zinc administration. The largest antidotal effect was observed 0.50 h after zinc administration. DTPA more effectively than CDTA prevented acute zinc poisoning.

Both EDTA and DTPA mobilize Zn in humans (Catsch & Harmuth-Hoehne, 1976). There is very limited knowledge about the efficiency of BAL in acute zinc poisoning. A limited number of clinical cases of chelation treatment of acute zinc intoxication have been published.

Chobanian (1981) described a 24-year-old man who accidentally drank a $ZnCl_2$ solution and presented with nausea, abdominal vomiting and pain, hyperamylasemia and hypocalcemia indicating acute pancreatitis. He had erosive pharyngitis and esophagitis and developed lethargy and confusion. Despite development of microhematuria his renal function did not deteriorate. Chelation therapy with i.v. CaNa2EDTA, 15 mg/kg every 12 h, was instituted, with reversal of the clinical and biochemical effects of zinc poisoning.

McKinney, Brent, and Kulig (1994) described a 16-month-old boy who was admitted vomiting in a lethargic state with progressing respiratory symptoms after ingestion of about one tablespoon of a $ZnCl_2$ soldering flux solution. He received supportive care with i.v. fluids, i.v. penicillin, and humidified oxygen pn. Peak measured plasma Zn was 11,99 μg/L. Progressing esophageal and gastric ulcerations with mucosal sloughing and coagulative necrosis developed over several days as observed by repeated endoscopy. Transfusion of packed erythrocytes was given due to decreasing hemoglobin values, likely caused by gastric bleeding. Transient pancreatic and hepatobiliary dysfunction with metabolic acidosis rapidly improved, while kidney function was not affected. Chelation therapy with i.v. EDTA and i.m. BAL started on day 4 leading to clinical improvement, however, without apparent increase in urinary zinc excretion The extensive esophageal and gastric scarring necessitated total parenteral nutrition upon discharge. Due to scarring in the gastric antrum an antrectomy was performed several weeks later reestablished gastric-duodenal passage.

Hantson et al. (1996) described a 86-year-old woman who accidentally drank a solution containing 3 g of each of $ZnSO_4$ and $CuSO_4$ ("Eau de Dalibour" used in diluted form to treat skin ulcers). At 90 min after ingestion, Zn and Cu peak plasma levels were 1.9790 and 2.090 mg/L, respectively, indicating high zinc absorption. The corrosive properties of the solution induced gastric and bronchial inflammation. She received gastric lavage and i.v. fluid, and 4 mg/kg BAL i.m. every 6 h and 250 mg DPA every 6 h via the nasogastric tube. This chelation was started less than 4 h after ingestion. She developed cardiovascular failure and renal insufficiency and her deteriorating condition necessitated intubation for mechanical ventilation on day 3. Her clinical condition gradually improved and she was extubated on day 16 and discharged on day 20 with normal renal and cardiac function. The patient made a complete recovery. According to the authors the chelation therapy apparently did not improve her condition based on available clinical and toxicokinetic data.

Hantson, Lula, Lievens, and Mahieu (1998) described a 20-year-old woman ingesting a metal scouring solution containing 385 g/L of $ZnCl_2$ for suicidal purpose. She rapidly developed extensive ulcerative and necrotic lesions in the gastric mucosa but only mild esophageal ulcerations. Bronchoscopy did not demonstrate damage in trachea or the bronchial tree. She received supportive care with i.v. fluid administration and mechanical ventilation. Chelation with i.m. BAL initiated 6 h after ingestion was associated with increased urinary Zn excretion. She was discharged on day 18 after a complete recovery.

It is difficult to assess whether Zn or Cu induced the major toxic insult in the case described by Hantson et al. (1996). The chelators BAL and DPA are both grossly ineffective in Zn poisoning, and it is fair to state that only the Cu poisoning was (if at all) affected by the chelation treatment. Also in the case described by Hantson et al. (1998) the chelation is unlikely to have enhanced recovery.

4.22.2 Conclusions

A potentially effective chelation treatment in acute human oral zinc poisoning would likely be immediate oral $CaNa_3DTPA$ administration after gastric decontamination followed by i.v. $CaNa_3DTPA$ chelation.

4.23 SUMMARY, CONCLUSIONS, AND PERSPECTIVES

The literature work associated with writing this chaper disclosed the surprising fact that despite the vast majority of acute metal poisonings are by the oral route due to accidental, suicidal or homicidal poisoning, by far the majority of experimental studies of effects of chelation in acute metal poisoning used parenteral (mainly intraperitoneal but also intramuscular or intravenous) administration of a metal salt and most often also parenteral administration of chelating agents intended to alleviate acute toxicity and enhance decorporation of absorbed metal. Only a couple of cases of suicidal i.v. injection of a metal salt and about a handful of i.v. injection of metallic mercury have been found in the clinical literature, while i.p. or i.m. accidental, homicidal or suicidal injection apparently never took place in humans.

The few examples of other administration routes in acute poisoning animal studies were a limited number using pulmonary exposure to, for example, nickel carbonyl or mercury vapor, or dermal exposure to, for example, nickel, and then a small number of animal studies using oral exposure to a metal salt to optimize acute chelation treatment preventing local toxicity including tissue damage and reducing systemic uptake. Based on experimental and clinical work, preliminary recommendations for chelating agents in acute poisonings with selected metals are:

- DFO for aluminum compounds, L1 and deferasirox are potential chelators.
- DMPS for acute and chronic poisonings by arsenic compounds.
- DFO for acute oral poisoning by iron compounds, L1 and deferasirox are potential chelators.
- DMSA for acute oral and chronic poisonings by lead compounds.
- DMPS for oral poisoning with inorganic mercury compounds and pulmonary poisoning with mercury vapor, DMSA may be superior for organic mercury compounds.

The classic chelators DPA, BAL, and EDTA have been used generally for decades in acute poisoning by several metals and are today outdated for most uses and even contraindicated in some situations. DMSA and DMPS are taking over, but still today clinical case reports of poisonings are seen where chelation with DPA, BAL, or EDTA was used despite they are suboptimal compared to DMSA or DMPS. This situation could be improved if experimental toxicologists would perform comparative studies of efficacies of the "old" clinical chelators compared to the "new" chelators, using administration routes that are relevant for human poisonings, that is, mainly oral.

Future development in clinical chelation will concentrate on further development of combined chelation schedules with lipophilic and hydrophilic chelators, further development of macromolecular chelators for gastrointestinal, dermal and extracorporal chelation, and continued development of new, often amphiphilic chelators including various esters of classic chelators, mainly DMSA, and amphiphilic chelators based on alkylation and carboxymethylation of DTPA being evaluated as decorporating agents for several metals. Kojic acid, hydroxypyridinone, catechole, bis-phosphonates calixarenes and triazoles are derivatized to form new chelating agents to be used both orally and poarenterally. In general, experimental chelating agents efficient in animal experiments cannot be used in humans except in cases, where the benefit clearly outweighs the potential toxicity of the agent, the same safety studies as for drugs in general are in principle required. Due to extensive experimental work by dedicated scientists establishing safety profiles, also some of the new compounds are on their way into clinical practice. This work can be is facilitated by giving orphan drug status to the moist promising compounds. The US Orphan Drug Act (ODA) administered by the USFDA can give orphan drug status to a drug to treat a rare disease or condition. This status offers various economic incentives to the developer: Tax credits for development expenses and marketing exclusivity in the US for 7 years after approval. In the European Union the European Medicines Agency (EMA) can give orphan drug status with developmental incentives and marketing exclusivity in the EU for 10 years after approval. DMSA (Chemet, succimer) was originally developed with orphan drug status by Bock Pharmaceutical Company (later sold to Sanofi) approved by the FDA, and in 1991, the FDA registered DMSA for lead poisoning in children providing exclusivity until 1998.

L1 (deferiprone, Ferriprox) was invented and developed for oral treatment of iron overload in UK academic institutions financed by thalassaemia patient organizations. L1 was licenced in EU in 2000 and has US orphan drug status for the treatment of iron overload in α and β thalassaemias, and sickle cell anemia (US licenced in 2011). Deferasirox (Exjade) by Novartis has been US licenced since 2005. It has EU orphan drug designation for oral chelation treatment of α and β thalassaemias, sickle cell anemia, and transfusional siderosis resulting from therapeutic palliation of sideroblastic anemia and other cases of myelodysplastic syndrome.

Important research needs for development of new chelating agents and further development of existing chelating agents:

- New oral chelators to reduce i.m./i.v. infusion based chelation (EDTA, DTPA, and DFO) in cases of mass poisoning.
- New oral chelators for protecting against metal induced GI tissue damage and for reducing GI absorption, for example, thiolated macromolecules.
- Further development of oral DTPA and oral Prussian Blue for iron and other oral poisonings.
- Further development of DTPA nebulizers and development of more efficient chelator preparations for inhalation in pulmonary metal poisonings protecting lung tissue and reducing systemic uptake.

Finally, despite a very large number of animal experimental studies have been published, comparative animal studies of efficacy of DMSA/DMPS versus BAL/NAPA/DPA/EDTA in acute As, Pb, Hg, and other poisonings are still lacking. Thus, should the BAL/EDTA combination still be used for acute Pb encephalopathy? In conclusion, lots of basic work are still needed!

REFERENCES

Aaseth, J. (1983). Recent advance in the therapy of metal poisonings with chelating agents. *Human and Experimental Toxicology*, *2*, 257–272.

Aaseth, J., & Friedheim, E. A. (1978). Treatment of methyl mercury poisoning in mice with 2,3-dimercaptosuccinic acid and other complexing thiols. *Acta Pharmacology and Toxicology*, *42*, 248–252.

Aaseth, J., Søli, N. E., & Førre, Ø. (1979). Increased brain uyptake of copper and zinc in mice caused by diethyldithiocarbamate. *Acta Pharmacology Et Toxicology*, *45*, 41–44.

Aaseth, J., Jellum, E., & Munthe, E. (1980). The effect of penicillamine and 2,3-dimercaptosuccinic acid on urinary excretion and tissue distribution of gold. *Scandenavian Journal of Reumathology*, *9*, 157–160.

Aaseth, J., Olsen, A., Halse, J., & Hovig, T. (1981). Argyria-tissue deposition of silver as selenide. *Scandinavian Journal of Clinical and Laboratory Investigation*, *41*, 247–251.

Aaseth, J., Haugen, M., & Førre, Ø. (1998). Rheumatoid arthritis and metal compounds—perspectives on the role of oxygen radical detoxification. *Analyst*, *123*, 3–6.

Ackrill, P., Ralston, A. J., Day, J. P., & Hodge, K. C. (1980). Successful removal of aluminium from a patient with dialysis encephalopathy. *Lancet*, *2*, 692–693.

Ahmed, S., Rahman, A., Saleem, M., Athar, M., & Sultana, S. (1999). Ellagic acid ameliorates nickel induced biochemical alterations: diminution of oxidative stress. *Human and Experimental Toxicology*, *18*, 691–698.

Aitio, A. I. O., Kiilunen, M., Santonen, T., & Nordberg, M. (2014). Gold and gold mining. In G. F. Nordberg, B. A. Fowler, & M. Nordberg (Eds.), *Handbook on the toxicology of metals* (4th ed., pp. 817–843). Amsterdam, NL: Elsevier/AP.

Akyildiz, B. N., Kondolot, M., Kurtoğlu, S., & Konuşkan, B. (2012). Case series of mercury toxicity among children in a hot, closed environment. *Pediatric Emergency Care*, *28*(3), 254–258.

Alexander, C. S. (1972). Cobalt-beer cardiomyopathy. A clinical and pathologic study of twenty-eight cases. *American Journal of Medicine*, *53*, 395–417.

Alexander, J., & Aaseth, J. (1981). Hepatobiliary transport and organ distribution of silver in the rat as influenced by selenite. *Toxicology*, *21*, 179–186.

Alfrey, A. C., & Froment, D. C. (1990). In M. E. de Broe, & J. W. Coburn (Eds.), *Aluminum and renal failure* (pp. 249–257). Dordrecht: Kluwer Academic Publishers.

Alfrey, A. C., Mishell, J. M., Burks, J., et al. (1972). Syndrome of dyspraxia and multifocal seizures associated with chronic hemodialysis. *Transactions—American Society for Artificial Internal Organs*, *18*, 257–261.

Alfrey, A. C., LeGendre, G. R., & Kaehny, W. D. (1976). The dialysis encephalopathy syndrome. Possible aluminum intoxication. *New England Journal of Medicine*, *294*, 184–188.

Alhamad, T., Rooney, J., Nwosu, A., MacCombs, J., Kim, Y. -S., & Shukla, V. (2012). Lessons learned from a fatal case of mercury intoxication. *International Urology and Nephrology*, *44*, 647–651.

Alhazzaa, S. A. F., & Krahn, P. M. (1995). Kohl—a hazardous eyeliner. *International Ophtalmology*, *19*, 83–88.

Allain, P., Krari, N., Chaleil, D., Lagier, G., & Jouglard, J. (1991). Effects of some chelating agents on bismuth absorption in the rat. *Fundamental & Clinical Pharmacology*, *5*, 39–45.

Allenby, C. F., & Goodwin, B. F. J. (1983). Influence of detergent washing powders on minimal eliciting patch test concentrations of nickel and chromium. *Contact Dermatitis*, *9*, 491–499.

Ambrus, C. M., Anthone, S., Stadler, A., Cameron, M. S., Wellsm, K., Stadlerm, I., & Ambrusm, J. L., Jr. (2001). Treatment of lead poisoning with an immobilized chelator comparison with conventional therapy. *Research Communications in Molecular Pathology and Pharmacology.*, *110*, 253–263.

Andersen, H. R., & Andersen, O. (1989). Effect of nickel chloride on hepatic lipid peroxidation and glutathione concentration in mice. *Journal of Trace Elements and Research*, *21*, 255–261.

Andersen, O. (1989a). Choice of chelating antidotes for acute cadmium intoxication. *Toxicological and Environmental Chemistry*, *23*, 105–120.

Andersen, O. (1989b). Oral cadmium exposure in mice: toxicokinetics and efficiency of chelating agents. *Critical Reviews in Toxicology*, *20*, 83–112.

Andersen, O. (1999). Principles and recent developments in chelation treatment of metal intoxication. *Chemical Reviews*, *99*, 2683–2710.

Andersen, O., & Aaseth, J. (2002). Molecular mechanisms of in vivo metal chelation: implications for clinical treatment of metal intoxications. *Environmental Health Perspectives*(110 Suppl.), 887–890.

Andersen, O., & Grandjean, P. (1989). Effects of tetraethylthiuram disulfide on the toxicokinetics of cadmium in mice. *Pharmacology and Toxicology*, *64*, 210–215.

Andersen, O., & Nielsen, J. B. (1989). Effects of diethyldithiocarbamate on the toxicokinetics of cadmium chloride in mice. *Toxicology*, *55*, 1–14.

Andersen, O., Nielsen, J. B., & Svendsen, P. (1988a). Oral cadmium chloride intoxication in mice: diethyldithiocarbamate enhances rather than alleviates acute toxicity. *Toxicology*, *52*, 331–342.

Andersen, O., Nielsen, J. B., & Svendsen, P. (1988b). Oral cadmium chloride intoxication in mice: effects of chelation. *Toxicology*, *52*, 65–79.

Andersen, O., Nielsen, J. B., & Svendsen, P. (1988c). Oral cadmium chloride intoxication in mice: effects of dose on tissue damage, intestinal absorption and relative organ distribution. *Toxicology*, *48*, 225–236.

Anderson, C. G. (2012). The metallurgy of antimony. *Chemie der Erde*, *72 S4*, 3–8.

Anderson, R. A., Bryden, N. A., & Waters, R. (1999). EDTA chelation therapy does not selectively increase chromium losses. *Biological Trace Element Research*, *70*, 265–272.

Andreini, C., Banci, L., Bertini, I., et al. (2006). Counting the zinc-proteins encoded in the human genome. *Journal of Proteome Research*, *5*, 196–201.

Anke, M., Groppel, B., Kronemann, H., et al. (1984). Nickel—an essential element. *IARC Scientific Publications*, *53*, 339–365.

Anthone, S., Ambrus, C. M., Kohli, R., Min, I., Anthone, R., Stadler, A., Stadler, I., & Vladutiu, A. (1995). Treatment of aluminum overload using a cartridge with immobilized desferrioxamine. *Journal of American Society of Nephrology*, *6*, 1271–1277.

Antonini, J. M., Roberts, J. R., Stone, S., et al. (2011). Persistence of deposited metals in the lungs after stainless steel and mild steel welding fume inhalation in rats. *Archives of Toxicology*, *85*, 487–498.

Aposhian, H. V., Tadlock, C. H., & Moon, T. E. (1981). Protection of mice against the lethal effects of sodium arsenite—a quantitative comparison of a number of chelating agents. *Toxicology and Applied Pharmacology*, *61*, 385–392.

Aposhian, H. V., Carter, D. E., Hoover, T. D., Hsu, C. -A., Mariano, R. M., & Stine, E. (1984). DMSA, DMPS, and DMPA—as arsenic antidotes. *Fundamental and Applied Toxicology*, *4*, S58–S70.

Aposhian, H. V., Bruce, D. C., Alter, W., Dart, R. C., Hurlbut, K. M., & Aposhian, M. M. (1992). Urinary mercury after administration of 2,3-dimercaptopropane-1-sulfonic acid: correlation with dental amalgam score. *The FASEB Journal*, *6*, 2472–2476.

Aposhian, M. M., Maiorino, R. M., Xu, Z. F., & Aposhian, H. V. (1996). Sodium 2,3-dimercapto-1-propanesulfonate (DMPS) treatment does not redistribute lead or mercury to the brain of rats. *Toxicology*, *109*, 49–55.

Aposhian, H. V., Arroyo, A., Cebrian, M. E., Del Razo, L. Z., Hurlbut, K. M., Dart, R. C., Gonzalez-Ramirez, D., Kreppel, H., Speisky, H., Smith, A., Gonsebatt, M. A., Strosky-Wegman, P., & Approshina, M. (1997). DMPSArsenic challenge test I. Increased urinary excretion of monomethylarsonic acid in humans given dimercaptopropane sulfonate. *Journal of Pharmacology and Experimental Therapeutics*, *282*, 192–200.

Appenroth, D., Winnefeld, K., Schröter, H., & Rost, M. (1993). Beneficial effect of acetylcysteine on cisplatin nephrotoxicity in rats. *Journal of Applied Toxicology*, *13*, 189–192.

Arakawa, T., Tamura, T., Igarashi, Y., et al. (1976). Zinc deficiency in two infants during total parenteral alimentation for diarrhea. *The American Journal of Clinical Nutrition*, *29*, 197–204.

Arenas, M. D., Malek, M. T., Gill, A., Moledus, C., Nunez, F., & Alvarez-Ude, F. (2008). Use of the aluminum phosphate-binders in hemodialysis in the ultrapure water era. *Nephrologia*, *28*, 168–173.

Artelt, S., Kock, H., Nachtigall, D., et al. (1998). Bioavailability of platinum emitted from automobile exhaust. *Toxicology Letters*, *96–97*, 163–167.

Artelt, S., Creutzenberg, O., Kock, H., et al. (1999). Bioavailability of fine dispersed platinum as emitted from automotive catalytic converters: a model study. *Science of the Total Environment*, *228*, 219–242.

Athar, M., Misra, M., & Srivastava, R. C. (1987). Evaluation of Chelating Drugs on the Toxicity, Excretion, and Distribution of Nickel in Poisoned Rats. *Fundamental and Applied Toxicology*, *9*, 26–33.

Atsmon, J., Taliansky, E., Landau, M., & Neufeld, M. Y. (2000). Thallium poisoning in Israel. *American Journal of Medical Sciences*, *320*, 327–330.

Atta, J. A., Faintuch, J. J., do Nascimento, L. O., Rocha, & Ados, S. (1992). Acute lethal intoxication caused by mercury vapor. *Revista do Hospital das Clínicas Universidade de São Paulo Hospital das Clínicas*, *47*, 34–37.

Bailly, R., Lauwerys, R., Buchet, J. P., Mahieu, P., & Konings, J. (1991). Experimental and human studies on antimony metabolism: their relevance for the biological monitoring of workers exposed to inorganic antimony. *British Journal of Industrial Medicine*, *48*, 93–97.

Baker, D. L., & Manno, C. S. (1988). Rapid excretion of gallium-67 isotope in an iron-overloaded patient receiving high-dose intravenous deferoxamine. *American Journal of Hematology*, *29*, 230–232.

Bakka, A., & Aaseth, J. (1979). Cadmium excretion in mice given dimercaptopropanesulphonate and some other complexing thiols. *Archives of Industrial Hygiene and Toxicology*(Suppl. 30), 183–189.

Bank, W. J., Pleasure, D. E., Suzuki, K., Nigro, M., & Katz, R. (1972). Thallium poisoning. *Archives of Neurology*, *26*, 456–464.

Banner, W., Jr., Koch, M., Capin, D. M., Hopf, S. B., Chang, S., & Tong, T. G. (1986). Experimental chelation therapy in chromium, lead, and boron intoxication with N-acetylcysteine and other compounds. *Toxicology and Applied Pharmacology*, *83*, 142–147.

Bansal, S. K., Haldar, N., Dhang, U. K., & Chopra, J. S. (1991). Phrenic neuropathy in arsenic poisoning. *Chest*, *100*, 878–880.

Barata, J. D., D'Haese, P. C., Pires, C., Lamberts, L. V., Simoes, J., & De Broe, M. E. (1996). Low-dose (5 mg/kg) desferrioxamine treatment in acutely aluminium-intoxicated haemodialysis patients using two drug administration schedules. *Nephrology Dialysis Transplantation*, *11*, 125–132.

Barceloux, D. G. (1999). Copper. *Journal of Toxicology: Clinical Toxicology*, *37*, 217–230.

Baresic, M., Gornik, I., Radonic, R., Zlopasa, O., Gubarev, N., & Gasparovic, V. (2009). Survival after severe acute chromic acid poisoning complicated with renal and liver failure. *Internal Medicine*, *48*, 711–715.

Barr, J., Berkovitch, M., Tavori, I., Kariv, N., Schejter, A., & Eshel, G. (1999). Acute iron intoxication: the efficacy of deferiprone and sodium biocarbonate in the prevention of iron absorption from the digestive tract. *Veterinary and Human Toxicology*, *41*, 308–311.

Barroso-Moguel, R., Villeda-Hernandez, J., Mendez-Armanta, M., Rios, C., & Monroy-Noyola, A. (1994). Combined D-penicillamine and prussian blue as antidotal treatment against thallotoxicosis in rats: evaluation of cerebellar lesions. *Toxicology*, *89*, 15–24.

Barry, P. S. I. (1975). A comparison of concentrations of lead in human tissues. *British Journal of Industrial Medicine*, *32*, 119–139.

Baselt, R. C., & Hanson, V. W. (1982). Efficacy of orally-administered chelating agents for nickel carbonyl toxicity in rats. *Research Communication in Chemical Pathology and Pharmacology*, *38*, 113–124.

Baselt, R. C., Sunderman, F. W., Jr., Mitchell, J., & Horak, E. (1977). Comparisons of antidotal efficacy of sodium diethyldithiocarbamate, D-penicillamine and triethylenetetramine upon acute toxicity of nickel carbonyl in rats. *Research Communication in Chemical Pathology and Pharmacology*, *18*, 677–688.

Basinger, M. A., & Jones, M. M. (1981b). Chelate antidotal efficacy in acute zinc intoxication. *Research Communication in Chemical Pathology and Pharmacology*, *33*, 263.

Basinger, M. A., Jones, M. M., & Tarka, M. P. (1980). Relative efficacy of chelating agents as antidotes for acute nickel(II) acetate intoxication. *Research Communication in Chemical Pathology and Pharmacology*, *30*, 133–141.

Basinger, M. A., & Jones, M. M. (1981a). Structural requirements for chelate antidotal efficacy in acute antimony(iii) intoxication. *Research Communications in Chemical Pathology and Pharmacology*, *32*, 355–363.

Basinger, M. A., Jones, M. M., & Shinobu, L. A. (1981a). Structural requirements for chelate antidotes for acute cadmium intoxication. *Journal of Inorganic and Nuclear Chemistry*, *43*, 3039–3042.

Basinger, M. A., Casas, J. S., Jones, M. M., Weaver, A. D., & Weinstein, N. H. (1981b). Structural Requirements for Hg(II) Antidotes. *Journal of Inorganic and Nuclear Chemistry*, *43*, 1419–1425.

Basinger, M. A., Johnson, J. E., Burka, L. T., & Jones, M. M. (1982). Antidotes for acute beryllium sulfate intoxication in mice. *Research Communications in Chemical Pathology and Pharmacology*, *6*, 519–522.

Basinger, M. A., Jones, M. M., & Mc. Croskey, S. A. (1983). Antidotes for acute bismuth intoxication. *Journal of Toxicology: Clinical Toxicology*, *20*, 159–165.

Basinger, M. A., Gibbs, S. J., Forti, R. L., Mitchell, W. M., & Jones, M. M. (1985). Antidotes for gold (sodium bis[thiosulfato]gold[I]) intoxication in mice. *Journal of Rheumatology*, *12*, 274–278.

Basinger, M. A., Jones, M. M., Gilbreath, G., IV, Walker, E. M., Fody, E. P., & Mayhue, M. A. (1989). Dithiocarbamate-induced biliary platinum excretion and the control of *cis*-platinum nephrotoxicity. *Toxicology and Applied Pharmacology*, *97*, 279–288, 1989.

Basinger, M. A., Jones, M. M., & Holscher, M. A. (1990). L-methionine antagonism of *cis*-platinum nephrotoxicity. *Toxicology and Applied Pharmacology*, *103*, 1–15.

Beasley, D. M., Schep, L. J., Slaughter, R. J., Temple, W. A., & Michel, J. M. (2014). Full recovery from a potentially lethal dose of mercuric chloride. *Journal of Medical Toxicology*, *10*, 40–44.

Behari, J. R., & Tandon, S. K. (1980). Chelation in metal intoxication. VIII. Removal of chromium from organs of potassium chromate administered rats. *Clinical Toxicology*, *16*, 33–40.

Bellés, M., Sánchez, D. J., Gómez, M., Domingo, J. L., Jones, M. M., & Singh, P. K. (1996). Assessment of the protective activity of monisoamyl meso-2,3-dimercaptosuccinate against methylmercury-induced maternal and embryo/fetal toxicity in mice. *Toxicology*, *106*, 93–97.

Bentham Science. (1996). The Antimonials. *Current Medicinal Chemistry*, 304–305.

Bentur, Y., Brook, J. G., Behar, R., & Taitelman, U. (1987). Meso-2,3-dimercaptosuccinic acid in the diagnosis and treatment of lead poisoning. *Clinical Toxicology*, *25*, 39–51.

Bentur, Y., Klein, J., Levy, M., Olivieri, N., McGuigan, M., & Koren, G. (1990). Methodological issues in studying the effect of the new oral chelator 1,2-dimethyl-3-hydroxypyrid-4-one (L1) on absorption of iron. *Veterinary Human Toxicology*, *32*, 159–161.

Berg, M., Tran, H. C., Nguyen, T. C., Pham, H. V., Schertenleib, R., & Giger, W. (2001). Arsenic contamination of groundwater and drinking water in vietnam: a human health threat. *Environmental and Science Technology*, *35*, 2621–2626.

Bergdahl, I. A., Schutz, A., & Grubb, A. (1996). Application of liquid chromatography–inductively coupled plasma mass spectrometry to the study of protein-bound lead in human erythrocytes. *Journal of Analytical Atomic Spectrometry*, *11*, 735–738.

Bergdahl, I. A., Schutz, A., Gerhardsson, L., & Skerfving, S. (1997). Lead concentrations in human plasma, urine and whole blood. *Scandinavian Journal of Work, Environment and Health, 23*, 359–363.

Bergdahl, I. A., Sheveleva, M., Schutz, A., Andrejs Schiitz, A., Volja, G., Artamonova, V. G., & Skerfving, S. (1998). Plasma and blood lead in humans: capacity-limited binding to 6-aminolevulinic acid dehydratase and other lead-binding components. *Toxicological Science, 46*, 247–253.

Berkovitch, M., Livne, A., Lushkov, G., Segal, M., Talmor, C., Bentur, Y., Klein, J., & Koren, G. (2000). The efficacy of oral deferiprone in acute iron poisoning. *American Journal of Emergency Medicine, 18*, 36–40.

Berlin, M., & Ullberg, S. (1963). Increased uptake of mercury in mouse brain caused by 2,3-dimercaptopropanol. *Nature, 197*, 84–85.

Berlin, M., Rudolfs, K., Zalups, R. K., & Fowler, B. A. (2014). Mercury. In F. Gunnar, G. F. Nordberg, B. A. Fowler, & M. Nordberg (Eds.), *Handbook on the toxicology of metals* (pp. 1013–1075). Amsterdam, NL: Elsevier/Academic Press.

Bernstein, L. R., Tanner, T., Godfrey, C., & Noll, B. (2000). Chemistry and pharmacokinetics of gallium maltolate, a compound with high oral gallium bioavailability. *Metal-Based Drugs, 7*, 33–47.

Besunder, J. B., Anderson, R. L., & Super, D. M. (1995). Short-term efficacy of oral dimercaptosuccinic acid in children with low to moderate lead intoxication. *Pediatrics, 96*, 683–687.

Besunder, J. B., Super, D. M., & Anderson, R. L. (1997). Comparison of dimercaptosuccinic acid and calcium disodium ethylenediaminetetraacetic acid versus dimercaptopropanol and ethylenediaminetetraacetic acid in children with lead poisoning. *Journal of Pediatrics, 130*, 966–971.

Beton, D. C., Andrews, G. S., Davies, H. J., Howells, L., & Smith, G. F. (1966). Acute Cadmium Fume Poisoning: Five Cases with one Death from Renal Necrosis. *British Journal of Industrial Medicine, 23*, 292–301.

Bhatt, K., & Flora, S. J. (2009). Oral co-administration of α-lipoic acid, quercetin and captopril prevents gallium arsenide toxicity in rats. *Environmental Toxicology and Pharmacology, 28*, 140–146.

Bhattacharya, R., & Mukherjee, P. (2008). Biological properties of "naked" metal nanoparticles. *Advanced Drug Delivery Reviews, 60*, 1289–1306.

Bhowmik, D., Mathur, R., Bhargava, Y., Dinda, A. K., Agarwal, S. K., Tiwari, S. C., & Dash, S. C. (2001). Chronic interstitial nephritis following parenteral copper sulfate poisoning. *Renal Failure, 23*, 731–735.

Bjerregaard, P., Andersen, C. B. I., & Andersen, O. (2014). Ecotoxicology of metals—sources, transport, and effects on the ecosystem. In G. F. Nordberg, B. A. Fowler, & M. Nordberg (Eds.), *Handbook on the toxicology of metals* (pp. 1013–1075). Amsterdam, NL: Elsevier/Academic Press.

Blaha, K., Nerudova, J., Jehlicova, H., Cikrt, M., Jones, M. M., & Singh, P. K. (1995). In vivo and in vitro efficacy of a new carbodithioate for the mobilization of cadmium. *Journal of Toxicology and Environmental Health, 44*, 87–100.

Blain, R., & Kazantzis, G. (2014). Thallium. In: Nordberg, G. F., Foøwler, B., & Nordberg, M. *Handbook on the toxicology of metals* (4th ed., pp. 1229-1240). Amsterdam NL: Elsevier/Academic Press.

Blanc, P. L., Saudin, F., Wilner, C., Gerard, M., Thomas, L., & Robert, D. (1980). A case of acute posisoning possibly related to antimony. *Medecine Legale Toxicologie, 23*, 637–642.

Blanusa, M., Prester, L., Varnai, V. M., Pavlovic, D., Kostial, K., Jones, M. M., & Singh, P. K. (2000). Chelation of aluminum by combining DFO and L1 in rats. *Toxicology, 147*, 151–156.

Blocka, K., Furst, D. E., Landaw, E., Dromgoole, S., Blomberg, A., & Paulus HE (1982). Single dose pharmacokinetics of auranofin in rheumatoid arthritis. *Journal of Rheumatology* (Suppl. 8), 110–119.

Bluhm, R. E., Bobbitt, R. G., Welch, L. W., Wood, A. J. J., Bonfiglio, J. F., Sarzen, C., Heath, A. J., & Branch, R. A. (1992). Elemental mercury vapour toxicity, treatment, and prognosis after acute, intensive exposure in chloralkali plant workers. Part I: history, neuropsychological findings and chelator effects. *Human and Experimental Toxicology*, *11*, 201–210.

Bokemeyer, C., Fels, L. M., Dunn, T., Voigt, W., Gaedeke, J., Schmoll, H. J., Stolte, H., & Lentzen, H. (1996). Silibinin protects against cisplatin-induced nephrotoxicity without compromising cisplatin or ifosfamide anti-tumour activity. *British Journal of Cancer*, *74*, 2036–2041.

Bolliger, C. T., van Zijl, P., & Louw, J. A. (1992). Multiple organ failure with the adult respiratory distress syndrome in homicidal arsenic poisoning. *Respiration*, *59*, 57–61.

Borch, R. F., Katz, J. C., Lieder, P. H., & Pleasants, M. E. (1980). Effect of diethyldithiocarbamate rescue on tumor response to *cis*-platinum in a rat model. *Proceedings of the Natural Academy of Sciences USA*, *77*, 5441–5444.

Bowden, C. A., & Krenzelok, E. P. (1997). Clinical applications of commonly used contemporary antidotes. A US perspective. *Drug Safety*, *16*, 9–47.

Bradberry, S. M. (2009). *The role of succimer (DMSA) in the treatment of inorganic lead poisoning*. Birmingham, UK: University of Birmingham.

Bradberry, S. M., & Vale, J. A. (1999). Therapeutic review: is ascorbic acid of value in chromium poisoning and chromium dermatitis? *Journal of Toxicology—Clinical Toxicology*, *37*, 195–200.

Bradberry, S., & Vale, A. (2009a). Dimercaptosuccinic acid (succimer; DMSA) in inorganic lead poisoning. *Clinical Toxicology*, *47*, 617–631.

Bradberry, S., & Vale, A. (2009b). Comparison of sodium calcium edetate (edetate calcium disodium) and succimer (DMSA) in the treatment of inorganic lead poisoning. *Clinical Toxicology*, *47*, 841–858.

Bradberry, S. M., Wilkinson, J. M., & Ferner, R. E. (2014). Systemic toxicity related to metal hip prostheses. *Clinical Toxicology (Philadelphia)*, *52*, 837–847.

Bradberry, S., Sheehan, T., & Vale, A. (2009). Use of oral dimercaptosuccinic acid (succimer) in adult patients with inorganic lead poisoning. *Quaterly Journal of Medicine*, *102*, 721–732.

Brannan, E. H., Su, S., & Alverson, B. K. (2012). Elemental mercury poisoning presenting as hypertension in a young child. *Pediatric Emergency Care*, *28*, 812–814.

Braun, H. A., Lusky, L. M., & Calvery, H. O. (1946). The efficacy of 2,3-dimercaptopropanol (BAL) in the therapy of poisoning by compounds of antimony, bismuth, chromium, mercury and nickel. *Journal of Pharmacology and Experimental Therapeutics*, *87*(Suppl.), 119–125.

Breeher, L., Gerr, F., & Fuortes, L. (2013). A case report of adult lead toxicity following use of ayurvedic herbal medication. *Journal of Occupational Medicine and Toxicology*, *8*, 26.

Brewer, G. J. (2009). Zinc and tetrathiomolybdate for the treatment of Wilson's disease and the potential efficacy of anticopper therapy in a wide variety of diseases. *Metallomics*, *1*, 199–206.

Brewer, G. J. (2012). Copper toxicity in Alzheimer's disease: Cognitive loss from ingestion of inorganic copper. *Journal of Trace Elements in Medicine and Biology*, *26*, 89–92.

Bronstein, A. C., Spyker, D. A., Cantilena, L. R., Jr., Green, J. L., Rumack, B. H., & Dart, R. C. (2010). Annual Report of the American Association of Poison Control Centers' National Poison Data System (NPDS): 28th Annual Report. *Clinical Toxicology (Philadelphia)*, *49*, 910–941.

Brown, M. A., Thom, J. V., Orth, G. L., Cova, P., & Juare, J. (1964). Food Poisoning involving Zinc Contamination. *Archives of Environmental Health*, *34*, 657–660.

Brydl, L. E., Hindsberger, C., Kyvik, K. O., Agner, T., & Menné, T. (2004). Genetic factors in nickel allergy evaluated in a population-based female twin sample. *Journal of Investigative Dermatology*, *123*, 1025–1029.

Buchet, J. P., & Lauwerys, R. R. (1989). Influence of 2,3-dimercaptopropane-1-sulfonate and dimercaptosuccinic acid on the mobilization of mercury from tissues of rats pretreated with mercuric chloride, phenylmercury acetate or mercury vapors. *Toxicology*, *54*, 323–333.

Bureau, Y., Barriere, H., Nicolas, G., & Leroux, M. J. (1962). Remarkable action of chelation in 2 cases of gold erythroderma. *Presse Med*, *70*, 1523–1525.

Butterman, W., Amey, E.R. (2005). Mineral commodity probiles—Gold. US Department of the Interior, US Geological Survey. http://pubs.usgs.gov/of/2002/of02-303/OFR_02-303.pdf

Campbell, G., Leitch, D., Lewington, A., Dargan, P. I., & Baker, R. J. (2009). Minimal-change nephrotic syndrome due to occupational mercury vapor inhalation. *Clinical Nephrology*, *72*, 216–219.

Canavese, C., Pacitti, A., Segoloni, G., Thea, A., D'Amicone, M., Stratta, P., Rossi, P., Sabbioni, E., Pietra, R., & Constantini, S. (1989). Clinical and histological results of long-term management of aluminium overloading in uraemic patients with desferrioxamine. *Journal of Trace Elements and Electrolytes in Health and Disease*, *3*, 17–23.

Canteros-Piccotto, M. A., Fernandez-Martin, J. L., Cannata-Ortiz, M. J., & Cannata-Andia, J. B. (1996). Effectiveness of deferiprone (L1) releasing the aluminium bound to plasma proteins in chronic renal failure. *Nephrology, Dialysis, Transplantation*, *11*, 1488–1489.

Cantilena, L. R., & Klaassen, C. D. (1981). Comparison of the effectiveness of several chelators after single administration on the toxicity, excretion, and distribution of cadmium. *Toxicology and Applied Pharmacology*, *58*, 452–460.

Cantilena, L.R., & Klaassen, C.D. (1982). Decreased effectiveness of chelation therapy with time after acute cadmium poisoning. *Toxicology and Applied Pharmacology*, *63*, 173–180.

Cao, Y., Chen, A., Jones, R. L., Radcliffe, J., Dietrich, K. N., Caldwell, K. L., Peddada, S., & Rogan, W. J. (2011). Efficacy of succimer chelation of mercury at background exposures in toddlers: a randomized trial. *Journal of Pediatrics*, *158*, 480–485.

Cao, Y., Chen, A., Bottai, M., Caldwell, K. L., & Rogan, W. J. (2013). The impact of succimer chelation on blood cadmium in children with background exposures: a randomized trial. *Journal of Pediatrics*, *163*, 598–600.

Carrier, P., Legros, R., Le Sidaner, A., Morel, A., Harry, P., Moesch, C., Sautereau, D., Ly, K. -H., & Loustaud-Ratti, V. (2012). Lead poisoning by fishing sinker ingestion. *Revue de Medicine interne*, *33*, 697–699.

Cash, R., Shapiro, R. I., Levy, S. H., & Hopkins, S. M. (1959). Chelating agents in the therapy of beryllium poisoning. *New England Journal of Medicine*, *260*, 683–686.

Catalani, S., Rizzetti, M. C., Padovani, A., & Apostoli, P. (2012). Neurotoxicity of cobalt. *Human and Experimental Toxicology*, *31*, 421–437.

Catsch, A., & Harmuth-Hoehne, A. E. (1976). Pharmacology and therapeutic applications of agents used in heavy metal poisoning. *Pharmacology and Therapeutics*, *1*, 1–118.

Cavanagh, J. B., & Gregson, L. (1978). Some effects of a thallium salt on the proliferation of hair follicle cells. *Journal of Pathology*, *125*, 179–191.

Cengiz, N., Uslu, Y., Gök, F., & Anarat, A. (2005). Acute renal failure after overdose of colloidal bismuth subcitrate. *Pediatric Nephrology*, *20*, 1355–1358.

Chalmin, E., Vignaud, C., Salomon, H., Farges, F., Susini, J., & Menu, M. (2006). Minerals discovered in paleolithic black pigments by transmission electron microscopy and micro-X-ray absorption near-edge structure. *Applied Physics A*, *83*, 213–218.

Chamberlain, P. H., Stavinoha, B., Davis, H., Kniker, W. T., & Panos, T. C. (1958). Thallium poisoning. *Pediatrics*, *22*, 1170–1176.

Charlier, C., Kintz, P., Dubois, N., & Plomteux, G. (2004). Fatal overdosage with cisplatin. *Journal of Analytical Toxicology*, *28*, 138–140.

Chaves, S., Dron, P. I., Danalache, F. A., Sacoto, D., Gano, L., & Santos, M. A. (2009). Combined chelation based on glycosyl-mono- and bis-hydroxypyridinones for aluminium mobilization: solution and biodistribution studies. *Journal of Inorganic Biochemistry*, *103*, 1521–1529.

Chen, H., Davidson, T., Singleton, S., Garrick, M. D., & Costa, M. (2005). Nickel decreases cellular iron level and converts cytosolic aconitase to iron-regulatory protein 1 in A549 cells. *Toxicology and Applied Pharmacology*, *206*, 275–287.

Chen, S. J., Zhou, G. B., Zhang, X. W., Mao, J. H., de The, H., & Chen, Z. (2011). From an old remedy to a magic bullet: molecular mechanisms underlying the therapeutic effects of arsenic in fighting leukemia. *Blood*, *117*, 6425–6437.

Cheney, K., Gumbiner, C., Benson, B., & Tenenbein, M. (1995). Survival after a severe iron poisoning treated with intermittent infusions of deferoxamine. *Journal of Toxicology: Clinical Toxicology*, *33*, 61–66.

Cherian, M. G. (1980). Biliary excretion of cadmium in rat. VI. Mobilization of cadmium from metallothionein by 2,3-dimercaptopropanol. *Journal of Toxicology and Environmental Health*, *6*, 393–401.

Chin, C. C. (1958). Detoxification of antimony potassium tartrate by Na-dimercaptopropanesulfonate. *Acta Physiologica Sinica*, *22*, 323–328.

Chisholm, J. J. (1968). The use of chelating agents in the treatment of acute and chronic lead intoxication in childhood. *Journal of Pediatrics*, *73*, 1–38.

Chisolm, J. J. (2000). Safety and efficacy of meso-2,3-dimercaptosuccinic acid (DMSA) in children with elevated blood lead concentrations. *Journal of Toxicology: Clinical Toxicology*, *38*, 365–375.

Chitambar, C. R. (2010). Medical applications and toxicities of gallium compounds. *International Journal of Environmental Research and Public Health*, *7*, 2337–2361.

Chobanian, S. J. (1981). Accidental ingestion of liquid zinc chloride: local and systemic effects. *Annals of Emergency Medicine*, *10*, 91–93.

Chou, C. J., Tsai, M. S., Tsai, J. L., Lee, H. H., & Lin, T. J. (2002). The chelating treatment is not useful in human's intoxication with acute herbicidal organic arsenic. *Human and Experimental Toxicology*, *21*, 631–634.

Christensen, J. D. (1982). Disulfiram treatment of three patients with nickel dermatitis. *Contact Dermatitis*, *8*, 105–108.

Christensen, O. B., & Kristensen, M. (1982). Treatment with disulfiram in chronic nickel hand dermatitis. *Contact Dermatitis*, *8*, 59–63.

Christopherson, J. B. (1918). The successful use of antimony in bilharziosis. *The Lancet*, *192*(4958), 325.

Chuttani, H. K., Gupta, P. S., Gulati, S., & Gupta, D. N. (1965). Acute copper sulfate poisoning. *American Journal of Medicine*, *39*, 849–854.

Cicek-Senturk, G., Altay, F. A., Ulu-Kilic, A., Gurbuz, Y., Tutuncu, E., & Sencan, I. (2014). Acute mercury poisoning presenting as fever of unknown origin in an adult woman: a case report. *Journal of Medical Case Reports*, *8*, 266.

Clarke, D., Buchanan, R., Gupta, N., & Haley, B. (2012). Amelioration of acute mercury toxicity by a novel, non-toxic lipid soluble chelator N,N′bis-(2-mercaptoethyl)isophthalamide: effect on animal survival, health, mercury excretion and organ accumulation. *Toxicology and Environmental Chemistry*, *94*, 616–640.

Cohen, M. A. (1988). Adverse reactions to gold compounds. *Adverse Drug Reactions and Acute Poisoning Reviews*, *7*, 163–178.

Collery, P., Domingo, J. L., & Keppler, B. K. (1996). Preclinical toxicology and tissue gallium distribution of a novel antitumour gallium compound: tris (8-quinolinolato) gallium (III). *Anticancer Research, 16*, 687–691.

Comar, C. L., & Davis, G. K. (1947). Cobalt metabolism studies. IV. Tissue distribution of radioactive cobalt administered to rabbits. swine and young calves. *Journal of Biological Chemistry, 170*, 379–389.

Cook, D. G., Fahn, S., & Brait, K. A. (1974). Chronic manganese intoxication. *Annals of Neurology, 30*, 59–64.

Corsello, S., Fulgenzi, A., Vietti, D., & Ferrero, M. E. (2009). The usefulness of chelation therapy for the remission of symptoms caused by previous treatment with mercury-containing pharmaceuticals: a case report. *Cases Journal, 18*(2), 1992009.

Cory-Slechta, D. A. (1988). Mobilization of lead over the course of DMSA chelation therapy and long-term efficacy. *Journal of Pharmacology and Experimental Therapeutics, 246*, 84–91.

Cory-Slechta, D. A., & Weiss, B. (1989). Efficacy of the chelating agent CaEDTA in reversing lead-induced changes in behavior. *Neurotoxicology, 10*, 685–698, 1989.

Cory-Slechta, D. A., Weiss, B., & Cox, C. (1987). Mobilization and redistribution of lead over the course of calcium disodium ethylenediamine tetraacetate chelation therapy. *Journal of Pharmacology and Experimental Therapeutics, 243*, 804–813.

Cousins, R. J. (2010). Gastrointestinal factors influencing zinc absorption and homeostasis. *International Journal for Vitamin and Nutrition Research, 80*, 243–248.

Craddock, P. T. (1978). The composition of copper alloys used by the Greek, Etruscan and Roman civilizations. The origins and early use of brass. *Journal of Archaeological Science, 5*, 1.

Cromwell, O., Pepys, J., Parish, W. E., & Hughes, E. G. (1979). Specific IgE antibodies to platinum salts in sensitized workers. *Clinical Allergy, 9*, 109–117.

Cullen, N. M., Wolf, L. R., & St. Clair, D. (1995). Pediatric arsenic ingestion. *American Journal of Emergency Medicine, 13*, 432–435.

Dalhamn, T., & Friberg, L. (1955). Dimercaprol (2, 3-dimercaptopropanol) in chronic cadmium poisoning. *Acta Pharmacology Toxicology, 11*, 68–71.

Dang, S., Rasmussen, C. A., & Levine, S. M. (1994). Immunocytochemical localization of desferrioxamine in the kidney, liver and brain of the developing and adult mouse: implications for drug processing and therapeutic mechanisms. *Research Communications in Chemical Pathology & Pharmacology, 86*, 43–57.

Daram, S. R., & Hayashi, P. H. (2005). Acute liver failure due to iron overdose in an adult. *Southern Medical Journal, 98*, 241–244.

Dargan, P. I., Giles, L. J., Wallace, C. I., House, I. M., Thomson, A. H., Beale, R. J., & Jones, A. L. (2003). Case report: severe mercuric sulphate poisoning treated with 2,3-dimercaptopropane-1-sulphonate and haemodiafiltration. *Critical Care, 7*, R1–R6.

Davison, S. (2003). *Conservation and restoration of glass*. Oxford: Butterworth-Heinemann.

Davis, P., & Barraclough, D. (1977). Interaction of D-penicillamine with gold salts: in vivo studies on gold chelation and in vitro studies on protein binding. *Arthritis & Rheumatology, 20*, 1413–1418.

Dean, B., Oehme, F. W., Krenzelok, E., & Hines, R. (1988). A study of iron complexation in a swine model. *Veterinary and Human Toxicology, 30*, 313–315.

Dean, B. S., Oehme, F. W., Krenzelok, E. P., Griffith, G. R., & Hines, R. H. (1996). Iron complexation with oral deferoxamine in a swine model. *Veterinary and Human Toxicology, 38*, 96–98.

DeGregorio, M. W., Gandara, D. R., Holleran, W. M., Perez, E. A., King, C. C., Wold, H. G., Montine, T. J., & Borch, R. F. (1989). High-dose cisplatin with diethyldithiocarbamate (DDTC) rescue therapy: preliminary pharmacologic observations. *Cancer Chemotherapy and Pharmacology, 23*, 276–278.

D'Haese, P. C., Couttenye, M. M., Goodman, W. G., Lemoniatou, E., Digenis, P., Sotornik, I., Fagalde, A., Barsoum, R. S., Lamberts, L. V., & De Broe, M. E. (1995). Use of the low-dose desferrioxamine test to diagnose and differentiate between patients with aluminium-related bone disease, increased risk for aluminium toxicity, or aluminium overload. *Nephrology, Dialysis, Transplantation, 10*, 1874–1884.

Dickey, D. T., Muldoon, L. L., Doolittle, N. D., Peterson, D. R., Kraemer, D. F., & Neuwelt, E. A. (2008). Effect of N-acetylcysteine route of administration on chemoprotection against cisplatin-induced toxicity in rat models. *Cancer Chemotherapy and Pharmacology, 62*, 235–241.

Ding, G. S., & Liang, Y. Y. (1991). Antidotal effects of dimercaptosuccinic acid. *Journal of Applied Toxicology, 11*, 7–14.

Domingo, J. L. (1989). Cobalt in the environment and its toxicological implications. *Reviews of Environmental Contamination and Toxicology, 108*, 105–132.

Domingo, J. L., & Llobet, J. M. (1984). Treatment of acute cobalt intoxication in rats with L-methionine. *Revista Española De Fisiología, 40*, 443–448.

Domingo, J. L., Llobet, J. M., & Corbella, J. (1983). The effects of EDTA in acute cobalt intoxication in rats. *Toxicological European Research, 5*, 251–255.

Domingo, J. L., Llobet, J. M., & Tomas, J. M. (1985). N-acetyl-L-cysteine in acute cobalt poisoning. *Archives of Pharmacology and Toxicology, 11*, 55–62.

Domingo, J. L., Llobet, J. M., & Corbella, J. (1987). Relative efficacy of chelating agents as antidotes for acute gallium nitrate intoxication. *Archives of Toxicology, 59*, 382–383.

Dong, H. Q., Wang, K. L., & Ma, Y. J. (1993). A clinical analysis of 117 cases of acute arsenic poisoning. *Zhonghua Nei Ke Za Zhi, 32*, 813–815.

Downs, W. L., Scott, J. K., Steadman, L. T., & Maynard, E. A. (1960). Acute and sub-acute toxicity studies of thallium compounds. *American Industrial Hygiene Association Journal, 21*, 399–406.

Dragsten, P. R., Hallaway, P. E., Hanson, G. J., Berger, A. E., Bernard, B., & Hedlund, B. E. (2000). First human studies with a high-molecular-weight iron chelator. *Journal of Laboratory and Clinical Medicine, 135*, 57–65.

Drake, P. L., & Hazelwood, K. J. (2005). Exposure-related health effects of silver and silver compounds: a review. *The Annals of Occupational Hygiene, 49*, 575–585.

Dresow, B., Nielsen, P., Fischer, R., Wendel, J., Gabbe, E. E., & Heinrich, H. C. (1991). Bioavailability of bismuth from ^{205}Bi-labelled pharmaceutical oral Bi-preparations in rats. *Archives of Toxicology, 65*, 646–650.

Dubowitz, M. N., Hughes, P. J., Lane, R. J., & Wade, J. P. (1991). Gold-induced neuroencephalopathy responding to dimercaprol. *Lancet, 337*(8745), 850–851.

Dvorak, P. (1970). Hexacyanoferrates (II) as thallium antidotes. Preparation and properties. *Arzneimittelforsch, 20*, 1886–1888.

Dvorak, P. (1971). Binding by hexacyanoferrates (II) of Thallium (I). *Zeitschrift für Naturforschung, 26*, 277–281.

Dwivedi, P. P., Athar, M., Hasan, S. K., & Srivastava, R. C. (1986). Removal of nickel by chelating drugs from the organs of nickel poisoned rats. *Chemosphere, 15*, 813–821.

Eagle, H., Germuth, F. G., Magnuson, H. J., & Fleischman, R. (1947). The protective action of bal in experimental antimony poisoning. *Journal of Pharmacology and Experimental Therapeutics, 89*, 196–204.

Eberl, H., & Altmann, H. (1970). The transport form of gold in the blood serum following intravenous or intramuscular administration of various gold salts]. *Zeitschrift für Klinische Chemie und Klinische Biochemie, 8*, 99–103.

EFSA (European Food Safety Authority). (2010). Scientific opinion on lead in food." European Food Safety Authority. EFSA Panel on Contaminants in the Food Chain (CONTAM). *EFSA Journal*, *8*, 1570–1717.

Eisler, R. (2006). *Mercury hazards to living organisms*. Oxford, UK: CRC Press/Taylor & Francis.

Ehrlich, H. L., & Newman, D. K. (2008). *Geomicrobiology*. Oxford, UK: CRC Press/Taylor & Francis, p. 265.

Ellingsen, D. G., Møller, L. B., & Aaseth, J. (2014). Copper. In G. F. Nordberg, B. A. Fowler, & M. Monica Nordberg (Eds.), *Handbook on the toxicology of metals* (4th ed., pp. 765–786). Amsterdam, NL: Elsevier/AP.

Ellis, E. N., Brouhard, B. H., Lynch, R. E., Dawson, E. B., Tisdell, R., Nichols, M. M., & Ramirez, F. (1982). Effects of hemodialysis and dimercaprol in acute dichromate poisoning. *Journal of Toxicology—Clinical Toxicology*, *19*, 249–258.

Ellis, L. S., Mullins, M. E., Galvin, N., Anthony, J., & Scalzo, A. J. (2009). Detection of Elemental Mercury in Abdominal Wall Soft Tissue. *Journal of Medical Toxicology*, *5*, 205–208.

Encyclopædia Britannica Online. Encyclopædia Britannica Inc., 2012. Web. 24 April 2012.

Erden, A., Karahan, S., Bulut, K., Basak, M., Aslan, T., Cetinkaya, A., Karagoz, H., & Avci, D. (2013). A case of bismuth intoxication with irreversible renal damage. *International Journal of Nephrology and Renovascular Disease*, *6*, 241–243.

Esparza, J. L., Gómez, M., Domingo, J. L., del Castillo, D., & Hernández, M. (2000). Age-related differences on aluminium mobilization by chelating agents in aluminium-loaded uraemic rats. *Pharmacology and Toxicology*, *87*, 33–38.

Eu-lex.europa.eu, 2003. Directive 2002/95/ec of the European Parliament and of the Council of 27 January 2003 on the restriction of the use of certain hazardous substances in electrical and electronic equipment. Official Journal of the European Union L 37/19.

Ewers, U. (1988). Environmental exposure to thalium. *Science of the Total Environment*, *71*, 285–292.

Eybl, V., Sykora, J., & Mertl, F. (1965). Effects of chelating agents on the excretion of cadmium in cadmium poisoning. *Naynun-Schmiedebergs Archives of Experimental Pathology and Pharmacology*, *252*, 85–93.

Eybl, V., Sykora, J., & Mertl, F. (1969). The effect of the Ca-complexes of the aminopolycarboxylic acids on the excretion and distribution of manganese during manganese poisoning. *International Archives of Commercial Path Commercial Hygiene*, *25*, 115–123, 1969.

Eybl, V., Sykora, J., & Mertl, F. (1970). [Influence of the Ca-complexes of aminopolycarboxylic acids on the excretion and distribution of zinc]. *Z. Ges. Exp. Med*, *152*, 274–283, 1970.

Eybl, V., Sykora, J., Koutensky, J., Caisova, D., Schwartz, A., & Mertl, F. (1984). Interaction of chelating agents with cadmium in mice and rats. *Environmental Health Perspectives*, *54*, 267–273.

Eybl, V., Koutensky, J., Koutenska, M., Sykora, J., Melsova, H., Majerova, S., & Mertl, F. (1985). The interaction of CaDTPA, DMPS and DMSA with zinc, cadmium, mercury and cobalt in acute experiments in mice. *Plzen Lek Sborn*(Suppl. 49), 53–57.

Eybl, V., Kotyzova, D., Koutensky, J., Jones, M. M., & Singh, P. K. (1995). Effect of chelators, monoisoamyl meso-2,3-dimercaptosuccinate and N-(4-methylbenzyl)-4-O-(beta-D-galactopyranosyl)-D-glucamine-N-carbodit hioate, on cadmium and essential element levels in mice. *Analyst*, *120*, 855–857.

Eybl, V., Kotyzova, D., Koutensky, J., Mickova, V., Jones, M. M., & Singh, P. K. (1998). Effect of cadmium chelating agents on organ cadmium and trace element levels in mice. *Analyst*, *123*, 25–26.

Eybl, V., Kotyzova, D., Kolek, M., Koutensky, J., & Nielsen, P. (2002). The influence of deferiprone (L1) and deferoxamine on iron and essential element tissue level and parameters of oxidative status in dietary iron-loaded mice. *Toxicology Letters*, *128*, 169–175.

Eyer, F., Felgenhauer, N., Pfab, R., Drasch, G., & Zilker, T. (2006). Neither DMPS nor DMSA is effective in quantitative elimination of elemental mercury after intentional IV injection. *Journal of Clinical Toxicology*, *44*, 395–397.

Fassos, F. F., Berkovitch, M., Daneman, N., Koren, L., Cameron, R. G., Klein, J., Falcitelli, C., Louis, P., St. Daneman, R., & Koren, G. (1996). Efficacy of deferiprone in the treatment of acute iron intoxication in rats. *Journal of Toxicology: Clinical Toxicology*, *34*, 279–287.

Fatemi, S. J., Saljooghi, A. S., Balooch, F. D., Iranmanesh, M., & Golbafan, M. R. (2011). Chelation of cadmium by combining deferasirox and deferiprone in rats. *Toxicology and Industrial Health*, *27*, 371–377.

Faure, A., Mathon, L., Poupelin, J. C., Allaouchiche, B., & Chassard, D. (2003). Acute cupric sulfate intoxication: pathophysiology and therapy about a case report. *Annales Françaises d'Anesthésie et de Réanimation*, *22*, 557–559.

Felicetti, S. W., Thomas, R. G., & McClellan, R. O. (1974). Metabolism of two valence states of inhaled antimony in hamsters. *American Industrial Hygiene Association Journal*, *355*, 292–300.

Felson, D. T., Anderson, J. J., & Meenan, R. F. (1990). The comparative efficacy and toxicity of second-line drugs in rheumatoid arthritis. Results of two metaanalyses. *Arthritis Rheumatology*, *33*, 1449–1461.

Ferrari, S., Smeland, S., Mercuri, M., Bertoni, F., Longhi, A., Ruggieri, P., Alvegard, T. A., Picci, P., Capanna, R., Bernini, G., Müller, C., Tienghi, A., Wiebe, T., Comandone, A., Böhling, T., Del, Prever, A. B., Brosjö, O., Bacci, G., Saeter, G., & Italian and Scandinavian Sarcoma Groups (2005). Neoadjuvant chemotherapy with high-dose Ifosfamide, high-dose methotrexate, cisplatin, and doxorubicin for patients with localized osteosarcoma of the extremity: a joint study by the Italian and Scandinavian Sarcoma Groups. *Journal of Clinical Oncology*, *23*, 8845–8852.

Flora, S. J., & Kumar, P. (1996). Biochemical and immunotoxicological alterations following repeated gallium arsenide exposure and their recoveries by meso-2,3-dimercaptosuccinic acid and 2,3-dimercaptopropane 1-sulfonate administration in rats. *Environment Toxicology and Pharmacology*, *20*, 315–320.

Flora, S. J. S., & Pachauri, V. (2010). Chelation in metal intoxication. *International Journal of Environmental Research and Public Health*, *7*, 2745–2788.

Flora, G. J. S., Seth, P. K., Prakash, A. O., & Mathur, R. (1995a). Therapeutic efficacy of combined meso 2,3-dimercaptosuccinic acid and calcium disodium edetate treatment during acute lead intoxication in rats. *Human and Experimental Toxicology*, *14*, 410–413.

Flora, S. J., Bhattacharya, R., & Vijayaraghavan, R. (1995b). Combined therapeutic potential of meso-2,3-dimercaptosuccinic acid and calcium disodium edetate on the mobilization and distribution of lead in experimental lead intoxication in rats. *Fundam Applied Toxicology*, *25*, 233–240, 1995.

Flora, S. J. S., Mathur, S., & Mathur, R. (1995c). Effects of meso-2,3-dimercaptosuccinic acid or 2,3-dimercaptopropane 1-sulfonate on beryllium-induced biochemical alterations and metal concentration in male rats. *Toxicology*, *95*, 167–175.

Flora, S. J., Dube, S. N., Arora, U., Kannan, G. M., Shukla, M. K., & Malhotra, P. R. (1995). Therapeutic potential of meso 2,3-dimercaptosuccinic acid or 2,3-dimercaptopropane 1-sulfonate in chronic arsenic intoxication in rats. *BioMetals*, *8*, 111–116.

Flora, S. J. S., Pant, B. P., Tripathi, N., Kannan, G. M. T., & Jaiswal, D. K. (1997). Therapeutic efficacy of a few diesters of meso 2,3-dimercaptosuccinic acid during sub-chronic arsenic intoxication in rats. *Journal of Occupational Health*, *39*, 119–123.

Flora, S. J., Dubey, R., Kannan, G. M., Chauhan, R. S., Pant, B. P., & Jaiswal, D. K. (2002a). Meso 2,3-dimercaptosuccinic acid (DMSA) and monoisoamyl DMSA effect on gallium arsenide induced pathological liver injury in rats. *Toxicology Letters*, *132*, 9–17.

Flora, S. J., Kannan, G. M., Pant, B. P., & Jaiswal, D. K. (2002b). Combined administration of oxalic acid, succimer and its analogue for the reversal of gallium arsenide-induced oxidative stress in rats. *Archives of Toxicology, 76*, 269–276.

Flora, S. J., Mehta, A., Rao, P. V., Kannan, G. M., Bhaskar, A. S., Dube, S. N., & Pant, B. P. (2004). Therapeutic potential of monoisoamyl and monomethyl esters of meso 2,3-dimercaptosuccinic acid in gallium arsenide intoxicated rats. *Toxicology, 195*, 127–146.

Flora, S. J., Bhatt, K., Dwivedi, N., Pachauri, V., & Kushwah, P. K. (2011). Co-administration of meso 2,3-dimercaptosuccinic acid monoesters reduces arsenic concentration and oxidative stress in gallium arsenide exposed rats. *Clinical and Experimental Pharmacology and Physiology, 38*, 423–429.

Flora, S. J., Bhadauria, S., Pachauri, V., & Yadav, A. (2012). Monoisoamyl 2, 3-dimercaptosuccinic Acid (MiADMSA) demonstrates higher efficacy by oral route in reversing arsenic toxicity: a pharmacokinetic approach. *Basic and Clinical Pharmacology and Toxicology, 110*, 449–459.

Florentine, M. J., & Sanfilippo, D. J., II (1991). Elemental mercury poisoning. *Clinical Pharmacology, 10*, 213–221.

Fortenberry, J. D. (1985). Gasoline sniffing. *American Journal of Medicine, 79*, 740–744.

Fournier, L., Thomas, G., Garnier, R., Buisine, A., Houze, P., Pradier, F., & Dally, S. (1988). 2,3-Dimercaptosuccinic acid treatment of heavy metal poisoning in humans. *Medical Toxicology, 3*, 499–504.

Fowler, B. A., & Sexton, M. J. (2014). Gallium and gallium semiconductor compounds. In G. F. Nordberg, A. Bruce, B. A. Fowler, & M. Nordberg (Eds.), *Handbook on the toxicology of metals* (4th ed., pp. 787–797). Amsterdam: Elsevier/AP.

Franchitto, N., Gandia-Mailly, P., Georges, B., Galinier, A., Telmon, N., Ducassé, J. L., & Rougé, D. (2008). Acute copper sulphate poisoning: a case report and literature review. *Resuscitation, 78*, 92–96.

Friedheim, E. A. H., DaSilva, J. R., & Martins, A. V. (1954). Treatment of schistosomiasis mansoni with antimony-a, a'-dimercapto-potassium succinate (twsb). *American Journal of Tropical Medicine and Hygiene, 3*, 714–727.

Friedheim, E. A. H., & Corvi, C. (1975). Meso-dimercaptosuccinic acid, a chelating agent for the treatment of mercury poisoning. *Journal of Pharmacy and Pharmacology, 27*, 624–626.

Friedheim, E., Corvi, C., & Wakker, C. H. J. (1976). Meso-dimercaptosuccinic acid a chelating agent for the treatment of mercury and lead poisoning. *Journal of Pharmacy and Pharmacology, 28*, 711–712.

Friedheim, E., Graziano, J. H., Popovac, D., Dragovic, D., & Kaul, B. (1978). Treatment of lead poisoning by 2,3-dimercaptosuccinic acid. *Lancet, 2*(8102), 1234–1236.

Froment, D. P., Molitoris, B. A., Buddington, B., Miller, N., & Alfrey, A. C. (1989). Site and mechanism of enhanced gastrointestinal absorption of aluminum by citrate. *Kidney International, 36*, 978–984.

Frost, D. V. (1967). Arsenicals in biology—retrospect and prospect. *Federation Proceedings, 26*, 194–208.

Furchner, J. E., Richmond, E. R., & Drake, G. A. (1968). Comparative metabolism of radionuclides in mammals-IV. Retention of silver-110m in the mouse, rat, monkey, and dog. *Health Physics, 15*, 505–514.

Gabard, B. (1976). The excretion and distribution of inorganic mercury in the rat as influenced by several chelating agents. *Archives of Toxicology, 35*, 15–24.

Gabard, B. (1980). Removal of internally deposited gold by 2,3-dimercaptopropane sodium sulphonate (Dimaval). *British Journal of Pharmacology, 68*, 607–610.

Gaetke, L. M., & Chow, C. K. (2003). Copper toxicity, oxidative stress, and antioxidant nutrients. *Toxicology*, *189*, 147–163.

Gale, G. R., Atkins, L. M., & Walker, E. M., Jr. (1982). Effects of diethyldithiocarbamate on organ distribution and excretion of cadmium. *Annals of Clinical and Laboratory Science*, *12*, 463–470.

Gale, G. R., Smith, A. B., Jones, M. M., & Singh, P. K. (1993). Meso-2,3-dimercaptosuccinic acid monoalkyl esters: effects on mercury levels in mice. *Toxicology*, *81*, 49–56.

Gandara, D. R., Nahhas, W. A., Adelson, M. D., Lichtman, S. M., Podczaski, E. S., Yanovich, S., Homesley, H. D., Braly, P., Ritch, P. S., Weisberg, S. R., et al. (1995). Randomized placebo-controlled multicenter evaluation of diethyldithiocarbamate for chemoprotection against cisplatin-induced toxicities. *Journal of Clinical Oncology*, *13*, 490–496.

Ganrot, P. O. (1986). Metabolism and possible health effects of aluminum. *Environment Health Perspectives*, *65*, 363–441.

Garg, S., Thyssen, J. P., Uter, W., Schnuch, A., Johansen, J. D., Menné, T., Belloni Fortina, A., Statham, B., & Gawkrodger, D. J. (2013). Nickel allergy following European Union regulation in Denmark, Germany, Italy and the U.K. *British Journal of Dermatology*, *169*, 854–858.

Garza-Orcanas, L., Torres-Alanis, O., & Pineyro-Lopez, A. (1997). Urinary mercury in twelve cases of cutaneous mercurous chloride (calomel) exposure: effect of sodium 2,3-dimercaptopropane-1-sulfonate (DMPS) therapy. *Journal of Toxicology: Clinical Toxicology*, *35*, 653–655.

Gastel, B. (Ed.), (1978). Clinical conferences at the Johns Hopkins Hospital. Thallium poisoning. *Johns Hopkins Medical Journal*, *142*, 27–31.

Gawkrodger, D. J., Healy, J., & Howe, A. M. (1995). The prevention of nickel contact dermatitis. A review of the use of binding agents and barrier creams. *Contact Dermatitis*, *32*, 257–265.

Gehring, P. J., & Hammond, P. B. (1966). The interrelationship between thallium and potassium in animals. *Journal of Pharmacology and Experimental Therapeutics*, *155*, 187–201.

Geller, R. (2001). Chromium. In J. B. Sullivan, Jr., & G. R. Krieger (Eds.), *Clinical environmental health and toxic exposures* (2nd ed.). Philadelphia, PA: Lippincott Williams & Wilkins.

Gemini observatory (2015). Gemini Mirror is First With Silver Lining. http://www.gemini.edu/project/announcements/press/2004-12.html

Gencpınar, P., Büyüktahtakın, B., Ibisoglu, Z., Genc, S., Yılmaz, A., & Mıhci, E. (2015). Mercury poisoning as a cause of intracranial hypertension. *Journal of Child Neurology*, *30*, 760–763.

Gerber, G. B., Maes, J., & Eykens, B. (1982). Transfer of antimony and arsenic to the developing organism. *Archives of Toxicology*, *49*, 159–168.

Gerhardsson, L., Borjesson, J., Grubb, A., Hultberg, B., Mattsson, S., Schütz, A., & Skerfving, S. (1998). In vivo XRF as a means to evaluate the risk of kidney effects in lead and cadmium exposed smelter workers. *Applied Radiation and Isotopes*, *49*, 711–712.

Gil, H., Kang, E., Lee, K., Yang, J., Le, E., & Hong, S. (2011). Effect of glutathione on the cadmium chelation of EDTA in a patient with cadmium intoxication. *Human and Experimental Toxicology*, *30*, 79–83.

Giordano, R., Ioppolo, A., Ciaralli, L., Rubbiani, M., Vernillo, I., & Costantini, S. (1989). Aluminum removal after chronic intoxication in rats. *Research Communications in Chemical Pathology and Pharmacology*, *63*, 119–127.

Gómez, M., Domingo, J. L., del Castillo, D., Llobet, J. M., & Corbella, J. (1994). Comparative aluminium mobilizing actions of several chelators in aluminium-loaded uraemic rats. *Human and Experimental Toxicology*, *13*, 135–139.

Gomez, M., Esparza, J. L., Domingo, J. L., Corbella, J., Singh, P. K., & Jones, M. M. (1998a). Aluminium distribution and excretion: a comparative study of a number of chelating agents in rats. *Pharmacology and Toxicology*, *82*, 295–300.

Gomez, M., Esparza, J. L., Domingo, J. L., Singh, P. K., & Jones, M. M. (1998b). Comparative aluminium mobilizing actions of deferoxamine and four 3-hydroxypyridin-4-ones in aluminium-loaded rats. *Toxicology*, *130*, 175–181.

Gong, Z., & Evans, H. L. (1997). Effect of chelation with meso-dimercaptosuccinic acid (DMSA) before and after the appearance of lead-induced neurotoxicity in the rat. *Toxicology and Applied Pharmacology*, *144*, 205–214.

Gonzales-Ramirez, D., Maiorino, R. M., Zuniga-Charles, M., Xu, Z., Hurlbut, K. M., Junco-Munoz, P., Aposhian, M. M., Dart, R. C., Gama, J. H. D., Echeverria, D., Woods, J. S., & Aposhian, H. V. J. (1995). Sodium 2,3-dimercaptopropane-1-sulfonate challenge test for mercury in humans: II. Urinary mercury, porphyrins and neurobehavioral changes of dental workers in Monterrey, Mexico. *Pharmacology and Experimental Therapeutics*, *272*, 264–272.

Gonzales-Ramirez, D., Zuniga-Charles, M., Narro-Juarez, A., Molina-Recio, Y., Hurlbut, K. M., Dart, R. C., & Aposhian, H. V. J. (1998). DMPS (2,3-dimercaptopropane-1-sulfonate, dimaval) decreases the body burden of mercury in humans exposed to mercurous chloride. *Pharmacology and Experimental Therapeutics*, *287*, 8–12.

Goodman, M., LaVerda, N., Clarke, C., Foster, E. D., Iannuzzi, J., & Mandel, J. (2002). Neurobehavioural testing in workers occupationally exposed to lead: systematic review and meta-analysis of publications. *Occupational and Environmental Medicine*, *59*, 217–223.

Gordon, R. A., Roberts, G., Amin, Z., Williams, R. H., & Paloucek, F. P. (1998). Aggressive approach in the treatment of acute lead encephalopathy with an extraordinarily high concentration of lead. *Archives of Pediatrics and Adolescent Medicine*, *152*, 1100–1104.

Graham, D. Y., Opekun, A. R., Belson, G., El-Zimaity, H. M., & Carlson, M. R. (2005). Novel bismuth-metronidazole-tetracycline triple-layer tablet for treatment of Helicobacter pylori. *Alimentary Pharmacology and Therapeutics*, *15*, 165–168.

Grandjean, P., Jacobsen, I. A., & Jørgensen, P. J. (1991). Chronic lead poisoning treated with dimercaptosuccinic acid. *Pharmacology and Toxicology*, *68*, 266–269, 1991.

Grasso, P., Abrahan, R., Hendy, R., et al. (1970). Hepatocellular necrosis from dietary silver in vitamin E-deficient rats. *Journal of Pathology*, *100*, ix.

Grazina, R., Gano, L., Sebestík, J., & Amelia Santos, M. (2009). New tripodal hydroxypyridinone based chelating agents for Fe(III), Al(III) and Ga(III): Synthesis, physico-chemical properties and bioevaluation. *Journal of Inorganic Biochemistry*, *103*, 262–273.

Graziano, J. H. (1993). Conceptual and practical advances in the measurement and clinical management of lead toxicity. *Neurotoxicology*, *14*, 219–224.

Graziano, J. H., Cuccia, D., & Friedheim, E. A. H. (1978a). The pharmacology of 2,3-dimercaptosuccinic acid and its potential use in arsenic poisoning. *Journal of Pharmacology and Experimental Therapeutics*, *207*, 1051–1055.

Graziano, J. H., Leong, J. K., & Friedheim, E. J. (1978b). 2,3-Dimercaptosuccinic acid: a new agent for the treatment of lead poisoning. *Pharmacology and Experimental Therapeutics*, *206*, 696–700, 1978B.

Graziano, J., Jones, B., & Pisciotto, P. (1981). The effect of heavy metal chelators on the renal accumulation of platinum after *cis*-dichlorodiammineplatinum II administration to the rat. *British Journal of Pharmacology*, *73*, 649–654.

Graziano, J. H., LoIacono, N., Molton, T., Mitchell, M. E., Slavcovich, V., & Zarate, C. J. (1992). Controlled study of meso-2,3-dimercaptosuccinic acid for the management of childhood lead intoxication. *Pediatrics*, *120*, 133–139.

Greenwood, N., & Earnshaw, A. (2011). *Chemistry of the Elements* (2nd ed.). Amsterdam, NL: Elsevier.

Greig, J., Thurtle, N., Cooney, L., Ariti, C., Ahmed, A. O., Ashagre, T., Ayela, A., Chukwumalu, K., Criado-Perez, A., Gómez-Restrepo, C., Meredith, C., Neri, A., Stellmach, D., Sani-Gwarzo, N., Nasidi, A., Shanks, L., & Dargan, P. I. (2014). Association of blood lead level with neurological features in 972 children affected by an acute severe lead poisoning outbreak in Zamfara State, northern Nigeria. *PLoS One*, *9*(4), e93716.

Griffith, E. A., Fallgatter, K. C., Tantama, S. S., Tanen, D. A., & Matteucci, M. J. (2011). Effect of deferasirox on iron absorption in a randomized, placebo-controlled, crossover study in a human model of acute supratherapeutic iron ingestion. *Annals of Emergency Medicine*, *58*(1), 69–732011.

Guha Mazumder, D.N. (1998). Chronic arsenic toxicity: dose related clinical effect, its natural history and therapy. *Proceedings of third international conference on arsenic exposure and health effects*. San Diego, CA.

Guha Mazumder, D. N., Ghoshal, U. C., Saha, J., Santra, A., De, B. K., Chatterjee, A., Dutta, S., Angle, C. R., & Centeno, J. A. (1998). Randomized Placebo-Controlled Trial of 2,3-Dimercaptosuccinic Acid in Therapy of Chronic Arsenicosis Due to Drinking Arsenic-Contaminated Subsoil Water. *Journal of Toxicology: Clinical Toxicology*, *36*, 683–690.

Guha Mazumder, D. N., De, B. K., Santra, A., Ghosh, N., Das, S., Lahiri, S., & Das, T. (2001). Randomized placebo-controlled trial of 2,3-dimercapto-1-propanesulfonate (DMPS) in therapy of chronic arsenicosis due to drinking arsenic-contaminated water. *Clinical Toxicology*, *39*, 665–674.

Gumber, M. R., Kute, V. B., Shah, P. R., Vanikar, A. V., Patel, H. V., Balwani, M. R., Ghuge, P. P., & Trivedi, H. L. (2013). Successful treatment of severe iron intoxication with gastrointestinal decontamination, deferoxamine, and hemodialysis. *Renal Failure*, *35*, 729–731.

Hagan, P. (2009). Schistosomiasis—a rich vein of research. *Parasitology*, *136*, 1611–1619.

Haider, F., De Carli, C., Dhanani, S., & Sweeney, B. (2009). Emergency laparoscopic-assisted gastrotomy for the treatment of an iron bezoar. *Journal of Laparoendoscopic and Advanced Surgical Techniques A*, *19*(Suppl. 1), S141–S143.

Hantson, P., Haufroid, V., Buchet, J. P., & Mahieu, P. (2003). Acute arsenic poisoning treated by intravenous dimercaptosuccinic acid (DMSA) and combined extrarenal epuration techniques. *Journal of Toxicology: Clinical Toxicology*, *41*, 1–6.

Hantson, P., Lievens, M., & Mahieu, P. (1996). Accidental ingestion of a zinc and copper sulfate preparation. *Journal of Toxicology: Clinical Toxicology*, *34*, 725–730.

Hantson, P., Lula, F., Lievens, M., & Mahieu, P. (1998). Extremely high plasma zinc following zinc chloride ingestion. *Journal of Toxicology: Clinical Toxicology*, *36*, 375–377, 1998.

Hantson, P., Van Caenegem, O., Decordier, I., Haufroid, V., & Lison, D. (2005). Hexavalent chromium ingestion: biological markers of nephrotoxicity and genotoxicity. *Clinical Toxicology*, *43*, 111–112.

Hassan, S., Shaikh, M. U., Ali, N., & Riaz, M. (2010). Copper sulphate toxicity in a young male complicated by methemoglobinemia, rhabdomyolysis and renal failure. *Journal of the College of Physicians and Surgeons (Pakistan)*, *20*, 490–491.

Haust, H. L., Inwood, M., Spence, D., Poon, H. C., & Peter, F. (1989). Intramuscular administration of iron during long-term chelation therapy with 2,3-dimercaptosuccinic acid in a man with severe lead poisoning. *Clinical Biochemistry*, *22*, 189–196.

Henretig, F., & Shannon, M. (1988). An 11-year-old boy develops vomiting,weakness, weight loss and a neckmass. *International Journal of Medicine and Toxicology*, *1*, 13–15.

Herrmann, M., & Schweinsberg, F. (1993). Biomonitoring for the evaluation of a mercury burden from amalgam fillings. Mercury determination in urine before and after oral doses of 2,3-dimercapto-1-propanesulfonic acid (DMPS) and in hair. *International Journal of Hygiene and Environmental Medicine*, *194*, 271–291.

Heydlauf, H. (1969). Ferric-cyanoferrate (II): an effective antidote in thallium poisoning. *European Journal of Pharmacology*, *1*, 340–344.

Hidaka, S., Tsuruoka, M., Funakoshi, T., Shimada, H., Kiyuzomi, M., & Kojima, S. (1994). Protective effects of dithiocarbamates against renal toxicity of *cis*-diamminedichloroplatinum in rats. *Renal Failure*, *16*, 337–349.

Hidaka, S., Funakoshi, T., Shimada, H., Tsuruoka, M., & Kojima, S. J. (1995). Comparative effects of diethyldithiocarbamate and N-benzyl-D-glucamine dithiocarbamate on *cis*-diamminedichloroplatinum-induced toxicity in kidney and gastrointestinal tract in rats. *Applied Toxicology*, *15*, 267–273.

Hiron, A., Posteraro, B., Carriere, M., Remy, L., Delporte, C., La Sorda, M., Sanguinetti, M., Juillard, V., & Borezée-Durant, E. (2010). A nickel ABC-transporter of Staphylococcus aureus is involved in urinary tract infection. *Molecular Microbiology*, *77*, 1246–1260.

Hoffman, R. S. (2003). Thallium toxicity and the role of Prussian blue in therapy. *Toxicological Reviews*, *22*, 29–40.

Hohage, H., Otte, B., Westerman, G., Witta, J., Welling, U., Zidek, W., & Heidenreich, S. (1997). Elemental mercurial poisoning. *Southern Medical Journal*, *90*, 1033–1036.

Holbrook, D. J., Jr., Washington, M. E., Leake, H. B., & Brubaker, P. E. (1975). Studies on the evaluation of the toxicity of various salts of lead, manganese, platinum, and palladium. *Environmental Health Perspectives*, *10*, 95–101.

Holleman, A.F., Wiberg, E., & Wiberg, N. (1985). Blei. Lehrbuch der Anorganischen Chemie (91–100 ed.) (pp. 801–810). Walter de Gruyter.

Holler, J. S., Fowler, B. A., & Nordberg, G. F. (2014). Silver. In G. F. Nordberg, B. A. Fowler, & M. Nordberg (Eds.), *Handbook on the Toxicology of Metals* (4th ed., pp. 1209–1216). Amsterdam, NL: Elsevier/AP 2014.

Horn, N., Tonnesen, T., & Tumer, Z. (1992). Menkes disease: an X-linked neurological disorder of the copper metabolism. *Brain Pathology*, *2*, 351–362.

Howell, S.B., Pfeifle, C.E., Wung, W.E., & Olshen, R.A. (1983). Intraperitoneal *cis*-diamminedichloroplatinum with systemic thiosulfate protection. *Cancer Research*, 43, 1426–1431.

Houeto, P., Sandouk, P., Baud, F. J., & Levillain, P. (1994). Elemental mercury vapour toxicity: treatment and levels in plasma and urine. *Human and Experimental Toxicology*, *13*, 848–852, 1994.

Hruz, P., Mayr, M., Löw, R., Drewe, J., & Huber, G. (2002). Fanconi's syndrome, acute renal failure, and tonsil ulcerations after colloidal bismuth subcitrate intoxication. *American Journal of Kidney Disorders*, *239*, E18.

Huang, Y., Savory, J., Herman, M. M., Nicholson, J. R., Reyes, J. C., Boyd, J. C., & Will, M. R. (1995). Quantitative evaluation of al maltolate-induced neurodegeneration with subsequent al removal by desferrioxamine treatment. *Neurotoxicology*, *16*, 291–296.

Huang, C., Zhang, X., Li, G., Jiang, Y., Wang, Q., & Tian, R. (2014). A case of severe thallium poisoning successfully treated with hemoperfusion and continuous veno-venous hemofiltration. *Human Experimental Toxicology*, *33*, 554–558.

Huffman, D. L., & O'Halloran, T. V. (2001). Function, structure, and mechanism of intracellular copper trafficking proteins. *Annual Review of Biochemistry*, *70*, 677–701.

Hunter, D., Milton, R., & Perry, K. (1945). Asthma caused by the complex salts of platinum. *British Journal of Industrial Medicine*, *2*, 92–98.

Hursh, J. B., Cherian, M. G., Clarkson, T. W., Vostal, J. J., & Mallie, R. V. (1976). Clearance of mercury (HG-197, HG-203) vapor inhaled by human subjects. *Archives of Environmental Health*, *31*, 302–309.

Hyun, C., & Filippich, L. C. (2004). Inherited Copper toxicosis with emphasis on copper toxicosis in Bedlington terriers. *Journal of Experimental Animal Science*, *43*, 39–64.

IARC (1990). IARC Monographs on the Evaluation of Carcinogenic Risks to Humans, vol. 49. Chromium, Nickel and Welding. International Agency for Research on Cancer, Lyon.

IARC (2006). IARC Monographs on the Evaluation of Carcinogenic Risks to Humans, vol. 87. Inorganic and Organic Lead Compounds. International Agency for Research on Cancer, Lyon, France.

IARC (2012). IARC Monographs on the Evaluation of Carcinogenic Risks to Humans, vol. 100C. Arsenic, Metals, Fibres, and Dusts. International Agency for Research on Cancer, Lyon.

Iffland, R., & Bösche, G. (1987). Therapy and clinicotoxicologic follow-up of tartar emetic poisoning caused by an ant insecticide in a small child. *Monatsschr. Kinderheilkd, 135*, 227–230.

Illner, N., Gerth, J., Pfeiffer, R., Bruns, T., & Wolf, G. (2009). Nearly a stairway to heaven"--severe dichromate intoxication in a young man. *Clinical Nephrology, 71*, 338–341.

Inns, R. H., & Rice, P. (1993). Efficacy of dimercapto chelating agents for the treatment of poisoning by percutaneously applied dichloro(2-chlorovinyl)arsine in rabbits. *Human and Experimental Toxicology, 12*, 241–246.

Inns, R. H., Rice, P., Bright, J. E., & Marrs, T. C. (1990). Evaluation of the efficacy of dimercapto chelating agents for the treatment of systemic organic arsenic poisoning in rabbits. *Human and Experimental Toxicology, 9*, 215–220.

International Lead and Zinc Study Group (2012). End uses of lead. http://www.ilzsg.org/static/enduses.aspx?from=5

International Lead Zinc Study Group (2013). World refined zinc supply and usage 2009-2013. www.ilzsg.org/static/home.aspx

Intoccia, A. P., Flanagan, T. L., Walz, D. T., Gutzait, L., Swagzdis, J. E., Flagiello, J., Jr., Hwang, B. Y., Dewey, R. H., & Noguchi, H. (1982). Pharmacokinetics of auranofin in animals. *Journal of Rheumatology Supplement, 8*, 90–98.

IPCS. (1991). *Environmental health criteria 125. Platinum. International programme on chemical safety*. Geneva: World Health Organization.

IPCS. (1992). *Environmental health criteria 134, Cadmium. international programme on chemical safety*. Geneva: World Health Organization.

Iranmanesh, M., Fatemi, S. J., Golbafan, M. R., & Balooch, F. D. (2013b). Treatment of mercury vapor toxicity by combining deferasirox and deferiprone in rats. *Biometals, 26*, 783–788.

Iranmanesh, M., Fatemi, S. J., Ebrahimpour, R., & Dahooee Balooch, F. (2013a). Chelation of chromium(VI) by combining deferasirox and deferiprone in rats. *Biometals, 26*, 465–471.

Isbister, G. K., Dawson, A. H., & Whyte, I. M. (2004). Arsenic trioxide poisoning: a description of two acute overdoses. *Human and Experimental Toxicology, 23*, 359–364.

Ivanovaa, J., Gluhchevab, Y. G., Kamenovac, K., Arpadjanc, S., & Mitewac, M. (2012). The tetraethylammonium salt of monensic acid—An antidote for subacute cadmium intoxication. A study using an ICR mouse model. *Journal of Trace Elements in Medicine and Biology, 26*, 279–284.

Izbicki, G., Chavko, R., Banauch, G. I., Weiden, M. D., Berger, K. I., Aldrich, T. K., et al. (2007). World Trade Center "sarcoid-like" granulomatous pulmonary disease in New York City Fire Department rescue workers. *CHEST Journal, 131*, 1414–1423.

Jackson, T. W., Ling, L. J., & Washington, V. (1995). The effect of oral deferoxamine on iron absorption. *Journal of Toxicology: Clinical Toxicology, 33*, 325–329.

Jain, D., & Zaret, B. L. (2005). Nuclear imaging in cardiovascular medicine. In C. Rosendorff (Ed.), *Essential cardiology: principles and practice* (2nd ed., pp. 221–222). Totowa, NJ, USA: Humana Press.

Jakubke, H. D., & Jeschkeit, H. (Eds.). (1994). *Concise encyclopedia chemistry*. Eagleson, Mary. Berlin: Walter de Gruyter.

Jakubowskij, J., & Palczynski, C. (2014). Beryllium. In F. Gunnar, G. F. Nordberg, A. Bruce, B. A. Fowler, & M. Nordberg (Eds.), *Handbook on the Toxicology of Metals* (4th ed., pp. 549–564). Amsterdam, NL: Elsevier/AP.

James, H. M., Hilburn, M. E., & Blair, J. A. (1985). Effects of meals and meal times on uptake of lead from the gastrointestinal tract in humans. *Human Toxicology*, *4*, 401–407.

Jantsch, W., Kulig, K., & Rumack, B. H. (1985). Massive copper sulfate ingestion resulting in hepatotoxicity. *Clinical Toxicology*, *22*, 585–588.

Jarich, R., Ballczo, H., & Richter, W. Z. (1975). Nickel allergy: removal of the allergen by means of cation exchangers & Nickel allergy: elimination of the noxa using a cation exchanger. *Hautkr.*, *50*, 33–39 & 53–57.

Jasim, S., Danielsson, B. R., Tjälve, H., & Dencker, L. (1985). Distribution of ^{64}Cu in foetal and adult tissues in mice: influence of sodium diethyldithiocarbamate treatment. *Acta Pharmacology Toxicology*, *57*, 262–270.

JECFA (2011). Joint FAO/WHO Expert Committee on Food Additives. Seventy-third report of the Joint FAO/WHO Expert Committee on Food Additives and Contaminants. Technical Report Series No. 960. Joint FAO/WHO Expert Committee on Food Additives and Contaminants. Evaluation of certain food additives and contaminants. World Health Organization, Geneva.

Jensen, L. S., Peterson, R. P., & Falen, L. (1974). Inducement of enlarged hearts and muscular dystrophy in turkey poults with dietary silver. *Poultry Science*, *53*, 57–64.

Jiang, Y. M., Mo, X. A., Du, F. O., Fu, X., Zhu, X. Y., Gao, H. Y., Xie, J. L., Liao, F. L., Pira, E., & Zheng, W. (2006). Effective treatment of manganese-induced occupational Parkinsonism with p-aminosalicylic acid: A case of 17-year follow-up study. *Journal of Occupational and Environmental Medicine*, *48*, 644–649.

Jin, Y., Yu, F., Liao, Y., Liu, S., Liu, M., Xu, J., & Yang, J. (2011). Therapeutic efficiency of succimer used with calcium and ascorbic acid in the treatment of mild lead-poisoning. *Environmental Toxicology and Pharmacology*, *31*, 137–142.

Johansen, J. B., Abildtrup, A., Ebbehøj, N. E., Kristensen, S. R., & Eshøj, O. (1996). Acute arsenic poisoning. *Ugeskr Laeger*, *158*, 4201–4202.

Johnson, P. E., Milne, D. B., & Lykken, G. I. (1992). Effects of age and sex on copper absorption, biological half-life, and status in humans. *American Journal of Clinical Nutrition*, *56*, 917–925.

Johnson, M. A., & Greger, J. L. (1982). Effects of dietary tin on tin and calcium metabolism of adult males. *American Journal of Clinical Nutrition*, *35*, 655–660.

Johri, S., Shukla, S., & Sharma, P. (2002). Role of chelating agents and antioxidants in beryllium induced toxicity. *Indian Journal of Experimental Biology*, *40*, 575–582.

Johri, S., Shrivastava, S., Sharma, P., & Shukla, S. (2004). Analysis of time-dependent recovery from beryllium toxicity following chelation therapy and antioxidant supplementation. *Indian Journal of Experimental Biology*, *42*, 798–802.

Jolliffe, D. M. (1993). A history of the use of arsenicals in man. *Journal of the Royal Society of Medicine*, *86*, 287–289.

Jolliffe, D. M., Budd, A. J., & Gwilt, D. J. (1991). Massive acute arsenic poisoning. *Anasthesia*, *46*, 288–290.

Jones, M. M. (1991). New developments in therapeutic chelating agents as antidotes for metal poisoning. *Critical Reviews of Toxicology*, *21*, 209–233.

Jones, M. M., & Basinger, M. A. (1989). Control of nephrotoxicity in the rat during repeated *cis*-platinum treatments. *Journal of Applied Toxicology*, *9*, 229–233.

Jones, M. M., & Cherian, M. G. (1990). The search for chelate antagonists for chronic cadmium intoxication. *Toxicology*, *62*, 1–25.

Jones, M. M., Weaver, A. D., & Weller, W. L. (1978). The relative effectiveness of some chelating agents as antidotes in acute cadmium poisoning. *Research Communications in Chemical Pathology and Pharmacology*, *22*, 581–588.

Jones, M. M., Basinger, M. A., Weaver, A. D., Davis, C. M., & Waughn, W. K. (1980). Comparison of standard chelating agents for acute mercuric chloride poisoning in mice. *Research Communications in Chemical Pathology and Pharmacology*, *27*, 363–372.

Jones, M. M., Cherian, M. G., Singh, P. K., Basinger, M. A., & Jones, S. G. (1991a). A comparative study of the influence of vicinal dithiols and a dithiocarbamate on the biliary excretion of cadmium in rat. *Toxicology and Applied Pharmacology*, *110*, 241–250.

Jones, M. M., Singh, P. K., Jones, S. G., & Holscher, M. A. (1991b). Dithiocarbamates of improved efficacy for the mobilization of retained cadmium from renal and hepatic deposits. *Pharmacology and Toxicology*, *68*, 115–120.

Jones, M. M., Weaver, A. D., & Basinger, M. A. (1981). Characteristics of chelate antidotes for acute Cu(II) intoxication. *Journal of Inorganic and Nuclear Chemistry*, *43*, 2175–2181.

Jones, M. M., Basinger, M. A., & Holscher, M. A. (1991c). Thioether suppression of cisplatin nephrotoxicity in the rat. *Anticancer Research*, *11*, 449–453.

Jones, M. M., Singh, P. K., Gale, G. R., Smith, A. B., & Atkins, L. M. (1992). Cadmium mobilization in vivo by intraperitoneal or oral administration of monoalkyl esters of meso-2,3-dimercaptosuccinic acid in the mouse. *Pharmacology and Toxicology*, *70*, 336–343.

Jones, M. M., Singh, P. K., Basinger, M. A., Gale, G. R., Smith, A. B., & Harris, W. R. (1994a). Design of in vivo cadmium-mobilizing agents: synthesis and properties of monobenzyl meso-2,3-dimercaptosuccinate. *Chemical Research and Toxicology*, *7*, 367–373.

Jones, M. M., Basinger, M. A., Gale, G. R., Atkins, L. M., Smith, A. B., & Stone, A. (1994b). Effect of chelate treatments on kidney, bone and brain lead levels of lead-intoxicated mice. *Toxicology*, *89*, 91–100.

Joshi, S.R., & Bhandari, R.P. (2008). Chronic arsenic toxicity: clinical features, epidemiology, and treatment: experience in Indo-Nepal border abstracts: ISEE 20th Annual Conference, Pasadena, California, October 12–16, 2008. *Epidemiology 19*, S349–S350.

Joshi, D., Mittal, D. K., Bhadauria, M., Nirala, S. K., Shrivastava, S., & Shukla, S. (2010). Role of micronutrients against dimethylmercury intoxication in male rats. *Environmental Toxicology and Pharmacology*, *29*, 97–103.

Joshi, D., Mittal, D. K., Shukla, S., Srivastav, A. K., & Srivastav, S. K. (2014). Methylmercury toxicity: amelioration by selenium and water-soluble chelators as N-acetyl cysteine and dithiothreitol. *Cell Biochemistry and Function*, *32*, 351–360.

Kaaber, K., Menne, T., Tjell, J. C., & Veien, N. (1979). Antabuse treatment of nickel dermatitis. Chelation—a new principle in the treatment of nickel dermatitis. *Contact Dermatitis*, *5*, 221–228.

Kaaber, K., Menne, T., Veien, V., & Hougaard, P. (1983). Treatment of nickel dermatitis with Antabuse; a double blind study. *Contact Dermatitis*, *9*, 297–299.

Kaaber, K., Mennem, T., Veien, N. K., & Baadsgaard, O. (1987). Some adverse effects of disulfiram in the treatment of nickel-allergic patients. *Derm Beruf Umwelt*, *35*, 209–211.

Kadikoylu, G., Bolaman, Z., Demir, S., Balkaya, M., Akalin, N., & Enli, Y. (2004). The effects of desferrioxamine on cisplatin-induced lipid peroxidation and the activities of antioxidant enzymes in rat kidneys. *Human and Experimental Toxicology*, *23*, 29–34.

Kalita, J., & Misra, U. K. (2006). Sequelae of thallium poisoning: clinical and neurophysiological follow-up. *European Neurology*, *56*, 253–255.

Kamerbeek, H. H., van Heijst, A. N., Rauws, A. G., & ten Ham, M. (1970). Therapeutic problems in thallium poisoning. Clinical trials with diethyl-dithiocarbamate. *Ned Tijdschr. Geneeskd*, *114*, 457–460.

Kamerbeek, H. H., Rauws, A. G., ten Ham, M., & van Heijst, A. N. (1971a). Dangerous redistribution of thallium by treatment with sodium diethyldithiocarbamate. *Acta Medica Scandinavia*, *189*, 149–154.

Kamerbeek, H. H., Rauws, A. G., ten Ham, M., & van Heijst, A. N. (1971b). Prussian blue in therapy of thallotoxicosis. An experimental and clinical investigation. *Acta Medica Scandinavia*, *189*, 321–324.

Kamijo, Y., Soma, K., Asari, Y., & Ohwada, T. (1998). Survival after massive arsenic poisoning self-treated by high fluid intake. *Journal of Toxicology: Clinical Toxicology*, *36*, 27–29.

Kan, W. C., Chien, C. C., Wu, C. C., Su, S. B., Hwang, J. C., & Wang, H. Y. (2010). Comparison of low-dose deferoxamine versus standard-dose deferoxamine for treatment of aluminium overload among haemodialysis patients. *Nephrology Dialysis Transplantation*, *25*, 1604–1608.

Kanluen, S., & Gottlieb, C. A. (1991). A clinical pathologic study of four adult cases of acute mercury inhalation toxicity. *Archives of Pathology and Laboratory Medicine*, *115*, 56–60.

Kapoor, S. C., Wielopolski, L., Graziano, J. H., & LoIacono, N. J. (1989). Influence of 2,3-dimercaptosuccinic acid on gastrointestinal lead absorption and whole-body lead retention. *Toxicology and Applied Pharmacology*, *97*, 525–529.

Kay, R. G., Tasman-Jones, C., Pybus, J., Whiting, R., & Black, H. (1976). A syndrome of acute zinc deficiency during total parenteral alimentation in man. *Annals of Surgery*, *183*, 331–340.

Kazantzis, G. (2000). Thallium in the environment and health effects. *Environmental Geochemistry and Health*, *22*, 275–280.

Kean, W. F., & Kean, I. R. (2008). Clinical pharmacology of gold. *Inflammopharmacology*, *16*, 112–125.

Keegan, G. M., Learmonth, I. D., & Case, C. P. (2007). Orthopaedic metals and their potential toxicity in the arthroplasty patient: a review of current knowledge and future strategies. *Journal of Bone and Joint Surgery. British Volume*, *89*, 567–573.

Kesteloot, H., Roelandt, J., Willems, J., Claes, J. H., & Joossens, J. V. (1968). An enquiry into the role of cobalt in the heart disease of chronic beer drinkers. *Circulation*, *37*, 854–864.

Khandelwal, S., Kachru, D. N., & Tandon, S. K. (1980). Chelation in metal intoxication. IX. Influence of amino and thiol chelators on excretion of manganese in poisoned rabbits. *Toxicology Letters*, *6*, 131–135.

Kharakwal, J.S. & Gurjar, L.K. (2006). Zinc and Brass in Archaeological Perspective I Kharakwal I Ancient Asia. Ancient-asia-journal.com.

Kiilunen, M., Kivisto, H., Ala-Laurila, P., Tossavainen, A., & Aitio, A. (1983). Exceptional pharmacokinetics of trivalent chromium during occupational exposure to chromium lignosulfonate dust. *Scandinavian Journal of Work, Environment & Health*, *9*, 265–271.

Kiilunen, M., Aitio, A., & Santonen, T. (2014). Platinum. In G. F. Nordberg, K. Nogawa, M. Nordberg, Cadmium, G. F. In: Nordberg, B. A. Fowler, & M. Nordberg (Eds.), *Handbook on the toxicology of metals* (4th ed., pp. 1125–1141). Amsterdam, NL: Elsevier/AP.

Kim, L. H., & Abel, S. J. (2009). Survival after a massive overdose of arsenic trioxide. *Critical Care Resuscitation*, *11*, 42–45.

Kim, B. E., Turski, M. L., Nose, Y., Casad, M., Rockman, H. A., & Thiele, D. J. (2010). Cardiac copper deficiency activates a systemic signaling mechanism that communicates with the copper acquisition and storage organs. *Cell Metabolism*, *11*, 353–363.

Kirschbaum, B. B., & Schoolwerth, A. C. (1989). Acute aluminum toxicity associated with oral citrate and aluminum-containing antacids. *American Journal of Medical Science*, *297*, 9–11.

Klaassen, C. (2006). Heavy metals and heavy-metal antagonists. In L. L. Brunton, J. S. Lazo, & K. L. Parker (Eds.), *Goodman & Gilman's The pharmacological basis of therapeutics* (11th ed., pp. 1753–1775). New York, USA: McGraw-Hill.

Klein, C., & Costa, M. (2014). Nickel. In G. F. Nordberg, A. Bruce, B. A. Fowler, & M. Nordberg (Eds.), *Handbook on the toxicology of metals* (4th ed., pp. 1091–1111). Amsterdam, NL: Elsevier/AP.

Kleinfeld, M., & Rosso, A. (1965). Ulcerations of the nasal septum due to inhalation of chromic acid mist. *Industrial Medicine and Surgery*, *34*, 242–243.

Kobidze, T., Urushadze, O., Afandiyev, I., Nemsadze, G., & Loladze, D. (2014). Clinical manifestation and management of intravenous mercury injection: a case report. *Georgian Medical News*, *226*, 11–16.

Kojima, S., Takahashi, Y., Kiyozumi, M., & Tagawa, Y. (1991). Protective effects of chelating agents against renal toxicity of gold sodium thiomalate in rats. *Archives of Toxicology*, *65*, 532–536.

Kolacinski, Z., Kostrzewski, P., Kruszewska, S., Razniewska, G., & Mielczarska, J. (1999). Acute potassium dichromate poisoning: a toxicokinetic case study. *Journal of Toxicology: Clinical Toxicology*, *37*, 785–791.

Kolanz, M. E. (2001). Introduction to beryllium: uses, regulatory history, and disease. *Applied Occupational and Environmental Hygiene*, *16*, 559–567.

Konstantopoulos, W. M., Ewald, M. B., & Pratt, D. S. (2012). Case 22-2012: A 34-year-old man with intractable vomiting after ingestion of an unknown substance antimony poisoning due to ingestion of tartar emetic (antimony potassium tartrate). *New England Journal of Medicine*, *367*, 259–268.

Kontoghiorges, G. J. (1995). Comparative efficacy and toxicity of desferrioxamine, deferiprone and other iron and aluminium chelating drugs. *Toxicology Letters*, *80*, 1–18.

Kontoghiorghes, G. J., Barr, J., & Baillod, R. A. (1994). Studies of aluminium mobilization in renal dialysis patients using the oral chelator 1,2-dimethyl-3-hydroxypyrid-4-one. *Arzneimittelforschung*, *44*, 522–526.

Koriakov, V. V., & Gol'dfarb, I. S. (1995). Acute grey mercury ointment poisoning. *Anesteziologiia i Reanimatologiia*, *3*, 59–60.

Korringa, P., & Hagel, P. 1974. Mercury pollution: A local problem. In Problems of contamination of man, his environment by mercury, cadmium, 279–293., Center for Information, Documentation (CID), C.E.C.: Luxembourg,

Kosta, L., Vyrne, A. R., & Zelenko, V. (1975). Correlation between selenium and mercury in man following exposure to inorganic mercury. *Nature (London)*, *254*, 238–239.

Kostial, K., Blanusa, M., Simonovic, I., Jones, M. M., & Singh, P. K. (1993). Decreasing 203Hg retention by intraperitoneal treatment with monoalkyl esters of meso-2,3-dimercaptosuccinic acid in rats. *Journal of Applied Toxicology*, *13*, 321–325.

Kostial, K., Kargacin, B., Blanusa, M., Piasek, M., Jones, M. M., & Singh, P. K. (1994). Monoisoamyl meso-2,3-dimercaptosuccinate as a delayed treatment for mercury removal in rats. *Environmental Health Perspectives*, *102*(Suppl. 3), 309–311.

Kostyniak, P. J. (1983). Methylmercury removal in the dog during infusion of 2,3-dimercaptosuccinic acid (DMSA). *Journal of Toxicology and Environmental Health*, *11*, 947–957.

Koutenský, J., Eybl, V., Koutenská, M., Sýkora, J., & Mertl, F. (1971). Influence of sodium diethyldithiocarbamate on the toxicity and distribution of copper in mice. *European Journal of Pharmacology*, *14*, 389–392.

Kravzov, J., Rios, C., Altagracia, M., Monroy-Noyola, A., & López, F. (1993). Relationship between physicochemical properties of prussian blue and its efficacy as antidote against thallium poisoning. *Journal of Applied Toxicology*, *13*, 213–216.

Kreppel, H., Reichl, F. X., Forth, W., & Fichtl, B. (1989). Lack of effectiveness of D-penicillamine in experimental arsenic poisoning. *Veterinary Human Toxicology*, *31*, 1–5.

Kreppel, H., Paepcke, U., Thiermann, H., Szinicz, L., Reichl, F. X., Singh, P. K., & Jones, M. M. (1993). Therapeutic efficacy of new dimercaptosuccinic acid (DMSA) analogues in acute arsenic trioxide poisoning in mice. *Archives of Toxicology*, *67*, 580–585.

Krewski, D., Yokel, R. A., Nieboer, E., Borchelt, D., Cohen, J., Harry, J., Kacew, S., Lindsay, J., Mahfouz, A. M., & Rondeau, V. (2007). Human health risk assessment for aluminium, aluminium oxide and aluminium hydroxide. *Journal of Toxicology and Environmental Health, Part B, 10*, 1–269.

Kreyberg, S., Torvik, A., Bjørneboe, A., Wiik-Larsen, W., & Jacobsen, D. (1992). Trimethyltin poisoning: report of a case with postmortem examination. *Clinical Neuropathology, 11*, 256–259.

Krigman, M. R., & Silverman, A. P. (1984). General toxicology of tin and its organic compounds. *Neurotoxicology, 5*, 129–139.

Kruck, T. P., Cui, J. G., Percy, M. E., & Lukiw, W. J. (2004). Molecular Shuttle Chelation: The Use of Ascorbate, Desferrioxamine and Feralex-G in Combination to Remove Nuclear Bound Aluminum. *Cellular and Molecular Neurobiology, 24*, 443–459.

Kruszewska, S., Wiese, M., Kołaciński, Z., & Mielczarska, J. (1996). The use of haemodialysis and 2,3 propanesulphonate (DMPS) to manage acute oral poisoning by lethal dose of arsenic trioxide. *International Journal of Occupational Medicine and Environmental Health, 9*, 111–115.

Kumar, A., Zhang, X., & Liang, X. J. (2013). Gold nanoparticles: emerging paradigm for targeted drug delivery system. *Biotechnology Advances, 31*, 593–606.

Kung, N. N., Sung, J. J., Yuen, N. W., Ng, P. W., Wong, K. C., Chung, E. C., Lim, B. H., Choi, C. H., Li, T. H., Ma, H. C., & Kwok, S. P. (1997). Anti-Helicobacter pylori treatment in bleeding ulcers: randomized controlled trial comparing 2-day versus 7-day bismuth quadruple therapy. *American Journal of Gastroenterology, 92*, 438–441.

Kuo, C. -H., Kuo, F. -C., Hu, H. -M., Liu, C. -J., Wang, S. W., Chen, Y. -H., Hsieh, M. C., Hou, M. -F., & Wu, D. -C. (2012). The optimal first-line therapy of helicobacter pylori infection in year 2012 gastroenterol. *Research and Practice, 2012*, 168361.

Kurtin, A., & Orentreich, N. J. (1954). Chelation deactivation of nickel ion in allergic eczematous sensitivity. *Investigative Dermatology, 22*, 441–445.

Lai, M. W., Boyer, E. W., Kleinman, M. E., Rodig, N. M., & Ewald, M. B. (2005). Acute arsenic poisoning in two siblings. *Pediatrics, 116*, 249–257.

Laine, L., Hunt, R., El-Zimaity, H., Nguyen, B., Osato, M., & Spénard, J. (2003). Bismuth-based quadruple therapy using a single capsule of bismuth biskalcitrate, metronidazole, and tetracycline given with omeprazole versus omeprazole, amoxicillin, and clarithromycin for eradication of Helicobacter pylori in duodenal ulcer patients: a prospective, randomized, multicenter, North American trial. *American Journal of Gastroenterology, 98*, 562–567.

Lansdown, A. B. (2006). Silver in health care: antimicrobial effects and safety in use. *Current Problems in Dermatology, 33*, 17–34.

Langård, S., & Costa, M. (2014). Chromium. In G. F. Nordberg, B. A. Fowler, & M. Monica Nordberg (Eds.), *Handbook on the Toxicology of Metals* (4th ed., pp. 717–742). Amsterdam, NL: Elsevier/AP.

Lanphear, B. P., Hornung, R., Khoury, J., Yolton, K., Baghurst, P., Bellinger, D. C., Canfield, R. L., Dietrich, K. N., Bornschein, R., Greene, T., Rothenberg, S. J., Needleman, H. L., Schnaas, L., Wasserman, G., Graziano, J., & Roberts, R. (2005). Low-level environmental lead exposure and children's intellectual function: an international pooled analysis. *Environmental Health Perspectives, 113*, 894–899.

Lauwers, L. F., Roelants, A., Rosseel, P. M., Heyndrickx, B., & Baute, L. (1990). Oral antimony intoxications in man. *Critical Care Medicine, 18*, 324–326.

Lee, B. K., Schwartz, B. S., Stewart, W., & Ahn, K. D. (1995). Provocative chelation with DMSA and EDTA: evidence for differential access to lead storage sites. *Occupational and Environmental Medicine, 52*, 13–19.

Lee, A. G. (1971). *The chemistry of thallium*. New York: Elsevier.

Leloux, M. S., Lich, N. P., & Claude, J. R. (1990). Experimental studies on thallium toxicity in rats. II--The influence of several antidotal treatments on the tissue distribution and elimination of thallium, after subacute intoxication. *Clinical and Experimental Toxicology Journal, 10,* 147–156, 1990.

Lentz, K., Hruby, K., Druml, W., Eder, A., Gaszner, A., Kleinberger, G., Pichler, M., & Weiser, M. (1981). 2,3-Dimercaptosuccinic acid in human arsenic poisoning. *Archives of Toxicology, 47,* 241–243.

Levin-Scherz, J. K., Patrick, J. D., Weber, F. H., & Garabedian, C., Jr. (1987). Acute arsenic ingestion. *Annals of Emergency Medicine, 16,* 702–704.

Lewis, R. (2004). Occupational Exposures: Metals. 439-441. In J. LaDou (Ed.), *Current Occupational & Environmental Medicine* (3rd ed.). New York: Lange Medical Books/McGraw-Hill Companies, Inc.

Licht, A., Oliver, M., & Rachmilewitz, E. A. (1972). Optic atrophy following treatment with cobalt chloride in a patient with pancytopenia and hypercellular marrow. *Israel Journal of Medical Sciences, 8,* 61–66.

Lide, D.R. (2007–2008). Platinum. In CRC., contributors, *CRC handbook of chemistry, physics* (Vol. 4). New York: CRC Press. (p. 26).

Lie, R., Thomas, R. G., & Scott, J. K. (1960). The distribution and excretion of thallium-204 in the rat, with suggested MPC's and a bio-assay procedure. *Health Physics, 2,* 334–340.

Liebelt, E. L., Shannon, M., & Graef, J. W. (1994). Efficacy of oral meso-2,3-dimercaptosuccinic acid therapy for low-level childhood plumbism. *Journal of Pediatrics, 124,* 313–317.

Lin, C. C., Wu, M. L., Yang, C. C., Ger, J., Tsai, W. J., & Deng, J. F. (2009). Acute severe chromium poisoning after dermal exposure to hexavalent chromium. *Journal of the Chinese Medical Association, 72,* 219–221.

Linder, M. C., & Hazegh-Azam, M. (1996). Copper biochemistry and molecular biology. *American Journal of Clinical Nutrition, 63,* 797S–811S.

Linder, M. C., Wooten, L., Cerveza, P., Cotton, S., Shulze, R., & Lomeli, N. (1998). Copper transport. *American Journal of Clinical Nutrition, 67,* 965–971.

Lison, D. (2014). Cobalt. In G. F. Nordberg, B. A. Fowler, & M. Nordberg (Eds.), *Handbook on the toxicology of metals* (4th ed., pp. 743–763). Amsterdam, NL: Elsevier/AP.

Litovitz, T., & Manoguerra, A. (1992). Comparison of pediatric poisoning hazards: an analysis of 3.8 million exposure incidents. A report from the American Association of Poison Control Centers. *Pediatrics, 89,* 999–1006.

Liu, K. J., & Shi, X. (2001). In vivo reduction of chromium (VI) and its related free radical generation. *Molecular and Cellular Biochemistry, 222,* 41–47.

Liu, P., Yao, Y. N., Wu, S. D., Dong, H. J., Feng, G. C., & Yuan, X. Y. (2005). The efficacy of deferiprone on tissues aluminum removal and copper, zinc, manganese level in rabbits. *Journal of Inorganic Biochemistry, 99,* 1733–1737.

Ljunggren, K. G., Lidums, V., & Sjögren, B. (1991). Blood and urine concentrations of aluminium among workers exposed to aluminium flake powders. *British Journal of Industrial Medicine, 48,* 106–109.

Llanos, R. M., & Mercer, J. F. B. (2002). The molecular basis of copper homeostasis copper-related disorders. *DNA and Cell Biology, 21,* 259–270.

Llobet, J. M., Domingo, J. L., & Corbella, J. (1985). Comparison of antidotal efficacy of chelating agents upon acute toxicity of Co(II) in mice. *Research Communications in Chemical Pathology and Pharmacology, 50,* 305–308.

Llobet, J. M., Domingo, J. L., & Corbella, J. (1986). Comparison of the effectiveness of several chelators after single administration on the toxicity, excretetion and distribution of cobalt. *Archives of Toxicology, 58,* 278–281.

Llobet, J. M., Domingo, J. L., & Corbella, J. (1988a). Comparative effects of repeated parenteral administration of several chelators on the distribution and excretion of cobalt. *Research Communications in Chemical Pathology and Pharmacology*, *60*, 225–233.

Llobet, J. M., Domingo, J. L., & Corbella, J. (1988b). Antidotes for zinc intoxication in mice. *Archives of Toxicology*, *61*, 321–323.

Llobet, J. M., Colomina, M. T., Domingo, J. L., & Corbella, J. (1989). Comparison of the antidotal efficacy of polyamincarboxylic acids (CDTA and DTPA) with time after acute zinc poisoning. *Veterinary and Human Toxicology*, *31*, 25–28.

Llobet, J. M., Domingo, J. L., Paternain, J. L., & Corbella, J. (1990). Treatment of acute lead intoxication. A quantitative comparison of a number of chelating agents. *Archives of Environmental Contamination and Toxicology*, *19*, 185–189.

Loehrer, P.J., & Einhorn, L.H. (1984). Drugs five years later. Cisplatin. *Annals of Internal Medicine, 100*, 704–713.

Love, C., & Palestro, C. J. (2004). Radionuclide imaging of infection. *Journal of Nuclear Medicine Technology*, *32*, 47–57.

Low, G. C. (1916). The history of the use of intravenous injections of tartar emetic (Antimonium tartaratum) in tropical medicine. *Transactions of the Royal Society of Tropical Medicine and Hygiene*, *10*, 37–47.

Lown, B. A., Morganti, J. B., Stineman, C. H., D'Agostino, R. B., & Massaro, E. J. (1980). Tissue organ distribution and behavioral effects of platinum following acute and repeated exposure of the mouse to platinum sulfate. *Environmental Health Perspectives*, *34*, 203–212.

Lu, C. S., Huang, C. C., Chu, N. S., & Calne, D. B. (1994). Levodopa failure in chronic manganism. *Neurology*, *44*, 1600–1602.

Lu, C. I., Huang, C. C., Chang, Y. C., Tsai, Y. T., Kuo, H. C., Chuang, Y. H., & Shih, T. S. (2007). Short-term thallium intoxication: dermatological findings correlated with thallium concentration. *Archives of Dermatology*, *143*(1), 93–98.

Lu, L. K., Warshaw, E. M., & Dunnick, C. A. (2009). Prevention of nickel allergy: the case for regulation? *Dermatologic Clinics*, *27*, 155–161.

Lucchini, R. G., Zoni, S., Guazzetti, S., Bontempi, E., Micheletti, S., Broberg, K., Parrinello, G., & Smith, D. R. (2012). Inverse association of intellectual function with very low blood lead but not with manganese exposure in Italian adolescents. *Environmental Research*, *118*, 65–71.

Lund, A. (1956a). The effect of various substances on the excretion and the toxicity of thallium in the rat. *Acta Pharmacology and Toxicology*, *12*, 260–268.

Lund, A. (1956b). Distribution of thallium in the organism and its elimination. *Acta Pharmacology and Toxicology*, *12*, 251–259.

Magdalan, J., Smolarek, M., Porebska, B., Zawadzki, M., & Dyś, P. (2007). Two different clinical cases of acute arsenic trioxide intoxication. *Przegl Lek*, *64*, 336–338.

Magos, L. (1976). The effects of dimercaptosuccinic acid on the excretion and distribution of mercury in rats and mice treated with mercuric chloride and methylmercury chloride. *British Journal of Pharmacology*, *56*, 479–484.

Mahoney, J. R., Jr., Hallaway, P. E., Hedlund, B. E., & Eaton, J. W. (1989). Acute iron poisoning. Rescue with macromolecular chelators. *Journal of Clinical Investigation*, *84*, 1362–1366.

Maillard, J. Y., & Hartemann, P. (2013). Silver as an antimicrobial: facts and gaps in knowledge. *Critical Reviews in Microbiology*, *39*, 373–383.

Maier, L., & Newman, L. S. (1998). Beryllium disease. In W. N. Rm (Ed.), *Environmental and occupational medicine* (3rd ed., pp. 1017–1031). Philadelphia: Lippincott-Raven.

Maiorino, R. M., & Aposhian, H. V. (1985). Dimercaptan metal binding agents influence the biotransformation of arsenite in the rabbit. *Toxicology and Applied Pharmacology*, *77*, 240–250.

Maiorino, R. M., Gonzales-Ramirez, D., Zuniga-Charles, M., Xu, Z., Hurlbut, K. M., Aposhian, M. M., Dart, R. C., Woods, J. S., Ostrosky-Wegman, P., Gonsebatt, M. E., & Aposhian, H. V. (1996). Sodium 2,3-dimercaptopropane-1-sulfonate challenge test for mercury in humans. III. Urinary mercury after exposure to mercurous chloride. *Journal of Pharmacology and Experimental Therapeutics*, *277*, 938–944.

Malbrain, M. L., Lambrecht, G. L., Zandijk, E., Demedts, P. A., Neels, H. M., Lambert, W., De Leenheer, A. P., Lins, R. L., & Daelemans, R. (1997). Treatment of severe thallium intoxication. *Clinical Toxicology*, *35*(1), 97–100.

Malfertheiner, P1, Megraud, F., O'Morain, C. A., Atherton, J., Axon, A. T., Bazzoli, F., Gensini, G. F., Gisbert, J. P., Graham, D. Y., Rokkas, T., El-Omar, E. M., Kuipers, E. J., & European Helicobacter Study Group (2012). Management of Helicobacter pylori infection—the Maastricht IV/ Florence Consensus Report. *Gut*, *61*, 646–664.

Malkani, R., Weinstein, J. M., Kumar, N., Victor, T. A., & Bernstein, L. (2011). Ataxia and cranial neuropathies from subcutaneously injected elemental mercury. *Clinical Toxicology*, *49*, 334–336.

Malluche, H. H., Smith, A. J., Abreo, K., & Faugere, M. C. (1984). The use of deferoxamine in the management of aluminum accumulation in bone in patients with renal-failure. *New England Journal of Medicine*, *311*, 140–144.

Maloof, C. C. (1955). Use of edathamil calcium in treatment of chrome ulcers of the skin. *AMA Archives of Industrial Health*, *11*, 123–125.

Mamdani, H., & Vettese, T. E. (2013). Pulmonary Emboli Caused by Mercury. *New England Journal of Medicine*, *369*, 2031.

Maret, W. (2013). Zinc biochemistry: from a single zinc enzyme to a key element of life. *Advances in Nutrition*, *4*, 82–91.

Markman, M. (2003). Toxicities of the platinum antineoplastic agents. *Expert Opinion on Drug Safety*, *2*, 597–607.

Markowitz, M. E., Bijur, P. E., Ruff, H., & Rosen, J. F. (1993a). Effects of calcium disodium versenate (CaNa2EDTA) chelation in moderate childhood lead poisoning. *Pediatrics*, *92*, 265–271.

Markowitz, M. E., Bijur, P. E., Ruff, H. A., Balbi, K., & Rosen, J. F. (1993b). Moderate lead poisoning: trends in blood lead levels in unchelated children. *Environmental Health Perspectives*, *104*, 968–972.

Martin-Bouyer, G. (1976). Poisoning by orally administered bismuth salts. Epidemiologic survey. *Thérapie*, *31*, 683–702.

Mason, R. W. (1983). Time course of gold-induced accumulation of copper and zinc and the effects of dimercaptosuccinate and cadmium on gold metabolism in rat kidney. *Chemico–Biological Interactions*, *43*, 199–208.

Mathieu, D., Mathieu-Nolf, M., Germain-Alonso, M., Neviere, R., Furon, D., & Wattel, F. (1992). Massive arsenic poisoning—effect of hemodialysis and dimercaprol on arsenic kinetics. *Intensive Care Medicine*, *18*, 47–50.

Mathur, S., Flora, S. J. S., Mathur, R., & Gupta, S. D. (1993). Mobilization and distribution of beryllium over the course of chelation therapy with some polyaminocarboxylic acids in the rat. *Human & Experimental Toxicology*, *12*, 19–24.

Mathur, S., Flora, S. J. S., Mathur, R., Kannan, G. M., & Gupta, S. D. (1994). Beryllium-induced biochemical alterations and their prevention following co-administration of meso-2,3-dimercaptosuccinic acid or 2,3-dimercaptopropane sulphonate in rats. *Journal of Applied Toxicology*, *14*, 263–267.

Matthey, J. (2004). Johnson Matthey Reviews, 2005. DeHavilland Information Services plc, 1998–2005.

McCallum, R. I. (1977). President's Address. Observations upon Antimony. *Proceedings of the Royal Society of Medicine*, *70*, 756–763.

McCallum, R. I. (2001). Captain James Cook's antimony cup. *Vesalius*, *7*, 62–64.

McCarthy, J. T., Milliner, D. S., & Johnson, W. J. (1990). Clinical experience with desferrioxamine in dialysis patients with aluminium toxicity. *Quarterly Journal of Medicine*, *74*, 257–276.

McCauley, J., & Sorkin, M. I. (1989). Exacerbation of aluminium encephalopathy after treatment with desferrioxamine. *Nephrology Dialysis Transplant*, *4*, 110–114.

Mccray, W. P. (1998). Glassmaking in renaissance Italy: the innovation of venetian cristallo. *Journal of the Minerals, Metals and Materials Society*, *50*, 14–19.

McKinney, P., Brent, J., & Kulig, K. (1994). Acute zinc chloride ingestion in a child: local and systemic effects. *Annals of Emergency Medicine*, *23*, 1383–1387, 1994.

McKinney, P. E., Brent, J., & Kulig, K. (1995). Zinc chloride ingestion in a child: exocrine pancreatic insufficiency. *Annals of Emergency Medicine*, *25*, 562.

Meggs, W. J., Cahill-Morasco, R., Shih, R. D., Goldfrank, L. R., & Hoffman, R. S. (1997). Effects of Prussian blue and N-acetylcysteine on thallium toxicity in mice. *Clinical Toxicology*, *35*, 163–166.

Memon, A. A., Molokhia, M. M., & Friedman, P. S. (1994). The inhibitory effects of topical chelating agents and antioxidants on nickel-induced hypersensitivity reactions. *Journal of American Academy of Dermatology*, *30*, 560–565.

Menne, T., & Kaaber, K. (1978). Treatment of pompholyx due to nickel allergy with chelating agents. *Contact Dermatitis*, *4*, 289–290.

Menne, T., Kaaber, K., & Tjell, C. (1980). Treatment of nickel dermatitis. (The influence of tetraethylthiuramdisulfide (Antabuse) on nickel metabolism). *Annals of Clinical and Laboratory Science*, *10*, 160–164.

Mercer, J. J., Bercovitch, L., & Muglia, J. J. (2012). Acrodynia and hypertension in a young girl secondary to elemental mercury toxicity acquired in the home. *Pediatric Dermatology*, *29*, 199–201.

Merget, R., Reineke, M., Rückmann, A., Bergmann, E. M., & Schultze-Werninghaus, G. (1994). Nonspecific and specific bronchial responsiveness in occupational asthma caused by platinum salts after allergen avoidance. *American Journal of Respiratory and Critical Care Medicine*, *150*, 1146–1149.

Merkord, J., Weber, H., Kröning, G., & Hennighausen, G. (2000). Antidotal effects of 2,3-dimercaptopropane-1-sulfonic acid (DMPS) and meso-2,3-dimercaptosuccinic acid (DMSA) on the organotoxicity of dibutyltin dichloride (DBTC) in rats. *Human and Experimental Toxicology*, *19*, 132–137.

Mesopotamia, The International History Project, 2003. http://history-world.org/mesopotamia_9000.htm

Michaux, I., Haufroid, V., Dive, A., Buchet, J. P., Bulpa, P., Mahieu, P., & Installé, E. (2000). Repetitive endoscopy and continuous alkaline gastric irrigation in a case of arsenic poisoning. *Journal of Toxicology: Clinical Toxicology*, *38*, 471–476.

Mikler, J., Banovcin, P., Jesenak, M., Hamzikova, J., & Statelova, D. (2009). Successful treatment of extreme acute lead intoxication. *Toxicology and Industrial Health*, *25*, 137–140.

Mills, K. C., & Curry, S. C. (1994). Acute iron poisoning. *Emergency Medicine Clinics of North America*, *12*, 397–413.

Milne, C., & Petros, A. (2010). The use of haemofiltration for severe iron overdose. *Archives of Disease in Childhood*, *95*, 482–483.

Molina, J. A., Calandre, L., & Bermejo, F. (1989). Myoclonic encephalopathy due to bismuth salts: treatment with dimercaprol and analysis of CSF transmitters. *Acta Neurologica Scandinavia*, *79*, 200–203.

Molina-Jijón, E., Zarco-Márquez, G., Medina-Campos, O. N., Zataraín-Barrón, Z. L., Hernández-Pando, R., Pinzón, E., Zavaleta, R. M., Tapia, E., & Pedraza-Chaverri, J. (2012). Deferoxamine pretreatment prevents Cr(VI)-induced nephrotoxicity and oxidant stress: role of Cr(VI) chelation. *Toxicology*, *291*, 93–101.

Moller, L. B., Ott, P., Lund, C., & Horn, N. (2005). Homozygosity for a gross partial gene deletion of the C-terminal end of ATP7B in a Wilson patient with hepatic and no neurological manifestations. *American Journal of Medical Genetics A*, *138*, 340–343.

Montes, S., Pérez-Barrón, G., Rubio-Osornio, M., Ríos, C., Diaz-Ruíz, A., Altagracia-Martínez, M., & Monroy-Noyola, A. (2011). Additive effect of DL-penicillamine plus Prussian blue for the antidotal treatment of thallotoxicosis in rats. *Environmental Toxicology and Pharmacology*, *32*, 349–355.

Moore, D. F., O'Callaghan, C. A., Berlyne, G., Ogg, C. S., Davies, H. A., House, I. M., & Henry, J. A. (1994). Acute arsenic poisoning: absence of polyneuropathy after treatment with 2,3-dimercaptopropanesulphonate (DMPS). *Journal of Neurology, Neurosurgery and Psychiatry*, *57*, 1133–1135.

Moore, W., Jr., Hysell, D., Hall, L., Campbell, K., & Stara, J. (1975a). Preliminary studies on the toxicity and metabolism of palladium and platinum. *Environmental Health Perspectives*, *10*, 63–71.

Moore, W., Jr., Hysell, D., Crocker, W., & Stara, J. (1975b). Biological fate of a single administration of 191Pt in rats following different routes of exposure. *Environmental Research*, *9*, 152–158.

Moore, W., Jr., Malanchuk, M., Crocker, W., Hysell, D., Cohen, A., & Stara, J. F. (1975c). Whole body retention in rats of different 191Pt compounds following inhalation exposure. *Environmental Health Perspectives*, *12*, 35–39.

Morin, Y., & Daniel, P. (1967). Quebec beer-drinkers' cardiomyopathy: etiological considerations. *Canadian Medical Association Journal*, *97*, 926–928.

Morris, C. C. (2000). Pediatric iron poisonings in the United States. *South Medical Journal*, *93*, 352–358.

Mostafazadeh, B., Kiani, A., Mohamadi, E., Shaki, F., & Shirazi, F. H. (2013). Mercury exposure of gold mining workers in the northwest of Iran. *Pakistan Journal of Pharmaceutical Sciences*, *26*, 1267–1270.

Mroz, M. M., Balkisson, R., & Newman, L. S. (2001). Beryllium. In E. Bingham, B. Cohrssen, & Ch. H. Powell (Eds.), *Patty's toxicology* (5th ed., pp. 177–220). New York: John Wiley and Sons, Inc.

Muckter, H., Liebl, B., Reichl, F. X., Hunder, G., Walther, U., & Fichtl, B. (1997). Are we ready to replace dimercaprol (BAL) as an arsenic antidote? *Human & Experimental Toxicology*, *16*, 460–465.

Mulkey, J. P., & Oehme, F. W. (2000). Are 2,3-dimercapto-1-propanesulfonic acid or prussian blue beneficial in acute thallotoxicosis in rats? *Veterinary and Human Toxicology*, *42*, 325–329.

Muñoz, A., & Costa, M. (2012). Elucidating the mechanisms of nickel compound uptake: a review of particulate and nano-nickel endocytosis and toxicity. *Toxicology and Applied Pharmacology*, *260*, 1–16.

Nakazawa, A., Ikeda, K., Ito, Y., Iwase, M., Sato, K., Ueda, R., & Dohi, Y. (2004). Usefulness of dual 67Ga and 99mTc-sestamibi single-photon-emission CT scanning in the diagnosis of cardiac sarcoidosis. *Chest*, *126*, 1372–1376.

Nagasawa, K., Ito, S., Kakuda, T., Nagai, K., Tamai, I., Tsuji, A., & Fujimoto, S. (2005). Transport mechanism for aluminum citrate at the blood-brain barrier: kinetic evidence implies involvement of system Xc- in immortalized rat brain endothelial cells. *Toxicology Letters*, *155*, 289–296.

Naha, K., Saravu, K., & Shastry, B. A. (2012). Blue vitriol poisoning: a 10-year experience in a tertiary care hospital. *Clinical Toxicology*, *50*, 197–201.

Nasemann, T., Rogge, T., & Schaeg, G. (1974). Light and electron microscopy studies of hydrargyrosis and argyrosis of the skin. *Hautarzt*, *25*, 534–540.

Neldner, K. H., Hambidge, K. M., & Walravens, P. A. (1978). Acrodermatitis enteropathica. *International Journal of Dermatology*, *17*, 380–387.

Newman, L. S., & Kreiss, K. (1992). Nonoccupational beryllium disease masquerading as sarcoidosis: identification by blood lymphocyte proliferative response to beryllium. *American Review of Respiratory Diseases*, *14*, 1212–1214.

Newton, D., & Holmes, A. (1966). A case of accidental inhalation of zinc-65 and silver-110m. *Radiation Research*, *29*, 403–412.

Ng, A. K., Bernardo, M. V., Silver, B., Van Den Abbeele, A., Stevenson, M. A., Fisher, D. C., & Mauch, P. M. (2005). Mid- and post-ABVD gallium scanning predicts for recurrence in early-stage Hodgkin's disease. *International Journal of Radiation Oncology Biology Physics*, *61*, 175–184.

Nicholson, P. (2009). Faience Technology. *UCLA encyclopedia of egyptology*. Los Angeles, California, USA: UCLA.

Nieboer, E., Gibson, B. L., Oxman, A. D., & Kramer, J. R. (1995). Health effects of aluminum: a critical review with emphasis on aluminum in drinking water. *Environmental Review*, *3*, 29–81.

Niehues, R., Horstkotte, D., Klein, R. M., Kühl, U., Kutkuhn, B., Hort, W., Iffland, R., & Strauer, B. E. (1995). Repeated ingestion with suicidal intent of potentially lethal amounts of thallium. *German Medical Weekly*, *120*, 403–408.

Nielsen, J. B., & Andersen, O. (1989). Oral mercuric chloride exposure in mice: effects of dose on intestinal absorption and relative organ distribution. *Toxicology*, *59*, 1–10.

Nielsen, J. B., & Andersen, O. (1991). Effect of four thiol-containing chelators on disposition of orally administered mercuric chloride. *Human and Experimental Toxicology*, *10*, 423–430.

Nielsen, G. D., & Andersen, O. (1994). Effect of tetraethylthiuramdisulphide and diethyldithiocarbamate on nickel toxicokinetics in mice. *Pharmacology and Toxicology*, *75*, 285–293.

Nielsen, G. D., Andersen, O., & Jensen, M. (1993). Toxicokinetics of nickel in mice studied with the γ-emitting isotope ^{57}Ni. *Fundamental Applied Toxicology*, *21*, 236–243.

Niezborala, M., & Garnier, R. (1996). Allergy to complex platinum salts: a historical prospective cohort study. *Occupational and Environmental Medicine*, *53*, 252–257.

Nirala, S. K., Bhadauria, M., Mathur, R., & Mathur, A. (2007). Amelioration of beryllium induced alterations in hepatorenal biochemistry and ultramorphology by co-administration of tiferron and adjuvants. *Journal of Biomedical Science*, *14*, 331–345.

Nirala, S. K., Bhadauria, M., Shukla, S., Agrawal, O. M., Mathur, A., Li, P. Q., & Mathur, R. (2008). Pharmacological intervention of tiferron and propolis to alleviate beryllium-induced hepatorenal toxicity. *Fundamental & Clinical Pharmacology*, *22*, 403–415.

No authors listed (1993). Diagnosis and treatment of aluminium overload in end-stage renal failure patients. Consensus conference. Paris, France, 27 June 1992. *Nephrology Dialysis Transplantation*, *1*(8 Suppl.), 1–54.

Nogue, S., Mas, A., Pares, A., Nadal, P., Bertrán, A., Millá, J., Carrera, M., To, J., Pazos, M. R., & Corbella, J. (1982). Acute thallium poisoning: an evaluation of different forms of treatment. *Journal of Toxicology: Clinical Toxicology*, *19*, 1015–1021.

Nordberg, G. F., Nogawa, K., & Nordberg, M. (2014). Cadmium. In G. F. Nordberg, B. A. Fowler, & M. Nordberg (Eds.), *Handbook on the toxicology of metals* (4th ed., pp. 667–715). Amsterdam, NL: Elsevier/AP.

Nowak-Wiaderek, W. (1975). Influence of various drugs on excretion and distribution of chromium-51 in acute poisoning in rats. *Polish Journal of Medicine and Pharmacy*, *7*, 308–310.

NRC (National Research Council) (1975). Nickel. National Academy of Sciences, Washington, DC.

Nriagu, J. O. (1996). A history of global metal pollution. *Science*, *272*, 223–224.

Nriagu, J. O. (1998). Tales told in lead. *Science*, *281*, 1622–1623.

Okonishnikova, I. E., Rozenberg, E. E., & Rezina, I. A. (1976). Therapeutic and prophylactic action of succimer in experimental subacute lead acetate poisoning. *Gig. Tr. Orof. Zabol*, *8*, 24–28.

Oldenburg, M., Wegner, R., & Baur, X. (2009). Severe cobalt intoxication due to prosthesis wear in repeated total hip arthroplasty. *Journal of Arthroplasty*, *24*, 820–825.

Oldenquist, G., & Salem, M. (1999). Parenteral copper sulfate poisoning causing acute renal failure. *Nephrology Dialysis Transplantation*, *14*, 441–443.

Oskarsson, A., & Tjälve, H. (1980). Effects of diethyldithiocarbamate and penicillamine on the tissue distribution of 63NiCl2 in mice. *Archives of Toxicology*, *45*, 45–52.

Ottaway, B. S., & Roberts, B. (2008). In A. Jones (Ed.), *The emergence of metalworking., prehistoric europe: theory and practice* (pp. 208). London: Wiley-Blackwell.

Ovaska, H., Wood, D. M., House, I., Dargan, P. I., Jones, A. L., & Murray, S. (2008). Severe iatrogenic bismuth poisoning with bismuth iodoform paraffin paste treated with DMPS chelation. *Clinical Toxicology*, *46*, 855–857.

Özbal, H. (2001). Ancient Anatolian Metallurgy. (pdf. Downloaded 4/11-2015). http://www.transanatolie.com/english/turkey/Turkey%20PDF/SOMP-05-Research-Ancient%20Metallurg-Ozbal.pdf

Pappas, J. B., Nuttall, K. L., Ahlquist, J. T., Allen, E. M., & Banner, W., Jr. (1995). Oral dimercaptosuccinic acid and ongoing exposure to lead: effects on heme synthesis and lead distribution in a rat model. *Toxicology and Applied Pharmacology*, *133*, 121–129.

Pau, P. W. (2000). Management of thallium poisoning. *Hong Kong Medical Journal*, *6*, 316–318.

Pawlas, N., Broberg, K., Olewinska, E., Prokopowicz, A., Skerfving, S., & Pawlas, K. (2012). Modification by the genes ALAD and VDR of lead-induced cognitive effects in children. *Neurotoxicology*, *33*, 37–43.

Pazzaglia, U. E., Apostoli, P., Congiu, T., Catalani, S., Marchese, M., & Zarattini, G. (2011). Cobalt, chromium and molybdenum ions kinetics in the human body: data gained from a total hip replacement with massive third body wear of the head and neuropathy by cobalt intoxication. *Archives of Orthopaedic and Trauma Surgery*, *31*, 1299–1308.

Peck, M. G., Rogers, J. F., & Rivenbark, J. F. (1982). Use of high doses of deferoxamine (Desferal) in an adult patient with acute iron overdosage. *Journal of Toxicology and Clinical Toxicology*, *19*, 865–869.

Pelclová, D., Urban, P., Ridzon, P., Senholdová, Z., Lukás, E., Diblík, P., & Lacina, L. (2009). Two-year follow-up of two patients after severe thallium intoxication. *Human and Experimental Toxicology*, *28*, 263–272.

Pelclova, D., Sklensky, M., Janicek, P., & Lach, K. (2012). Severe cobalt intoxication following hip replacement revision: clinical features and outcome. *Clinical Toxicology*, *50*, 262–265.

Pélissier-Alicot, A. L., Salério, G., Marquet FP., Panteix, G., & Léonetti, G. (2003). Acute poisoning caused by intravenous arsenic. *Medical Press*, *32*, 1849–1851.

Peters, R. A., Stocken, L. A., & Thompson, R. H. S. (1945). British anti-lewisite (BAL). *Nature*, *156*, 616–619.

Peterson, R. P., Jensen, L. S., & Harrison, P. C. (1973). Effect of silver-induced enlarged hearts during the first four weeks of life on subsequent performance of turkeys. *Avian Diseases*, *17*, 802–806.

Petracca, M., Scafa, F., Boeri, R., Flachi, D., & Candura, S. M. (2013). Imported occupational lead poisoning: report of four cases. *Medicina del Lavoro*, *104*, 428–433.

Petris, M. J., Smith, K., Lee, J., & Thiele, D. J. (2003). Copper-stimulated endocytosis and degradation of the human copper transporter, hCtr1. *Journal of Biological Chemistry*, *278*, 9639–9646.

Pitsillides, C. M., Joe, E. K., Wei, X., Anderson, R. R., & Lin, C. P. (2003). Selective cell targeting with light-absorbing microparticles and nanoparticles. *Biophysical Journal*, *84*, 4023–4032.

Pfab, R., Müchter, H., Roider, G., & Zilker, T. (1996). Clinical course of severe poisoning with thiomersal. *Clinical Toxicology*, *34*, 453–460.

Pfister, G., Catsch, A., & Nigrović, V. (1967). Antidotes in acute iron poisoning. Animal experimental studies. *Arzneimittelforschung*, *17*, 748–751.

Planas-Boehne, F. J. (1981). The influence of chelating agents on the distribution and biotransformation of methylmercuric chloride in rats. *Journal of Pharmacology and Experimental Therapeutics*, *217*, 500–504.

Planas-Boehne, F., Shand, E., & Taylor, D. M. (1982). The effects of dimercaptosuccinic acid and other chelating agents on the retention of platinum in the rat kidney after treatment with cisplatin. *Cancer Chemotherapy and Pharmacology*, *9*, 120–121.

Playford, R. J., Matthews, C. H., Campbell, M. J., Delves, H. T., Hla, K. K., Hodgson, H. J., & Calam, J. (1990). Bismuth induced encephalopathy caused by tri potassium dicitrato bismuthate in a patient with chronic renal failure. *Gut*, *31*, 359–360.

Polyzois, I., Nikolopoulos, D., Michos, I., Patsouris, E., & Theocharis, S. (2012). Local and systemic toxicity of nanoscale debris particles in total hip arthroplasty. *Journal of Applied Toxicology*, *32*, 255–269.

Ponka, P., Tenenbeim, M., & Eaton, J. W. (2014). Iron. In G. F. Nordberg, B. A. Fowler, & M. Nordberg (Eds.), *Handbook on the toxicology of metals* (4th ed., pp. 879–902). Amsterdam, NL: Elsevier/AP.

POISINDEX (2004). Poisindex System, Thomson Micromedex Health Care Series 2004. (monograph on CD-ROM), Vol. 122.

Priest, N. D. (2004). The biological behaviour and bioavailability of aluminium in man, with special reference to studies employing aluminium-26 as a tracer: review and study update. *Journal of Environmental Monitoring*, *6*, 375–403.

Priest, N. D., Talbot, R. J., Newton, D., Day, J. P., King, S. J., & Fifield, L. K. (1998). Uptake by man of aluminium in a public water supply. *Human and Experimental Toxicology*, *17*, 296–301.

Quarles, C. D., Jr., Marcus, R. K., & Brumaghim, J. L. (2011). Competitive binding of Fe3+, Cr3+, and Ni2+ to transferrin. *Journal of Biological Inorganic Chemistry*, *16*, 913–921.

Quevauviller, P., Lavigne, R., Pinel, R., & Astruc, M. (1989). Organo-tins in sediments and mussels from the Sado estuarine system (Portugal). *Environmental Pollution*, *57*, 149–166.

Rabinowitz, M. B., Kopple, J. D., & Wetherill, G. D. (1980). Effect of food intake and fasting on gastrointestinal lead absorption in humans. *American Journal of Clinical Nutrition*, *33*, 1784–1788.

Rae, T. D., Schmidt, P. J., Pufahl, R. A., Culotta, V. C., & O'Halloran, T. V. (1999). Undetectable intracellular free copper: the requirement of a copper chaperone for superoxide dismutase. *Science*, *284*, 805–808.

Raedsch, R., Walter-Sack, I., Weber, E., & Blessing, J. (1990). Pharmacokinetics of bismuth preparatio ns in patients with gastritis and ulcer disease. *Klin Wochenschr*, *68*, 488.

Rauws, A. G. (1974). Thallium pharmacokinetics and its modification by Prussian Blue. *Naunyn Schmiedebergs Archives of Pharmacology*, *284*, 294–306.

Rauws, A. G., ten Ham, M., & Kamerbeek, H. H. (1969). Influence of the antidote dithiocarb on distribution and toxicity of thallium in the rat. *Archives of International Pharmacodynamics and Therapy*, *182*, 425–426.

Rehani, B., & Wissman, R. (2011). Lead Poisoning from a Gunshot Wound. *Southern Medical Journal*, *104*, 57–58.

Reynolds, P. T., Abalos, K. C., Hopp, J., & Williams, M. E. (2012). Bismuth toxicity: a rare cause of neurologic dysfunction. *International Journal of Clinical Medicine*, *3*, 46–48.

Richeson, E. M. (1958). Industrial thallium intoxication. *Industrial Medicine and Surgery*, *27*, 607–619.

Riedel, S., & Kaupp, M. (2009). The highest oxidation states of the transition metal elements. *Coordination Chemistry Reviews*, *25*, 606–624.

Rios, C., & Monroy-Noyola, A. (1992). D-penicillamine and prussian blue as antidotes against thallium intoxication in rats. *Toxicology*, *74*, 69–76.

Riyaz, R., Pandalai, S. L., Schwartz, M., & Kazzi, Z. N. (2013). A fatal case of thallium toxicity: challenges in management. *Journal of Medical Toxicology*, *9*, 75–78.

Roberts, E. A., & Schilsky, M. L. (2003). A practice guideline on Wilson disease. *Hepatology*, *37*, 1475–1492.

Roberts, A. (1951). Platinosis; a five-year study of the effects of soluble platinum salts on employees in a platinum laboratory and refinery. *Archives of Industrial Hygiene and Occupational Medicine*, *4*, 549–559.

Roels, H. A., Boeckx, M., Ceulemans, E., & Lauwerys, R. R. (1991). Urinary excretion of mercury after occupational exposure to mercury vapour and influence of the chelating agent meso-2,3-dimercaptosuccinic acid (DMSA). *British Journal of Industrial Medicine*, *48*, 247–253.

Rogan, W. J., Bornschein, R. L., Chisholm, J. J., et al. (1998). *Pediatric and Perinatal Epidemiology*, *12*, 313–333.

Rogan, W. J., Dietrich, K. N., Ware, J. H., Dockery, D. W., Salganik, M., Radcliffe, J., Jones, R. L., Ragan, N. B., Chisolm, J. J., Jr., & Rhoads, G. G. (2001). Treatment of Lead-Exposed Children Trial Group. The effect of chelation therapy with succimer on neuropsychological development in children exposed to lead. *New England Journal of Medicine*, *344*, 1421–1426.

Roses, O. E., Garcia Fernandes, J. C., Villaamil, E. C., Camussa, N., Minetti, S. A., Martinez de Marco, M., Quiroga, P. N., Rattay, P., Sassone, A., Valle, Garecca, B. S., Lopez, C. M., Olmos, V., Pazos, P., Pineiro, P., & Todrigues Lenci, J. (1991). Mass poisoning by sodium arsenite. *Journal of Toxicology: Clinical Toxicology*, *29*, 209–213.

Roskams, A. J., & Connor, J. R. (1990). Aluminum access to the brain: a role for transferrin and its receptor. *Proceedings of National Academy of Sciences of the USA*, *87*, 9024–9027.

Rosner, M. H., & Carter, D. E. (1987). Metabolism and excretion of gallium arsenide and arsenic oxides by hamsters following intratracheal instillation. *Fundamental Applied Toxicology*, *9*, 730–737.

Rossi, L. S., Clemente, G. F., & Santaroni, G. (1976). Mercury and selenium distribution in a defined area and in its population. *Archives of Environmental Health*, *31*, 160–165.

Rowens, B., Guerrero-Betancourt, D., Gottlieb, C. A., Boyes, R. J., & Eichenhorn, M. S. (1991). Respiratory failure and death following acute inhalation of mercury vapor. A clinical and histologic perspective. *Chest*, *99*, 185–190.

Rubin, M., Sliwinski, A., Photias, M., Feldman, M., & Zvaifler, N. (1967). Influence of chelation on gold metabolism in rats. *Proceedings of the Society for Experimental Biology and Medicine*, *124*, 290–296.

Ruprecht, J. (2008). Dimaval. *Scientific Product Monograph*. Berlin: Heyl.

Rusyniak, D. E., Kao, L. W., Nanagas, K. A., Kirk, M. A., Furbee, R. B., Brizendine, E. J., & Wilmot, P. E. (2003). Dimercaptosuccinic acid and Prussian Blue in the treatment of acute thallium poisoning in rats. *Journal of Toxicology: Clinical Toxicology*, *41*, 137–142.

Rytuba, J. J. (2003). Mercury from mineral deposits and potential environmental impact. *Environmental Geology*, *43*, 326–338.

Sakai, T., Ushio, K., & Ikeya, Y. (1998). Mobilized plasma lead as an index of lead body burden and its relation to the heme-related indices. *Industrial Health*, *36*, 240–246.

Saljooghi, A. S. (2012). Chelation of aluminum by combining deferasirox and deferiprone in rats. *Toxicology and Industrial Health*, *28*, 740–745.

Saljooghi, A. S., & Fatemi, S. J. A. (2010). Clinical evaluation of Deferasirox for removal of cadmium ions in rat. *Biometals*, *23*, 707–712.

Sallsten, G., Barregard, L., & Schutz, A. (1994). Clearance half life of mercury in urine after the cessation of long term occupational exposure: influence of a chelating agent. *Occupational and Environmental Medicine*, *51*, 337–342 (DMPS) on excretion of mercury in urine.

Salvator, H., Gille, T., Hervé, A., Bron, C., Lamberto, C., & Valeyre, D. (2013). Chronic beryllium disease: azathioprine as a possible alternative to corticosteroid treatment. *European Respiratory Journal*, *41*, 234–236.

Samitz, M. H., & Pomerantz, H. (1958). Studies of the effects on the skin of nickel and chromium salts. *Archives of Industrial Health*, *18*, 473–479.

Sampson, B., & Hart, A. (2012). Clinical usefulness of blood metal measurements to assess the failure of metal-on-metal hip implants. *Annals of Clinical Biochemistry*, *49*, 118–131.

Sanchez, D. J., Gomez, M., Llobet, J. M., & Domingo, J. L. (1993). Effects of meso-2,3-dimercaptosuccinic acid (DMSA) on methyl mercury-induced teratogenesis in mice. *Ecotoxicology and Environmental Safety*, *26*, 33–39.

Sandstrom, B. (1997). Bioavailability of zinc. *European Journal of Clinical Nutrition*, *51*(Suppl. 1), S17–S19.

Sandstrom, B., Cederblad, A., Kivisto, B., Stenquist, B., & Andersson, H. (1986). Retention of zinc and calcium from the human colon. *American Journal of Clinical Nutrition*, *44*, 501–504.

Sangvanich, T., Morry, J., Fox, C., Ngamcherdtrakul, W., Goodyear, S., Castro, D., Fryxell, G. E., Addleman, R. S., Summers, A. O., & Yantasee, W. (2014). Novel oral detoxification of mercury, cadmium, and lead with thiol-modified nanoporous silica. *ACS Applied Materials and Interfaces*, *23*, 5483–5493.

Sankar, J., Shukla, A., Khurana, R., & Dubey, N. (2013). Near fatal iron intoxication managed conservatively. *BMJ Case Reports*, *2013*, ii.

Santos, M. A., Gil, M., Marques, S., Gano, L., Cantinho, G., & Chaves, S. (2002). N-Carboxyalkyl derivatives of 3-hydroxy-4-pyridinones: synthesis, complexation with Fe(III), Al(III) and Ga(III) and in vivo evaluation. *Journal of Inorganic and Biochemistry*, *92*, 43–54.

Saric, M. M., Blanusa, M., Juresa, D., Saric, M., Marija Varnai, V. M., & Kostial, K. (2004). Combined early treatment with chelating agents DMSA and CaDTPA in acute oral cadmium exposure. *Basic & Clinical Pharmacology & Toxicology*, *94*, 119–123.

Sarikaya, S., Karcioglu, O., Ay, D., Cetin, A., Aktas, C., & Serinken, M. (2010). Acute mercury poisoning: a case report. *BMC Emergency Medicine*, *10*, 7.

Sasan, M. S., Hadavi, N., Afshari, R., Mousavi, S. R., Alizadeh, A., & Balali-Mood, M. (2012). Metal mercury poisoning in two boys initially treated for brucellosis in Mashhad, Iran. *Human and Experimental Toxicology*, *31*, 193–196.

Sastry, J., & Kellie, S. J. (2005). Severe neurotoxicity, ototoxicity and nephrotoxicity following high-dose cisplatin and amifostine. *Pediatric Hematology and Oncology*, *22*, 441–445.

Sayre, E. V., & Smith, R. W. (1961). Compositional Categories of Ancient Glass. *Science*, *133*(3467), 1824–1826.

Schäfer, B., Kreppel, H., Reichl, F. X., Fichtl, B., & Forth, W. (1991). Effect of oral treatment with Bal, DMPS or DMSA arsenic in organs of mice injected with arsenic trioxide. *Archives of Toxicology* (Suppl. 14), 228–230.

Schell, H., & Hornstein, O. P. (1974). Histochemical demonstration of silver in argyria. *Journal of Dermatology*, *49*, 1023–1030.

Scheuplein, R., Charnley, G., & Dourson, M. (2002). Differential sensitivity of children and adults to chemical toxicity. I. Biological basis. *Regulatory Toxicology and Pharmacology*, *35*, 429–447.

Schiffle, H., Weidmann, P., Weiss, M., & Massry, S. G. (1982). Dialysis treatment of acute chromium intoxication and comparative efficacy of peritoneal versus hemodialysis in chromium removal. *Mineral and Electrolyte Metabolism*, *7*, 28–35.

Schirrmacher, U. O. (1967). Case of cobalt poisoning. *British Medical Journal, 1*, 544–545.

Schmidt, M., & Goebeler, M. (2011). Nickel allergies: paying the Toll for innate immunity. *Journal of Molecular Medicine, 89*, 961–970.

Schubert, J., & Lindenbaum, A. (1954). Studies on the mechanism of protection by aurintricarboxylic acid in beryllium poisoning ii. Equilibria involving alkaline phosphatase. *Journal of Biological Chemistry, 208*, 359–368.

Schultze-Werninghaus, G., Roesch, A., Wilhelms, O. H., Gonsior, E., & Meir-Sydow, J. (1978). Bronchial asthma due to occupation allergy of immediate type (I) to platinum salts. *Dtsch Med Wochenschr, 103*, 972–975.

Schwetz, B. A., O'Neil, P. V., Voelker, F. A., & Jacobs, D. W. (1967). Effects of diphenylthiocarbazone and diethyldithiocarbamate on the excretion of thallium by rats. *Toxicology and Applied Pharmacology, 10*, 79–88.

Scott, L. K., Grier, L. R., Arnold, T. C., & Conrad, S. A. (2002). Respiratory failure from inhalational nickel carbonyl exposure treated with continuous high-volume hemofiltration and disulfiram. *Inhalation Toxicology, 14*, 1103–1109.

Sears, D. A. (1988). History of the treatment of chronic myelocytic leukaemia. *American Journal of Medical Science, 296*, 85–86.

Seeber, A., Meyer-Baron, M., & Schaper, M. (2002). A summary of two meta-analyses on neurobehavioural effects due to occupational lead exposure. *Archives of Toxicology, 76*, 137–145.

Seymour, R.J., & O'Farrelly, J.I. (2001). Platinum-Group Metals. *Kirk-Othmer Encyclopedia of Chemical Technology.*

Shah Syed, G. M., Younis, M. N., Usmani, G. N., & Zafar, N. (2004). Pretherapy Gallium-67 scanning in paediatric patients with Hodgkin's disease. *Medical Principles and Practice, 13*, 74–77.

Shaik, Z. A., & Lucis, O. J. (1972). Biological differences in cadmium and zinc turnover. *Archives of Environmental Health, 24*, 410.

Shakhashiri, B.Z. (2008). Chemical of the Week: Aluminum. *Sci.Fun.org.* University of Wisconsin.

Shannon, M., Graef, J., & Lovejoy, F. H., Jr. (1988). Efficacy and toxicity of D-penicillamine in low-level lead poisoning. *Journal of Pediatrics, 112*, 799–904.

Sharma, B. L., Kachru, D. N., Singh, S., & Tandon, S. K. (1986). Chelation in metal intoxication. XIX. alpha-Mercapto-beta-aryl acrylic acid as antidotes to nickel and lead toxicity. *Journal of Applied Toxicology, 6*, 253–257.

Sharma, B. L., Khandelwal, S., Kachru, D. N., Singh, S., & Tandon, S. K. (1987). Chelation in metal intoxication XXV: mercaptoacrylic acids as antidotes of lead and nickel toxicity. *Japanese Journal of Pharmacology, 45*, 295–302.

Sharma, P., Johri, S., & Shukla, S. (2000). Beryllium-induced toxicity and its prevention by treatment with chelating agents. *Journal of Applied Toxicology, 20*, 313–318.

Shi, Z. (1986). Acute nickel carbonyl poisoning: a report of 179 cases. *British Journal of Industrial Medicine, 43*, 422–424.

Shortland, A. J. (2006). Application of lead isotope analysis to a wide range of late bronze age egyptian materials. *Archaeometry, 48*, 657.

Shum, S., Whitehead, J., Vaughn, L., Shum, S., & Hale, T. (1995). Chelation of organoarsenate with dimercaptosuccinic acid. *Veterinary and Human Toxicology, 37*, 239–242.

Sidhu, P., Garg, M. L., Morgenstern, P., Vogt, J., Butz, T., & Dhawan, D. K. (2004). Role of zinc in regulating the levels of hepatic elements following nickel toxicity in rats. *Biological Trace Elements Research, 102*, 161–172.

Simon-Hettich, B., Wibbertmann, A., Wagner, D., Tomaska, L., & Malcolm, H. (2001). Zinc. Environmental Health Criteria. Report 221. World Health Organization, Geneva.

Simonse, E., Valk-Swinkels, C. G., van 't Veer, N. E., Ermens, A. A., & Veldkamp, E. J. (2013). Iron autointoxication in a 16-year-old girl: a protective role for hepcidin? *Annals of Clinical Biochemistry, 50*, 76–79.

Singer, A. J., Mofenson, H. C., Carracio, T. R., & Ilasi, J. (1994). Mercu*ric chloride poisoning due to ingestion of a stool fixative. Journal of Toxicology: Clinical Toxicology, 32*, 577–582.

Singh, P. K., Jones, M. M., Kostial, K., Blanusa, M., Piasek, M., & Restek-Samarzija, N. (1996). Meso-2,3-dimercaptosuccinic acid mono-N-alkylamides: syntheses and biological activity as novel in vivo cadmium mobilizing agents. *Chemical Research in Toxicology, 9*, 965–969.

Singh, S., Khodr, H., Tayler, M. I., & Hider, R. C. (1995). Therapeutic iron chelators and their potential side-effects. *Biochemical Society Symposium, 61*, 127–137.

Singhi, S. C., & Baranwal, A. K. (2003). Acute iron poisoning: clinical picture, intensive care needs and outcome. *Indian Pediatrics, 40*, 1177–1182.

Sinkovic, A., Strdin, A., & Svensek, F. (2008). Severe acute copper sulphate poisoning: a case report. *Archives of Industrial Hygiene and Toxicology, 59*, 31–35.

Sjögren, B., Elinder, C. G., Lidums, V., & Chang, G. (1988). Uptake and urinary excretion of aluminum among welders. *International Archives of Occupational and Environmental Health, 60*, 77–79.

Sjögren, B., Iregren, A., Montelius, J., & Yokel, R. A. (2014). Aluminum. In G. F. Nordberg, B. A. Fowler, & M. Nordberg (Eds.), *Handbook on the toxicology of metals* (4th ed., pp. 549–564). Amsterdam, NL: Elsevier/AP 2014.

Skerfving, S., & Bergdahl, I. A. (2014). Lead. In G. F. Nordberg, B. A. Fowler, & M. Nordberg (Eds.), *Handbook on the toxicology of metals* (4th ed., pp. 911–967). Amsterdam, NL: Elsevier/AP.

Skerfving, S., Ahlgren, L., Cristoffersson, J., Haeger-Aronsen, B., Mattsson, S., Schutz, A., & Lindberg, G. (1985). Metabolism of inorganic lead in men. *Nutrition Research*(Suppl. I), 601–607.

Skoczynska, A., Kwiecinska, D., Kielbinski, M., & Lukaszewski, M. (2007). Acute iron poisoning in adult female. *Human and Experimental Toxicology, 26*, 663–666.

Slikkerveer, A., & de Wolff, F. A. (1989). Pharmacokinetics and toxicity of bismuth compounds. *Medical Toxicology and Adverse Drug Experience, 4*, 303–323.

Slikkerveer, A., Jong, H. B., Helmich, R. B., & De Wolff, F. A. (1992). Development of a therapeutic procedure for bismuth intoxication with chelating agents. *Journal of Laboratory and Clinical Medicine, 119*, 529–537.

Slikkerveer, A., Van der Voet, G. B., De Wolff, F. A., Leslie, A., Noach, L. A., & Tytgat, G. N. J. (1998). Comparison of enhanced elimination of bismuth in humans after treatment with *meso*-2,3-dimercaptosuccinic acid and D,L-2,3-dimercaptopropane-1-sulfonic acid. *Analyst, 123*, 91–92.

Smith, D. R., Markowitz, M. E., Crick, J., Rosen, J. F., & Flegal, A. R. (1994). The effects of succimer on the absorption of lead in adults determined by using the stable isotope 204Pb. *Environmental Research, 67*, 39–53.

Smith, D., Bayer, L., & Strupp, B. J. (1998). Efficacy of succimer chelation for reducing brain Pb levels in a rodent model. *Environmental Research, 78*, 168–176.

Smith, D. R., Calacsan, C., Woolard, D., Luck, M., Cremin, J., & Laughlin, N. K. (2000). Succimer and the urinary excretion of essential elements in a primate model of childhood lead exposure. *Toxicological Sciences, 54*, 473–480.

Smyth, L. T., Ruhf, R. C., Whitman, N. E., & Dugan, T. J. (1973). Clinical manganism and exposure to manganese in the production and processing of ferromanganese alloy. *Occupational Medicine, 15*, 101–109.

Solomons, N. W. (1982). Biological availability of zinc in humans. *American Journal of Clinical Nutrition, 35*, 1048–1075.

Sosabowsky, J., Melendez-Alfort, L., & Mather, S. (2003). Radiolabelling of peptides for diagnosis and therapy of non-oncological diseases. *Quaterly Journal of Nuclear Medicine, 47*, 223–237.

Spruit, D., Bongaarts, P. J. M., & Jongh, G. J. D. (1978). Dithiocarbamate therapy for nickel dermatitis. *Contact Dermatitis*, *4*, 350–358.

Stenehjem, A. E., Vahter, M., Nermell, B., Aasen, J., Lierhagen, S., Mørland, J., & Jacobsen, D. (2007). Slow recovery from severe inorganic arsenic poisoning despite treatment with DMSA (2.3-dimercaptosuccinic acid). *Clinical Toxicology*, *45*, 424–428.

Stephanopoulos, D. E., Willman, D. A., Shevlin, D., Pinter, L., & Gummin, D. D. (2002). Treatment and toxicokinetics of acute pediatric arsenic ingestion: danger of arsenic insecticides in children. *Pediatric Critical Care Medicine*, *3*, 74–80.

Stevens, W., van Peteghem, C., Heyndrickx, A., & Barbier, F. (1974). Eleven cases of thallium intoxication treated with Prussian blue. *International Journal of Clinical Pharmacology*, *10*, 1–22.

Stevens, P. E., Moore, D. F., House, I. M., Volans, G. N., & Rainford, D. J. (1995). Significant elimination of bismuth by haemodialysis with a new heavy-metal chelating agent. *Nephrology Dialysis Transplantation*, *10*, 696–698.

Stewart, P. W., Burright, R. G., & Donovick, P. J. (1995). DMSA chelation during co-exposure to lead: increased locomotor activity in lead-exposed mice but not controls. *Physiological Behaviour*, *57*, 863–867.

Stewart, P. W., Blaine, C., Cohen, M., Burright, R. G., & Donovick, P. J. (1996). Acute and longer term effects of meso-2,3 dimercaptosuccinic acid (DMSA) on the behavior of lead-exposed and control mice. *Physiological Behaviour*, *59*, 849–855.

Straus, L.G., Gonzalez Morales, M.R., & Carretero, J.M. (2011). Lower Magdalenian secondary human burial in El Mirón Cave, Cantabria, Spain. *Antiquity 85*, 1151–1164.

Sun, T. W., Xu, Q. Y., Zhang, X. J., Wu, Q., Liu, Z. S., Kan, Q. C., Sun, C. Y., & Wang, L. (2012). Management of thallium poisoning in patients with delayed hospital admission. *Clinical Toxicology*, *50*, 65–69.

Sunderman, F. W. (1979). Efficacy of sodium diethyldithiocarbamate (dithiocarb) in acute nickel carbonyl poisoning. *Annals of Clinical and Laboratory Science*, *9*, 1–10.

Sunderman, F. W. (1981). Chelation therapy in nickel poisoning. *Annals of Clinical and Laboratory Science*, *11*, 1–8.

Sunderman, F. W. (1990). Use of sodium diethyldithiocarbamate in the treatment of nickel carbonyl poisoning. *Annals of Clinical and Laboratory Science*, *20*, 12–21.

Sunderman, F. W., Jr., Hopfer, S. M., Sweeney, K. C., Marcus, A. H., Most, B. M., & Creason, J. (1989). Nickel absorption and kinetics in human volunteers. *Proceedings of the Society for Experimental Biology and Medicine*, *191*, 5–11.

Taguchi, T., Nazneen, A., Abid, M. R., & Razzaque, M. S. (2005). Cisplatin-associated nephrotoxicity and pathological events. *Contributions to Nephrology*, *148*, 107–121.

Takahashi, Y., Funakoshi, T., Shimada, H., & Kojima, S. (1994). Comparative effects of chelating agents on distribution, excretion, and renal toxicity of gold sodium thiomalate in rats. *Toxicology*, *90*, 39–51.

Takahashi, Y., Funakoshi, T., Shimada, H., & Kojima, S. (1995). The utility of chelating agents as antidotes for nephrotoxicity of gold sodium thiomalate in adjuvant-arthritic rats. *Toxicology*, *97*, 151–157.

Takeda, T., Yukioka, T., & Shimazaki, S. (2000). Cupric sulfate intoxication with rhabdomyolysis, treated with chelating agents and blood purification. *Internal Medicine*, *39*, 253–255.

Tallkvist, J., Bowlus, C. L., & Lonnerdal, B. (2003). Effect of iron treatment on nickel absorption and gene expression of the divalent metal transporter (DMT1) by human intestinal Caco-2 cells. *Pharmacology Toxicology*, *92*, 121–124.

Tandon, S. K. (1978). Chelation in metal intoxication. VI. Influence of PAS and CDTA on the excretion of manganese in rabbits given MnO_2. *Toxicology*, *9*, 379–785.

Tandon, S. K., & Mathur, A. K. (1976). Chelation in metal intoxication. III. Lowering of nickel content in poisoned rat organs. *Acta Pharmacology and Toxicology*, *38*, 401–408.

Tandon, S. K., & Gaur, J. S. (1977). Chelation in metal intoxication. IV. Removal of chromium from organs of experimentally poisoned animals. *Clinical Toxicology*, *11*, 257–264.

Tandon, S. K., & Khandelwal, S. (1982a). Chelation in metal intoxication X: Influence of different polyaminocarboxylic acids and thiol chelators in the excretion and tissue distribution of ^{54}Mn in rat. *Research Communications in Chemical Pathology and Pharmacology*, *36*, 337–340.

Tandon, S. K., & Khandelwal, S. (1982b). Chelation in metal intoxication. XII. Antidotal efficacy of chelating agents on acute toxicity of manganese. *Archives in Toxicology*, *50*, 19–25.

Tandon, S. K., Chandra, S. V., Singh, J., Husain, R., & Seth, P. K. (1975). Chelation in metal intoxication. I. In vivo effect of chelating agents on liver and testis of manganese administered rats. *Environmental Research*, *9*, 18–25.

Tandon, S. K., Hashmi, N. S., & Kachru, D. N. (1990). The lead-chelating effects of substituted dithiocarbamates. *Biomedical and Environment Science*, *3*, 299–305.

Tandon, S. K., Singh, S., Jain, V. K., & Prasad, S. (1996). Chelation in metal intoxication. XXXVIII: effect of structurally different chelating agents in treatment of nickel intoxication in rat.Fundam. *Applied Toxicology*, *31*, 141–148.

Tandon, S. K., Singh, S., Prasad, S., & Mathur, N. (1998). Mobilization of lead by calcium versenate and dimercaptosuccinate in the rat. *Clinical and Experimental Pharmacology and Physiology*, *25*, 686–692.

Tang, H. L., Mak, Y. F., Chu, K. H., Lee, W., Fung, S. K., Chan, T. Y., & Tong, K. L. (2013). Minimal change disease caused by exposure to mercury-containing skin lightening cream: a report of 4 cases. *Clinical Nephrology*, *79*, 326–329.

Tapiero, H., Townsend, D. M., & Tew, K. D. (2003). Trace elements in human physiology and pathology. Copper. *Biomedicine and Pharmacotherapy*, *57*, 386–398.

Tasende, M. S., Gale, G. R., Smith, A. B., Jones, M. M., & Singh, P. K. (1992). Monoisoamyl meso-2,3-dimercaptosuccinate: interaction with metallothionein-bound cadmium in vitro and evidence of active transport into renal and hepatic cells in vivo. *Research Communications in Chemical Pathology and Pharmacology*, *76*, 323–339.

Taylor, D. M. (1962). The absorption of cobalt from the gastrointestinal tract of the rat. *Physics in Medicine and Biology*, *6*, 445–451.

Taylor, A., & Marks, V. (1978). Cobalt:a review. *Journal of Human Nutrition*, *32*, 165–177.

Tell, I., Somervaille, L. J., Nilsson, U., Bensryd, I., Schütz, A., Chettle, D. R., Scott, M. C., & Skerfving, S. (1992). Chelated lead and bone lead. *Scandinavian Journal of Work Environment and Health*, *18*, 113–119.

Tenenbein, M. (1997). Leaded gasoline abuse: the role of tetraethyl lead. *Human Experimental Toxicology*, *16*, 217–222.

Tenenbein, M. (2005). Unit-dose packaging of iron supplements and reduction of iron poisoning in young children. *Archives of Pediatrics and Adolescent Medicine*, *159*, 557–560.

Tezer, H., Erkoçog˘lu, M., Kara, A., Bayrakcı, B., Düzova, A., Teks¸am, Ö., & Aysun, S. (2011). Household poisoning cases from mercury brought from school. *European Journal of Pediatrics*, *170*, 397–400.

Thakor, A. S., Jokerst, J., Zavaleta, C., Massoud, T. F., & Gambhir, S. S. (2011). Gold nanoparticles: a revival in precious metal administration to patients. *Nano Letters*, *11*, 4029–4036.

The Silver Institute (2015). "Silver in windows and glass". https://www.silverinstitute.org/site/silver-in-technology/silver-in-green/energy-reduction-windows/

Thompson, D. M., Pegelow, C. H., Singsen, B. H., Powars, D. R., & Hanson, V. (1978). Neutropenia associated with chrysotherapy for juvenile rheumatoid arthritis. *Journal of Pediatrics*, *93*, 871–875.

Thurtle, N., Greig, J., Cooney, L., Amitai, Y., Ariti, C., Brown, M. J., Kosnett, M. J., Moussally, K., Sani-Gwarzo, N., & Akpan, H. (2014). More Description of 3,180 courses of chelation with dimercaptosuccinic acid in children <= 5 y with severe lead poisoning in zamfara, northern nigeria: a retrospective analysis of programme data. *Plos Medicine*, *11*(10), e1001739.

Tilbrook, G. S., & Hider, R. C. (1998). Iron chelators for clinical use. *Metal Ions in Biological Systems*, *35*, 691–730.

Tjälve, H., & Borg-Neczak, K. (1994). Effects of lipophilic complex formation on the disposition of nickel in experimental animals. *Science of Total Environment*, *148*, 217–242.

Tjälve, H., Jasim, S., & Oskarsson, A. (1984). Nickel mobilization by sodium diethyldithiocarbamate in nickel-carbonyl-treated mice. *IARC Science Publications*, *53*, 311–320.

TLC Trial Group. (2000). Safety and efficacy of succimer in toddlers with blood lead levels 20-44 mcg/dL. *Pediatric Research*, *48*, 593–599.

Toet, A. E., van Dijk, A., Savelkoul, T. J., & Meulenbelt, J. (1994). Mercury kinetics in a case of severe mercuric chloride poisoning treated with dimercapto-1-propane sulphonate (DMPS). *Human and Experimental Toxicology*, *13*, 11–16.

Tondel, M., Rahman, M., Magnuson, A., Chowdhury, I. A., Faruquee, M. H., & Ahmad, S. A. (1999). The relationship of arsenic levels in drinking water and the prevalence rate of skin lesions in Bangladesh. *Environment and Health Perspectives*, *107*, 727–729.

de la Torre, A., Belles, M., Llobet, J. M., Mayayo, E., & Domingo, J. L. (1998). Comparison of the effectiveness of 2,3-dimercaptopropanol (BAL) and meso-2,3-dimercaptosuccinic acid (DMSA) as protective agents against mercuric chloride-induced nephrotoxicity in rats. *Biological Trace Element Research*, *63*, 1–10.

Torres-Alanis, O., Garza-Ocanas, L., & Pineyro-Lopez, A. J. (1995). Evaluation of urinary mercury excretion after administration of 2,3-dimercapto-1-propane sulfonic acid to occupationally exposed men. *Journal of Toxicology: Clinical Toxicology*, *33*, 717–720.

Torres-Alanis, O., Garza-Ocanas, L., & Pineyro-Lopez, A. (1997). Intravenous self-administration of metallic mercury: report of a case with a 5-year follow-up. *Journal of Toxicology: Clinical Toxicology*, *35*, 83–87.

Torres-Alanis, O., Garza-Ocanas, L., Bernal, M. A., & Pineyro-Lopez, A. (2000). Urinary excretion of trace elements in humans after sodium 2,3-dimercaptopropane-1-sulfonate challenge test. *Journal of Toxicology: Clinical Toxicology*, *38*, 697–700.

Torres-Alanís, O., Garza-Ocañas, L., & Piñeyro-López, A. (2002). Effect of meso-2,3-dimercaptosuccinic acid on urinary lead excretion in exposed men. *Human and Experimental Toxicology*, *21*, 573–577.

Tossavainen, A., Nurminen, M., Mutanen, P., & Tola, S. (1980). Application of mathematical modelling for assessing the biological half-times of chromium and nickel in field studies. *British Journal of Industrial Medicine*, *37*, 285–291.

Tozman, E. C., & Gottlieb, N. L. (1987). Adverse reactions with oral and parenteral gold preparations. *Journal of Medical Toxicology*, *2*, 177–189.

Tsai, C. Y., Shiau, A. L., Chen, S. Y., Chen, Y. H., Cheng, P. C., Chang, M. Y., Chen, D. H., Chou, C. H., Wang, C. R., & Wu, C. L. (2007). Amelioration of collagen-induced arthritis in rats by nanogold. *Arthritis Rheumatology*, *56*, 544–554.

Tubafard, S., & Fatemi, S. J. (2008). Chelation of bismuth by combining desferrioxamine and deferiprone in rats. *Toxicology and Industrial Health*, *24*, 235–240.

Tuli, M. M., Al-Shemmari, S. H., Ameen, R. M., Al-Muhanadi, S., Al-Huda, F. A., Ballani, N., Khoshi, M., Al-Enezi, F., Bajciova, V., & Mottl, H. (2004). The use of gallium-67 scintigraphy to monitor tumor response rates and predict long-term clinical outcome in patients with lymphoma. *Clinical Lymphoma*, *5*, 56–61.

Tylenda, C. A., Sullivan, D. W., Jr., & Fowler, b. A. (2014). Antimony. In G. F. Nordberg, B. A. Fowler, & M. Nordberg (Eds.), *Handbook on the toxicology of metals* (4th ed., pp. 565–579). Amsterdam, NL: Elsevier/AP.

USGS, 2014. US Geological Survey. Mineral commodity summaries 2014. http://minerals.usgs.gov/minerals/pubs/mcs/2014/mcs2014.pdf

US National Toxicology Program, 2012. NTP monograph on health effects of low-level lead. June 2012. https://ntp.niehs.nih.gov/pubhealth/hat/noms/lead/index.html

USGS (2015). US Geological Survey. http://minerals.usgs.gov/minerals/pubs/commodity/mercury/

Vallant, B., Deutsch, J., Muntean, M., & Goessler, W. (2008). Intravenous injection of metallic mercury: case report and course of mercury during chelation therapy with DMPS. *Clinical Toxicology*, *46*, 566–569.

van den Berghe, P. V. E., & Klomp, L. W. J. (2009). New developments in the regulation of intestinal copper absorption. *Nutrition Reviews*, *67*, 658–672.

Van der Linde, A. A., Pillen, S., Gerrits, G. P., & Bouwes Bavinck, J. N. (2008). Stevens-Johnson syndrome in a child with chronic mercury exposure and 2,3-dimercaptopropane-1-sulfonate (DMPS) therapy. *Clinical Toxicology*, *46*, 479–481.

van der Merwe, C. F. (1972). The treatment of thallium poisoning. A repeort of 2 cases. *South African Medical Journal*, *46*, 560–561.

van der Stock, J., & de Schepper, J. (1978). The effect of Prussian blue and sodium-ethylenediaminetetraacetic acid on the faecal and urinary elimination of thallium by the dog. *Research in Veterinary Science*, *25*, 337–342.

van Ketel, W. G., & Bruynzeel, D. P. (1982). The possible chelating effect of sodium diethyldithiocarbamate (DDC) in nickel allergic patients. Patch test procedures with nickel on DDC pretreated skin. *Derm Beruf Umwelt*, *30*, 198–202.

Vantroyen, B., Heilier, J. F., Meulemans, A., Michels, A., Buchet, J. P., Vanderschueren, S., Haufroid, V., & Sabbe, M. (2004). Survival after a lethal dose of arsenic trioxide. *Journal of Toxicology: Clinical Toxicology*, *42*, 889–895.

Verpooten, G. A., D'Haese, P. C., Boelaert, J. A., Because, I., Lamberts, L. V., & De Broe, M. E. (1992). Pharmacokinetics of aluminoxamine and ferrioxamine and dose-finding of desferrioxamine in haemodialysis patients. *Nephrology Dialysis Transplantation*, *7*, 931–938.

Vogelsang, U. (1994). Aluminum poisoning in dialysis patients—diagnosis and therapy. *Revue Suisse de Medecine Praxis*, *83*, 738–756.

Wade, K., & Banister, A. J. (1973). The chemistry of aluminium, gallium, indium and thallium. *Pergamon texts in inorganic chemistry* (vol. 12). New York: Pergamon Press.

Wainwright, A. P1, Kox, W. J., House, I. M., Henry, J. A., Heaton, R., & Seed, W. A. (1988). Clinical features and therapy of acute thallium poisoning. *Quaterly Journal Medicine*, *69*(259), 939–944.

Wallpole, I. R., Johnston, K., Clarkson, R., Wilson, G., & Bower, G. (1985). Acute Chromium Poisoning in a 2 year old child. *Australian Paedriatric Journal*, *21*, 65–67.

Walshe, J. M. (1956). Penicillamine, a new oral therapy for Wilson's disease. *American Journal of Medicine*, *21*, 487–495.

Walshe, J. M. (1973). Copper chelation in patients with Wilson's disease. A comparison of penicillamine and triethylene tetramine dihydrochloride. *Quarterly Journal of Medicine*, *42*, 441–452.

Walshe, J. M. (1982). Treatment of Wilson's disease with trientine (triethylene tetramine) dihydrochloride. *Lancet*, *1*, 643–647.

Wang, X. -P., Yang, R. -M., Ren, M. -S., & Sun, B. -S. (2003). Anticopper efficacy of captopril and sodium dimercaptosulphonate in patients with Wilson's disease. *Functional Neurology*, *18*, 149–153.

Wang, S. -C., Ting, K. -S., & Wu, C. -C. (1965). Chelating therapy with Na-DMS in occupational lead and mercury intoxications. *Chinese Medical Journal*, *84*, 437–439.

Wang, E. E., Mahajan, N., Wills, B., & Leikin, J. (2007). Successful treatment of potentially fatal heavy metal poisonings. *Journal of Emergency Medicine*, *32*, 289–294.

Wang, B. J., Guo, Y. L., Chang, H. Y., Sheu, H. M., Pan, M. H., Lee, Y. H., & Wang, Y. J. (2010). N-acetylcysteine inhibits chromium hypersensitivity in coadjuvant chromium-sensitized albino guinea pigs by suppressing the effects of reactive oxygen species. *Experimental Dermatology*, *19*, e191–e200.

Wang, Y., He, Y. Z., & Zhang, X. G. (2012). Detoxification effects of two drugs in thallium -poisoned mice. *Zhongguo Wei Zhong Bing Ji Jiu Yi Xue*, *24*, 338–341.

Ward, J. M., Young, D. M., Fauvie, K. A., Wolpert, M. K., Davis, R., & Guarino, A. M. (1976). Comparative nephrotoxicity of platinum cancer chemotherapeutic agents. *Cancer Treatment Reports*, *60*, 1675–1678.

Waters, R. S., Bryden, N. A., Patterson, K. Y., Veillon, C., & Anderson, R. A. (2001). EDTA chelation effects on urinary losses of cadmium calcium, chromium, cobalt, copper, lead, magnesium, and zinc. *Biological Trace Element Research*, *83*, 207–221.

Watson, W. A., Litovitz, T. L., Klein-Schwartz, W., Rodgers, G. C., Jr., Youniss, J., Reid, N., Rouse, W. G., Rembert, R. S., & Borys, D. (2004). 2003 annual report of the American Association of Poison Control Centers Toxic Exposure Surveillance System. *American Journal of Emergency Medicine*, *22*, 335–404.

Wax, P. M., & Thornton, C. A. (2000). Recovery from Severe Arsenic-Induced Peripheral Neuropathy with 2,3-Dimercapto-1-propanesulphonic Acid. *Clinical Toxicology*, *38*, 777–780.

Wehner, A. P., & Craig, D. K. (1972). Toxicology of inhaled NiO and CoO in Syrian golden hamsters. *American Journal of Industrial Hygiene Association*, *33*, 146–155.

Wheate, N. J., Walker, S., Craig, G. E., & Oun, R. (2010). The status of platinum anticancer drugs in the clinic and in clinical trials. *Dalton Transactions*, *39*, 8113–8127.

Whitlock, C. M., Amuso, S. J., & Bittenbender, J. B. (1966). Chronic neurological disease in two manganese steel workers. *American Journal of Industrial Hygiene Association*, *27*, 454–459.

WHO/IPCS (1997). World Health Organization International Programme on Chemical Safety. Aluminium. Environmental health criteria 194. Geneva.

WHO/IPCS (2000). World Health Organization International Programme on Chemical Safety. Safety evaluation of certain food additives and contaminants. *Fifty-third meeting of the joint FAO/WHO expert committee on food additives (JEFCA)*. Lead. WHO Food Additives Series: 44. Geneva.

WHO (2001). World Health Organization. Food additives series 46.

WHO (2006). World Health Organization. Report Series 930.

Wieczorek, H., & Oberdörster, G. (1989). Effects of selected chelating agents on organ distribution and excretion of manganese after inhalation exposure to 54MnCl2. I. Injection of chelating agents. *Polish Journal of Occupational Medicine*, *2*, 261–267.

Wijmenga, C., & Klomp, L. W. J. (2004). Molecular regulation of copper excretion in the liver. *Proceedings of the Nutrition Society*, *63*, 31–39.

Willhite, C. C., Karyakina, N. A., Yokel, R. A., Yenugadhati, N., Wisniewski, T. M., Arnold, I. M. F., Momoli, F., & Krewski, D. (2014). Systematic review of potential health risks posed by pharmaceutical, occupational and consumer exposures to metallic and nanoscale aluminum, aluminum oxides, aluminum hydroxide and its soluble salts. *Critical Reviews in Toxicology*, *44*(S4), 1–80.

Winship, K. A. (1988). Toxicity of tin and its compounds. *Adverse Drug Reactions and Acute Poisoning Reviews*, *7*, 19–38.

Wirth, A., Seymour, J. F., Hicks, R. J., Ware, R., Fisher, R., Prince, M., MacManus, M. P., Ryan, G., Januszewicz, H., & Wolf, M. (2002). Fluorine-18 fluorodeoxyglucose positron emission tomography, gallium-67 scintigraphy, and conventional staging for Hodgkin's disease and non-Hodgkin's lymphoma. *The American Journal of Medicine*, *112*, 262–268, 2002.

Wu, M. L., Deng, J. F., Lin, K. P., & Tsai, W. J. (2013). Lead, mercury, and arsenic poisoning due to topical use of traditional chinese medicines. *The American Journal of Medicine*, *126*, 451–454.

Wyatt, C. J., Fimbres, C., Romo, L., Méndez, R. O., & Grijalva, M. (1998a). Incidence of heavy metal contamination in water supplies in northern Mexico. *Environmental Research*, *76*, 114–119.

Wyatt, C. J., Lopez Quiroga, V., Olivas Acosta, R. T., & Olivia Méndez, R. (1998b). Excretion of arsenic (As) in urine of children, 7-11 years, exposed to elevated levels of As in the city water supply in Hermosillo, Sonora, México. *Environmental Research*, *78*, 19–24.

Xi, C., Ping, L., Wushide, Shue, W., & Benjie, W. (1997). Influence of the chelator 1,2-dimethyl-3-hydroxypyrid-4-one on aluminum elimination in aluminum-loaded rabbits. *Trace Elements and Electrocytes*, *14*, 130–133.

Xiao, Z., & Laplante, A. R. (2004). Characterizing and recovering the platinum group minerals—a review. *Minerals Engineering*, *17*, 961–979.

Xie, J., Funakoshi, T., Shimada, H., & Kojima, S. (1994). Effects of chelating agents on tissue distribution and excretion of nickel in mice. *Research Communications in Molecular Pathology and Pharmacology*, *86*, 245–255.

Xie, J., Funakoshi, T., Shimada, H., & Kojima, S. (1995). Effects of chelating agents on testicular toxicity in mice caused by acute exposure to nickel. *Toxicology*, *103*, 147–155.

Xie, J., Funakoshi, T., Shimada, H., & Kojima, S. J. (1996). Comparative effects of chelating agents on pulmonary toxicity of systemic nickel in mice. *Applied Toxicology*, *16*, 317–324.

Xu, Z. F., & Jones, M. M. (1988). Comparative mobilization of lead by chelating agents. *Toxicology*, *53*, 277–288.

Yamauchi, H., Takahashi, K., & Yamamura, Y. (1986). Metabolism and excretion of orally and intraperitoneally administered gallium arsenide in the hamster. *Toxicologist*, *40*, 237–246.

Yan, X. M., Li, L., Liang, Y. Y., Tao, Z. Q., Xu, X. H., Chen, Z. J., & Zhang, J. S. (1993). Effects of dimercaptosuccinic acid per os on copper excretion in rat. *Zhongguo Yao Li Xue Bao*(14 Suppl.), S34–S37.

Yang, H. -J., He, S. -Y., & Yang, H. -Y. (2014). Self-seeded growth of five-fold twinned copper nanowires: mechanistic study, characterization, and SERS applications. *Langmuir*, *30*, 602–610.

Yang, Y., Faustino, P. J., Progar, J. J., Brownell, C. R., Sadrieh, N., May, J. C., Leutzinger, E., Place, D. A., Duffy, E. P., Yu, L. X., Khan, M. A., & Lyon, R. C. (2008). Quantitative determination of thallium binding to ferric hexacyanoferrate: Prussian blue. *International Journal of Pharmaceutics*, *353*, 187–194.

Yarris, J. P., Caravati, E. M., Horowitz, Z. B., Stromness, J. R., Crouch, B. I., & Mckeown, N. J. (2008). Acute arsenic trioxide ant bait ingestion by toddlers. *Clinical Toxicology*, *46*, 785–789.

Yeoh, B., Woolfenden, S., Lanphear, B., Ridley, G.F., Livingstone, N., & Jorgensen, E. 2014. Household interventions for preventing domestic lead exposure in children. *Cochrane Database of Systematic Reviews*. *12*. Article number CD006047.

Yilmaz, Y., Armagan, E., Olmez, O., Esen, M., Alkis, N., & Dolar, E. (2009). Acute arsenic self-poisoning for suicidal purpose in a dentist: a case report. *Human and Experimental Toxicology*, *28*, 63–65.

Yokel, R. A. (2002). Aluminum chelation principles and recent advances. *Coordination chemistry reviews*, *228*, 97–113.

Yokel, R. A. (2006). Blood-brain barrier flux of aluminum, manganese, iron and other metals suspected to contribute to metal-induced neurodegeneration. *Journal of Alzheimers Disease*, *10*, 223–253.

Yokel, R. A. (2012). Aluminum in food-The nature and contribution of food additives. In Y. El-Samragy (Ed.), *Food additive* (pp. 203–228). Croatia: Intech, Rijeka.

Yokel, R. A., & McNamara, P. J. (2001). Aluminium toxicokinetics: an updated mini review. *Pharmacology & Toxicology*, *88*, 159–167.

Yokel, R. A., Ackrill, P., Burgess, E., Day, J. P., Domingo, J. L., Flaten, T. P., & Savory, J. (1996a). Prevention and treatment of aluminum toxicity including chelation therapy: status and research needs. *Journal of Toxicology and Environmental Health*, *48*, 667–683.

Yokel, R. A., Meurer, K. A., Skinner, T. L., & Fredenburg, A. M. (1996b). The 3-hydroxypyridin-4-ones more effectively chelate aluminum in a rabbit model of aluminum intoxication than does desferrioxamine. *Drug Metabolism and Disposition*, *24*, 105–111.

Yokel, R. A., Rhineheimer, S. S., Sharma, P., Elmore, D., & McNamarqa, P. J. (2001). Entry, half-life, and desferrioxamine clearance of brain aluminum after a single ^{26}Al exposure. *Toxicology Science*, *64*, 77–82.

Yoshida, M., Satoh, H., Igarashi, M., Akashi, K., Yamamura, Y., & Yoshida, K. (1997). Acute mercury poisoning by intentional ingestion of mercuric chloride. *Tohoku Journal of Experimental Medicine*, *182*, 347–352.

Zander, D., Ewers, U., Frier, I., & Brockhaus, A. (1992). The mercury exposure of the population. III. Mercury mobilisation by DMPS (Dimaval) in subjects with and without amalgam fillings. *Zentralbl Hyg.Umweltmed*, *192*, 447–454.

Zhang, G. J., & Ye, Z. (1962). Cardiac dysfunction and toxic hepatitis from a single intravenious injection of superhigh dose of potassium antimony tartrate miataken fort glucose solution in 2 cases. *Chinese Journal of Internal Medicine*, *10*, 535–536.

Zhang, B., Georgiev, O., Hagmann, M., Günes, C., Cramer, M., Faller, P., Vasák, M., & Schaffner, W. (2003). Activity of metal-responsive transcription factor 1 by toxic heavy metals and H2O2 in vitro is modulated by metallothionein. *Molecular and Cell Biology*, *23*, 8471–8485.

Zheng, W., Jiang, Y. -M., Zhang, Y., Jiang, W., Wang, X., & Cowan, D. M. (2009). Chelation therapy of manganese intoxication with para-aminosalicylic acid (PAS) in Sprague-Dawley rats. *Neurotoxicology*, *30*, 240–248.

Chapter 5

Decorporation of Radionuclides

Ole Andersen

Chapter Outline

5.1 INTRODUCTION

Metal radionuclides occur naturally in the environment, however, most radionuclides categorized as harmful are of anthropogenic origin, released from military, industrial, or medical processes. The USEPA (2010) classified radionuclides as "heavy" radionuclides (elements with over 83 protons, thus also categorized as unstable) or "light" nuclides (elements with fewer than 83 protons). The uses of metal radionuclides for energy production, medicinal, industrial, and military purposes often generate wastes with extensively long decay half-times and potential for environmental pollution.

Major pathways to hazardous radionuclides exposures are through inhalation (eg, uranium and radon), food contamination (eg, radium), and through occupational exposure at mining and processing sites. Radionuclides can be released to the environment through accidents, by poor working standard or waste disposal, or by other means. Accidents or low working standards at nuclear facilities can lead to contamination of employees with radionuclides due to ingestion, inhalation of gases or particulates, or contamination of skin or wounds, as well as contamination of the surroundings. The most frequent exposure situation is contamination of skin or hair during work with radionuclides. Other potential sources for radionuclide exposure are terrorist actions via production of "dirty bombs" or deliberate contamination of infrastructure key facilities,

Chelation Therapy in the Treatment of Metal Intoxication. http://dx.doi.org/10.1016/B978-0-12-803072-1.00005-5

for example, drinking water reservoirs, situations fortunately not realized yet but feared by authorities. Exposure can be to one main metal compound or to complicated mixtures.

Due to decay of parent radionuclides, the effects of exposure are in some cases caused by combined effects of parent and daughter radionuclides. The health effects of metal radionuclides exposures are a combination of radiation increasing cancer risk in chronic exposure and toxicity of the metals. Acute health effects after extensive radiation exposure starts with nausea, vomiting, and headaches. Further exposure leads to weakness and fatigue, fever, hair loss, disorientation and dizziness, diarrhea with bloody stools, decreased blood pressure, and ultimately death.

The major hazards associated with internal contamination are associated with α-emitting isotopes with slow decay (long physical $t_{1/2}$) combined with prolonged body retention (long biological $t_{1/2}$) which gives larger radiation doses where all energy is delivered to tissues close to the isotope's depot, which is often bone from where the radionuclide is not easily removed.

Along with the development of radionuclide technology an extensive amount of research has been carried out to develop methods for decorporation of internalized radionuclides, mainly by chelation. The compounds most widely used are diethylene triamine pentaacetic acid (DTPA) and Prussian blue. The effectiveness of DTPA falls however rapidly with time after contamination.

As described later, an extensive number of other chelating agents have been studied in experimental animals, both experimental compounds and drugs licensed for metal storage diseases. Several of these compounds were highly effective in decorporating radionuclides (Cassatt et al., 2008).

The clinical experience with Ca or Zn DTPA chelation of contaminated nuclear workers is formed by a large number of cases with one or few exposed individuals, where aggressive chelation has reduced systemic uptake and promoted excretion of internalized systemic radionuclides, mainly americium, plutonium, and uranium, in theory reducing the risk of developing cancer. In fact, several life-time animal experiments in rats and mice injected with carcinogenic doses of plutonium showed that repeated daily chelation by Ca-DTPA or Zn-DTPA reduced both the body burden of Pu and the frequency of bone cancers (reviewed by Taylor et al. 2000). In a long-term study in ^{241}Am citrate exposed beagles), > 6 years chelation with Zn DTPA reduced both the skeleton Am burden and the incidence of bone tumors by 71%, and slightly more than doubled survival time (Lloyd, Taylor, & Mays, 1998). In a small study in beagles exposed to poly-disperse 239Pu colloids by i.v. injection, daily Zn-DTPA injection reduced the skeletal Pu burden by 95%, more than doubled survival time without reducing bone tumor incidence (100% in control and chelated beagles), however, the latency time for tumor formation was about 2.6 times longer (Bruenger, Taylor, Taylor, & Lloyd, 1991). The radioactive Pu dose in this experiment was about 3 times higher than the radioactive Am dose in the study by Lloyd et al. (1998).

5.2 AMERICIUM

Americium (Am, atomic number 95 in group 9 of the periodic table of elements, standard atomic weight 243, density 13.67 g/cm^3, most common oxidation number +3) is a silver-white, crystalline transuranic actinide. Am is a man-made metal produced from uranium or plutonium by neutron absorption in nuclear reactors and in nuclear weapons. All Americium isotopes are radioactive. The only Am isotope with widespread commercial use is ^{241}Am with $t_{½}$ 432.7 years. ^{241}Am is primarily an α-emitter but also emits γ rays, the decay product is ^{237}Np. The largest and most widespread uses of ^{241}Am are in household and industrial smoke detectors. Other uses are in medical diagnostic devices, fluid-density, thickness, and aircraft fuel gauges, and distance-sensing devices. A ^{241}Am-Be mixture is a neutron source for industrial devices, for example, for nondestructive testing of machinery and measuring product thickness. ^{241}Am formed by β decay of ^{241}Pu in spent nuclear fuel is a major contributor to long-lived nuclear waste. Inhaled/absorbed ^{241}Am concentrates in lungs, bone, liver, and muscle with very long elimination halftime. The most important health effect risk induced by internally deposited ^{241}Am is cancer.

On Aug. 30, 1976 an explosion in a ^{241}Americium ion exchange column in a Hanford Site nuclear waste management facility resulted in extensive contamination of a male worker. The internal dose received via skin and inhalation was calculated to be more than 1 mCi (Robinson, Heid, Aldrig, & Glenn, 1983). The man underwent medical treatment for acid burns and wound debridement, extensive skin decontamination, and Ca-DTPA chelation therapy for an extended time period. Initial intensive Ca-DTPA therapy was calculated to prevent 99% of ^{241}Am in blood from being deposited in internal organs (Robinson et al., 1983). Analysis of trace element levels in urine during 3 years of Ca-DTPA chelation indicated that only zinc excretion was enhanced, this was corrected by administration of oral $ZnSO_4$ or use of Zn-DTPA (Kalkwarf, Thomas, Nielson, & Mauch, 1983). The patient died 11 years after the accident from preexisting cardiovascular disease. Postmortem examinations of tissues demonstrated acellularity of bone marrow, peritrabecular fibrosis, and lack of bone surface remodeling. Tissue levels of ^{241}Am indicated liver and bone as primary deposition organs. The distribution of ^{241}Am in soft tissues was in agreement with data from animal experiments (Toohey & Kathren, 1995; Thompson, 1983).

Cohen, Sasso, and Wrenn (1979) reported a case of accidental contamination of a 50 year old man and his 4 year old son by ^{241}Am by inhalation in the home. Chelation with Ca-DTPA for 8 years was effective in reducing body burdens of ^{241}Am, more effectively in the child than in the father.

Volf (1986) compared the ^{241}Am mobilizing effectiveness of the tetracarboxycatecholate ligand, 3,4,3-LICAM(C) (N1,N5,N10,N14-tetrakis(2,3-dihydroxy-4-carboxybenzoyl-tetraaza tetradecane, tetra sodium salt) with those of chelators approved for clinical use, Ca-DTPA and deferoxamine (DFO). When administered early after ^{241}Am exposure and at clinical doses used for actinide decorporation with DTPA (30 μmol/kg b.w.), LICAM(C) was superior to DFO while Ca-DTPA was superior to LICAM(C). The best result 1 day after injection of ^{241}Am was combined single injection of LICAM(C) and DTPA followed by continuous administration of Ca-DTPA in drinking water. The data indicated that about 3% of orally administered LICAM(C) was absorbed.

Schoeters, Maisin, and Vanderborght (1991) found that injection of $ZnNa_3$DTPA intraperitoneal (i.p.) once a week for 8 weeks starting 4 days after injection of 58 or 373 kBq ^{241}Am/kg in mice effectively protected against long-term radiation damage. $ZnNa_3$DTPA reduced bone levels of ^{241}Am between 33% and 45% and liver levels by 97% at both dose levels of ^{241}Am. Chelation therapy significantly reduced the incidences of liver carcinomas and bone tumors and the total number of malignant tumors after the low ^{241}Am dose, proportional to the decreased ^{241}Am level and reduced cumulative radiation dose due to chelation therapy.

Bruenger, Kuswik-Rabiega, and Miller (1992) synthesized and characterized chelating agents, suitable for oral administration for decorporation of heavy metals. The partially lipophilic polyamino carboxylic acids (PACA) synthesized from triethylenetetraminepentaacetic acid by monoalkylation of a primary amino group and carboxymethylation of remaining amino groups had extensive intestinal absorption and can be administered orally in contrast to the nonlipophilic chelators ethylenediaminetetraacetic acid (EDTA) and DTPA. Increasing length of the alkyl chain in C12- and C22-triethylenetetraminepentaacetic acid directed these chelators to the liver, an important target organs for actinide contamination. Daily feeding of 200 μmol/kg b.w. of C12 or C22 derivatives to rats for 10 days reduced whole body levels of Am by 29 and 44%, respectively. The liver levels were reduced by 71 and 89%.

Volf et al. (1993, 1996) tested siderophore analogue chelating agents for the removal of injected ^{241}Am in rats. The effectiveness of early single chelate injections on ^{241}Am tissue retention decreased in the order 3,4,3-LIHOPO (a linear tetrahydroxypyridinone) > DTPA-DX (a dihydroxamic derivative of DTPA) > DTPA>>DFO-HOPO (a hydroxypyridone derivative of DFO). DTPA-DX effectively removed ^{241}Am from the liver. Injected 3,4,3-LIHOPO decreased the Am-241Am levels in bone and liver to 30 and 6%, respectively, of levels in unchelated controls. Continuous infusion of 3,4,3-LIHOPO had a superior effect at chelate doses slightly higher than those given by injection. The bone retention of ^{241}Am was reduced to 10% of controls. The liver level was < 2% of controls. DFO-HOPO and 3,4,3-LIHOPO did not increase the renal retention of ^{241}Am. The Am mobilizing effect of LIHOPO on liver Am levels decreased with time. The mobilized fractions of skeletal and renal Am decreased rapidly from the first day.

Paquet, Chazel, Houpert, Guilmette, and Muggenburg (2003) investigated the Am mobilizing efficacy of 3,4,3-LIHOPO after intramuscular injection of 1 mg (U-Pu)O_2 particles (MOX) in rats. Rats received LIHOPO (30 or 200 μmol/kg) or Ca-DTPA (30 μmol/kg) daily for 7 days. LIHOPO was inefficient for removing Am from the wound site. However, it reduced Am retention in carcass and liver by factors of 10 and 30. The results indicate LIHOPO as a chelating candidate after MOX contamination.

Miller, Liu, Bruenger, and Lloyd (2006) compared the ^{241}Am mobilizing efficacies of orally administered triethylenetetraminepentaacetic acids (TTs) with varying lipophilic properties with parenteral Zn-DTPA chelation. 30 days chelation treatment was started 2 weeks after ^{241}Am administration to rats. ^{241}Am levels were significantly reduced during the first week, Zn-DTPA being most effective. After 30 days, reductions in organ levels of ^{241}Am correlated with increasing lipophilicity of the TT chelators, and oral docosyl-triethylenetetraminepentaacetic acid (C22TT) was as effective as Zn-DTPA in reducing liver and bone Am levels. Amphipathic TT chelators could be developed to oral alternatives to parenteral DTPA for removal of actinides.

Taylor, Hodgson, and Stradling (2007) reviewed the available experimental data on effects of oral Ca or Zn DTPA on decorporation of inhaled actinides in rats. Orally administered Zn-DTPA was found to be as effective as repeated i.v. injection for decorporation of inhaled Am nitrate, although higher doses are required. Oral Zn-DTPA appears to be an effective treatment after AmO_2 exposure. The authors conclude that oral administration of an aqueous Zn-DTPA solution offers an important treatment in accident or emergency situations after exposure to pure chemical forms of Am, which are highly or moderately soluble in biological fluids.

Grémy et al. (2010) investigated effects of pulmonary administration of Ca-DTPA dry powder on pulmonary kinetics of Am after inhalation of Am containing PuO_2 in rats. Epithelial lining fluid (ELF) was demonstrated as an early compartment for both actinides. Higher levels of Am than of Pu were found in ELF and urine because Am is more soluble than Pu. Am was chelated more effectively than Pu by Ca-DTPA, preferentially inhibiting extrapulmonary Am deposition and increasing urinary Am excretion compared to Pu. Early local Ca-DTPA chelation is recommended after inhalation of PuO_2 aerosols with high Am levels as in aged compounds.

Bunin et al. (2013) studied the ^{241}Am decorporating potentials of the hydroxypyridinone-containing chelators, 3,4,3-LI(1,2-HOPO) and 5-LIO(Me-3,2-HOPO). Both compounds mobilized ^{241}Am at substantially higher rates than the clinically approved chelator DTPA. Both chelators were nongenotoxic in Salmonella/Escherichia coli/microsome plate incorporation tests and in Chinese hamster ovary cell chromosome aberration assays with or without metabolic activation. Maximum tolerated dose studies in rats confirmed the safety of presumed efficacious doses for both chelators. This study adds to the growing evidence that 3,4,3-LI(1,2-HOPO) and 5-LIO(Me-3,2-HOPO) are effective decorporating agents with promising toxicological safety profiles.

Griffiths et al. (2014) investigated combinations of chelation/resection protocols in anesthetized rats contaminated with moderately soluble Am or Pu nitrate or insoluble mixed U and Pu oxide in hind leg muscle wounds. DTPA treatment (30 μmol/kg) reduced bone and liver Am levels even if DTPA treatment was started after 7 days. Surgery increased urinary Am excretion indicating release from the wound, however, increased bone or liver levels were not observed.

Sueda et al. (2014) investigated the penta-ethyl ester of DTPA as potential oral prodrug chelating antidote for inhaled ^{241}Am. Oral administration of the DTPA penta-ethyl ester in rats gave a sustained plasma concentration and lower clearance. Hydrolysis to DTPA was extensive but incomplete. The urinary excretion of ^{241}Am in rats given a single oral dose of the prodrug after pulmonary exposure to ^{241}Am nitrate aerosols was 19% higher than in controls. Consistent with prior reports of DTPA chelation in Am exposure, the prodrug was most effective when administered rapidly after Am exposure.

The clinically recommended Am-antidote is still DTPA administered as its Ca- or Zn- salt by intravenous or intramuscular routes, or by inhalation—depending on the Am exposure route.

5.3 CESIUM

Cesium (Cs, atomic number 55, in group 1 of the periodic table of elements, standard atomic weight 132.9, density 1.9 g/cm^3, occurring as Ce^+ in chemical compounds) has 40 known isotopes with atomic masses from 112 to 151. Only ^{133}Cs is stable. The longest lived isotopes are ^{135}Cs, $t_{½}$ 2.3 million years, ^{137}Cs, $t_{½}$ 30.167 years, and ^{134}Cs, $t_{½}$ 2.065 years. All other isotopes have $t_{½}$ of some days, most below 1 h. Cesium is a soft, malleable, silvery white metal, one of 3 metals liquid near room temperature (melting point 28.44°C). Fission of uranium and plutonium in nuclear reactors and nuclear weapons due to neutron absorption create numerous fission products, including ^{134}Cs and ^{137}Cs. ^{134}Cs decays to either ^{134}Xe or ^{134}Ba with β and γ emission, neither of which is radioactive. ^{137}Ce decays by β and γ emissions to ^{137m}Ba, which is also not radioactive. ^{134}Cs and especially ^{137}Cs were among the most important environmental pollutants after the Chernobyl and the Fukushima nuclear accidents. ^{137}Ce has a wide range of industrial uses, for example, in moisture-density gauges, leveling gauges, thickness gauges, and well-logging devices in the drilling industry. ^{137}Ce is also used in cancer radiation therapy. Absorbed ^{137}Ce is uniformly distributed in soft tissues, with slightly higher levels in muscles and slightly lower levels in bone and fat. ^{137}Ce is excreted in urine, initially with a biological half-time around 3 days. The major part of absorbed Ce is excreted with $t_{½}$ 65 days (women) and 90 days (men) (Melo et al., 1997).

Nielsen, Dresow, Fischer, and Heinrich (1991) studied effects of two Prussian blue derivatives, $KFe[Fe(CN)_6]$ (KFeHCF) and $Fe_4[Fe(CN)_6]_3$ (FeHCF), on intestinal absorption of ^{134}Cs in two male volunteers. Administration of 500–1000 mg KFeHCF or FeHCF 10 min before a ^{134}Cs-labelled test meal reduced the ^{134}Cs absorption from 100% to 3–10%. Administration of HFC preparations simultaneously with the test meal decreased ^{134}Cs uptake to 38–63%. Daily administration of 3×0.5 g KFeHCF decreased the elimination $t_{½}$ of previously absorbed ^{134}Cs from 106 (73) to 44 (46) days.

Brandão-Mello, Oliveira, Valverde, Farina, and Cordeiro (1991) and Farina, Brandão-Mello, Oliveira (1991) described results of the treatment of some of the patients exposed to ^{137}Cs in the Goiânia accident in Brazil on Sep. 13, 1987, where a radiotherapy source containing an estimated 50.9 TBq (1,380 Ci) of ^{137}Cs was stolen from an abandoned hospital and broken open, resulting in four deaths. Among 112,000 people examined for radioactive contamination, 249 had significant internal or external radioactive contamination (IAEA, 1988). Internal contamination was verified by the analysis of urine and fecal samples and in a whole-body counter installed in Goiânia in Nov. 1987. The first report described 14 patients developing severe bone marrow depression with neutropenia and thrombocytopenia, 8 received intravenous granulocyte-macrophage colony-stimulating factor, none had bone marrow transplantation. Four died from hemorrhage and infection. Patients with extensive internal contamination were chelated by Prussian blue at doses from 1.5 to 10 g/day. Other measures to increase ^{137}Cs decorporation included diuretics, water overload, and ergometric exercises. The second report described the decorporation of ^{137}Cs in patients less severely affected. Oral Prussian blue was administered to 46 patients, 17 patients received oral diuretics. Induced perspiration was also used to increase ^{137}Cs elimination. The doses of Prussian blue were about 6.5 times the doses previously reported in the literature.

Melo, Lundgren, Muggenburg, and Guilmette (1996) investigated the effect of age on the decorporation effectiveness of Prussian blue for ^{137}Cs injected into immature (4.7 months), young adult (2.4 years), and aged (13.5 years) male beagles. The ^{137}Cs excretion rates decreased with increasing age of the dogs. Prussian blue changed the ratio of fecal to urinary ^{137}Cs excretion from 0.8 in untreated dogs to 2.2 in treated animals. Tissue levels of ^{137}Cs were similar in Prussian blue-treated and untreated dogs after 6-week chelation, with highest levels in skeletal muscle, kidneys, and spleen. The hepatic ^{137}Cs levels were reduced in chelated dogs. The reductions in whole-body levels from Prussian blue chelation were 51% in immature, 31% in young adult, and 38% in aged dogs.

Le Gall, Taran, Renault, Wilk, and Ansoborlo (2006) compared the ^{137}cesium decorporating efficacies of apple-pectin and Prussian Blue in rats intravenously injected with 5 kBq per rat of ^{137}Cs. Apple-pectin or Prussian blue were administered in the drinking water at a concentration corresponding to 400 mg/kg per day during 11 days starting immediately after Cs injection. Prussian blue increased the fecal Cs excretion by fivefold, resulting in reduced Cs levels in main organs. In contrast, differences in Cs elimination and organ levels between rats treated with apple-pectin and untreated rats were not observed.

Timchalk et al. (2010) investigated novel actinide sorbents, self-assembled monolayers on mesoporous supports (SAMMS), which are hybrid materials where differing organic moieties are grafted onto mesoporous silica. A ferrocyanide copper (FC-Cu-EDA)-SAMMS was compared with insoluble Prussian Blue in groups of jugular cannulated rats given 40 μg/kg ^{137}Cs chloride by i.v. injection or oral gavage. Orally administered ^{137}Cs was rapidly and approximately

100% absorbed compared to i.v. administration, with pharmacokinetics (blood, urine, feces, and tissue levels) very similar to that after i.v. administration, with urine and feces elimination of 20 and 3% of the dose, respectively. Preformed ^{137}Cs-SAMMS chelate was retained in feces (72% of the dose), with approximately 1.4% in urine, indicating that ^{137}Cs was bound to SAMMS. Both Prussian blue and SAMMS administered independently of ^{137}Cs chelated available ^{137}Cs in the gut, fecal elimination accounting for 80–88% of the administered dose with less than 2% in urine.

Levitskaia et al. (2011) investigated the ^{137}Cs decorporating efficacies of D-penicillamine (DPA) and triethylenetetramine (trien) in rats given radionuclide solutions by i.v. injection followed by single i.v. doses of either DPA or Trien. DPA and Trien were modestly effective in decorporation of ^{137}Cs.

The clinically recommended ^{137}Cs antidote is still Prussian blue given orally early after poisoning. In addition, acute cases may require intravenous infusion with appropriate fluids accompanied by adequate biochemical monitoring, including measurements of electrolytes—and in particular maintenance of adequate potassium levels in blood.

5.4 ^{60}COBALT

Cobalt (Co, atomic number 27 in group 9 of the periodic table of elements, standard atomic weight 58.933, density 8.9 g/cm^3) is a hard, brittle, gray metal with a bluish tint. The most common radioactive isotope of cobalt is ^{60}Co produced in linear accelerators for commercial use. It is also formed as a by-product when structural materials, such as steel, are exposed to neutron radiation in nuclear reactor operations. ^{60}Co decays by strong γ and also β emission with $t_{1/2}$ 5.27 years. ^{60}Co is used in leveling devices and thickness gauges, for industrial metal radiography to detect structural errors, and in cancer radiotherapy, for example, for the treatment of otherwise inoperable deformities of blood vessels and brain tumors. Large ^{60}Co irradiation sources are used for sterilization of spices and certain foods, "cold pasteurization." Intentional ^{60}Co exposures occur during medical uses, but accidental exposures may occur via loss of or improper disposal of medical and industrial ^{60}Co sources. Though rare, exposures have occurred by accidental mishandling a ^{60}Co source at a steel mill or metal recycling facility. The major health concern of ^{60}Co is external exposure from a source because of the high energy γ emission. Cobalt can exist in vivo as Co(I), Co(II), and Co(III). Absorbed Co is rapidly excreted mainly in urine (Lison, 2014).

Levitskaia et al. (2009) investigated the ^{60}Co decorporating efficacy of the low molecular weight random polymer chitosan (acetyl-β-(1-4)-D-glucosamine *N*-acetyl-D-glucosamine) in rats given a single oral dose of ^{60}Co followed by a single oral or repeated intravenous chitosan administration over 5 days. Oral chitosan increased fecal and decreased urinary ^{60}Co elimination and reduced renal, hepatic, and skeleton ^{60}Co levels compared to controls. Intravenous chitosan slightly reduced tissue ^{60}Co levels.

Levitskaia et al. (2010a) compared decorporation efficacies of L-glutathione (GSH), L-cysteine (Cys), and a liposomal GSH formulation (ReadiSorb) administered orally after i.v. administration of GSH or Cys in rats given ^{60}Co by i.v. injection followed by intravenous or oral chelator administration each 24 h for 5 days. GSH and Cys were potent ^{60}Co decorporating agents after i.v. administration reducing ^{60}Co tissue levels and increasing ^{60}Co excretion compared to controls. Liposomal encapsulation markedly enhanced the oral bioavailability of GSH compared to free GSH. Oral liposomal GSH reduced ^{60}Co levels in most tissues by 12–43% compared to oral free GSH. Oral Cys was slightly less efficacious compared to i.v. Cys.

Levitskaia et al. (2010b) compared the decorporating effects of a single oral dose of DPA or trien on i.v. injected Co in rats. Trien increased urinary Co elimination and bone Co levels. DPA had little effect on Co excretion but reduced renal, hepatic, muscle, stomach, and bone Co levels compared to control animals. DPA effectively reduced spleen Co levels, and trien reduced spleen and bone Co levels compared to control.

Levitskaia et al. (2011) investigated the ^{60}Co decorporating efficacies of DPA and trien in rats given radionuclide solutions by i.v. injection followed by a single i.v. dose of either DPA or trien. DPA was effective in decorporating ^{60}Co within the time frame evaluated.

Animal experiments and clinical cases of nonradioactive cobalt poisoning offer considerably more information on the effectiveness of chelating agents in cobalt poisoning. In humans, EDTA and dimercaptopropane sulfonate (DMPS) enhanced Co excretion in Co poisoning, and in animals EDTA, DTPA, and DMPS both reduced mortality and enhanced Co excretion (reviewed by Andersen, 1999).

In severe clinical cobalt poisonings, for example, due to wear after hip replacement (Pelclova, Sklensky, Janicek, & Lach, 2012), DMPS appears to be the antidote of choice.

5.5 PLUTONIUM

Plutonium (Pu, atomic number 94 in group 7 of the periodic table of elements, standard atomic weight 244, density 19.86 g/cm^3) is a silvery-gray transuranic actinide. Plutonium metal becomes yellowish when exposed to air. Plutonium has at least 15 different radioactive isotopes, the most common are ^{238}Pu, α decay with $t_{1/2}$ 87.7 years to ^{234}U, ^{239}Pu, α decay with $t_{1/2}$ 24,100 years to ^{235}U, ^{240}Pu, α decay with $t_{1/2}$ 6,560 years to ^{236}U, and ^{241}Pu, β decay with $t_{1/2}$ 14 years to ^{241}Am. Trace amounts of plutonium have been naturally produced during spontaneous fission in rocks with very high local uranium levels. Further, the most stable plutonium isotope, ^{244}Pu, α decay with $t_{1/2}$ 8.08×10^7 years to ^{240}U, just makes Pu a primordial element. Despite these special cases, plutonium is considered a man-made element. Plutonium is formed in nuclear reactors by neutron absorption by uranium. Different U isotopes and different combinations of neutron absorptions and radioactive decay create different Pu isotopes. ^{239}Pu is used to produce nuclear weapons. ^{238}Pu generates significant heat during decay making it a long-lived power source, for example, in thermocouples converting heat into electric power in satellites and in heart pacemakers. Very low levels of plutonium was dispersed around the world during the 1950s and 1960s from fallout from atmospheric testing of nuclear weapons. In vivo, Pu is believed to exist as Pu(IV) (Taylor et al., 2000). Absorbed plutonium is mainly deposited in bones and liver and is eliminated very slowly, t½ for bone Pu is estimated to be more than 8000 days (Taylor et al., 2000). Plutonium may cause damage to the kidneys.

Volf (1986) compared the ^{238}Pu mobilizing capacity of the carboxylated catecholamide 3,4,3-LICAM(C) with effects of Ca-DTPA and DFO. After early administration at doses used for actinide decorporation with Ca-DTPA (30 μmol/kg b.w.), LICAM(C) was more effective than DFO. Only in bone LICAM(C) was more effective than Ca-DTPA in reducing Pu levels since only 1 μmol LICAM(C)/kg was as effective as 30 μmol Ca-DTPA/kg. However, LICAM(C) treatment extensively increased the renal ^{238}Pu levels. Single injection of LICAM(C) and Ca-DTPA 1 day after injection of ^{238}Pu followed by continuous administration of Ca-DTPA in drinking water most effectively reduced Pu retention. Orally administered LICAM(C) also reduced ^{238}Pu retention. After delayed treatment LICAM(C) was equally or less effective than Ca-DTPA on bone ^{238}Pu retention, but still increased renal ^{238}Pu levels.

Volf, Burgada, Raymond, and Durbin (1993) investigated mobilizing effects of various chelating agents on injected ^{238}Pu in rats. The effect on ^{238}Pu retention in tissues after single early single chelator injections decreased in the order 3,4,3-LIHOPO > DTPA-DX > DTPA >> DFO-HOPO. Injected 3,4,3-LIHOPO decreased ^{238}Pu levels in bone and liver to 9 and 3% of levels in controls. Continuous infusion of 3,4,3-LIHOPO reduced ^{238}Pu levels in bone to < 5%, a superior effect with total chelate doses only slightly higher than that given by single injection. The hepatic level was < 2% of controls.

Miller, Bruenger, Kuswik-Rabiega, Liu, and Lloyd (1993) investigated the ^{239}Pu decorporating effect of the amphipathic chelator, docosyltriethylenetetramine pentaacetic acid (C22TT) in rats injected with ^{239}Pu. 30 days of treatment induced dose-related reductions in the Pu levels in soft tissues and bones. All C22TT dose levels substantially reduced hepatic Pu levels. The largest reductions in organ Pu levels occurred during the first 30 days of treatment, particularly in the liver, but further reductions occurred at 60 or 90 days compared to controls. Neutron-induced autoradiography indicated that C22TT reduced the incorporation of Pu into new bone and into bone marrow. There were no signs of overt toxicity in the experiment. The study indicates that oral C22TT is a potential chelator reducing soft and hard tissue levels of Pu.

Guilmette and Muggenberger (1993) gave dogs exposed to a polydisperse aerosol of $^{238}Pu(NO_3)_4$ by inhalation a single injection of 30 μmol/kg CaDTPA followed by repeated i.v. injections of 30 μmol/kg ZnDTPA or by subcutaneous infusion of 30 or 120 μmol/kg ZnDTPA per day, starting 1 h after aerosol exposure and continuing for 64 days. The different DTPA treatments did not result in significant differences in ^{238}Pu, removing about 85% of initial pulmonary ^{238}Pu burden compared to 24% removed in unchelated control dogs. The authors explain the lack of additional effectiveness of continuous infusion of DTPA by high in vivo solubility of the Pu aerosol resulting in rapid systemic Pu uptake and translocation to soft tissues and reducing the long-term effect of DTPA.

Volf, Burgada, Raymond, and Durbin (1996) investigated the siderophore analogues DFO-HOPO (a hydroxypyridone derivative of desferrioxamine) and 3,4,3-LIHOPO as ^{238}Pu mobilizing agents in rats. A single oral administration of 100 μmol/kg of these chelators had the same effect on Pu mobilization as subcutaneous (s.c.) injection of 30 μmol/kg if the oral dose was administered earlier. 3,4,3-LIHOPO reduced hepatic and skeletal Pu levels to < 10% of control values. No increase in renal Pu retention was observed. The Pu mobilizing effects of the injected ligands decreased exponentially with time between exposure and treatment. The $t_{1/2}$ for decreased Pu mobilization from bone and liver was 5 and 12 h for DFO-HOPO. The Pu mobilizing effect of 3,4,3-LIHOPO decreased more slowly, with $t_{1/2}$ 3–4 weeks.

Paquet et al. (2003) investigated the Pu mobilizing efficacy of 3,4,3-LIHOPO after intramuscular injection of 1 mg (U-Pu)O_2 particles (MOX) in rats. Rats received 3,4,3-LIHOPO (30 or 200 μmol/kg) or Ca-DTPA (30 μmol/kg) daily for 7 days. 3,4,3-LIHOPO was inefficient for removing Pu from the injection site. However, it reduced Pu retention in carcass and liver by factors of 2 and 6 respectively indicating that 3,4,3-LIHOPO is a potential chelating agent after MOX contamination.

Ramounet-Le Gall et al. (2003) compared the ^{238}Pu decorporating efficacies of DTPA, 3,4,3-LIHOPO and a newly synthesized molecule, 4,4,4-LIHOPO in rats. 30 μmol/kg DTPA or 0.3 or 30 μmol/kg 3,4,3-LIHOPO or 4,4,4-LIHOPO were injected at 1, 6, 24, and 48 h after i.v. injection of ^{238}Pu citrate. 4,4,4-LIHOPO and 3,4,3-LIHOPO had similar decorporating efficacies for Pu, much higher than that of DTPA. 0.3 μmol/kg of these LIHOPO analogs was as efficient as 30 μmol/kg DTPA.

Phan et al. (2004) investigated the Pu mobilizing effects of ^{14}C-DTPA encapsulated in conventional and stealth liposomes in rats given as a single i.v. injection 2 h after administration of colloidal ^{239}Pu phytate or soluble ^{238}Pu citrate. ^{14}C-DTPA accumulated mainly in the liver and with stealth liposomes in bone and spleen. Both liposomal preparations increased urinary Pu elimination and decreased skeletal Pu deposition. After administration of Pu phytate, 6 μmol/kg DTPA in conventional liposomes was as efficient as 30 μmol/kg free Ca-DTPA in maintaining the femur Pu level below 4.3% of the injected dose after 16 days, corresponding to a 3.6-fold reduction compared to administration of 4 μmol/kg free Ca-DTPA and to unchelated controls. This study indicates that liposome formulation could be a powerful tool to improve the efficiency of Pu chelating agents in vivo.

Miller et al. (2006) compared the ^{239}Pu mobilizing efficacies of orally administered TTs with varying lipophilic properties with parenteral Zn-DTPA chelation. Chelation treatment was started 2 weeks after ^{239}Pu administration to rats. After 30 days, reductions in organ levels of ^{239}Pu correlated with increasing lipophilicity of the TT chelators, and oral administration of docosyltriethylenetetramine pentaacetic acid (C22TT) was as effective as Zn-DTPA in reducing liver and bone Pu levels. The removal of ^{239}Pu from the liver and reduction of redeposition of ^{239}Pu in newly formed bone by C22TT was confirmed by neutron-induced autoradiographs. Amphipathic TT chelators could be developed to oral alternatives to parenteral DTPA for removal of actinides.

Sérandour et al. (2007) investigated the Pu decorporating effects of pulmonary administration of a formulation of Ca-DTPA dry powder with improved aerodynamic properties after pulmonary exposure of rats to different Pu compounds. A delayed intratracheal administration of 18 μmol/kg b.w. DTPA dry powder could not significantly reduce the pulmonary Pu retention after PuO_2 inhalation exposure, but limited Pu transfer to liver and bones. Early insufflation of DTPA powder after pulmonary administration of Pu nitrate was 2 times more efficient than i.v. injection of 30 μmol/kg Ca-DTPA in reducing pulmonary Pu retention, and was as effective as i.v. Ca-DTPA administration in limiting extrapulmonary Pu deposition while delayed DTPA powder administration did not reduce the lung or extrapulmonary Pu retention. The improvement of aerodynamic properties of DTPA powder increased the DTPA deposition in the lungs and enhanced Pu decorporation.

Taylor et al. (2007) reviewed the available experimental data on effects of oral Ca or Zn DTPA on decorporation of inhaled actinides in rats. Orally administered Zn-DTPA was found to be as effective as repeated i.v. injection for decorporation of inhaled Pu nitrate, although higher doses were required. Oral Zn-DTPA appears not to be effective for inhaled PuO_2. Effective Pu decorporation by oral or i.v. DTPA administration required an extensive molar excess of DTPA over Pu. Oral or injected Zn-DTPA is unlikely to mobilize Pu oxides. The authors conclude that oral administration of an aqueous Zn-DTPA solution offers an important treatment in accident or emergency situations after exposure to pure chemical forms of Pu which are highly or moderately soluble in biological fluids.

Carbaugh et al. (2010) described 24 years of follow-up on a puncture wound in a worker's right index finger, contaminated with 48 kBq of primarily $^{239+240}Pu$ and ^{241}Am in an accident in the Hanford facility in 1985. Surgical excisions reduced the residual activity in the wound to 5.4 kBq. DTPA chelation in 164 courses during 17 months mobilized about 7 kBq via urine. Annual in vivo measurements of ^{241}Am and plutonium in urine, and ^{241}Am in wound, lung, liver, axillary lymph nodes, and skeleton showed relatively stable ^{241}Am levels in the wound site and gradually increasing levels of ^{241}Am in the skeleton. Urine Pu excretion after termination of DTPA chelation ranged from 10 to 20 mBq per day, Am excretion being about 10% of $^{239+240}Pu$ excretion. Annual medical examinations have not revealed adverse health effects associated with the contamination.

Grémy, Tsapis, Bruel, Renault, and Van der Meeren (2012) compared the Pu decorporating efficacy of pulmonary administration of DTPA dry powder with intravenous injection of DTPA and with combined administration of DTPA via both routes in rats after pulmonary exposure to plutonium nitrate. Insufflated DTPA was more effective than i.v. injected DTPA in reducing the plutonium lung burden both after early and late administration. Early treatment with DTPA powder was more effective in reducing extrapulmonary Pu depositions by removing transportable Pu from lungs prior to absorption into blood. The efficacy of DTPA dry powder was further increased by combined i.v. DTPA administration reducing extrapulmonary Pu deposition and increasing renal Pu excretion. The most effective protocol for plutonium decorporation was early pulmonary DTPA powder insufflation combined with i.v. administration of DTPA.

Bunin et al. (2013) studied the ^{238}Pu decorporating potentials of the hydroxypyridinone-containing chelators, 3,4,3-LIHOPO and 5-LIO(Me-3,2-HOPO). Both compounds mobilized ^{238}Pu at substantially higher rates than the clinically approved chelator DTPA. Genotoxicity tests and acute toxicity tests confirmed the safety of presumed efficacious doses for both chelators adding to the growing evidence that 3,4,3-LIHOPO and 5-LIO(Me-3,2-HOPO) are effective decorporators with promising toxicological safety profiles.

An et al. (2014) investigated the Pu decorporating efficacy of 3,4,3-LIHOPO after delayed postexposure treatment. Male and female mice given soluble ^{238}Pu citrate received one of six doses from 1–300 μmol/kg of 3,4,3-LIHOPO parenterally 24 h later. Pu decorporation was dose-dependent in the dose range at several investigated time-points, with some significant reductions in tissue and body Pu levels. The highest dose induced mild toxicity with a short recovery period, which delayed Pu excretion. While some sex differences were observed, sustained dose-dependent enhancement of ^{238}Pu elimination by 3,4,3-LIHOPO was observed in all experimental groups.

Griffiths et al. (2014) investigated different chelation/resection protocols after contamination of rats with plutonium (Pu) nitrate or mixed oxide (MOX); uranium (U), Pu oxide in hind leg muscle wounds. Immediate or delayed, systemic or local treatment with 30 μmol/kg DTPA was combined or not with wound resection. A more heterogeneous localization of MOX particles than of Pu nitrate was observed at the wound site. In all cases DTPA chelation reduced bone and liver Pu levels even when DTPA chelation was delayed for 7 days. Surgery increased urinary Pu excretion without increased Pu retention in bone and liver. The combination of surgery and DTPA increased Pu excretion and reduced tissue levels markedly.

5.6 POLONIUM

Polonium (Po, atomic number 84 in group 16 of the periodic table of elements, standard atomic weight 209, density 9.142 g/cm^3) is a rare metal occurring in low amounts in uranium ores. All 33 known Po isotopes with masses ranging from 188 to 220 are radioactive (Ansoborlo et al., 2012). Polonium was discovered by Mme Curie in 1898 during her seek for the cause of the higher radioactivity of the uranium ore pitchblende from Joachimsthal (uraninite) and other uranium and thorium ores than in purified uranium. The element is named after Poland, Mme Curie's native country. Polonium's most stable isotope ^{209}Po (α-emitter, $t_{½}$ 102 years) decays into ^{205}Pb. The most prominent naturally occurring and most widely available polonium isotope ^{210}Po (α-emitter with very low γ-emission, $t_{½}$ 138.4 days) is constantly produced from decay of ^{238}U, which contributes more than 99% of all uranium. It decays into stable ^{206}Pb. Po occurs as Po(II), Po(IV), and Po (VI) in chemical compounds. ^{210}Po is probably the most toxic compound known: From the LD_{50} for acute radiation exposure, 8.8×10^{6} Bq (Strom, 2003), and the very high specific activity of ^{210}Po, 1.7×10^{14} Bq/g, the LD_{50} to an average 75 kg adult can be calculated to be about 52 ng or 0.7 ng ^{210}Po per kg b.w. after ingestion and about 0.13 ng/kg after inhalation. Due to excretion of Po (the biological half-time life of Po is 30 to 50 days in humans; Naimark, 2015) the effective LD_{50} of ^{210}Po is somewhat higher, still less than 1.3 ng/kg b.w. To compare, the LD_{50} of TCDD is 100 ng/kg and that of butolinum toxin is 10 ng/kg (Eaton & Klaassen, 2001). The former Soviet and Russian spy Alexander Litvinenko died from radiation sickness after ^{210}Po poisoning from drinking tea during a meeting in London with two Russian men.

^{210}Po has been produced in significant amounts in the former USSR. Due to the intensive heat generated by ^{210}Po α decay it is used as atomic heat source in thermoelectric generators. Alpha particles emitted by polonium can be converted to neutrons in Po-BeO alloys used as neutron source in the neutron trigger of nuclear weapons (Rhodes, 2002). Alpha particles from polonium ionize air molecules that in turn neutralize charges on the nearby surfaces, allowing the use of polonium in tools eliminating static charges in various industrial processes (ThermoCahn, 2015). Due to the high toxicity of its α irradiation and high cost, ^{210}Po has been replaced by less dangerous β emitters in some applications, however, ^{210}Po has still important industrial uses. Like other soft metals polonium has a high affinity for SH groups. Important storage organs for polonium are erythrocytes, bone marrow, and soft organs. Fecal excretion dominates.

^{210}Po is a severe health hazard only when internalized. Fifty to ninety percent of ingested ^{210}Po is excreted in feces depending on diet composition (Ansoborlo et al., 2012). Initially after oral intake ^{210}Po concentrates in erythrocytes, later in liver, kidneys, gastrointestinal tract, bone marrow, spleen, and gonads. ^{210}Po is excreted in urine, bile, sweat, and is deposited in hair (Jefferson, Goans, Blain, & Thomas, 2009). The chronic toxicity of ^{210}Po is related to the internal radiation dose, depending on the exposure route. There is no information about the chemical toxicity of polonium.

Yuile, Berke, & Hull (1967) exposed groups of rats to NaCl aerosols with small amounts of ^{210}Po added corresponding to accumulated lung doses of 538, 202, and 71 rads after 280 days. 87% of animals in the highest dose group died within one year after exposure, compared to 35% in controls and the other experimental groups. Mortality was mainly due to acute pneumonia. 41 primary lung tumors, mainly squamous cell carcinoma, were found in 288 exposed rats dying spontaneously during the 96-week experiment. Over 70% of the squamous cell tumors occurred in rats exposed to the highest dose of ^{210}Po, none were observed in control rats.

Little, Kennedy, and McGandy (1975) gave Syrian golden hamsters multiple intratracheal instillations of ^{210}Po corresponding to lifetime exposures of 15–300 rads to the lungs resulting in dose related induction of lung cancers (9–53% of exposed hamsters).

Due to the softness character of Po, EDTA, and DTPA are of no use for Po decorporation, and Po has high affinity for HS-containing compounds. The chelator of choice for ^{210}Po decorporation among clinically established chelators is DMPS. Ruprecht (2008) presented an extensive review of early Soviet/Russian animal studies on the effect of DMPS after acute ^{210}Po poisoning in different animal species. In essence, DMPS chelation increased the survival, increased the excretion, and reduced ^{210}Po levels and thereby radiation loads in several organs including critical organs as brain and bone marrow. Early administration and high doses for extended time were effective. In some studies, the renal levels were increased by DMPS chelation increasing the risk of pathological changes including kidney tumors.

Volf (1973) investigated effects of intraperitoneal or oral administration of chelators on the distribution of ^{210}Po in rats. Again DMPS was the most effective chelator followed by DDC>2-mercaptopropionyl-glycin > D-penicillamine while DTPA was without effects.

Aposhian et al. (1987) investigated effects of dimercaptosuccinic acid (DMSA), DMPS, and N-(2,3-dimercaptopropyl)phthalamidic acid (DMPA) on median survival time in rats after i.p. injection of 40 μCi/kg ^{210}Po. Repeated s.c. injections of DMSA, DMPS, or DMPA increased the 39 days median survival time in controls to106 days. Repeated s.c. injections of DMPA in rats given 0.4 μCi ^{210}Po s.c. reduced kidney levels of ^{210}Po to 28% and spleen levels to 25% of those in the untreated controls, significantly lower than in rats injected with DMSA or DMPS. DMPA is, however, yet not a licensed or commercially available antidote for human use.

Bogdan and Aposhian (1990) injected 0.20 mmol/kg DMPA or DMSA s.c. 1 h after and then daily for 12 days in male rats injected 3.33×10^7 cpm/kg ^{210}Po i.p. DMPA and DMSA increased the urinary excretion of ^{210}Po 8× and 5× compared to controls. DMPA increased the fecal excretion of ^{210}Po and decreased the level of ^{210}Po in the spleen compared to the other treatments. In another experiment, intravenous administration of DMPA, 0.20 mmol/kg, increased the biliary excretion of ^{210}Po fivefold compared to controls.

Rencova, Volf, Jones, and Singh (1993) evaluated 9 different sulfur-based chelators, including dithiols and dithiocarbamates, for ability to decorporate ^{210}Po in rats. Most compounds induced a redistribution of ^{210}Po in the body and decreased ^{210}Po levels in spleen and muscle. Diethyldithiocarbamate (DDC), dimercaptopropanol (BAL), and DMPA most effectively reduced blood levels of ^{210} Po, however, DDC and BAL substantially increased the deposition of ^{210}Po in the brain while DMPA, DMPS, and DMSA increased ^{210} Po deposition in kidneys. The DMSA derivative Mi-ADMS reduced ^{210} Po levels in blood, bone, and muscle more effectively than DMSA, but increased ^{210} Po deposition in kidneys. Combination of BAL or DDC with other agents induced larger reductions in whole-body retention of ^{210} Po. Removal of ^{210} Po from the bone, spleen, and kidneys by BAL was increased by repeated treatment. None of the chelating agents could reduce the whole-body retention of ^{210} Po below 85% of the retention in untreated controls.

Volf, Rencova, Jones, and Singh (1995) investigated decorporation of ^{210}Po from wounds simulated in rats by intramuscular injection. Chelators in clinical use (BAL, DMPS, DMSA, and DDC) as well as 10 newly synthesized compounds with vicinal sulfhydryl and carbodithioate groups were used. Two injections of DMPS at the injection site starting 2 h after injection of ^{210}Po completely removed ^{210}Po from the injection site. Some compounds translocated ^{210}Po from the injection site to other tissues. Two weeks DMPS administration combined with repeated s.c. administration during of NN′-di-(2-hydroxyethyl)ethylenediamine-*NN′*-biscarbodithioate (HOEtTTC, a derivative of DDC) increased the excretion of ^{210}Po from 8 to 54%, mainly via faeces, and reduced the estimated total body retention of ^{210}Po to about one-third of that in unchelated controls.

Rencová, Volf, Jones, Singh, and Filgas (1995) investigated the effect of single or repeated administration of DDC and three bis-dithiocarbamates: N,N′-dimethylethylenediamine-N,N′-biscarbodithioate (MeTTC), N,N′-diethylethylenediamine-N,N′biscarbodithioate (EtTTC), and HOEtTTC on organ distribution and excretion of i.v. injected ^{210}Po. HOEtTTC was most effective, both after s.c. injection immediately after Po-210 and after 1 h delay. DDC increased ^{210}Po deposition in brain and transiently in liver. HOEtTTC increased fecal excretion of ^{210}Po. MeTTC, EtTTC, and DMPA were ineffective when the treatment started 1 h after injection of ^{210}Po.

Rencova, Volf, Jones, and Singh (2000) compared the efficiency of repeated subcutaneous injection of chelators (0.4 mmol/kg) of racemic or meso-DMSA, or its derivatives mono-isoamyl-meso-2,3-dimercapto succinate (Mi-ADMS) and mono-N-(i-butyl)-meso-2,3-dimercapto succinamide (Mi-BDMA)) for decorporation of intravenously injected ^{210}Po, 11 kBq/animal. Mi-BDMA and Mi-ADMS but not DMSA increased fecal excretion while all 3 compounds increased the urinary excretion of ^{210}Po. The total excretion was increased most (about 3×) by Mi-BDMA, while meso-DMSA was without effect on excretion compared to controls. However, the detoxification efficacy of Mi-BDMA was less than that of HOEtTTC (Rencová et al., 1995).

Also in the study by Rencova, Vlkova, Curik, Holusa, and Vesela (2004) s.c. injection of DMPS for 5 days in animals injected with ^{210}Po increased the excretion of ^{210}Po in urine and feces and reduced ^{210}Po levels in all organs investigated as well as the total body burden of ^{210}Po.

Levitskaia et al. (2010b) investigated the decorporating effects of oral DPA or trien for i.v. administered Po. Rats received a total of 5 doses given at 24 h intervals. DPA reduced spleen Po levels compared to controls, and trien reduced Po levels in spleen and skeletal tissues compared to controls.

Despite extensive literature search, cases of clinical chelation in polonium poisoning have not been found. Some experimental chelators not registered for human use, notably HOEtTTC were highly efficacious in acute experimental ^{210}Po poisoning. However, DMPS remains the choice for chelation in potential cases of human ^{210}Po poisoning. The effects of DMPS are most likely due, both to chelation of ^{210}Po, and to radiotoxicity protection via antioxidative properties.

5.7 RADIUM

Radium (Ra, atomic number 88 in group 2 of the periodic table of elements, standard atomic weight 226, density 5.5 g/cm^3) is a naturally occurring silvery-white metal which blackens when exposed to air. Metallic radium is highly chemically reactive. Ra has 33 known isotopes, the most common are ^{224}Ra (α decay with $t_{1/2}$ 3.63 days to radon-220), ^{226}Ra (α decay with $t_{1/2}$ 1600 years to radon-222), and ^{228}Ra (β decay with $t_{1/2}$ 5.57 years goes through several decays to radium-224 before forming radon-220). The various Ra isotopes are formed by decay of uranium or thorium, ^{226}Ra in the ^{238}U decay series, and ^{228}Ra and ^{224}Ra in the ^{232}Th decay series. Ra occurs at very low levels in virtually all water, soil, rock, animals, and plants. Radium salts and phosphors were used for clock dials and gauges before the risks of radium exposure were realized. Radium is used as radiation source in industrial radiography instruments to inspect for defects in metal parts. Radium-beryllium alloy is a potent neutron source, for example, for well logging devices. Radium has been used in lightening rods, since it ionizes air. The intestinal uptake of radium is about 20%. Absorbed Ra is mainly deposited in bones with a long $t_{1/2}$ increasing the risk of developing bone cancer, lymphoma, leukemia, or aplastic anemia. Chronic inhalation exposure to radium can lead to leukopenia and increased risk for contracting infections.

Schoeters, Van Puymbroeck, and Vanderborght, (1980); Schoeters, Luz, and Vanderborght, (1983) investigated effects of long-term alginate treatment on ^{226}Ra induced depression of multipotent bone marrow stem cells in mice. Mice fed a diet containing 6% Na-alginate every second day starting 12 days after injection of $^{226}RaCl_2$ had significant reduction of stem-cell depression at 8 and 12 weeks after ^{226}Ra injection compared to groups, where nonalginate-fed controls had manifest radiation effects on the stem cells. Further, Schoeters et al. (1980) investigated the effectiveness of daily dietary administration of Na-alginate in removing ^{226}Ra from bone and reducing osteosarcoma incidence. Although alginate feeding substantially increased ^{226}Ra decorporation, the incidence of osteosarcoma was not reduced.

5.8 STRONTIUM

Strontium (Sr, atomic number 38, in group 2 of the periodic table of elements, standard atomic weight 226, density 5.5 g/cm^3) is a soft silver-white chemically highly reactive metal turning yellowish on exposure to air. Metallic strontium is not found naturally. Strontium has 16 known isotopes, 4 stable (^{84}Sr, ^{86}Sr, ^{87}Sr, and ^{88}Sr) and 12 radioactive isotopes. ^{85}Sr is used in industry and medicine, ^{89}Sr occurs as pollutant around nuclear facilities, ^{90}Sr is formed as a by-product during fission of plutonium and uranium and in nuclear reactors and nuclear weapons and is an important highly hazardous pollutant in waste from nuclear reactors. Large amounts of ^{90}Sr were dispersed worldwide during atmospheric nuclear weapons tests in the 1950s and 1960s. ^{90}Sr decays with $t_{½}$ 29.1 years by β decay to ^{90}Y. Heat from ^{90}Sr decay is used in thermocouples as long-lived electric power supplies in weather stations, navigational beacons, and space vehicles. ^{90}Sr is used in electron tubes, in industrial thickness gauges, and in cancer radiation therapy, for example, in bone cancer. The intestinal uptake of Sr is 20–30%. Absorbed Sr is mainly deposited in bone with a very long $t_{½}$, increasing risk of bone cancer, soft tissue cancer, and leukemia.

Varga et al. (1994) synthesized various water soluble N,N′-disubstituted derivatives of the crown ether 1,4,10,13-tetraoxa-7,16-diaza-cyclooctadecane, cryptand (2.2) and tested their capacity for mobilizing ^{85}Sr 30–60 min after i.p. injection or pulmonary instillation of ^{85}Sr in mice. The unsubstituted cryptand (2.2) had no ^{85}Sr mobilizing effect while the dimalonate of cryptand (2.2) had a moderate mobilizing effect, achieving 80–95% decorporation of the initial ^{85}Sr body burden compared to 20–30% in controls. The agents were effectively resorbed from the lung, and cryptand (2.2) derivatives inhibited ^{85}Sr deposition in bone. The decorporating effectiveness depended upon the time lag between ^{85}Sr and chelator administration.

Jagtap et al. (2003) compared the ^{85}Sr mobilizing effects of Ca gluconate (CaG), Ca lactate (CaL), Ca carbonate (CaC), and Ca phosphate (CaP) with that of Ca alginate (CaA), normally advised for Sr decorporation. Rats given ^{85}Sr i.p. or orally were given one of the Ca salts 2 h after ^{85}Sr administration and thereafter once daily. Ca salts were administered orally except for CaG which was administered i.p. in the i.p. Sr group. The diet of experimental subgroups was supplemented with the respective Ca salts to 2% elemental Ca. Administration of Ca salts significantly reduced the ^{85}Sr whole-body retention (WBR) from 50–60% at 24 h to 20–30% after 15 days compared with 70–80% at 24 h to 50–60% after 15 days in controls. The results indicate that any commonly used Ca salts could replace CaA for reducing ^{85}Sr WBR.

In a subsequent study, Sonawane, Jagtap, Pahuja, Rajan, and Samuel, (2004) were unsuccessful in mobilizing the remaining 20–30% ^{85}Sr after Ca salt treatment by administering various compounds (Ca pyrophosphate, magnesium sulfate, sodium citrate, the bioabsorbent chitin, a crown ether, or ammonium chloride) in drinking water for another 4 week. The remaining ^{85}Sr burden is fixed in bone and difficult to mobilize.

The use of commercial alginate for ^{85}Sr decorporation is limited by low solubility and gel formation. Levitskaia et al. (2010c) increased the solubility of alginate using a low molecular weight polyethylene glycol (PEG) sodium chloride/sodium bicarbonate buffer. Oral administration of this alginate/electrolyte/PEG solution removed internal ^{85}Sr in rats compared to sodium alginate/electrolyte or electrolyte/PEG solutions. These nontoxic compounds are readily available for oral administration to humans in emergency cases of exposure of large population numbers.

Levitskaia et al. (2011) investigated the ^{85}Sr decorporating efficacies of DPA and trien in rats given radionuclide solutions by i.v. injection followed by single i.v. doses of either DPA or trien. DPA and trien were modestly effective in decorporation of ^{85}Sr. The present clinical recommendation for strontium decorporation may be long-term dietary alginates, and enhancement of alginate solubility may increase decorporating efficacy. However, oral calcium salts may be as effective as alginates. The antidote trien may be added.

5.9 TECHNETIUM

Technetium (Tc, atomic number 43 in group, in group 7 of the periodic table of elements, standard atomic weight 98, density 11.5 g/cm^3) is a silver-gray transition metal occurring naturally in very small amounts in the earth's crust, but Tc is primarily a man-made metal. All Tc isotopes are radioactive. ^{99}Tc ($t_{½}$ 212,000 years) is a major product of fission of ^{235}U in nuclear reactors and detonation of nuclear weapons. ^{99}Tc and ^{99m}Tc are the most common Tc isotopes. ^{99}Tc has no important uses and is mainly found in the radioactive wastes from nuclear reactor and fuel cycle facilities, hospitals, and academic research institutions. ^{99m}Tc is the most widely used isotope for medical diagnostic studies. Molybdenum/technetium generators are used to produce ^{99m}Tc for diagnostic tests or research. The nuclear reactor produces ^{99}Mo which decays with $t_{½}$ 66 h to ^{99m}Tc which decays with $t_{½}$ 6.01 h to ^{99}Tc primarily by γ emission. ^{99}Tc decays by beta and gamma radiation to stable ^{99}Ru. Technetium has several nuclear isomers. ^{97m}Tc is the most stable ($t_{½}$ 91 days) followed by ^{95m}Tc ($t_{½}$ 61 days) and ^{99m}Tc ($t_{½}$ 6.01 h). Human exposure to ^{99}Tc is mainly due to use of ^{99m}Tc in nuclear medicine. Absorbed ^{99m}Tc is mainly deposited in the thyroid gland and the gastrointestinal tract but is excreted with $t_{½}$ 60 h. Experiences from nuclear medicine have revealed that ^{99m}Tc is chelated by DMSA, and this chelate is transported to kidneys and subsequently into urine (Gorla, Agrawal, Sood, Bhattacharya, & Mittal, 2014).

5.10 THORIUM

Thorium (Th, atomic number 90, in group 3 of the periodic table of elements, standard atomic weight 232, density 11.78 g/cm^3) is the first member of the actinide series. Thorium is a naturally occurring soft, silvery white radioactive metal present in very low levels in water, soils, rocks, plants, and animals. The thorium ores monazite, thorite, and thorianite are mined for the metal. All of thoriums several isotopes are radioactive. The most common thorium isotope is ^{232}Th, $t_{½}$ 14x10^9 years by α decay with accompanying γ radiation. ^{232}Th is the top element of a long decay series ending with stable ^{208}Pb, ^{228}Ra is the first decay product as described above. Most thorium is natural, but thorium isotopes are produced by decay processes in nuclear reactors. ^{230}Th, $t_{½}$ 75,400 years, and ^{228} Th, $t_{½}$ 1.9 years, both by α decay with accompanying γ radiation, are environmentally important Th isotopes. Thorium oxide has previously been used in lantern mantles due to its bright white glow when heated, alternatives are replacing this use. Thorium is added in small amounts to welding rods to improve burning. Thorium is used in alloys in the aerospace industry and in ophthalmic lenses. Thorium is used as coloring agent in ceramic glazes. Inhaled thorium compounds of low solubility have long pulmonary halftimes. In vivo, Thorium exists as Th(IV). The intestinal uptake of Th is low, absorbed systemic Th is mainly deposited in bones increasing bone cancer risk. Inhaled thorium dust increases lung and pancreatic cancer risk. The biological halftime of Th deposited in bone is several years (Taylor et al., 2000).

Stradling et al. (1995) compared the ^{228}Th decorporating potential of the siderophore analog 3,4,3-LIHOPO with that of DTPA after s.c. or i.m. injection of ^{228}Th nitrate in rats to simulate wound contamination. Treatment started 30 min, 6 h or 1 day after ^{228}Th nitrate administration. 3,4,3-LIHOPO was considerably more effective than DTPA for ^{228}Th decorporation. The efficacy of treatment decreased rapidly with delay after ^{228}Th injection. For both chelators, local administration at 30 min followed by repeated i.p. injection 6 h, 1, 2, and 3 days later resulted in optimum ^{228}Th decorporation, reducing the ^{228}Th body burden to 20% of controls after s.c. injection and 15% after i.m. injection, compared to 80% and 54%, respectively, after DTPA injection. 3,4,3-LIHOPO potentially offers a considerable advantage over DTPA, the agent of choice for treatment of ^{228}Th contaminated wounds.

Rencova, Vlková, and Veselá, (2003) compared the translocation and retention of ^{234}Th (46 ng) + ^{232}Th (5 μg) injected i.m. in rats as preformed complexes with citrate, CaDTPA or citrate + CaDTPA. Thorium in mixed-ligand solution was completely translocated from muscle with the majority excreted. In 2 days the whole-body Th retention decreased to 16% of injected Th with 13% retained in the skeleton. When citrate + CaDTPA were injected i.m. after i.m. injection of ^{234}Th + ^{232}Th as the nitrate, the whole-body Th retention at 2 days was 30, 37, and 55% of injected Th when chelators were injected immediately, 1 h or 24 h, after Th injection. Only a slight reduction in whole body Th retention occurred in unchelated control rats.

Kumar, Sharma, Ali, Pandey, and Mishra (2012) examined the effect ^{99m}Tc-labeled DTPA encapsulated in neutral liposomes (dipalmitoylphosphatidylcholine and cholesterol) and encapsulated in positively charged liposomes (dipalmitoylphosphatidylcholine, cholesterol, and stearylamine) on DTPA organ distribution and effects on ^{232}Th accumulation and Th induced liver toxicity in rats given 600 μg/kg ^{232}Th-nitrate. ^{99m}Tc-DTPA in neutral liposomes had higher uptake into liver, spleen, and blood than ^{99m}Tc-DTPA in positively charged liposomes and free ^{99m}Tc-DTPA. Administration of ^{232}Th-nitrate significantly increased the levels of liver toxicity markers, which were found to be restored more significantly by neutral liposomal-DTPA than by free-DTPA. Neutral liposomal-DTPA decreased blood and hepatic ^{232}Th accumulation and reduced ^{232}Th induced liver toxicity and oxidative injury more effectively than free DTPA.

Thus, although CaDTPA is the commercially available clinically recommended antidote for ^{232}Th, liposomal encapsulation of DTPA offers a potential for future improvement of the effects of DTPA chelation in some situations.

5.11 URANIUM

Uranium (U, atomic number 92, in group 5 of the periodic table of elements, standard atomic weight 238, density 19.05 g/cm^3) is a naturally occurring actinide. Uranium is present in very small amounts in water, soil, rocks, plants, and animals. High concentrations of uranium can occur in phosphate rock deposits, and uraninite (mainly UO_2) in uranium-rich ores. Natural Uranium has 3 isotopes, ^{238}U contributing more than 99% to natural U metal, ^{235}U, and ^{234}U. Because these uranium U isotopes have long $t_{1/2}$ (^{238}U 4.47×10^9 years, ^{235}U 7×10^8 years, ^{234}U 2.46×10^5 years), the amount of uranium on earth remains almost constant. Pure uranium metal is silvery white and weakly radioactive. Uranium mining and nuclear reactors are sources of radionuclides primarily contained in wastes. Long-lived radionuclides as ^{230}Th and ^{226}Ra are not removed by uranium extraction leaving 85% of the initial radioactivity of the ore in waste sludges (Diehl, 2004). Uranium processing generates ^{137}Cs and ^{90}Sr with very long $t_{1/2}$. ^{238}uranium decays to ^{226}Ra which has $t_{1/2}$ 1600 years. Uranium mining often uses ores with uranium content as low as 0.1–0.2%. Primary mining processes are open-pit mining with drilling and blasting and crushing methods and in situ leaching where liquid is injected into the ore and then pumped to the surface. Both extraction processes yield "yellow cake" mainly used to produce fuel for nuclear power plants. 76% of the global uranium production is used for power generation, and the demand for uranium is increasing (World Nuclear Organization, 2015). About 63% of global uranium production comes from Kazakhstan, Canada, and Australia. Other uranium producing countries are Namibia, Russia, Niger, and Uzbekistan (World Nuclear Organization, 2015). Uranium enriched with ^{235}U to 2–3% is used as fuel in nuclear power reactors. This produces large quantities of ^{238}U ("depleted uranium") used as protective shielding and in munition and missiles, in helicopters and airplanes as counter weights, and for coloring ceramic glazes.

The toxicokinetics of uranium depend on the chemical form, for inhaled particles, also on the physical, aerodynamic, and thermodynamic properties. Uranium absorption is low by inhalation, oral, and dermal exposures. The intestinal U uptake is very low, about 1%. The distribution and excretion of systemic uranium are considered independent of the exposure route, but determined by compound solubility (Keith et al., 2014). The biological halftime of soluble U compounds is short, excretion is mainly via urine, however, a small fraction is deposited in bone with a biological halftime around 30 days (Taylor et al 2000). Uranium salts are toxic to kidneys and liver and increases cancer risk (Keith et al., 2014).

Domingo, Ortega, Llobet, and Corbella (1990) investigated the U mobilizing effects of DTPA, Gallic acid, 5-aminosalicylic acid (5-AS), and 4,5-dihydroxy-1,3- benzenedisulfonic acid (Tiron) administered i.p. at doses equal to one-fourth of their respective LD_{50} values immediately after or 0.25, 1, 4, or 24 h after s.c. injection of 10 mg/kg of uranyl acetate dihydrate in mice. The U excretion was rapid in the first 24 h. Tiron or gallic acid administered 0, 0.25, or 1 h after U increased U excretion significantly. Only Tiron at 0, 0.25, or 1 h, and gallic acid at 1 h after U injection significantly reduced renal and bone U levels 4 days after U injection. Chelation 4 or 24 h after U injection was without effect on U and organ levels of U.

Ubios, Braun, and Cabrini (1994) evaluated the antidotal effect of ethane-1-hydroxy-1,1-bisphosphonate (EHBP) on uranyl nitrate induced renal damage and mortality in rats. A single i.p. injection of 10 mg/kg b.w. EHBP prevented mortality due to injection of 2 mg/kg b.w. uranyl nitrate compared to 50% mortality in unchelated U injected controls. Animals injected only with U had renal histological damage not observed in U injected chelated animals. EHBP is in use as a therapeutic agent in osteoporotic diseases with a well-studied toxicity profile, and therefore is a candidate for use in human U contamination.

Henge-Napoli, Archimbaud, Ansoborlo, Metivier, and Gourmelon (1995) compared the siderophore analog 3,4,3-LIHOPO and sodium bicarbonate for uranium decorporating capacity in rats after i.v. or i.m. injection of uranium nitrate. Single i.m. or i.v. injection of 30 μmol/kg of 3,4,3-LIHOPO immediately after U injection extensively enhanced the urinary U excretion and reduced renal and bone U levels 24 h later to about 20 and 50% of levels in controls, while 640 μmol/kg sodium bicarbonate reduced renal and bone U levels only to about 90 and 70% of controls with lower U excretion. When 3,4,3-LIHOPO and sodium bicarbonate were injected i.p. after 30 min delay, there was no difference in U excretion and organ levels between the two treatments.

Durbin, Kullgren, Xu, and Raymond, (1997) and Durbin, Kullgren, Ebbe, Xu, and Raymond (2000) found that chelating agents containing 2, 3, or 4 bidentate catecholate or hydroxypyridinonate metal binding groups effectively chelated U(VI) in vivo in mice. The most effective compounds had 2 bidentate groups attached to linear 4- or 5-carbon backbones (4-LI, butylene; 5-LI, pentylene; 5-LIO, diethyl ether). The bidentate groups, sulfocatechol [CAM(S)], carboxycatechol [CAM(C)], methylterephthalamide (MeTAM), 1,2-hydroxypyridinone (1,2-HOPO), or 3,2-hydroxypyridinone (Me-3,2-HOPO), were attached to the two linear backbones (4-LI and 5-LI or 5-LIO). Those ten tetradentate ligands and octadentate 3,4,3-LI(1,2-HOPO) were evaluated in mice for in vivo chelation of $^{233}U(VI)$ or ^{232} + U^{235}. Chelators were injected i.p. 3 min after i.v. injection of ^{233}U or ^{232} + U^{235} as UO_2Cl_2 at chelator/U molar ratios between 75 and 92. All 10 chelators reduced renal U levels significantly compared with controls or mice given $CaNa_3DTPA$, regardless of backbone structure, denticity, or binding unit, and 4 CAM(S) or CAM(C) chelators significantly reduced bone U levels. Several chelators reduced renal U levels when injected 1 or 24 h after U. 5-LIO(Me-3,2-HOPO) and TREN-(Me-3,2-HOPO) reduced renal U levels to about 10% of control levels when injected at 300 or larger molar ratios, and also after oral administration to fasting mice at 300 or larger molar ratios, they significantly reduced renal U levels. Intraperitoneal administration of 100 μmol/kg of these Me-3,2-HOPO ligands daily for 10 days starting 1 h after i.v. injection of 42 μmol/kg ^{235}U reduced the renal U level extensively, and histological renal injury was not observed. The efficacy screening identified 5-LICAM(S) and 5-LIO(Me-3,2-HOPO) as the most effective low-toxicity chelators, binding circulating U(VI) at chelator/U molar ratios ≥ 20, effectively decorporating newly deposited U(VI) from bone and kidneys at molar ratios ≥ 100 and reducing renal U(VI) levels significantly at molar ratios ≥ 100 after oral administration. 5-LICAM(S) had greater affinity for bone U(VI), and 5-LIO(Me-3,2-HOPO) had greater affinity for renal U(VI). An 1:1 mixture at total molar ratio 91 reduced kidney and bone U(VI) to 15 and 58% of control levels, more than equimolar amounts of either ligand alone.

Henge-Napoli et al. (1999) investigated the U mobilizing efficacy of EHBP in rats at EHBP doses of 50–100 μmol/kg and chelator/U ratios 2500–5000. One injection of EHBP immediately after i.m. U injection reduced renal U levels by a factor of 5 and reduced the whole-body U levels to 70% of control levels. EHBP injection 30 min after U injection reduced the renal U level by a factor of two.

Martinez, Cabrini, and Ubios (2000) examined whether oral administration of 350, 500, or 700 mg/kg or s.c. administration of 50 mg/kg EHBP could reduce the lethal effect of a single oral dose of 350 mg/kg uranyl nitrate in mice, which killed 100% of mice after 3 days. At day 14 the survivals in uranyl nitrate poisoned mice given 50 mg/kg EHBP orally or s.c. were 45.0 and 49.6%, respectively. In uranyl nitrate poisoned mice killed after 2 days, tubular necrotic lesions were less severe in EHBP chelated mice than in unchelated mice.

Paquet et al. (2003) investigated the uranium mobilizing efficacy of 3,4,3-LIHOPO after intramuscular injection of 1 mg $(U\text{-}Pu)O_2$ particles (MOX) in rats. Rats received LIHOPO (30 or 200 μmol/kg) or DTPA (30 μmol/kg) daily for 7 days. LIHOPO was inefficient for removing U from the wound site. However, it reduced the renal retention of U by a factor of 75. The results indicate LIHOPO as a chelating candidate after MOX contamination.

Fukuda, Iida, Ikeda, Yan, and Xie (2005) investigated effects of Catechol-3,6-bis(methyleiminodiacetic acid) (CBMIDA) and EHBP on the acute toxicity of uranyl nitrate and on decorporation of uranium (99.3% ^{238}U, 0.7% ^{235}U) after i.m. injection into the femoral muscles to simulate wound contamination in rats. Rats injected i.m. with 2 mg/kg uranium were injected i.p. with 240 or 480 mg/kg CBMIDA or with 10 mg/kg EHBP once daily for 28 days, beginning 1 h after uranium injection. The survivals at 28 days were 80 and 40% in the 240 and 480 mg/kg CBMIDA groups, 50% in the EHBP group, and 20% in the nonchelated control group. Administration of CBMIDA or EHBP decreased the renal, hepatic, and bone levels of uranium.

Xu et al. (2008) investigated the potential of DTPA and bisphosphonate-containing supramolecular hydrogels as decorporation agent for uranium-contaminated wounds. Mice with wounds on the back contaminated with a toxic dose of uranium were treated with supramolecular hydrogels with DTPA or the bisphosphonate pamidronate added. Hydrogel-treatment of Pu contaminated mice significantly increased the survival rate compared to untreated mice and hydrogel-treated mice had significant recovery in body weights after 10 days compared to mice without hydrogel treatment where the b.w. decreased. Organ uranium levels (mainly in kidneys) were reduced in hydrogel-treated mice compared to mice without hydrogel treatment. The pamidronate-based hydrogel was most effective in reducing mortality and decorporating uranium.

Bergeron, Wiegand, and Singh (2009) compared the uranium decorporating potentials of 9 desferrithiocin related analogues to that of DTPA in bile duct-cannulated rats. Oral administration of the 2 most effective compounds (S)-4,5-dihydro-2-[2-hydroxy-4-(3,6,9-trioxadecyloxy)phenyl]-4-methyl-4-thiazolecarboxylic acid [(S)-4′-(HO)-DADFT-PE] and (S)-4,5-dihydro-2-[2-hydroxy-3-(3,6,9-trioxadecyloxy)phenyl]-4-methyl-4-thiazolecarboxylic acid [(S)-3′-(HO)-DADFT-PE] reduced renal U levels by 57 and 62%, respectively, mainly by enhancing biliary uranium excretion, thus further reducing kidney uranium exposure.

Spagnul, Bouvier-Capely, Phan, Rebiere, and Fattal (2010) and Phan et al. (2013) investigated the potential use for decontaminating uranium contaminated skin of an oil-in-water nanoemulsion containing a tricarboxylic calixarene with high uranium affinity and selectivity. Ex vivo experiments on pig ear skin explants showed that immediate application of the calixarene nanoemulsion on uranyl nitrate contaminated intact or excoriated skins reduced the transcutaneous uranium diffusion by about 98%. In a second experiment the effectiveness of the calixarene emulsion was compared with that of DTPA and EHBP solutions. The calixarene emulsion reduced the uranium diffusion flux by 87% in the pig ear skin explants model compared to 50 and 55% reduction of uranium permeation, respectively, for EHBP and DTPA solutions. Application of the emulsion without calixarene did not reduce transdermal uranium flux. This calixarene nanoemulsion potentially offers an emergency system for uranium skin decontamination.

Bao et al. (2013) evaluated the efficacy of the chelator BPCBG containing two catechol groups and two aminocarboxylic acid groups for decorporation of U(VI) and protection against acute U(VI) nephrotoxicity in rats. BPCBG injections at various times before or after injections of U(VI) in rats increased 24 h-urinary U(VI) excretion and decreased renal and bone U(VI) levels. BP-CBG injection reduced the severity of the U(VI)-induced histological renal damage parallel with amelioration indicated by serum urea, and creatinine, and urine protein markers of U(VI) nephrotoxicity.

Belhomme-Henry et al. (2014) further developed the formulation of the calixarene-oil-in-water nanoemulsion developed by Spagnul et al. (2010) by modifying the external phase of the nanoemulsion with the gelifying polymers hydroxypropylmethylcellulose (HPMC) or methylcellulose (MC). In the pig ear skin explant model both HPMC and MC nanoemulsions limited the diffusion of uranyl ions to less than 5%.

5.12 DEVELOPMENT OF NEW CHELATORS AND OFF-LABEL USE OF CHELATING AGENTS

In general, drugs can only be used for purposes for which they are licensed. The USFDA has established regulatory pathways for the use of unlicensed medical countermeasures in radionuclide exposure situations. Chelating agents not licensed must have sufficient data on safety and efficacy filed at the FDA to be administered under an Investigational New Drug protocol or an Emergency Use Authorization. Because human experimentation is not possible, the FDA has established the Animal Efficacy Rule allowing that pivotal efficacy testing can be done in animals under certain circumstances: (1) the mechanisms of injury and radionuclide elimination as a result of the treatment are reasonably well understood; (2) efficacy is demonstrated under Good Laboratory Practice (GLP) conditions in more than one animal species, unless one species has a very well-understood response that is known to be characteristic for humans; (3) the study end point is related to the benefit in humans; (4) an effective human dose can be determined by human and animal pharmacokinetic and pharmacodynamics studies.

FDA guidelines for testing decorporating agents state that efficacy can demonstrated as "direct measurement of the elimination of the radioactive contaminant through feces and/or urine (or exhalation as appropriate) at various time points after administration of the decorporation agent. Alternatively, the residual body burden may be measured." This could support drug approval by showing that the candidate countermeasure drug offers a "clinically-meaningful reduction in whole-body committed radiation dose." Since human data on the counter measure compound may be limited to phase I safety studies, the usual number of test subjects may be increased. Thus, "for products that (1) are intended to treat conditions for which there are no available therapies; (2) meet an unmet medical need; (3) are intended for short-term use; or (4) have a well-defined and acceptable toxicity profile in animals, 200 to 300 subjects may be sufficient to support approval, if those subjects have been exposed to the decorporation agent at doses and durations comparable to those anticipated in marketed use and have had an adequate battery of safety testing (in animals, authors note)." The animal data and human testing requirements would be determined on a case-by-case basis for each decorporating agent. (US Department of Health and Human Services, Food and Drug Administration, Center for Drug Evaluation and Research, 2015). Cassat et al. (2008) offer an excellent discussion on the entire subject of research and development of new decorporating agents.

5.13 CONCLUSIONS AND PERSPECTIVES

The main purpose of radionuclide decorporation is to minimize the radiation dose (eg, polonium) and chemical insult (eg, uranium) received by exposed individuals. Since some of the important metal radionuclides have very long biological half-times after deposition in bone, liver, or kidneys, rapid initiation of chelation treatment is imperative after a contamination event, to reduce uptake from skin or wounds, lungs, or gastrointestinal tract, and to promote excretion of circulating radionuclide in blood before tissue deposition.

Major strategies in the acute phase involve physical decorporation of wounds by wound resection or by using various preparations containing chelating compounds to clean wounds or skin. In oral exposures, oral PB and other macromolecular chelators can reduce systemic absorption. In the chronic phase, long-term systemic or oral chelation can promote renal or biliary/fecal excretion of circulating radionuclides. Important examples are:

For Am decorporation, i.v. administered DTPA remains the standard treatment choice, but even oral DTPA effectively reduced internal Am deposits, and pulmonary DTPA powder reduced systemic uptake of pulmonary deposited Am dust.

For Cs decorporation, oral Prussian Blue is the choice, extensively used in highly contaminated individuals from the Goiania accident and resulting in reduction of whole-body radiation by a factor of about 2 (Farina, Brandão-Mello, Oliveira, 1991; Melo, Lipsztein, de Oliveira, & Bertelli, 1994).

For cobalt, information on cobalt chelation in general indicates that EDTA, DTPA, and presumably DMPS as first choice, stand out as effective Co mobilizing agents. For low-level Co exposure as in ^{60}Co contamination, several experimental chelators have been evaluated with good results in animal experiments.

For plutonium, DTPA is the standard chelating agent, again several experimental chelators have been evaluated.

For polonium, DMPS is the present choice.

For strontium the present treatment is long term dietary alginates, however, oral calcium salts may be as effective as alginates, and enhancement of alginate solubility may increase decorporating efficacy.

For thorium the present treatment is DTPA chelation.

For uranium DTPA is the choice, but an extensive amount of research has tested numerous experiment chelators. DTPA chelation should be started immediately after contamination.

The USFDA has approved Ca- and Zn-DTPA for administration i.v. or by nebulizer for decorporation of the transuranic radionuclides, americium, curium and plutonium, and Prussian blue capsules for internal contamination with cesium. Numerous nuclear workers have been chelated with DTPA after exposure to americium and plutonium (Cassat et al., 2008).

Several amphipathic chelators including esters of polyaminopolycarboxylic acids, DDC and DMSA are under development both for general chelation and for decorporation of radionuclides. Both for general chelation and for radionuclide decorporation development of macromolecular chelators for oral use and high molecular weight renally filtrable chelators for i.v. use is a high priority research subject.

REFERENCES

An, D. D., Villalobos, J. A., Morales-Rivera, J. A., Rosen, C. J., Bjornstad, K. A., Gauny, S. S., Choi, T. A., Sturzbecher-Hoehne, M., & Abergel, R. J. (2014). (238)Pu elimination profiles after delayed treatment with 3,4,3LI(1,2HOPO) in female and male Swiss-Webster mice. *Internal Journal of Radiation Biology*, *90*, 1055–1061.

Andersen, O. (1999). Principles and recent developments in chelation treatment of metal intoxication. *Chemical Reviews*, *99*, 2683–2710.

Ansoborlo, E., Berard, P., Den Auwer, C., Leggett, R., Menetrier, F., Younes, A., Montavon, G., & Moisy, P. (2012). Review of chemical and radiotoxicological properties of polonium for internal contamination purposes. *Chemical Research in Toxicology*, *25*, 1551–1564.

Aposhian, H. V., Dart, R. C., Aposhian, M. M., & Dawson, B. V. (1987). Tissue decorporation of polonium-210 in rats by DMPA. *Research Communication in Chemical Pathology and Pharmacology*, *58*, 157–171.

Bao, Y., Wang, D., Li, Z., Hu, Y., Xu, A., Wang, Q., Shao, C., & Chen, H. (2013). Efficacy of a novel chelator BPCBG for removing uranium and protecting against uranium-induced renal cell damage in rats and HK-2 cells. *Toxicology and Applied Pharmacology*, *269*, 17–24.

Belhomme-Henry, C., Phan, G., Huang, N., Bouvier, C., Rebiere, F., Agarande, M., & Fattal, E. (2014). Texturing formulations for uranium skin decontamination. *Pharmaceutical Development and Technology*, *19*, 692–701.

Bergeron, R. J., Wiegand, J., & Singh, S. (2009). Desferrithiocin analogue uranium decorporation agents. *Internal Journal of Radiation Biology*, *85*, 348–361.

Bogdan, G. M., & Aposhian, H. V. (1990). N-(2,3-dimercaptopropyl)phthalamidic acid (DMPA) increases polonium-210 excretion. *Biology of Metals*, *3*, 232–236.

Brandão-Mello, C. E., Oliveira, A. R., Valverde, N. J., Farina, R., & Cordeiro, J. M. (1991). Clinical and hematological aspects of 137Cs: the Goiânia radiation accident. *Health Physics*, *60*, 31–39.

Bruenger, F. W., Taylor, D. M., Taylor, G. N., & Lloyd, R. D. (1991). Effectiveness of DTPA treatments following the injection of particulate plutonium. *Internal Journal of Radiation Biology*, *60*, 803–881.

Bruenger, F. W., Kuswik-Rabiega, G., & Miller, S. C. (1992). Decorporation of aged americium deposits by oral administration of lipophilic polyamino carboxylic acids. *Journal of Medicinal Chemistry*, *35*, 112–118.

Bunin, D. I., Chang, P. Y., Doppalapudi, R. S., Riccio, E. S., An, D., Jarvis, E. E., Kullgren, B., & Abergel, R. J. (2013). Dose-dependent efficacy and safety toxicology of hydroxypyridinonate actinide decorporation agents in rodents: towards a safe and effective human dosing regimen. *Radiation Research*, *179*, 171–182.

Carbaugh, E. H., Lynch, T. P., Antonio, C. L., & Medina-Del Valle, F. (2010). Twenty-four years of follow-up for a Hanford plutonium wound case. *Health Physics*, *99*, 483–494.

Cassatt, D. R., Kaminski, J. M., Hatchett, R. J., DiCarlo, A. L., Benjamin, J. M., & Maidment, B. W. (2008). Medical countermeasures against nuclear threats: radionuclide decorporation agents. *Radiation Research*, *170*, 540–548.

Cohen, N., Sasso, T. L., & Wrenn, M. E. (1979). Metabolism of americium-241 in man: an unusual case of internal contamination of a child and his father. *Science*, *206*(4414), 64–66.

Diehl, P. 2004. Uranium mining and milling wastes: An introduction. WISE Uranium Project. Available from: http://www.wise-uranium.org/uwai.html

Domingo, J. L., Ortega, A., Llobet, J. M., & Corbella, J. (1990). Effectiveness of chelation therapy with time after acute uranium intoxication. *Fundamental and Applied Toxicology*, *14*, 88–95.

Durbin, P. W., Kullgren, B., Xu, J. D., & Raymond, K. N. (1997). New agents for in vivo chelation of uranium(VI): efficacy and toxicity in mice of multidentate catecholate and hydroxypyridinonate ligands. *Health Physics*, *72*, 865–879.

Durbin, P. W., Kullgren, B., Ebbe, S. N., Xu, J., & Raymond, K. N. (2000). Chelating agents for uranium(VI): 2 efficacy and toxicity of tetradentate catecholate and hydroxypyridinonate ligands in mice. *Health Physics*, *78*, 511–521.

Eaton, D. L., & Klaassen, C. D. (2001). Principles of toxicology. In C. D. Klaassen (Ed.), *Casarett and Doull's Toxicology* (6th ed.). New York: McGraww-Hill.

Farina, R., Brandão-Mello, C. E., & Oliveira, A. R. (1991). Medical aspects of 137Cs decorporation: the Goiânia radiological accident. *Health Physics*, *60*, 63–66.

Fukuda, S., Iida, H., Ikeda, M., Yan, X. M., & Xie, Y. Y. (2005). Toxicity of uranium and the removal effects of CBMIDA and EHBP in simulated wounds of rats. *Health Physics*, *89*, 81–88.

Gorla, A. K. R., Agrawal, K., Sood, A., Bhattacharya, A., & Mittal, B. R. (2014). Differential uptake of Tc-99m DMSA and Tc-99m EC in renal tubular disorders: report of two cases and review of the literature. *Indian Journal of Nuclear Medicine*, *29*, 160.

Grémy, O., Tsapis, N., Chau, Q., Renault, D., Abram, M. C., & Van der Meeren, A. (2010). Preferential decorporation of americium by pulmonary administration of DTPA dry powder after inhalation of aged PuO(2) containing americium in rats. *Radiation Research*, *174*, 637–644.

Grémy, O., Tsapis, N., Bruel, S., Renault, D., & Van der Meeren, A. (2012). Decorporation approach following rat lung contamination with a moderately soluble compound of plutonium using local and systemic Ca-DTPA combined chelation. *Radiation Research*, *178*, 217–223.

Griffiths, N. M., Coudert, S., Renault, D., Wilk, J. C., Van der, & Meeren, A. (2014). Actinide handling after wound entry with local or systemic decorporation therapy in the rat. *Internal Journal of Radiation Biology*, *90*, 989–995.

U.S. Department of Health and Human Services, Food and Drug Administration, Center for Drug Evaluation and Research (CDER), March 2006. Available from: http://www.fda.gov/downloads/drugs/guidancecomplianceregulatoryinformation/guidances/ucm071944.pdf

Guilmette, R. A., & Muggenburg, B. A. (1993). Decorporation therapy for inhaled plutonium nitrate using repeatedly and continuously administered DTPA. *Internal Journal of Radiation Biology*, *63*, 395–403.

Henge-Napoli, M. H., Archimbaud, M., Ansoborlo, E., Metivier, H., & Gourmelon, P. (1995). Efficacy of 3,4,3-LIHOPO for reducing the retention of uranium in rat after acute administration. *Internal Journal of Radiation Biology*, *68*, 389–393.

Henge-Napoli, M. H., Ansoborlo, E., Chazel, V., Houpert, P., Paquet, F., & Gourmelon, P. (1999). Efficacy of ethane-1-hydroxy-1,1-bisphosphonate (EHBP) for the decorporation of uranium after intramuscular contamination in rats. *Internal Journal of Radiation Biology*, *75*, 1473–1477.

IAEA (1988). The radiological accident in goiania. International Atomic Energy Agency, Vienna. sti/pub/815, isbn 92-0-129088-8

Jagtap, V. S., Sonawane, V. R., Pahuja, D. N., Rajan, M. G., Rajashekharrao, B., & Samuel, A. M. (2003). An effective and better strategy for reducing body burden of radiostrontium. *Journal of Radiological Protection*, *23*, 317–326.

Jefferson, R. D., Goans, R. E., Blain, P. G., & Thomas, S. H. (2009). Diagnosis and treatment of polonium poisoning. *Clinical Toxicology*, *47*, 379–392.

Kalkwarf, D. R., Thomas, V. W., Jr., Nielson, K. K., & Mauch, M. L. (1983). 1976 Hanford americium exposure incident: urinary excretion of trace metals during DTPA treatments. *Health Physics*, *45*, 937–947.

Keith, L.S., Faroon, O.M., Fowler, B.A. (2014) Uranium. In Nordberg, G.F., Fowler, B.A., Nordberg, M., (Eds.). *Handbook on the toxicology of metals*, (4th ed.) Elsevier/AP Amsterdam, pp. 1307–1345.

Kumar, A., Sharma, P., Ali, M., Pandey, B. N., & Mishra, K. P. (2012). Decorporation and therapeutic efficacy of liposomal-DTPA against thorium-induced toxicity in the Wistar rat. *Internal Journal of Radiation Biology*, *88*, 223–229.

Le Gall, B., Taran, F., Renault, D., Wilk, J. C., & Ansoborlo, E. (2006). Comparison of Prussian blue and apple-pectin efficacy on 137Cs decorporation in rats. *Biochimie*, *88*, 1837–1841.

Levitskaia, T. G., Creim, J. A., Curry, T. L., Luders, T., Morris, J. E., Sinkov, S. I., Woodstock, A. D., & Thrall, K. D. (2009). Investigation of chitosan for decorporation of 60Co in the rat. *Health Physics*, *97*, 115–124.

Levitskaia, T. G., Morris, J. E., Creim, J. A., Woodstock, A. D., Luders, T., Curry, T. L., & Thrall, K. D. (2010a). Aminothiol receptors for decorporation of intravenously administered (60)Co in the rat. *Health Physics*, *98*, 53–60.

Levitskaia, T. G., Creim, J. A., Curry, T. L., Luders, T., Morris, J. E., Woodstock, A. D., Levinson, B., & Thrall, K. D. (2010b). Evaluation of Cuprimine and Syprine for decorporation of (60)Co and (210)Po. *Health Physics*, *98*, 471–479.

Levitskaia, T. G., Creim, J. A., Curry, T. L., Luders, T., Morris, J. E., Peterson, J. M., & Thrall, K. D. (2010c). Biomaterials for the decorporation of (85)Sr in the rat. *Health Physics*, *99*, 394–400.

Levitskaia, T. G., Creim, J. A., Curry, T. L., Luders, T., Peterson, J. M., Thrall, K. D., & Levinson, B. (2011). Evaluation of Cuprimine(R) and Syprine(R) for decorporation of radioisotopes of cesium, cobalt, iridium and strontium. *Health Physics*, *101*, 118–127.

Lison, D. (2014). Cobalt. In Nordberg, G.F., Fowler, B.A., Nordberg, M., (Eds.). *Handbook on the toxicology of metals*, 4th ed., Elsevier/AP Amsterdam, pp. 743–763.

Little, B., Kennedy, A. R., & McGandy, R. B. (1975). Lung cancer induced in hamsters by low doses of alpha radiation from polonium-210. *Science*, *188*(4189), 737–738.

Lloyd, R. D., Taylor, G. N., & Mays, C. W. (1998). ^{241}Am removal by DTPA vs occurrence of skeletal malignancy. *Health Physics*, *75*, 640–645.

Martinez, A. B., Cabrini, R. L., & Ubios, A. M. (2000). Orally administered ethane-1-hydroxy-1,1-biphosphonate reduces the lethal effect of oral uranium poisoning. *Health Physics*, *78*, 668–671.

Melo, D. R., Lipsztein, J. L., de Oliveira, C. A., & Bertelli, L. (1994). ^{137}Cs internal contamination involving a Brazilian accident, and the efficacy of Prussian Blue treatment. *Health Physics*, *66*, 245–252.

Melo, D. R., Lundgren, D. L., Muggenburg, B. A., & Guilmette, R. A. (1996). Prussian Blue decorporation of 137Cs in beagles of different ages. *Health Physics*, *71*, 190–197.

Melo, D. R., Lipzstein, J. L., Oliviera, C. A. N., Lundgren, D. L., Muggenberg, B. A., & Guilmette, R. A. (1997). A biokinetic model for ^{137}Cs. *Health Physics*, *73*, 320–332.

Miller, S. C., Bruenger, F. W., Kuswik-Rabiega, G., Liu, G., & Lloyd, R. D. (1993). Duration and dose-related effects of an orally administered, partially lipophilic polyaminocarboxylic acid on the decorporation of plutonium and americium. *The Journal of Pharmacology and Experimental Therapeutics*, *267*, 548–554.

Miller, S. C., Liu, G., Bruenger, F. W., & Lloyd, R. D. (2006). Efficacy of orally administered amphipathic polyaminocarboxylic acid chelators for the removal of plutonium and americium: comparison with injected Zn-DTPA in the rat. *Radiation Protection Dosimetry*, *118*, 412–420.

Naimark, D.H. (2015). Effective half-life of polonium in the human. Technical Report MLM-272/XAB, Mound Lab., Miamisburg, OH. http://www.osti.gov/scitech/biblio/7162390.

Nielsen, P., Dresow, B., Fischer, R., & Heinrich, H. C. (1991). Inhibition of intestinal absorption and decorporation of radiocaesium in humans by hexacyanoferrates(II). *International Journal of Radiation Application and Instrumentation*, *18*, 821–826.

Paquet, F., Chazel, V., Houpert, P., Guilmette, R., & Muggenburg, B. (2003). Efficacy of 3,4,3-LI(1,2-HOPO) for decorporation of Pu, Am and U from rats injected intramuscularly with high-fired particles of MOX. *Radiation Protection Dosimetry*, *105*, 521–525.

Pelclova, D., Sklensky, M., Janicek, P., & Lach, K. (2012). Severe cobalt intoxication following hip replacement revision: clinical features and outcome. *Clinical Toxicology*, *50*(4), 262–265.

Phan, G., Ramounet-Le Gall, B., Manceau, J., Fanet, M., Benech, H., Fritsch, P., Fattal, E., & Deverre, J. R. (2004). Targeting of diethylene triamine pentaacetic acid encapsulated in liposomes to rat liver: an effective strategy to prevent bone deposition and increase urine elimination of plutonium in rats. *Internal Journal of Radiation Biology*, *80*, 413–422.

Phan, G., Semili, N., Bouvier-Capely, C., Landon, G., Mekhloufi, G., Huang, N., Rebiere, F., Agarande, M., & Fattal, E. (2013). Calixarene cleansing formulation for uranium skin contamination. *Health Physics*, *105*, 382–389.

Ramounet-Le Gall, B., Grillon, G., Rateau, G., Burgada, R., Bailly, T., & Fritsch, P. (2003). Comparative decorporation efficacy of 3,4,3-LIHOPO, 4 4,4-LIHOPO and DTPA after contamination of rats with soluble forms of 238Pu and 233U. *Radiation Protection Dosimetry*, *105*, 535–538.

Rencová, J., Volf, V., Jones, M. M., & Singh, P. K. (1993). Relative effectiveness of dithiol and dithiocarbamate chelating agents in reducing retention of polonium-210 in rats. *Internal Journal of Radiation Biology*, *63*, 223–232.

Rencová, J., Volf, V., Jones, M. M., Singh, P. K., & Filgas, R. (1995). Bis-dithiocarbamates: effective chelating agents for mobilization of polonium-210 from rat. *Internal Journal of Radiation Biology*, *67*, 229–234.

Rencova, J., Volf, V., Jones, M. M., & Singh, P. K. (2000). Mobilization and detoxification of polonium-210 in rats by 2,3-dimercaptosuccinic acid and its derivatives. *International Journal of Radiation Biology*, *76*, 1409–1415.

Rencová, J., Vlková, A., & Veselá, G. (2003). Improved chelation therapy of intramuscularly deposited thorium by CaDTPA in the rat. *Radiation Protection Dosimetry*, *105*, 513–516.

Rencova, J., Vlkova, A., Curik, R., Holusa, R., & Vesela, G. (2004). Influence of heavy metals upon the retention and mobilization of polonium-210 in rats. *Internal Journal of Radiation Biology*, *80*, 769–776.

Rhodes, R. (2002). *Dark sun: The making of the hydrogen bomb*. New York: Walker & Company, 187–188.

Robinson, B., Heid, K. R., Aldrig, T. L., & Glenn, R. D. (1983). 1976 Hanford americium exposure incident: organ burden and radiation dose estimates. *Health Physics*, *45*, 911–921.

Ruprecht, D.J. (2008). Dimaval. Scientific Product Monograph Edition 7.1. Heyl GmbH & Co. Berlin, Germany.

Schoeters, G., Van Puymbroeck, S., & Vanderborght, O. (1980). Influence of ^{226}Ra on bone marrow stem cells in mice: effect of radium decorporation by a long-term treatment with Na-alginate on stem-cell damage. *Radiation Research*, *82*, 74–80.

Schoeters, G. E., Luz, A., & Vanderborght, O. L. (1983). 226Ra induced bone-cancers: the effects of a delayed Na-alginate treatment. *Internal Journal of Radiation Biology and Related Studies in Physics Chemistry and Medicine*, *43*, 231–247.

Schoeters, G. E., Maisin, J. R., & Vanderborght, O. L. (1991). Protracted treatment of C57B1 mice with Zn-DTPA after 241Am injection reduces the long-term radiation effects. *Internal Journal of Radiation Biology*, *59*, 1027–1038.

Sérandour, A. L., Tsapis, N., Gervelas, C., Grillon, G., Fréchou, M., Deverre, J. R., Bénech, H., Fattal, E., Fritsch, P., & Poncy, J. L. (2007). Decorporation of plutonium by pulmonary administration of Ca-DTPA dry powder: a study in rat after lung contamination with different plutonium forms. *Radiation Protection Dosimetry*, *127*, 472–476.

Sonawane, V. R., Jagtap, V. S., Pahuja, D. N., Rajan, M. G., & Samuel, A. M. (2004). Difficulty in dislodging in vivo fixed radiostrontium. *Health Physics*, *87*, 46–50.

Spagnul, A., Bouvier-Capely, C., Phan, G., Rebiere, F., & Fattal, E. (2010). A new formulation containing Calixarene molecules as an emergency treatment of uranium skin contamination. *Health Physics*, *99*, 430–434.

Stradling, G. N., Gray, S. A., Pearce, M. J., Wilson, I., Moody, J. C., Burgada, R., Durbin, P. W., & Raymond, K. N. (1995). Decorporation of thorium-228 from the rat by 3,4,3-LIHOPO and DTPA after simulated wound contamination. *Human & Experimental Toxicology*, *14*, 165–169.

Strom, D.J. (2003). Health impacts from acute radiation exposure. *Pacific Northwest* National Laboratory. Pdf.

Sueda, K., Sadgrove, M. P., Huckle, J. E., Leed, M. G., Weber, W. M., Doyle-Eisele, M., Guilmette, R. A., & Jay, M. (2014). Orally administered DTPA penta-ethyl ester for the decorporation of inhaled (241)Am. *Journal of Pharmaceutical Sciences*, *103*, 563–571.

Taylor, D. M., Hodgson, S. A., & Stradling, N. (2007). Treatment of human contamination with plutonium and americium: would orally administered Ca- or Zn-DTPA be effective? *Radiation Protection Dosimetry*, *127*, 469–471.

Taylor, D. M., Stradling, G. N., & Hengé-Napoli, M.-H. (2000). The scientific background to decorporation. *Radiation Protection Dosimetry*, *87*, 11–17.

ThermoCahn, 2015. Static control for electronic balance systems. (PDF).

Thompson, R. C. (1983). 1976 Hanford americium exposure incident: overview and perspective. *Health Physics*, *45*, 837–845.

Timchalk, C., Creim, J. A., Sukwarotwat, V., Wiacek, R., Addleman, R. S., Fryxell, G. E., & Yantasee, W. (2010). In vitro and in vivo evaluation of a novel ferrocyanide functionalized nanopourous silica decorporation agent for cesium in rats. *Health Physics*, *99*, 420–429.

Toohey, R. E., & Kathren, R. L. (1995). Overview and dosimetry of the Hanford Americium accident case. *Health Physics*, *69*, 310–317.

Ubios, A. M., Braun, E. M., & Cabrini, R. L. (1994). Lethality due to uranium poisoning is prevented by ethane-1-hydroxy-1,1-biphosphonate (EHBP). *Health Physics*, *66*, 540–544.

USEPA (2010). U SEnvironmental Protection Agency. Commonly encountered radionuclides. Available from: http://www.epa.gov/rpdweb00/radionuclides/index.html

Varga, L. P., Sztanyik, L. B., Rónai, E., Bodó, K., Brücher, E., Györi, B., Emri, J., & Kovács, Z. (1994). Mobilization of radioactive strontium from mouse and rat using dicarboxylic acid derivatives of cryptand (2.2). *Internal Journal of Radiation Biology*, *66*, 399–405.

Volf, V. (1973). The effect of chelating agents on the distribution of^{210}Po in rats. *Experientia*, *29*, 307–308.

Volf, V. (1986). Chelation therapy of incorporated plutonium-238 and americium-241: comparison of LICAM(C), DTPA and DFOA in rats, hamsters and mice. *Internal Journal of Radiation Biology Related Studies in Physics Chemistry and Medicine*, *49*, 449–462.

Volf, V., Burgada, R., Raymond, K. N., & Durbin, P. W. (1993). Early chelation therapy for injected Pu-238 and Am-241 in the rat: comparison of 3,4,3-LIHOPO, DFO-HOPO, DTPA-DX, DTPA and DFOA. *Internal Journal of Radiation Biology*, *63*, 785–793.

Volf, V., Rencova, J., Jones, M. M., & Singh, P. K. (1995). Combined chelation treatment for polonium after simulated wound contamination in rat. *Internal Journal of Radiation Biology*, *68*, 395–404.

Volf, V., Burgada, R., Raymond, K. N., & Durbin, P. W. (1996). Chelation therapy by DFO-HOPO and 3,4,3-LIHOPO for injected Pu-238 and Am-241 in the rat: effect of dosage, time and mode of chelate administration. *Internal Journal of Radiation Biology*, *70*, 765–772.

World Nuclear Organization (2015). http://www.world-nuclear.org/info/Nuclear-Fuel-Cycle/Mining-of-Uranium/World-Uranium-Mining-Production/

Xu, K., Ge, W., Liang, G., Wang, L., Yang, Z., Wang, Q., Hsing, I. M., & Xu, B. (2008). Bisphosphonate-containing supramolecular hydrogels for topical decorporation of uranium-contaminated wounds in mice. *Internal Journal of Radiation Biology*, *84*, 353–362.

Yuile, C. L., Berke, H. L., & Hull, T. (1967). Lung cancer following polonium-210 inhalation in rats. *Radiation Research*, *31*, 760–774.

Chapter 6

Chelating Therapy in Metal Storage Diseases

Petr Dusek, Jan Aaseth

Chapter Outline

Chelation Therapy in the Treatment of Metal Intoxication. http://dx.doi.org/10.1016/B978-0-12-803072-1.00006-7

6.1 INTRODUCTION

Considering the importance of metal ions in the normal functions of the human brain, it is not surprising that dysregulation of metal homeostasis should have harmful effects on brain function (Dusek, Litwin, & Czlonkowska, 2015). A growing body of data supports the view that the redox-active metals, iron and copper can generate oxidative stress and inflammation, accelerating protein misfolding and aggregation associated with neurodegenerative diseases. There is increasing evidence that disruption of cerebral iron regulation plays a role in the etiology of Alzheimer's disease, Parkinson's disease, Friedreich's ataxia, and other neurological disorders. The therapeutic utilization of iron chelators in neurodegenerative diseases is still in its infancy. However, advances in noninvasive techniques, notably MRI have enabled us to quantify brain iron content in specific brain regions, which allows us to evaluate the effects of chelation therapy in removing iron.

In cases of general siderosis, precipitated by hereditary thalassemia, or other diseases requiring regular blood transfusions, orally administered chelating agents deferiprone and/or deferasirox to mobilize iron, have now emerged as a life-saving treatment of choice.

6.2 WILSON'S DISEASE

Wilson's disease is a hereditary chronic copper toxicosis, first defined in 1912 (Wilson, 1912). It results from mutations in the gene for an ATP-ase on chromsome 13, responsible for copper transport and efflux from liver cells (Tanzi et al., 1993). This protein, ATP7B copper transporter in the hepatocytes, pumps copper into the secretory compartment for the introduction of the element into ceruloplasmin and secretion into the bile. As a result of a defective function of ATP7B in Wilson's disease, the copper export from liver cells is blocked and the metal accumulates in the hepatocytes. The circulating levels of ceruloplasmin are low in this disease, whereas the circulating fraction of nonceruloplasmin bound low-molecular weight (toxic) copper compounds is characteristically increased. Copper inappropriately released from the liver as low-molecular weight compounds is deposited in various organs including in loci in the brain, explaining the neurological abnormalities. Acute release of high amounts of copper from the liver to the blood may also give rise to hemolytic crisis. High amounts of copper are filtered through the kidneys, and the increased urinary copper in combination with the high liver copper and low blood ceruloplasmin provide useful diagnostic markers (Dusek et al., 2015a). In addition, genetic testing for the *ATP7B* mutations is increasingly available to confirm the clinical diagnosis of Wilson's disease. Results from biochemical and genetic prevalence studies suggest that Wilson's disease might be much more common than previously estimated (Coffey et al., 2013).

Early diagnosis of Wilson's disease is crucial to ensure that patients can be started on an adequate treatment regimen. The drug treatment of Wilson's disease is based on establishing a negative copper balance, using copper chelators to promote copper excretion from the body, or administration of a zinc salt to reduce copper absorption, or on both. Best treatment options and the potency and side effects of available copper chelators are currently discussed. Unfortunately, no comparative study of treatment efficacy with penicillamine, trientine, and zinc has been conducted. Instead, there are reports with conflicting data about the superiority of different drugs based on the retrospective studies from individual WD centers (Ala, Aliu, & Schilsky, 2015; Askari, Greenson, Dick, Johnson, & Brewer, 2003; Czlonkowska et al., 2014; Weiss et al., 2011; Wiggelinkhuizen, Tilanus, Bollen, & Houwen, 2009).

6.2.1 Penicillamine in Wilson's Disease

The classical works by John Walshe clearly demonstrated the antidotal effect of D-penicillamine, a metabolite of penicillin (Walshe, 1956). The antidotal effect of penicillamine toward copper toxicity presumably involves formation of a mixed valence Cu(I)-/Cu(II)-complex, through an interaction that is referred to as reductive chelation. This complex chelate is probably implied in the copper elimination by penicillamine into urine (Sugiura & Tanaka, 1972).

Unfortunately, D-penicillamine may give rise to allergic and immunological side effects, that may be related to its interactions with aldehydes and thiol groups on proteins and other macromolecules (Friedman, 1977). Thus, penicillamine can act as a hapten eliciting allergy and autoimmunity. Skin rashes, thrombocytopenia, granulocytopenia, and pemphigus have been reported (Hennemann, Hubertus, & Stocker, 1975; Hewitt, Benveniste, & Lessana-Leibowitch, 1975). Among the more serious side reactions are Goodpasture's syndrome, systemic lupus erythematosus, and immune complex nephritis (Bacon et al., 1976; Dische, Swinson, Hamilton, & Parsons, 1976). To avoid early side effects, including worsening of neurological symptoms, a low initial dose of D-penicillamine is recommended, 250–500 mg/day, given in divided doses. The treatment is best taken 1 h before or 2 h after food. Absorption might only be 50% if it is taken with a meal. Monitoring of blood count and urinary protein is recommended because of the possible adverse effects, which occur in 10–20% of patients and can lead to the treatment being stopped. The penicillamine molecule can occupy the aldehyde group of pyridoxine, and vitamin B6 supplementation is therefore recommended (50 mg weekly). The clinical benefits of penicillamine in Wilson's disease are well documented. However, the adverse effects, including initial neurological deterioration reported in 20–50% of patients with a neurological presentation, in some cases irreversible, may change the recommendations. In recent years other agents, preferably trientine, has been recommended for the first line treatment (Andersen, 1999; Weiss et al., 2013).

6.2.2 Trientine Treatment—The Treatment of Choice Today?

Since some patients do not tolerate penicillamine, triethylenetetramine (trientine or Trien) was introduced as an alternative chelator in 1969 (Walshe, 1969).

Trientine or penicillamine has remained the mainstay of chelation treatment for patients with Wilson's disease. As evidence grows for the effectiveness of trientine, with fewer side effects than penicillamine, trientine is by several experts regarded as a preferred first drug for initial treatment of Wilson's disease (Schilsky, 2001). Trientine has a polyamine structure, which chelates copper by the formation of stable complexes with the four nitrogens in a planar ring. The initial dose is 1200–1800 mg/day in two to three divided doses. Maintenance therapy is 900–1200 mg/day. As in the case of penicillamine, the timing of oral administration in relation to food is important.

The frequency of neurological deterioration is thought to be less with trientine than with penicillamine, but could still arise (Brewer, 2006; Brewer et al., 2006). Data on its efficacy and side effects in patients with severe liver disease have been reported. Askari et al. (2003) studied nine adults with severe liver disease identified over a 10 year period, who received initial treatment with trientine (1000 mg/day) and zinc (150 mg/day). Only one patient had hepatic encephalopathy. One patient developed mild neurological symptoms and was given ammonium tetrathiomolybdate and zinc after 2 weeks of the original treatment. In the eight patients receiving trientine and zinc, the combination was given for at least 4 months and then maintenance zinc treatment was used. Over the first 12 months of treatment, prothrombin time and raised bilirubin and albumin concentrations returned to normal, and ascites disappeared. Benefit of the treatment was maintained during follow-up lasting up to 14 years, which are encouraging results (Askari et al., 2003).

6.2.3 Ammonium Tetrathiomolybdate—an Alternative Agent?

Since few patients might develop side effects also from trientine, a third copper chelating drug, ammonium tetrathiomolybdate, has been suggested as an alternative drug (Brewer et al., 1991). This agent can reduce the copper absorption from the gut. Ammonium tetrathiomolybdate was originally used by veterinarians for treating copper poisoning in animals. It is still under investigation in the United States, predominantly for the treatment of patients with neurological Wilson's disease (Brewer et al., 2003). This chelator remains an investigational drug, and it is yet not commercially available in Europe. Ammonium tetrathiomolybdate is reported to form a ternary complex with copper and protein. Taken with meals, the drug forms complexes with copper in the food, thus preventing its absorption. Taken between meals, the drug is to some extent absorbed, and it appears to complex circulating copper together with albumin. The resulting complex is metabolized in the liver and copper is excreted in bile. A randomized trial (Brewer et al., 2006) compared the efficacy of ammonium tetrathiomolybdate in patients with neurological Wilson's disease with that of trientine (both groups also received zinc). In the ammonium tetrathiomolybdate group, one of 27 patients had neurological deterioration, compared with five of 27 patients in the trientine group. Anemia or leukopenia occurred in three patients in the ammonium tetrathiomolybdate group, and four patients had increased circulating levels of liver enzymes.

6.2.4 Zinc—An Agent for Maintenance Therapy

Zinc salts were first introduced in treatment around 1970. This approach, given as monotherapy or combined with a chelator, has been studied in the United States. Today, zinc has gained recognition as maintenance therapy after an initial period of treatment with a chelator (Brewer et al., 1998). It has been shown to be effective in mild liver disease (Ranucci, Di Dato, Spagnuolo, Vajro, & Iorio, 2014) while it may be not sufficient in patients with more severe liver disease (Weiss et al., 2011). Zinc induces intestinal synthesis of metallothionein, which preferentially binds to copper within the intestinal enterocytes. Thus, copper absorption into the circulation is reduced, and copper is lost into feces when the enterocytes are shed during physiological cell turnover. The reduced copper absorption combined with physiological copper losses results in a negative copper balance. In addition, zinc can induce hepatic synthesis of metallothionein, thereby reducing the damaging effects of free copper. The dose of elemental zinc (given as sulfate) for adults is 150 mg/day administered in three doses. To some extent food may interfere with the zinc absorption. Dyspepsia can be a side effect, but timing of administration and use of alternative zinc salts, usually acetate or gluconate, can help (Roberts, Schilsky, & American Association for Study of Liver Diseases, 2008). Maintenance therapy with zinc has been reported to be effective, after an initial period of treatment with trientine (Askari et al., 2003). Presymptomatic patients can be successfully managed by zinc monotherapy (Brewer, Dick, Yuzbasiyan-Gurkan, Johnson, & Wang, 1994; Mizuochi et al., 2011).

6.2.5 Dimercaptosuccinic Acid (DMSA)—Useful in Wilson's Disease?

In China, there is substantial experience with the use of dimercaptosuccinic acid (DMSA, Succimer) in the treatment of Wilson's disease (Aaseth, Skaug, Cao, & Andersen, 2015; Andersen, 1999; Cao, Skaug, Andersen, & Aaseth, 2015; Ding, Xie, & Kang, 2011; Li, Wang, & Wang, 2013). Comparing long-term therapeutic effects, it has been claimed that DMSA is superior to penicillamine, because side effect incidence of DMSA was lower than that of penicillamine (Ren & Yang, 1997; Wang, Yang, Ren, & Sun, 2003). And DMSA appeared to have comparable short and long-term therapeutic efficacy as penicillamine, implicating that DMSA might even be recommended as initial therapy, and in reduced dosage as maintenance therapy of Wilson's disease. A usual initial oral dose to adult individuals is 100 mg three times daily. It might be relevant that the DMSA molecule, which has a dithiol structure, can embrace and shield the deleterious and "soft" Cu(I)-species, whereas trientine according to the basic chemical concepts, presumably will prefer Cu(II). Combined therapy with trientine and DMSA, given at lower doses than usual, could be a promising approach to the treatment of Wilson's disease, but this combination has, to the authors' knowledge, yet not been investigated.

6.2.6 Liver Transplantation

In some cases of severe or advanced Wilson's disease, liver transplantation may be the therapy of choice. Although transplantation may be an effective cure, there are risks associated with this procedure and the subsequent obligatory immunosuppressive drugs (Eghtesad et al., 1999). Liver transplantation is clearly indicated for patients with acute fulminant hepatic failure from Wilson's disease. There are only few reports of cure by medical therapy of the rare patients who have acute liver disease and hemolytic anemia caused by Wilson's disease.

Liver transplantation is also indicated for the patients with Wilson's disease when medical therapy is ineffective, as defined by a failure to stabilize or prevent progressive hepatic insufficiency (Roberts et al., 2008). These candidates include patients with a late diagnosis, when manifestations of cirrhosis or severe hepatic insufficiency are already present. Usually, this group includes a subset of patients who have both neurological and hepatic disease, but with predominantly hepatic symptoms. However, the delay between the initiation of medical treatment and measurable objective laboratory response may be at least two months. Therefore, a 2-month trial with medical treatment could be indicated before surgery, although some patients will deteriorate before this time has elapsed. Consequently, careful monitoring is essential to detect the individuals for whom transplantation might be more urgently needed. However, if the patient stabilizes during a period of two or three months, there is hope for the long-term use of medical therapy and avoidance of liver transplantation.

6.2.7 Conlusive Guidelines for Therapeutic Monitoring of Wilson's Disease

Previously, D-penicillamine (Cuprimine) has been the first treatment of choice in Wilson's disease, on the basis of clinical data and many years of experience. However, its side effects and neurological deterioration in some patients after initiation of this treatment have led to the suggestion that trientine is at least as effective as penicillamine and it is a safer alternative for initial therapy (Weiss et al., 2013). After initial chelation therapy, when significant clinical improvement has been achieved, the choice for maintenance therapy is between reduction in the dose of the chelator or zinc monotherapy. However, the best therapeutic approach remains controversial, as there is still no universally accepted regimen. Two aspects to obtain optimized outcome should be emphasized, namely, proper monitoring of the patient, and support to ensure compliance with the regimen used.

Patients on initial chelator therapy should have a close clinical follow-up with regard to the severity of their neurological or hepatic features. Neurological assessment and monitoring of liver function tests should be done, and signs of hepatic decompensation assessed. During chelation therapy, 24 h urinary copper excretion is measured and an output of 3–8 μmol/day (200–500 μg) denotes adequate treatment. During zinc therapy, 24 h copper excretion is also measured with a target of less than 2.0 μmol/day (less than 125 μg). During all treatments, whether with a chelator or with zinc, or both, an estimation of nonceruloplasmin bound serum copper is made from the measurements of total copper and ceruloplasmin. The target is a nonceruloplasmin copper concentration below 50–150 μg/L (Roberts et al., 2008).

6.3 OTHER NEURODEGENERATIVE DISEASES

6.3.1 Friedreich's Ataxia

Friedreich's ataxia is the most common of the hereditary ataxias. It is caused by a trinucleotide repeat extension or point mutations in a gene on chromosome 9, responsible for the iron chaperone frataxin. Friedreich's ataxia is a progressive neurodegenerative disease. The first symptoms usually develop during childhood or puberty with a life expectancy between 40 and 50 years. The most common mutation in the frataxin gene is an expanded GAA trinucleotide repeat in intron 1 of the frataxin gene which occurs in approximately 96% of Friedreich patients. Pathological amounts of iron accumulate in the mitochondria in Friedreich's ataxia, apparently leading to a deficiency of mitochondrial Fe-S cluster-containing proteins, such as aconitase. The respiratory chain electron transporters involving complex I-III are inhibited, resulting in oxidative stress and free radical accumulation (Marmolino, 2011). Physiologically, the highest concentration of frataxin is found in the heart and spinal cord, especially in dorsal root ganglia. The essential role of frataxin in mitochondrial iron metabolism is still poorly understood, although this chaperone apparently regulates iron handling in mitochondria, and thereby prevents iron from generating oxidative stress. Abnormal iron deposits were detected in cerebellar dentate nuclei by MRI by some groups (Bonilha da Silva et al., 2014), while others could not confirm this finding (Solbach et al., 2014) suggesting that iron quantification in dentate nuclei may not be a reliable biomarker of disease progression. Similarly, the question whether and to what extent iron accumulates in cardiomyocytes in Friedreich's ataxia is unsettled (Michael et al., 2006; Ramirez, Qian, Santambrogio, Levi, & Koeppen, 2012).

The first investigation on the efficacy of deferiprone in the treatment of these patients were done by Boddaert et al. (2007). They found that treatment with deferiprone, 20 or 30 mg/kg per day, for 6 months in 9 of the patients aged between 14 and 23 years, reduced the iron content of the dentate nuclei, which was associated with significant neurological improvements in speech fluency, neuropathy, and ataxic gait, particularly in the youngest patients. This occurred relatively rapidly, 2 months after commencing deferiprone treatment. And the larger the pretreatment iron deposits, the more changes appeared to be obtained by the chelation. In contrast to the reduced iron in dentate nuclei, no other brain region investigated, that is, the pallidal nuclei, the thalamus, and cerebellar white matter region, showed any significant changes in iron accumulation, as detected by T2* measurements over the period of the chelation therapy (Boddaert et al., 2007). In another study by Velasco-Sanchez et al. (2011) deferiprone, 20 mg/kg per day, together with the antioxidant idebenone was administered to 20 patients aged 8–25 years, suffering from Friedreich's ataxia. The chelation of iron from the dentate nuclei had occurred after 11 months of treatment, as assessed by T2* MRI, which was associated with a significant recovery of kinetic functions, although gait and postural scores worsened (Velasco-Sanchez et al., 2011). In a study comparing deferiprone dosage from 20 to 60 mg/kg per day for 6 months in a double-blind design patients receiving the highest dose (60 mg/kg per day) had to be discontinued due to worsening of ataxia while the lower dose (40 mg/kg per day) improved cardiac parameters but also led to milder clinical worsening of ataxia. The lowest dose (20 mg/kg per day) improved cardiac parameters and did not produce any changes in neurological status. Posthoc subgroup analyses in patients with less severe disease suggested a benefit of deferiprone 20mg/kg per day on ataxia and neurological function (Pandolfo et al., 2014). Another study have confirmed the observations of a mild positive response of a low-dose iron chelation therapy (Arpa et al., 2014); for review see Kolnagou, Kontoghiorghe, & Kontoghiorghes, 2014; Pandolfo & Hausmann, 2013).

6.3.2 Aceruloplasminemia

Aceruloplasminemia is caused by mutation in the gene coding for ceruloplasmin protein (Harris et al., 1995). Systemic iron accumulation is a consequence of lack of ceruloplasmin ferroxidase activity preventing cellular iron efflux. Among the neurodegeneration with brain iron accumulation (NBIA) group of disorders, aceruloplasminemia is associated with the highest iron accumulation affecting liver, pancreas, retina and many brain regions (Miyajima, 2015; Morita et al., 1995). Brain iron accumulation, reaching values 5–10 times higher than normal levels in patients (Morita et al., 1995), can be frequently detected even in presymptomatic subjects (Chen et al., 2008). Given the profound iron accumulation, chelating treatment in aceruloplasminemia is well advocated. Since aceruloplasminemia is a very rare orphan disease, treatment effects of deferasirox, desferrioxamine and deferiprone were reported only in case studies (Table 6.1). Deferasirox and desferrioxamine treatments lead to serum ferritin normalization, decrease of hepatic iron loading, and symptomatic improvement of anemia and diabetes in majority of patients (Badat, Kaya, & Telfer, 2015; Finkenstedt et al., 2010; Lindner et al., 2015; McNeill, Pandolfo, Kuhn, Shang, & Miyajima, 2008). Its effect on the removal of brain iron stores and neurological symptoms is variable.

Several weeks to months treatment with deferasirox 500–1000 mg/day led to neurological improvement in several cases (Skidmore et al., 2008; Suzuki et al., 2013), while no improvement after treatment lasting up to 48 months was

TABLE 6.1 Studies Examining Effect of Chelating Therapy on Neurological Symptoms in Aceruloplasminemia

Study (year)	Duration of neurosymptoms (yrs)	Age (yrs)	Medication (dose)	Duration of treatment	Outcome
Miyajima et al. (1997)	10	61	Desferrioxamine (500 mg/twice wk)	10 mo	Moderate clinical improvement; T2* increase in striatum/thalamus
Yonekawa et al. (1999)	5	54	Desferrioxamine (1000 mg/d)	6 wk	Mild clinical improvement; no change in MRI
Loreal et al. (2002)	3	62	Desferrioxamine (2000 mg/5× wk)	12 mo	No change in MRI
Haemers et al. (2004)	2	59	Desferrioxamine (2400 mg/d 5× wk)	6 mo	No clinical improvement
Mariani et al. (2004)	0	40	Deferiprone (75 mg/kg/d)+ Desferrioxamine (20 mg/kg/d 5× wk)	6+8 mo	Remained asymptomatic; no change in MRI
Skidmore et al. (2008)	4	54	Deferasirox (1000 mg/d)	3 mo	Moderate clinical improvement
Finkenstedt et al. (2010)	4; n.a.	47; 39	Deferasirox (15–20 mg/kg/day)	3;5 mo	No clinical improvement; no change in MRI
Hida et al. (2010)	7	58	Desferrioxamine (dose n.a.)	12 mo	Mild clinical improvement
Pan et al. (2011)	6	52	Desferrioxamine (500 mg/wk)	4 yrs	No clinical improvement; 10–30% T2* increase in BG/ SN
Roberti et al. (2011)	1; 0	57; 61	Deferasirox 5–20 mg/kg/d	16; 9 mo	Mild improvement; remains asymptomatic; no change in MRI in both

(Continued)

TABLE 6.1 Studies Examining Effect of Chelating Therapy on Neurological Symptoms in Aceruloplasminemia (*cont.*)

Study (year)	Duration of neurosymptoms (yrs)	Age (yrs)	Medication (dose)	Duration of treatment	Outcome
Tai et al. (2014)	0	35	Deferasirox 500–1000 mg/d	2 yrs	Remains asymptomatic; no change in MRI
Suzuki et al. (2013)	6	59	Deferasirox (500 mg/d)	10 d	Improvement of chorea and gait instability, no change of cognitive disorder
Lindner et al. (2015)	0	24; 39;43	Deferasirox 4–15 mg/kg/d	4 yrs	All remain asymptomatic; no change in MRI
Rusticeanu et al. (2014)	0	39	Deferasirox (500 mg/d)	2 yrs	Remains asymptomatic; no change in MRI
Badat et al. (2015)	0	28	Deferiprone 75 mg/kg/d Desferrioxamine 45 mg/kg/d	6 yrs	Remains asymptomatic; no change in MRI
Doyle et al. (2015)	0	20	Deferasirox (dose n.a.)	18 mo	Remains asymptomatic
Fasano et al. (2008); Bove and Fasano (2015)	0	58	Desferrioxamine (500 mg/d) Deferiprone 2500 mg 2–7 d/wk)	10 yrs	Remains asymptomatic; no change in MRI

Note: 0 yrs of neurologic symptoms denotes asymptomatic subjects.
Abbreviations: d, day; wk, week; mo, month; yrs, years; n.a., not available; BG, basal ganglia; SN, substantia nigra; MRI, magnetic resonance imaging.

reported by others (Bethlehem, van Harten, & Hoogendoorn, 2010; Finkenstedt et al., 2010; Roberti Mdo, Borges Filho, Goncalves, & Lima, 2011). Similarly, treatment with intravenous desferrioxamine up to 1000 mg daily led to partial improvement in several case studies (Hida et al., 2010; Miyajima et al., 1997; Yonekawa, Okabe, Asamoto, & Ohta, 1999), whereas other reports did not find any clinical improvement on doses of 500–2000 mg given 2–5 times weekly (Loreal et al., 2002; Pan, Tang, Chen, Song, & Shang, 2011). The desferrioxamine therapy is often associated with the decrease in hemoglobin and serum iron level suggesting sequestration of iron available for erythropoiesis. Thus, anemia, along with skin rash, are the most common side effects leading to discontinuation of the drug. Deferiprone 75 mg/kg per day administered for 6 months failed to remove iron from tissues in one case study (Mariani et al., 2004), while it prevented neurological symptoms to occur in a long-term treatment of an asymptomatic case (Bove & Fasano, 2015).

Most importantly, patients who started chelating treatment in the presymptomatic phase, remained free of neurologic symptoms during follow-up lasting up to 10 years (Badat et al., 2015; Bove & Fasano, 2015; Doyle, Rusli, & Bhathal, 2015; Fasano et al., 2008; Lindner et al., 2015; Mariani et al., 2004; Rusticeanu et al., 2014; Tai et al., 2014). The majority of aceruloplasminemia patients can be diagnosed before neurological impairment appears in a routine clinical setting since type 1 diabetes mellitus and anemia precede the neurological symptoms by a median of 12 years (Vroegindeweij et al., 2015).

Other treatment strategies tried in individual patients with only moderate positive effects include oral zinc therapy expected to decrease iron absorption and improve antioxidative defense (Kuhn et al., 2007) and administration of fresh frozen plasma expected to restore ceruloplasmin levels (Skidmore et al., 2008; Yonekawa et al., 1999).

In conclusion, long-term, probably life-long, iron chelation treatment should be initiated in every aceruloplasminemia patient, preferentially before neurologic symptoms appear. Chelation treatment should be monitored by regular examination of blood tests to exclude worsening of anemia, and monitor serum ferritin values. And 24 h urinary iron excretion tests are of importance to confirm the efficacy of treatment. Quantitative MRI can be used to document iron removal from liver and brain, although neurological improvement may not be directly related to brain iron concentration decrease.

6.3.3 Pantothenate Kinase Associated Neurodegeneration

Pantothenate kinase-associated neurodegeneration (PKAN) caused by mutation in the *PANK2* gene is the most prevalent disorder from the NBIA group (Schneider et al., 2013). The affected gene is involved in coenzyme A synthesis and the underlying mechanism of iron accumulation is unknown. In PKAN patients, iron is deposited focally in globus pallidus (GP) reaching 3–4 times higher concentration compared to healthy subjects (Dusek et al., 2014).

TABLE 6.2 Studies Examining Effect of Chelating Therapy in PKAN

Study (year)	Disease duration (yrs)	Number of patients (age-yrs)	Medication (dose)	Duration of treatment (months)	Outcome
Zorzi et al. (2011)	4–25	9 (7–39)	Deferiprone (25 mg/kg/d)	6	No clinical improvement; 30% T2* increase in GP
Pratini et al. (2013)	10	1 (15)	Deferiprone (1000 mg/d)	12	Moderate improvement
Cossu et al. (2014) Abbruzzese et al. (2011)	6–27	5 (22–40)	Deferiprone (30 mg/kg/d)	36–48	Clinical stabilization of dystonia in 4 pts; 20–50% T2* increase in GP

Abbreviations: d, day; pts, patients; n.a., not available; GP, globus pallidus.

A phase-II pilot study with 25 mg/kg per day deferiprone treatment lasting six months showed no clinical benefit in nine PKAN patients despite 30% reduction of iron content in the GP (Zorzi et al., 2011) (Table 6.2). In another study, 30 mg/kg per day deferiprone treatment led to clinical stabilization in 4 of 5 PKAN patients, persistent at a 4-year follow-up (Abbruzzese et al., 2011; Cossu et al., 2014). Other case study reported beneficial effect of 1000 mg/day deferiprone given together with baclofen pump in a PKAN patient (Pratini, Sweeters, Vichinsky, & Neufeld, 2013). Taken together, chelation treatment proved to be able to remove iron from GP. And, provided that long-term therapy is given, chelation may be a promising approach to retard the disease progression in the PKAN disorder.

6.3.4 Other Neurodegenerations with Brain Iron Accumulation

The clinical experience with chelation treatment in other NBIA yielded mixed results so far (Table 6.3). Hereditary ferritinopathy, also known as neuroferritinopathy, is a rare autosomal dominant disorder caused by mutations in the *ferritin light chain (FTL)* gene. It is manifested by low serum ferritin along with pathological iron deposits localized in various brain regions, namely GP, substantia nigra (SN), putamen, caudate, dentate nucleus, and cerebral cortex (Batla et al., 2015; Ohta & Takiyama, 2012). Brain iron deposition can be documented long before neurological symptoms appear (Keogh, Jonas, Coulthard, Chinnery, & Burn, 2012). In symptomatic patients with neuroferritinopathy, 4000 mg desferrioxamine weekly for 14 months, 2000 mg deferiprone for 2 months and

TABLE 6.3 Studies Examining Effect of Chelating Therapy in Other Neurodegenerative Disorders with Iron Accumulation

Study (year)	Type of NBIA	Disease duration (yrs)	Age (yrs)	Medication (dose)	Duration of treatment (months)	Outcome
Forni et al. (2008)	Idiopathic NBIA	5	61	Deferiprone (30 mg/kg/d)	6	Moderate clinical improvement; reduced T2 hypointensities in BG
Abbruzzese et al. (2011)	Idiopathic NBIA	9	65	Deferiprone (30 mg/kg/d)	12	No improvement
Kwiatkowski et al. (2012)	Idiopathic NBIA	5	52	Deferiprone (30 mg/kg/d)	32	Moderate improvement; T2* increase in SN/dentate nuclei
Cossu et al. (2014) Abbruzzese et al. (2011)	Idiopathic NBIA	7	52	Deferiprone (30 mg/kg/d)	48	Moderate improvement of dystonia and parkinsonism
Chinnery et al. (2007)	NFP	n.a.	n.a.	Desferrioxamine (4000 mg weekly) Deferiprone (2000 mg tid)	<14 2	No improvement
Loebel et al. (2014)	MPAN	6	13	Deferiprone (15–30 mg/kg/d)	24	No improvement; T2* increase in SN, no change in GP

Abbreviations: d, day; n.a., not available; BG, basal ganglia; GP, globus pallidus; SN, substantia nigra; MPAN, mitochondrial protein-associated neurodegeneration; NFP, neuroferritinopathy; NBIA, neurodegeneration with brain iron accumulation.

regular monthly venesections for 6 months did not lead to clinical improvement (Chinnery et al., 2007). Monthly venesections showed no effect in another case study (Kubota et al., 2009). There are no studies examining chelation treatment in the presymptomatic phase of this disease which may be the preferential approach given that iron deposition can be detected in the basal ganglia decades before the onset of clinical symptoms (Keogh, Morris, & Chinnery, 2013).

Patients with brain iron accumulation documented on MRI without mutation in genes causing NBIA are diagnosed as "idiopathic NBIA." Typically, focal siderosis in GP and later age at onset is observed in the idiopathic NBIA group. Mild to moderate clinical benefit and stabilization during follow-up lasting 6–48 months was observed in 3 out of 4 documented idiopathic NBIA patients treated with 30 mg/kg per day deferiprone (Abbruzzese et al., 2011; Cossu et al., 2014; Forni et al., 2008; Kwiatkowski et al., 2012).

Mitochondrial protein associated neurodegeneration (MPAN) is another disorder from the NBIA group caused by mutation in the *C19orf12* gene. Its physiological function and the mechanism of iron accumulation are unknown (Venco et al., 2015). Abnormal iron deposits are located into GP and SN in this disorder. Single case study reported no change in clinical status after 2 years long chelation therapy with 30 mg/kg per day deferiprone (Loebel et al., 2014).

6.3.5 Parkinson's Disease

Changes in brain iron homeostasis occur in Parkinson's disease (PD) patients, with elevated levels of iron bound to ferritin and neuromelanin, identified in neurons and glial elements in SN. In PD, focal siderosis of SN reaching iron concentrations about 2 times higher than normal, although no changes in iron content of other brain regions have been noted. From the early stages of PD, neuroinflammation and neurodegeneration occurs in the SN, probably due to the presence of aggregated alpha-synuclein and Lewy bodies. These misfolded proteins and extracellular neuromelanin released from dying neurons may activate microglia, which further accumulate iron (Sian-Hulsmann, Mandel, Youdim, & Riederer, 2011). One of the main pathological hallmarks of PD is the preferential degeneration of dopaminergic neurons, which supports a direct role of dopamine itself or dopamine production pathway in promoting the disorder. The oxidative chemistry of dopamine may ultimately lead to the formation of free radicals via the presence of reactive quinone species and activation of the indolamine deoxygenase enzyme. Dopamine-derived quinones may react with several cellular targets which could foster the processes involved in the pathogenesis of PD and contribute to the progression of the disorder (Dusek et al., 2015b; Ward, Dexter, & Crichton, 2015).

Two clinical trials have investigated the efficacy and safety of deferiprone in double-blind placebo studies for the treatment of PD, but results were published so far in one. T2* relaxation MRI techniques were utilized, motor scores were analyzed, and serum ferritin, a marker of iron stores and inflammation, was also measured. Results indicated that deferiprone, 30 mg/kg per day, slightly improved motor symptoms after 12 months of treatment, decreased motor handicap progression, and the iron content in SN was significantly decreased after one year. Three of the 40 patients in the study developed neutropenia or agranulocytosis which resolved rapidly with cessation of the oral therapy (Devos et al., 2014). Response to deferiprone treatment in PD may be modified by ceruloplasmin since patients with the lower ceruloplasmin activity in cerebrospinal fluid appeared to respond better to iron chelation (Grolez et al., 2015).

A low dose regimen of chelator therapy is consistent with the conservative mode of iron chelation approach. Its aim is to clear local siderosis from aberrant labile iron pools, thus redeploying it to physiological cell acceptors or to transferrin without interfering with essential local functions or with hematological parameters (Cabantchik, Munnich, Youdim, & Devos, 2013).

6.3.6 Demyelinating Disorders and Neuroinflammation

MRI and histological studies have shown global alterations in iron levels in the brains of multiple sclerosis (MS) patients in the white matter lesions and deep grey matter structures, which are associated with increased disability and grey matter atrophy (Bagnato et al., 2011; Haider et al., 2014; Hametner et al., 2013; Ropele et al., 2014). In addition, increases in the iron stored by macrophages and microglia are also evident, which may indicate that iron is involved in the pathogenic process. Iron overload evident in macrophages may promote a proinflammatory M1 activation state. Such increases in iron have generally been thought to be detrimental. The possible causes of iron accumulation and deposition in the CNS include degeneration of oligodendrocytes and myelin, infiltration of immune cells into sites of neurodegeneration, release of haem following vascular hemorrhage, dysregulation of iron transport proteins, or other regulatory molecules (Keogh & Chinnery, 2012; Stephenson, Nathoo, Mahjoub, Dunn, & Yong, 2014; Williams, Buchheit, Berman, & LeVine, 2012). Oligodendrocytes are the most metabolically active cells in the brain probably owing to their role in myelination, and contain an abundance of iron-requiring enzymes that are important for oxidative metabolism (Connor, Menzies, St Martin, & Mufson, 1990; Todorich, Pasquini, Garcia, Paez, & Connor, 2009). In addition, oligodendrocytes and myelin are rich in transferrin receptors. In actively demyelinating MS lesions, these are obviously a potential source of the iron accumulation observed in activated macrophages and microglia. Another demyelinating disease called Skogholt's disease is characterized by a substantial increase in iron and copper levels in the cerebrospinal fluid (Aspli et al., 2015).

Neuroinflammation appears to be involved in the pathogenesis of several neurodegenerative diseases, including PD and Alzheimer's disease (Ward et al., 2015). Inflammation may be induced by the presence of misfolded proteins which act as catalysts for the activation of glial cells. Microglia is vital for maintaining normal CNS function, as they are controlling brain homeostasis through their constant scanning ramifications and functions. They are involved in the maintenance of synapses and their receptors for a wide variety of neurotransmitters (Loreal et al., 2002).

Data from animal studies using chelators in experimental autoimmune encephalomyelitis, a model of MS, support the rationale for examining this treatment approach in MS (Choi et al., 2013; Weigel, Lynch, & LeVine, 2014; Zanella & Roberti di Sarsina, 2013). A pilot trial examined the effect of repeated two week courses of desferrioxamine (total dose 21 grams/2 weeks) applied during two years in 9 MS patients. During this treatment 5 patients worsened, 3 remained stable and 1 improved, suggesting that iron chelation may not be particularly helpful in MS (Lynch, Fonseca, & LeVine, 2000; Lynch, Peters, & LeVine, 1996). But here, future research is of importance.

6.4 TRANSFUSIONAL AND HEREDITARY SIDEROSIS—INCLUDING THALASSEMIAS

Chronic iron overload occurs in transfusional siderosis. This condition is frequently seen in patients with severe chronic anemias, particularly in those with thalassemia and also in patients suffering from sickle cell disease. Several of the patients with these diseases may need treatment with repetitive blood transfusions. But such treatment is a double-edged sword, since each unit of transfused blood contains 200 mg of iron. As the body has no mechanism for excretion of excess iron, chronic iron overload is a usual consequence, causing damage to the heart, liver, endocrine organs, and other tissues. Thalassemias are inherited autosomal recessive blood disorders characterized by abnormal formation of hemoglobin. The disorders occur most often among people of Italian, Greek, Middle Eastern, Southern Asian, and African descent. Normally, the majority of adult hemoglobin (HbA) is composed of four protein chains, two α- and two β-globin chains arranged into a tetramer. Patients or carriers of thalassemia have defects in either α- or the β-globin chains. In contrast, the mutation in sickle cell anemia affects specifically β-globin. Thalassemias are classified according to which chain of the hemoglobin molecule that is affected. In α-thalassemia, production of the α-globin chain is affected, while in β-thalassemia, production of the β-globin chain is affected. The β-globin chains are encoded by a single gene on chromosome 11; α-globin chains are encoded by two closely linked genes on chromosome 16. Specific variants or missing genes on these chromosomes causes thalassemias. Both α-and β-thalassemia are inherited in a recessive manner. People with a thalassemia mutation only in one gene is said to have thalassemia minor, and they are carriers. Thalassemia minor results in no or very slight anemia. If both parents are thalassemia carriers, there is a one in four (25%) chance that the child will have thalassemia major. Four genes (two from each parent) are needed to make appropriate α-globin protein chains. If one or two of the four genes for α-globin formation are missing, α-thalassemia traits occur. If more than two genes are missing, moderate to severe anemia occurs. The most severe form of α-thalassemia is called α-thalassemia major. Babies who have α-thalassemia major usually die before or shortly after birth. Babies with β-thalassemia major will usually grow up, but with abnormal hemoglobin. The abnormal hemoglobin results in continuous destruction of red blood cells (hemolytic anemia). Consequently, β-thalassemia major will cause several complications, such as iron overload and subsequent cardiomyopathia with heart failure. An estimated 60–80 million people in the world carry the β-thalassemia trait, but the actual number of those with overt thalassemia major is unknown due to the prevalence of thalassemia in less-developed countries. Today, concern is increasing that thalassemia may become a serious global problem in the next 50 years, one that will burden the world's blood bank supplies, and require specialized chelation therapy and burden the general health systems (Weatherall & Clegg, 2001).

Another group of patients that may require frequent blood transfusions is people suffering from myelodysplastic syndromes (often referred to as MDS), including those with sideroblastic anemia. The MDS are hematological medical conditions with ineffective production (dysplasia) of all blood cells. Patients with MDS can develop severe anemia and require regular blood transfusions, leading to siderosis.

6.4.1 Deferoxamine (Desferrioxamine) in Transfusional Siderosis

Iron chelation therapy has played a vital role in the management of patients with transfusional siderosis since the introduction of the parenterally administered chelator deferoxamine (desferal) more than 50 years ago. Chelation therapy has been extensively used in thalassemia major patients who have developed transfusional siderosis, and also in some other hemoglobinopathies. This disease group is characterized by structural changes of the hemoglobin molecule, leading to reduced half-life of the red cells, and consequently to a hemolytic type of anemia.

Chronic hereditary anemias are still rare in the Nordic countries, with currently only about less than 100 transfusion-requiring cases in Norway and Sweden totally. However, WHO estimates that about 7% of the population worldwide are carriers of hemoglobinopathy (Weatherall & Clegg, 2001). Thus, it is the most common hereditary disease in the world. More than 400,000 children are born yearly with a severe hemoglobinopathy, including the thalassemias.

Whatever the cause, serious anemia cases usually require transfusions, often every third week. There exists no consensus as to the follow-up and therapy of the resulting iatrogenic siderosis. Most of the patients will rapidly reach serum ferritin values above 2000 μg/L, which constitute obvious indication for the chelation therapy. The classical deferoxamine protocol involves the parenteral use of 25 mg/kg per day for a 5–7 day period after each blood transfusion. Obviously, such treatment is inconvenient and very stressful to patients. Therefore, an urgent need for an efficient long-term oral iron chelation therapy in outpatients has precipitated the development of an orally efficient iron chelator suited for in-home treatment.

6.4.2 Deferiprone Therapy

Deferiprone (Ferriprox) has now been used clinically in over 25,000 patients worldwide, and offers an alternative to rather unpleasant subcutaneous infusions of deferoxamine in the treatment of transfusional iron overload in thalassemia, both due to its low price compared to deferoxamine and because it can be administered orally (Kontoghiorghes, Neocleous, & Kolnagou, 2003).

Since leukopenia is a possible side effect, leukocyte counts are recommended weekly. And Ferriprox is not approved for the treatment of siderosis in patients with MDS, because of its potential side effects on leukocytes.

Deferiprone is rapidly absorbed in the gastrointestinal tract and normally appears in serum few minutes after oral administration. The main excretion route of the Fe-chelate is into urine. Deferiprone is a bidentate iron chelator forming a 3:1 complex with iron (Aaseth et al., 2015). This chelator is likely to act intracellularly. Here, it should be commented that cardiac disease apparently is the primary cause of death in thalassemia major patients. Importantly, Piga, Gaglioti, Fogliacco, and Tricta (2003) found that during an average follow-up period of 6 years, both mortality and worsening of cardiac dysfunction were significantly lower in patients treated with deferiprone than in patients treated with subcutaneous deferoxamine, indicating that deferiprone can chelate iron in myocardial cells and reduce cardiac iron (Piga et al., 2003). When monitoring the chelation treatment in thalassemic cases of siderosis, it is recommended to use cardiac MRI in addition to frequent determination of serum ferritin. This is because the iron-induced cardiomyopathy is asymptomatic until late stages, when the prognosis is poor (Modell et al., 2008). The cardiac toxicity is often undetectable on echocardiograms.

Combined chelation therapy with deferoxamine and deferiprone are now often used in Scandinavia (Flaten, Aaseth, Andersen, & Kontoghiorghes, 2012). Mourad et al. (2003) demonstrated that combined treatment with deferoxamine and deferiprone at doses lower than normally used, efficiently removed iron from thalassemic patients, indicating a potentiation of the iron chelation efficiency (Mourad et al., 2003). The advantages of combined chelation have precipitated the hypothesis that the two agents have different pools of chelation: deferiprone may chelate intracellularly whereas deferoxamine operates in the extracellular space. Thus, the oral chelator is presumed to act as a "shuttling" agent (Aaseth et al., 2015). It seems reasonable to recommend adjuvant treatment with ubiquinone, as free radical scavenger to cover the first months of the regimen (Alehagen & Aaseth, 2015).

6.4.3 Deferasirox

A relatively new alternative in iron chelation therapy is deferasirox (Exjade). This is an orally active tridentate chelator forming a 2:1 complex with iron, that is excreted via bile. Several phase II and phase III clinical trials with this agent have reported its convincing efficacy in mobilizing iron deposits in siderosis (Cappellini et al., 2006; Nisbet-Brown et al., 2003; Pennell et al., 2010; Wood et al., 2010). Reported side effects are gastrointestinal discomfort, elevated liver transaminases and erythematous maculopapular rashes. Renal failure is a seldom complication. A daily dose of 20 mg/kg was considered as efficacious as the traditional deferoxamine treatment in controlling iron stores, and 40 mg/kg resulted in a variable but positive net iron excretion. Maintenance therapy can be achieved by one daily dose. In a metaanalysis of available randomized clinical trials on iron chelators, Xia et al. (2013) concluded that seven selected trials found that deferiprone given as monotherapy or combined with deferoxamine were more effective in improving cardiac function than deferiprone alone. Although several nonrandomized trials suggest that deferasirox is effective to remove cardiac iron in patients with siderosis, they suggested that further randomized clinical trials are of importance to verify this observation. As indicated from this metaanalysis, deferasirox seemed to have a reasonable safety compared with deferoxamine.

It is of particular relevance that deferasirox can be combined with deferiprone in the treatment of iron overload (Totadri et al., 2015). This combination is preferable compared to the deferoxamine-deferiprone combination in β-thalassemia major patients in developing countries, due to the high costs associated with the continuous deferoxamine infusion. Monotherapy with either deferiprone or deferasirox may not always attain optimal control, especially not in heavily iron-loaded patients. The oral deferoxamine-deferiprone combination has been reported to be safe and efficacious in thalassemic patients with suboptimal response to monotherapy (Totadri et al., 2015).

Deferasirox therapy is also associated with reduced cardiac iron overload and reduced mortality in regularly transfused MDS patients (Bowen, Hellstrom-Lindberg, & Steensma, 2014; Zeidan et al., 2015).

6.4.4 Bone Marrow Transplantation in Thalassemia

In some cases of thalassemia bone marrow transplantation may be a preferred therapy. This approach may offer the possibility of a cure in young people who have an HLA-matched donor. Success rates have been in the 80–90% range. There are no randomized controlled trials, which have tested the safety and efficacy of nonidentical donor bone marrow transplantation in persons with β- thalassemia who are dependent on blood transfusion. If the person does not have an HLA-matched compatible donor, a method called bone marrow transplantation from haploidentical mother to child (mismatched donor) may be used. In a study of 31 people, the thalassemia-free survival rate 70%, rejection 23%, and mortality 7%. The best results are with very young people (Sodani et al., 2011).

6.4.5 Hemochromatosis—and Therapeutic Elimination by the Endogenous "Heme chelate"

Primary hemochromatosis constitutes another kind of chronic iron overload, being an autosomal recessive disease that is more common than previously thought. It is usually transferred by a gene mutation on the short arm of chromosome 6 (the *HFE* gene), in north-western Europe most often the C282Y mutation.

The symptoms of primary hemochromatosis are caused by progressive systemic iron deposition. The first clinical symptoms may become apparent during the 3rd to 6th decade of life, men usually being affected earlier than women whose iron stores are continuously depleted by menstruation. An unspecific asthenia may be present before other symptoms such as damage to the liver, heart, endocrine organs, and other tissues. Clinical symptoms rarely occur before the total body burden of iron exceeds 15 g, compared to a level below 5 g in healthy humans. Hemochromatosis should be suspected in any case with serum ferritin values above 300 μg/L if the transferrin saturation is 50% or higher. If primary hemochromatosis is suspected from traditional examination, genetic testing should be carried out.

Phlebotomy that involves removal of the *endogenous iron chelate of heme*, is the metal depletion treatment of choice in hemochromatosis. Such removal of the endogenous physiological chelate markedly improves survival and prevents most of the complications. The body burden of iron can be reduced by maximally 10–15 g during 1 year by using weekly phlebotomies. Some patients, however, apparently have body stores above 20–25 g of iron. For patients whose extensive iron depots need to be mobilized rapidly, combined treatment with phlebotomy and a chelating agent may be an option. Adjuvant therapy to mobilize iron deposits into hemoglobin for removal might be provided by erythropoietin (EPO) that indirectly speeds up the ferrochelatase activity and thus accelerates the encapsulation of tissue iron into protoporphyrin and subsequently into hemoglobin.

6.5 CONCLUDING REMARKS

Metal storage diseases include Wilson's disease with copper deposition in various organs, as well as some other neurodegenerative diseases characterized by localized deposits of iron. In addition, some chronic anemic conditions requiring frequent blood transfusions frequently give rise to siderosis with pathological deposition of iron in several organs, including liver and heart. Thalassemia and sickle cell anemia are examples of such anemias affecting hundreds of thousands of individuals worldwide. Orally administered chelating agents, such as deferiprone and/or deferasirox to mobilize iron, and D-penicillamine or triethylenetetramine to mobilize copper, are life-saving agents in these serious conditions.

ACKNOWLEDGMENTS

This work was supported by Charles University in Prague, PRVOUK P26/LF1/4 and Czech Ministry of Health, NV15-25602A.

REFERENCES

Aaseth, J., Skaug, M. A., Cao, Y., & Andersen, O. (2015). Chelation in metal intoxication—principles and paradigms. *Journal of Trace Elements in Medicine and Biology*, *31*, 260–266.

Abbruzzese, G., Cossu, G., Balocco, M., Marchese, R., Murgia, D., Melis, M., & Forni, G. L. (2011). A pilot trial of deferiprone for neurodegeneration with brain iron accumulation. *Haematologica*, *96*(11), 1708–1711.

Ala, A., Aliu, E., & Schilsky, M. L. (2015). Prospective pilot study of a single daily dosage of trientine for the treatment of Wilson disease. *Digestive Diseases and Sciences*, *60*(5), 1433–1439.

Alehagen, U., & Aaseth, J. (2015). Selenium and coenzyme Q10 interrelationship in cardiovascular diseases—a clinician's point of view. *Journal of Trace Elements in Medicine and Biology*, *31*, 157–162.

Andersen, O. (1999). Principles and recent developments in chelation treatment of metal intoxication. *Chemical Reviews*, *99*(9), 2683–2710.

Arpa, J., Sanz-Gallego, I., Rodriguez-de-Rivera, F. J., Dominguez-Melcon, F. J., Prefasi, D., Oliva-Navarro, J., & Moreno-Yanguela, M. (2014). Triple therapy with deferiprone, idebenone and riboflavin in Friedreich's ataxia—open-label trial. *Acta Neurologica Scandinavica*, *129*(1), 32–40.

Askari, F. K., Greenson, J., Dick, R. D., Johnson, V. D., & Brewer, G. J. (2003). Treatment of Wilson's disease with zinc. XVIII. Initial treatment of the hepatic decompensation presentation with trientine and zinc. *The Journal of Laboratory and Clinical Medicine*, *142*(6), 385–390.

Aspli, K. T., Flaten, T. P., Roos, P. M., Holmoy, T., Skogholt, J. H., & Aaseth, J. (2015). Iron and copper in progressive demyelination—new lessons from Skogholt's disease. *Journal of Trace Elements in Medicine and Biology*, *31*, 183–187.

Bacon, P. A., Tribe, C. R., Mackenzie, J. C., Verrier-Jones, J., Cumming, R. H., & Amer, B. (1976). Penicillamine nephropathy in rheumatoid arthritis. A clinical, pathological and immunological study. *The Quarterly Journal of Medicine*, *45*(180), 661–684.

Badat, M., Kaya, B., & Telfer, P. (2015). Combination-therapy with concurrent deferoxamine and deferiprone is effective in treating resistant cardiac iron-loading in aceruloplasminaemia. *British Journal of Haematology*, *171*(3), 430–432.

Bagnato, F., Hametner, S., Yao, B., van Gelderen, P., Merkle, H., Cantor, F. K., & Duyn, J. H. (2011). Tracking iron in multiple sclerosis: a combined imaging and histopathological study at 7 Tesla. *Brain*, *134*(Pt 12), 3599–3612.

Batla, A., Adams, M. E., Erro, R., Ganos, C., Balint, B., Mencacci, N. E., & Bhatia, K. P. (2015). Cortical pencil lining in neuroferritinopathy: a diagnostic clue. *Neurology*, *84*(17), 1816–1818.

Bethlehem, C., van Harten, B., & Hoogendoorn, M. (2010). Central nervous system involvement in a rare genetic iron overload disorder. *The Netherlands Journal of Medicine*, *68*(10), 316–318.

Boddaert, N., Le Quan Sang, K. H., Rotig, A., Leroy-Willig, A., Gallet, S., Brunelle, F., & Cabantchik, Z. I. (2007). Selective iron chelation in Friedreich ataxia: biologic and clinical implications. *Blood*, *110*(1), 401–408.

Bonilha da Silva, C., Bergo, F. P., D'Abreu, A., Cendes, F., Lopes-Cendes, I., & Franca, M. C., Jr. (2014). Dentate nuclei T2 relaxometry is a reliable neuroimaging marker in Friedreich's ataxia. *European Journal of Neurology*, *21*(8), 1131–1136.

Bove, F., & Fasano, A. (2015). Iron chelation therapy to prevent the manifestations of aceruloplasminemia. *Neurology*, *85*(12), 1085–1086.

Bowen, D. T., Hellstrom-Lindberg, E., & Steensma, D. P. (2014). Cardiac iron overload assessed by T2* magnetic resonance imaging and cardiac function in regularly transfused myelodysplastic syndrome patients. *British Journal of Haematology*, *164*(4), 610–611.

Brewer, G. J. (2006). Novel therapeutic approaches to the treatment of Wilson's disease. *Expert Opinion on Pharmacotherapy*, *7*(3), 317–324.

Brewer, G. J., Askari, F., Lorincz, M. T., Carlson, M., Schilsky, M., Kluin, K. J., & Sitterly, J. (2006). Treatment of Wilson disease with ammonium tetrathiomolybdate: IV. Comparison of tetrathiomolybdate and trientine in a double-blind study of treatment of the neurologic presentation of Wilson disease. *Archives of Neurology*, *63*(4), 521–527.

Brewer, G. J., Dick, R. D., Johnson, V. D., Brunberg, J. A., Kluin, K. J., & Fink, J. K. (1998). Treatment of Wilson's disease with zinc: XV long-term follow-up studies. *The Journal of Laboratory and Clinical Medicine*, *132*(4), 264–278.

Brewer, G. J., Dick, R. D., Yuzbasiyan-Gurkan, V., Johnson, V., & Wang, Y. (1994). Treatment of Wilson's disease with zinc. XIII: therapy with zinc in presymptomatic patients from the time of diagnosis. *The Journal of Laboratory and Clinical Medicine*, *123*(6), 849–858.

Brewer, G. J., Dick, R. D., Yuzbasiyan-Gurkin, V., Tankanow, R., Young, A. B., & Kluin, K. J. (1991). Initial therapy of patients with Wilson's disease with tetrathiomolybdate. *Archives of Neurology*, *48*(1), 42–47.

Brewer, G. J., Hedera, P., Kluin, K. J., Carlson, M., Askari, F., Dick, R. B., & Fink, J. K. (2003). Treatment of Wilson disease with ammonium tetrathiomolybdate: III. Initial therapy in a total of 55 neurologically affected patients and follow-up with zinc therapy. *Archives of Neurology*, *60*(3), 379–385.

Cabantchik, Z. I., Munnich, A., Youdim, M. B., & Devos, D. (2013). Regional siderosis: a new challenge for iron chelation therapy. *Frontiers in Pharmacology*, *4*, 167.

Cao, Y., Skaug, M. A., Andersen, O., & Aaseth, J. (2015). Chelation therapy in intoxications with mercury, lead and copper. *Journal of Trace Elements in Medicine and Biology*, *31*, 188–192.

Cappellini, M. D., Cohen, A., Piga, A., Bejaoui, M., Perrotta, S., Agaoglu, L., & Alberti, D. (2006). A phase 3 study of deferasirox (ICL670), a once-daily oral iron chelator, in patients with beta-thalassemia. *Blood*, *107*(9), 3455–3462.

Coffey, A. J., Durkie, M., Hague, S., McLay, K., Emmerson, J., Lo, C., & Bandmann, O. (2013). A genetic study of Wilson's disease in the United Kingdom. *Brain*, *136*(Pt 5), 1476–1487.

Connor, J. R., Menzies, S. L., St Martin, S. M., & Mufson, E. J. (1990). Cellular distribution of transferrin, ferritin, and iron in normal and aged human brains. *Journal of Neuroscience Research*, *27*(4), 595–611.

Cossu, G., Abbruzzese, G., Matta, G., Murgia, D., Melis, M., Ricchi, V., & Forni, G. L. (2014). Efficacy and safety of deferiprone for the treatment of pantothenate kinase-associated neurodegeneration (PKAN) and neurodegeneration with brain iron accumulation (NBIA): results from a four years follow-up. *Parkinsonism and Related Disorders*, *20*(6), 651–654.

Czlonkowska, A., Litwin, T., Karlinski, M., Dziezyc, K., Chabik, G., & Czerska, M. (2014). D-penicillamine versus zinc sulfate as first-line therapy for Wilson's disease. *European Journal of Neurology*, *21*(4), 599–606.

Devos, D., Moreau, C., Devedjian, J. C., Kluza, J., Petrault, M., Laloux, C., & Bordet, R. (2014). Targeting chelatable iron as a therapeutic modality in Parkinson's disease. *Antioxidants & Redox Signaling*, *21*(2), 195–210.

Ding, X., Xie, H., & Kang, Y. J. (2011). The significance of copper chelators in clinical and experimental application. *The Journal of Nutritional Biochemistry*, *22*(4), 301–310.

Dische, F. E., Swinson, D. R., Hamilton, E. B., & Parsons, V. (1976). Immunopathology of penicillamine-induced glomerular disease. *The Journal of Rheumatology*, *3*(2), 145–154.

Doyle, A., Rusli, F., & Bhathal, P. (2015). Aceruloplasminaemia: a rare but important cause of iron overload. *BMJ Case Reports*, *2015*, ii.

Dusek, P., Litwin, T., & Czlonkowska, A. (2015a). Wilson disease and other neurodegenerations with metal accumulations. *Neurologic Clinics*, *33*(1), 175–204.

Dusek, P., Roos, P. M., Litwin, T., Schneider, S. A., Flaten, T. P., & Aaseth, J. (2015b). The neurotoxicity of iron, copper and manganese in Parkinson's and Wilson's diseases. *Journal of Trace Elements in Medicine and Biology*, *31*, 193–203.

Dusek, P., Tovar Martinez, E. M., Madai, V. I., Jech, R., Sobesky, J., Paul, F., & Schneider, S. A. (2014). 7-Tesla magnetic resonance imaging for brain iron quantification in homozygous and heterozygous PANK2 mutation carriers. *Movement Disorders Clinical Practice*, *1*(4), 329–335.

Eghtesad, B., Nezakatgoo, N., Geraci, L. C., Jabbour, N., Irish, W. D., Marsh, W., & Rakela, J. (1999). Liver transplantation for Wilson's disease: a single-center experience. *Liver Transplant and Surgery*, *5*(6), 467–474.

Fasano, A., Colosimo, C., Miyajima, H., Tonali, P. A., Re, T. J., & Bentivoglio, A. R. (2008). Aceruloplasminemia: a novel mutation in a family with marked phenotypic variability. *Movement Disorders*, *23*(5), 751–755.

Finkenstedt, A., Wolf, E., Hofner, E., Gasser, B. I., Bosch, S., Bakry, R., & Zoller, H. (2010). Hepatic but not brain iron is rapidly chelated by deferasirox in aceruloplasminemia due to a novel gene mutation. *Journal of Hepatology*, *53*(6), 1101–1107.

Flaten, T. P., Aaseth, J., Andersen, O., & Kontoghiorghes, G. J. (2012). Iron mobilization using chelation and phlebotomy. *Journal of Trace Elements in Medicine and Biology*, *26*(2–3), 127–130.

Forni, G. L., Balocco, M., Cremonesi, L., Abbruzzese, G., Parodi, R. C., & Marchese, R. (2008). Regression of symptoms after selective iron chelation therapy in a case of neurodegeneration with brain iron accumulation. *Movement Disorders*, *23*(6), 904–907.

Friedman, M. (1977). Chemical basis for pharmacological and therapeutic actions of penicillamine. *Advances in Experimental Medicine and Biology*, *86B*, 649–673.

Grolez, G., Moreau, C., Sablonniere, B., Garcon, G., Devedjian, J. C., Meguig, S., & Devos, D. (2015). Ceruloplasmin activity and iron chelation treatment of patients with Parkinson's disease. *BMC Neurology*, *15*, 74.

Haemers, I., Kono, S., Goldman, S., Gitlin, J. D., & Pandolfo, M. (2004). Clinical, molecular, and PET study of a case of aceruloplasminaemia presenting with focal cranial dyskinesia. *J Neurol Neurosurg Psychiatry*, *75*(2), 334–337.

Haider, L., Simeonidou, C., Steinberger, G., Hametner, S., Grigoriadis, N., Deretzi, G., & Frischer, J. M. (2014). Multiple sclerosis deep grey matter: the relation between demyelination, neurodegeneration, inflammation and iron. *Journal of Neurology, Neurosurgery, and Psychiatry*, *85*(12), 1386–1395.

Hametner, S., Wimmer, I., Haider, L., Pfeifenbring, S., Bruck, W., & Lassmann, H. (2013). Iron and neurodegeneration in the multiple sclerosis brain. *Annals of Neurology*, *74*(6), 848–861.

Harris, Z. L., Takahashi, Y., Miyajima, H., Serizawa, M., MacGillivray, R. T., & Gitlin, J. D. (1995). Aceruloplasminemia: molecular characterization of this disorder of iron metabolism. *Proceedings of the National Academy of Sciences of the Unites States of America*, *92*(7), 2539–2543.

Hennemann, H. H., Hubertus, H., & Stocker, W. G. (1975). Severe side-effects of treatment with D-penicillamine. *Deutsche Medizinische Wochenschrift*, *100*(32), 1634–1638.

Hewitt, J., Benveniste, M., & Lessana-Leibowitch, M. (1975). Letter: pemphigus induced by D-penicillamine. *British Medical Journal*, *3*(5979), 371.

Hida, A., Kowa, H., Iwata, A., Tanaka, M., Kwak, S., & Tsuji, S. (2010). Aceruloplasminemia in a Japanese woman with a novel mutation of CP gene: clinical presentations and analysis of genetic and molecular pathogenesis. *Journal of the Neurological Sciences*, *298*(1–2), 136–139.

Chen, Q., Chen, X. P., Zou, L., Zhou, D., Gong, Q. Y., Burgunder, J. M., & Shang, H. F. (2008). High brain iron level in asymptomatic carriers of heterozygous ceruloplasmin gene mutations. *Movement Disorders*, *23*(6), 916–917.

Chinnery, P. F., Crompton, D. E., Birchall, D., Jackson, M. J., Coulthard, A., Lombes, A., & Burn, J. (2007). Clinical features and natural history of neuroferritinopathy caused by the FTL1 460InsA mutation. *Brain*, *130*(Pt 1), 110–119.

Choi, B. Y., Jang, B. G., Kim, J. H., Seo, J. N., Wu, G., Sohn, M., & Suh, S. W. (2013). Copper/zinc chelation by clioquinol reduces spinal cord white matter damage and behavioral deficits in a murine MOG-induced multiple sclerosis model. *Neurobiology of Diseases*, *54*, 382–391.

Keogh, M. J., & Chinnery, P. F. (2012). Current concepts and controversies in neurodegeneration with brain iron accumulation. *Seminar in Pediatric Neurology, 19*(2), 51–56.

Keogh, M. J., Jonas, P., Coulthard, A., Chinnery, P. F., & Burn, J. (2012). Neuroferritinopathy: a new inborn error of iron metabolism. *Neurogenetics, 13*(1), 93–96.

Keogh, M. J., Morris, C. M., & Chinnery, P. F. (2013). Neuroferritinopathy. *International Review of Neurobiology, 110*, 91–123.

Kolnagou, A., Kontoghiorghe, C. N., & Kontoghiorghes, G. J. (2014). Transition of thalassaemia and Friedreich ataxia from fatal to chronic diseases. *World Journal of Methodology, 4*(4), 197–218.

Kontoghiorghes, G. J., Neocleous, K., & Kolnagou, A. (2003). Benefits and risks of deferiprone in iron overload in thalassaemia and other conditions: comparison of epidemiological and therapeutic aspects with deferoxamine. *Drug Safety, 26*(8), 553–584.

Kubota, A., Hida, A., Ichikawa, Y., Momose, Y., Goto, J., Igeta, Y., & Tsuji, S. (2009). A novel ferritin light chain gene mutation in a Japanese family with neuroferritinopathy: description of clinical features and implications for genotype-phenotype correlations. *Movement Disorder, 24*(3), 441–445.

Kuhn, J., Bewermeyer, H., Miyajima, H., Takahashi, Y., Kuhn, K. F., & Hoogenraad, T. U. (2007). Treatment of symptomatic heterozygous aceruloplasminemia with oral zinc sulphate. *Brain & Development, 29*(7), 450–453.

Kwiatkowski, A., Ryckewaert, G., Jissendi Tchofo, P., Moreau, C., Vuillaume, I., Chinnery, P. F., & Devos, D. (2012). Long-term improvement under deferiprone in a case of neurodegeneration with brain iron accumulation. *Parkinsonism & Related Disorder, 18*(1), 110–112.

Li, W. J., Wang, J. F., & Wang, X. P. (2013). Wilson's disease: update on integrated Chinese and Western medicine. *Chinese Journal of Integrative Medicine, 19*(3), 233–240.

Lindner, U., Schuppan, D., Schleithoff, L., Habeck, J. O., Grodde, T., Kirchhof, K., & Stoelzel, U. (2015). Aceruloplasminaemia: a family with a novel mutation and long-term therapy with deferasirox. *Hormone and Metabolic Research, 47*(4), 303–308.

Loebel, U., Schweser, F., Nickel, M., Deistung, A., Grosse, R., Hagel, C., & Sedlacik, J. (2014). Brain iron quantification by MRI in mitochondrial membrane protein-associated neurodegeneration under iron-chelating therapy. *Annals of Clinical and Translational Neurology, 1*(12), 1041–1046.

Loreal, O., Turlin, B., Pigeon, C., Moisan, A., Ropert, M., Morice, P., & Brissot, P. (2002). Aceruloplasminemia: new clinical, pathophysiological and therapeutic insights. *Journal of Hepatology, 36*(6), 851–856.

Lynch, S. G., Fonseca, T., & LeVine, S. M. (2000). A multiple course trial of desferrioxamine in chronic progressive multiple sclerosis. *Cellular and Molecular Biology, 46*(4), 865–869.

Lynch, S. G., Peters, K., & LeVine, S. M. (1996). Desferrioxamine in chronic progressive multiple sclerosis: a pilot study. *Multiple Sclerosis, 2*(3), 157–160.

Mariani, R., Arosio, C., Pelucchi, S., Grisoli, M., Piga, A., Trombini, P., & Piperno, A. (2004). Iron chelation therapy in aceruloplasminaemia: study of a patient with a novel missense mutation. *Gut, 53*(5), 756–758.

Marmolino, D. (2011). Friedreich's ataxia: past, present and future. *Brain Research Reviews, 67*(1-2), 311–330.

McNeill, A., Pandolfo, M., Kuhn, J., Shang, H., & Miyajima, H. (2008). The neurological presentation of ceruloplasmin gene mutations. *European Neurology, 60*(4), 200–205.

Michael, S., Petrocine, S. V., Qian, J., Lamarche, J. B., Knutson, M. D., Garrick, M. D., & Koeppen, A. H. (2006). Iron and iron-responsive proteins in the cardiomyopathy of Friedreich's ataxia. *Cerebellum, 5*(4), 257–267.

Miyajima, H. (2015). Aceruloplasminemia. *Neuropathology, 35*(1), 83–90.

Miyajima, H., Takahashi, Y., Kamata, T., Shimizu, H., Sakai, N., & Gitlin, J. D. (1997). Use of desferrioxamine in the treatment of aceruloplasminemia. *Annals of Neurology, 41*(3), 404–407.

Mizuochi, T., Kimura, A., Shimizu, N., Nishiura, H., Matsushita, M., & Yoshino, M. (2011). Zinc monotherapy from time of diagnosis for young pediatric patients with presymptomatic Wilson disease. *Journal of Pediatric Gastroenterology and Nutrition*, *53*(4), 365–367.

Modell, B., Khan, M., Darlison, M., Westwood, M. A., Ingram, D., & Pennell, D. J. (2008). Improved survival of thalassaemia major in the UK and relation to T2* cardiovascular magnetic resonance. *Journal of Cardiovascular Magnetic Resonance*, *10*, 42.

Morita, H., Ikeda, S., Yamamoto, K., Morita, S., Yoshida, K., Nomoto, S., & Yanagisawa, N. (1995). Hereditary ceruloplasmin deficiency with hemosiderosis: a clinicopathological study of a Japanese family. *Annals of Neurology*, *37*(5), 646–656.

Mourad, F. H., Hoffbrand, A. V., Sheikh-Taha, M., Koussa, S., Khoriaty, A. I., & Taher, A. (2003). Comparison between desferrioxamine and combined therapy with desferrioxamine and deferiprone in iron overloaded thalassaemia patients. *British Journal of Haematology*, *121*(1), 187–189.

Nisbet-Brown, E., Olivieri, N. F., Giardina, P. J., Grady, R. W., Neufeld, E. J., Sechaud, R., & Nathan, D. G. (2003). Effectiveness and safety of ICL670 in iron-loaded patients with thalassaemia: a randomised, double-blind, placebo-controlled, dose-escalation trial. *Lancet*, *361*(9369), 1597–1602.

Ohta, E., & Takiyama, Y. (2012). MRI findings in neuroferritinopathy. *Neurology Research International*, *2012*, 197438.

Pan, P. L., Tang, H. H., Chen, Q., Song, W., & Shang, H. F. (2011). Desferrioxamine treatment of aceruloplasminemia: long-term follow-up. *Movement Disorder*, *26*(11), 2142–2144.

Pandolfo, M., Arpa, J., Delatycki, M. B., Le Quan Sang, K. H., Mariotti, C., Munnich, A., & Tricta, F. (2014). Deferiprone in Friedreich ataxia: a 6-month randomized controlled trial. *Annals of Neurology*, *76*(4), 509–521.

Pandolfo, M., & Hausmann, L. (2013). Deferiprone for the treatment of Friedreich's ataxia. *Journal of Neurochemistry*, *126*(Suppl. 1), 142–146.

Pennell, D. J., Porter, J. B., Cappellini, M. D., El-Beshlawy, A., Chan, L. L., Aydinok, Y., & Taher, A. (2010). Efficacy of deferasirox in reducing and preventing cardiac iron overload in beta-thalassemia. *Blood*, *115*(12), 2364–2371.

Piga, A., Gaglioti, C., Fogliacco, E., & Tricta, F. (2003). Comparative effects of deferiprone and deferoxamine on survival and cardiac disease in patients with thalassemia major: a retrospective analysis. *Haematologica*, *88*(5), 489–496.

Pratini, N. R., Sweeters, N., Vichinsky, E., & Neufeld, J. A. (2013). Treatment of classic pantothenate kinase-associated neurodegeneration with deferiprone and intrathecal baclofen. *American Journal of Physical Medicine & Rehabilitation*, *92*(8), 728–733.

Ramirez, R. L., Qian, J., Santambrogio, P., Levi, S., & Koeppen, A. H. (2012). Relation of cytosolic iron excess to cardiomyopathy of Friedreich's ataxia. *The American Journal of Cardiology*, *110*(12), 1820–1827.

Ranucci, G., Di Dato, F., Spagnuolo, M. I., Vajro, P., & Iorio, R. (2014). Zinc monotherapy is effective in Wilson's disease patients with mild liver disease diagnosed in childhood: a retrospective study. *Orphanet Journal of Rare Diseases*, *9*(1), 41.

Ren, M., & Yang, R. (1997). Clinical curative effects of dimercaptosuccinic acid on hepatolenticular degeneration and the impact of DMSA on biliary trace elements. *Chinese Medical Journal*, *110*(9), 694–697.

Roberti Mdo, R., Borges Filho, H. M., Goncalves, C. H., & Lima, F. L. (2011). Aceruloplasminemia: a rare disease—diagnosis and treatment of two cases. *Revista Brasileria de Hematologia e Hemoterapia*, *33*(5), 389–392.

Roberts, E. A., & Schilsky, M. L. American Association for Study of Liver Diseases. (2008). Diagnosis and treatment of Wilson disease: an update. *Hepatology*, *47*(6), 2089–2111.

Ropele, S., Kilsdonk, I. D., Wattjes, M. P., Langkammer, C., de Graaf, W. L., Frederiksen, J. L., & Fazekas, F. (2014). Determinants of iron accumulation in deep grey matter of multiple sclerosis patients. *Multiple Sclerosis*, *20*(13), 1692–1698.

Rusticeanu, M., Zimmer, V., Schleithoff, L., Wonney, K., Viera, J., Zimmer, A., & Lammert, F. (2014). Novel ceruloplasmin mutation causing aceruloplasminemia with hepatic iron overload and diabetes without neurological symptoms. *Clinical Genetics*, *85*(3), 300–301.

Schilsky, M. L. (2001). Treatment of Wilson's disease: what are the relative roles of penicillamine, trientine, and zinc supplementation? *Current Gastroenterology Reports*, *3*(1), 54–59.

Schneider, S. A., Dusek, P., Hardy, J., Westenberger, A., Jankovic, J., & Bhatia, K. P. (2013). Genetics and pathophysiology of neurodegeneration with brain iron accumulation (NBIA). *Current Neuropharmacology*, *11*(1), 59–79.

Sian-Hulsmann, J., Mandel, S., Youdim, M. B., & Riederer, P. (2011). The relevance of iron in the pathogenesis of Parkinson's disease. *Journal of Neurochemistry*, *118*(6), 939–957.

Skidmore, F. M., Drago, V., Foster, P., Schmalfuss, I. M., Heilman, K. M., & Streiff, R. R. (2008). Aceruloplasminaemia with progressive atrophy without brain iron overload: treatment with oral chelation. *Journal of Neurology, Neurosurgery and Psychiatry*, *79*(4), 467–470.

Sodani, P., Isgro, A., Gaziev, J., Paciaroni, K., Marziali, M., Simone, M. D., & Lucarelli, G. (2011). T cell-depleted hla-haploidentical stem cell transplantation in thalassemia young patients. *Pediatric Reports*, *3*(Suppl. 2), e13.

Solbach, K., Kraff, O., Minnerop, M., Beck, A., Schols, L., Gizewski, E. R., & Timmann, D. (2014). Cerebellar pathology in Friedreich's ataxia: atrophied dentate nuclei with normal iron content. *Neuroimage Clinical*, *6*, 93–99.

Stephenson, E., Nathoo, N., Mahjoub, Y., Dunn, J. F., & Yong, V. W. (2014). Iron in multiple sclerosis: roles in neurodegeneration and repair. *Nature Reviews Neurology*, *10*(8), 459–468.

Sugiura, Y., & Tanaka, H. (1972). Evidence for a ternary complex containing albumin, copper, and penicillamine. *Molecular Pharmacology*, *8*(2), 249–255.

Suzuki, Y., Yoshida, K., Aburakawa, Y., Kuroda, K., Kimura, T., Terada, T., & Yahara, O. (2013). Effectiveness of oral iron chelator treatment with deferasirox in an aceruloplasminemia patient with a novel ceruloplasmin gene mutation. *Internal Medicine*, *52*(13), 1527–1530.

Tai, M., Matsuhashi, N., Ichii, O., Suzuki, T., Ejiri, Y., Kono, S., & Harada, M. (2014). Case of presymptomatic aceruloplasminemia treated with deferasirox. *Hepatology Research*, *44*(12), 1253–1258.

Tanzi, R. E., Petrukhin, K., Chernov, I., Pellequer, J. L., Wasco, W., & Ross, B. (1993). The Wilson disease gene is a copper transporting ATPase with homology to the Menkes disease gene. *Nature Genetics*, *5*(4), 344–350.

Todorich, B., Pasquini, J. M., Garcia, C. I., Paez, P. M., & Connor, J. R. (2009). Oligodendrocytes and myelination: the role of iron. *Glia*, *57*(5), 467–478.

Totadri, S., Bansal, D., Bhatia, P., Attri, S. V., Trehan, A., & Marwaha, R. K. (2015). The deferiprone and deferasirox combination is efficacious in iron overloaded patients with beta-thalassemia major: a prospective, single center, open-label study. *Pediatric Blood & Cancer*, *62*(9), 1592–1596.

Velasco-Sanchez, D., Aracil, A., Montero, R., Mas, A., Jimenez, L., O'Callaghan, M., & Pineda, M. (2011). Combined therapy with idebenone and deferiprone in patients with Friedreich's ataxia. *Cerebellum*, *10*(1), 1–8.

Venco, P., Bonora, M., Giorgi, C., Papaleo, E., Iuso, A., Prokisch, H., & Tiranti, V. (2015). Mutations of C19orf12, coding for a transmembrane glycine zipper containing mitochondrial protein, cause mis-localization of the protein, inability to respond to oxidative stress and increased mitochondrial Ca(2)(+). *Frontiers in Genetics*, *6*, 185.

Vroegindeweij, L. H., van der Beek, E. H., Boon, A. J., Hoogendoorn, M., Kievit, J. A., Wilson, J. H., & Langendonk, J. G. (2015). Aceruloplasminemia presents as type 1 diabetes in non-obese adults: a detailed case series. *Diabetic Medicine*, *32*(8), 993–1000.

Walshe, J. M. (1956). Wilson's disease; new oral therapy. *Lancet, 270*(6906), 25–26.

Walshe, J. M. (1969). Management of penicillamine nephropathy in Wilson's disease: a new chelating agent. *Lancet, 2*(7635), 1401–1402.

Wang, X. P., Yang, R. M., Ren, M. S., & Sun, B. M. (2003). Anticopper efficacy of captopril and sodium dimercaptosulphonate in patients with Wilson's disease. *Functional Neurology, 18*(3), 149–153.

Ward, R. J., Dexter, D. T., & Crichton, R. R. (2015). Neurodegenerative diseases and therapeutic strategies using iron chelators. *Journal of Trace Elements in Medicine and Biology, 31*, 267–273.

Weatherall, D. J., & Clegg, J. B. (2001). Inherited haemoglobin disorders: an increasing global health problem. *Bulletin of the World Health Organization, 79*(8), 704–712.

Weigel, K. J., Lynch, S. G., & LeVine, S. M. (2014). Iron chelation and multiple sclerosis. *ASN Neurochemistry, 6*(1), e00136.

Weiss, K. H., Gotthardt, D. N., Klemm, D., Merle, U., Ferenci-Foerster, D., Schaefer, M., & Stremmel, W. (2011). Zinc monotherapy is not as effective as chelating agents in treatment of Wilson disease. *Gastroenterology, 140*(4), 1189–1198.

Weiss, K. H., Thurik, F., Gotthardt, D. N., Schafer, M., Teufel, U., Wiegand, F., & Consortium, E. (2013). Efficacy and safety of oral chelators in treatment of patients with Wilson disease. *Clinical Gastroenterology and Hepatology, 11*(8), 1028–1035.

Wiggelinkhuizen, M., Tilanus, M. E., Bollen, C. W., & Houwen, R. H. (2009). Systematic review: clinical efficacy of chelator agents and zinc in the initial treatment of Wilson disease. *Alimentary Pharmacology & Therapeutics, 29*(9), 947–958.

Williams, R., Buchheit, C. L., Berman, N. E., & LeVine, S. M. (2012). Pathogenic implications of iron accumulation in multiple sclerosis. *Journal of Neurochemistry, 120*(1), 7–25.

Wilson, S. A. K. (1912). Progressive lenticular degeneration: a familial nervous disease associated with cirrhosis of the liver. *Brain, 34*(4), 295–507.

Wood, J. C., Kang, B. P., Thompson, A., Giardina, P., Harmatz, P., Glynos, T., & Coates, T. D. (2010). The effect of deferasirox on cardiac iron in thalassemia major: impact of total body iron stores. *Blood, 116*(4), 537–543.

Xia, S., Zhang, W., Huang, L., & Jiang, H. (2013). Comparative efficacy and safety of deferoxamine, deferiprone and deferasirox on severe thalassemia: a meta-analysis of 16 randomized controlled trials. *PloS One, 8*(12), e82662.

Yonekawa, M., Okabe, T., Asamoto, Y., & Ohta, M. (1999). A case of hereditary ceruloplasmin deficiency with iron deposition in the brain associated with chorea, dementia, diabetes mellitus and retinal pigmentation: administration of fresh-frozen human plasma. *European Neurology, 42*(3), 157–162.

Zanella, S. G., & Roberti di Sarsina, P. (2013). Personalization of multiple sclerosis treatments: using the chelation therapy approach. *Explore: The Journal of Science and Healing, 9*(4), 244–248.

Zeidan, A. M., Hendrick, F., Friedmann, E., Baer, M. R., Gore, S. D., Sasane, M., & Davidoff, A. J. (2015). Deferasirox therapy is associated with reduced mortality risk in a medicare population with myelodysplastic syndromes. *Journal of Comparative Effectiveness Research, 4*(4), 327–340.

Zorzi, G., Zibordi, F., Chiapparini, L., Bertini, E., Russo, L., Piga, A., & Nardocci, N (2011). Iron-related MRI images in patients with pantothenate kinase-associated neurodegeneration (PKAN) treated with deferiprone: results of a phase II pilot trial. *Movement Disorder, 26*(9), 1756–1759.

Chapter 7

Guidance for Clinical Treatment of Metal Poisonings—Use and Misuse of Chelating Agents

Lars Gerhardsson, Jan Aaseth

Chapter Outline

Chelation Therapy in the Treatment of Metal Intoxication. http://dx.doi.org/10.1016/B978-0-12-803072-1.00007-9

7.1 INTRODUCTION

The management of acute metal poisoning requires emergency resuscitative procedures that may need to be started in the work or home environment and continued in an intensive care unit at a hospital. The principles for the management of the acute cases of poisoning and relevant aspects of emergency medicine are briefly discussed in this chapter. More detailed guidelines are presented in other reviews (Dreisbach, 1983; Vale & Meredith, 1981; Marx et al., 2014). Specific guidelines related to the therapy of metal poisonings have been outlined previously by Gerhardsson and Kazantzis (2014), and these principles will be discussed more in detail in the present chapter.

7.2 REDUCING THE ABSORBED DOSE

7.2.1 Removal From Exposure

Absorption of a toxic metal may follow inhalation, ingestion, or contamination of skin or wounds. In occupational settings, the dominant exposure route is via inhalation. If high-level inhalation exposure has taken place, the patient should immediately be removed from the contaminated area. This can be the case after exposure to volatile metal compounds such as stibine, arsine, alkyl mercury, inorganic mercury vapor, alkyl tin, and alkyl lead compounds. After contamination of the skin with lipid-soluble metal compounds, contaminated clothing should be removed as soon as possible, and the contaminated area must be irrigated and washed, but not rubbed, with large quantities of cold water. Decontamination procedures may also be required for hair and fingernails.

In chronic, cumulative metal poisoning, it may be enough to remove the subject from further exposure. This can be the case for a worker with mild poisoning after exposure to inorganic mercury vapor or to lead fume or dust. The normal excretory mechanisms will thereafter give a gradual recovery from the mild toxic effects.

A review of possible routes of absorption in the individual case at a workplace should also include consideration of the possibility of exposure by contamination of food, drink, cigarettes, or clothing. When this possibility exists, food, drinks, and cigarettes at the work site should be prohibited. Facilities should be provided for taking a shower followed by a complete change of clothing after each shift.

7.2.2 Removal of Toxic Element From the Gastrointestinal Tract

Up to about 4 h after ingestion, some of the poison may be recovered by emptying the stomach. If the patient is fully conscious, this may be accomplished by inducing vomiting. In a child, pharyngeal stimulation may be tried as a first-aid measure immediately after ingestion. Ipecacuanha mixture 10–15 mL for a child, 30 mL for an adult, may be effective in inducing vomiting.

Gastric lavage can be carried out through a gastric tube, but this should be avoided after the ingestion of corrosives or petroleum products and in drowsy or comatose patients. In the latter case, there is danger of inhalation of stomach contents unless adequate medical precautions are followed. Gastric lavage requires access to qualified medical personnel and should only be undertaken in a properly equipped emergency department, again within about 4 h after ingestion. If the cough reflex is absent or if the level of consciousness is lowered, the patient should be intubated to protect the lungs from inhalation of stomach contents.

7.2.3 Use of Gastric Lavage, Activated Charcoal, or Unabsorbed Resins

Gastric lavage with warm water can be an effective treatment in some cases. Some poisons, however, require treatment with a specific antidote given after lavage, to be inactivated in the stomach. Lavage, however, should not be delayed if the antidote is not immediately available. In such an emergency situation, alternative treatments with egg white or milk may help to partly inactivate mercury and other heavy metals by precipitation of protein complexes in the stomach. Another option is activated charcoal that will effectively adsorb many poisons still present in the stomach, and it will also decrease the enterohepatic circulation. This treatment, however, is not effective in iron poisoning. As a first-aid measure, sodium bicarbonate will partly precipitate soluble iron salts in the stomach. Then gastric lavage should be combined with deferoxamine mesylate, 2 g in 1 L of water. A solution of deferoxamine, 10 g in 50 mL water, should subsequently be left in the stomach to inhibit further iron absorption. Effective inactivation of the toxic barium ion in the stomach can be obtained by oral administration or gastric lavage with a 10% solution of sodium or magnesium sulfate. After the ingestion of chromic acid, lavage should be performed with magnesium carbonate. After ingestion of either thallium or cesium, Prussian blue (ferric hexacyanoferrate) will inactivate the poison. A colloidal solution of Prussian blue given by duodenal tube at a rate of 250 mg/kg per day in divided doses, totally about 15 g during the first day, is recommended. In cases of radioactive cesium-137 intake, Prussian blue (commercially available as Radiogardase) is recommended at a dose of 3 g × 3 the next days. This agent will trap cesium in the gut and reduce the body burden, since it interrupts enterohepatic circulation. The same regimen is also effective in thallium poisonings. The possible need for extensive, long-term human use of Prussian blue due to nuclear facility accidents and radioactive environmental pollution such as the Goiânia accident in Brazil in 1987, make data on toxicity of Prussian blue important to evaluate. In his review on Prussian blue toxicity, Pearce (1994) concluded from available animal and human data, that this agent was without any important toxic effects, even in long-term use.

7.3 GENERAL SUPPORTIVE THERAPY

In acute poisoning situations, resuscitative measures of the patient have the highest priority. If the severely poisoned patient can be kept alive, and excretory physiological mechanisms are functioning, the administration of specific antidotes, if such agents exist, should immediately be undertaken to facilitate elimination of the poison. Additional symptomatic medical care is always necessary, with an awareness of possible delayed undesired effects and complications.

7.3.1 Maintenance of Respiration and Circulation

Maintenance of respiration and circulation should have the highest priority. The patient must have a clear airway during the transport from the site of the accident to the treatment center, and artificial respiration may be necessary. At the treatment center, tracheobronchial intubation may be required. The arterial oxygen and carbon dioxide levels should be checked immediately.

Oxygen therapy may be required as well as mechanical ventilation. Treatment for acute pulmonary edema may be needed, especially after exposure to beryllium or cadmium fumes or nickel carbonyl.

A conscious patient in chock with a lowered systolic blood pressure around 80–90 mm Hg should be kept supine with the legs elevated and covered with blanks. When the patient has been transported to the treatment center, the blood volume can be restored with intravenous fluids. In severe cases of hemolytic anemia, for example, after exposure to arsine gas, blood transfusions may be necessary.

7.3.2 Maintenance of Water and Electrolyte Balance

Several factors such as vomiting, diarrhea, tissue damage, or treatment procedures to eliminate the poison may affect the water and electrolyte balance. In such cases intravenous infusion with appropriate fluids accompanied by adequate biochemical monitoring, including measurements of electrolytes, osmolality, and acid-base balance in blood, is required. In less severe cases it may be sufficient to give fluids by mouth to prevent dehydration. An adequate urinary flow should be ensured, and a catheter may be necessary to monitor urinary flow.

Acute tubular necrosis may give rise to anuria with retention of creatinine, carbamide and potassium, and dialysis may then be necessary. Careful water and electrolyte balance has to be maintained until regeneration of the tubular epithelium leads to recovery.

7.3.3 Control of Cerebral Functions

The general supportive treatment outlined earlier is usually adequate for the management of the patient whose level of consciousness is moderately depressed. Treatment with analeptic drugs is not indicated in acute metal poisoning. Convulsions, however, can be treated with diazepam, 5–30 mg, given parenterally. Complications such as cerebral edema may occur in, for example, acute lead poisoning. This should be treated with dexamethasone given intravenously. To overcome the hyperactivity and other behavioral disorders that may develop in poisoning with alkyl lead compounds, prolonged sedation with diazepam may be necessary.

7.4 ELIMINATION OF ABSORBED POISON

7.4.1 Diuresis

Forced diuresis will decrease the passive reabsorption from the proximal renal tubules, thereby increasing the clearance of many poisons. This can be achieved by combining the fluid load with osmotic agents like mannitol or by administration of a diuretic, for example, furosemide. The excretion of some poisons is affected by the pH of the urine, because passive tubular reabsorption is less effective with increased ionization of the solute in the tubular fluid. Excretion of toxic metals, for example, in acute inorganic mercury or lead poisoning, can generally be accelerated if a high urinary flow is maintained. Forced alkaline diuresis is of some value in aiding the elimination of lithium salts. Severe poisonings with lithium may require dialysis to achieve therapeutic elimination of the toxic metal.

7.4.2 Biliary Excretion

Toxic metals that have an enterohepatic circulation could have a prolonged effect in the human body as the excretion in the bile can occur against a high concentration gradient followed by intestinal reabsorption. The reabsorption can be decreased by the use of activated charcoal. Another way of diminishing the enterohepatic circulation has been described by Clarkson, Small, and Norseth (1973). By supplying a complex-binding agent perorally that will bind with the metal compound that has been excreted in the bile, the reabsorption of the metal is prevented, and an enhanced fecal excretion of those heavy metal compounds that undergo an extensive enterohepatic circulation will take place. A synthetic polystyrene resin containing fixed sulfhydryl groups, doubled the rate of excretion of methylmercury from mice and lowered blood and tissue levels compared with untreated controls, when added to food in a concentration of 1%. In man, mercury levels in blood were reduced and the fecal excretion of methylmercury increased upon treatment with the resin (Bakir et al., 1973). This resin however, is not commercially available. Presumably, this resin would also have inhibited the absorption of copper in cases of Wilson's disease, and reduced the absorption of lead and arsenic in contaminated areas.

7.4.3 Dialysis

Hemodialysis causes usually a more efficient clearance of toxic metals not irreversible bound to tissues, than forced diuresis. In general, however, the yield of metal ion in the dialysate is low. Metals that may be dialyzable are arsenic, copper, iron, lead, lithium, magnesium, mercury, potassium, sodium, strontium, and zinc. Hemodialysis is indicated when a potentially fatal dose has been absorbed, when the clinical condition is deteriorating despite adequate treatment by other means, and when a complication occurs, such as aspiration pneumonia or renal insufficiency. Prolonged hemodialysis is required in cases of severe poisoning with lithium salts, where this treatment may be lifesaving. In severe acute inorganic mercury poisoning, hemodialysis may be performed after giving DMPS (dimercaptopropanesulfonate), to remove the mercury chelate (Dargan et al., 2003). Peritoneal dialysis may be tried if hemodialysis is not available.

7.4.4 Exchange Transfusion

If the toxic compound is poorly dialyzable or if there are no facilities for hemodialysis, exchange transfusion may be lifesaving in severe poisoning by agents that remain in the blood in high concentrations. Exchange transfusion is the treatment of choice in severe poisonings with arsine or stibine.

7.5 DETOXIFICATION BY INACTIVATION OF THE ABSORBED POISON

To counteract the effects of an absorbed toxic metal, a limited number of therapeutic agents may be administered. Such specific antidotes have different mechanisms of action. The antidote may combine with the toxic agent to form a less toxic or a nontoxic compound, which may be excreted more effectively in the urine. Furthermore, it may compete with the toxic agent and displace it from its receptor site; or it may displace the poison into a tissue where it cannot exert its toxic effects. One example is the treatment of lead intoxication by the intravenous administration of calcium gluconate. The agent will displace lead from its site of action and will thereby temporarily relieve the intense pain of lead colic. An infusion of potassium has been shown to counteract the potassium-displacing capacity of absorbed soluble barium salts (Berning, 1975). Intravenous infusions of potassium in appropriate amounts are also an efficient treatment of thallium intoxication by accelerating the elimination of thallium from the cells and whole body. Certain antidotes have been designed specifically to compete with toxic metals that interact with chemical groups that are essential for normal physiological functions. These metal antidotes, also referred to as chelating agents, form a stable complex with the metal in the form of a heterocyclic ring (Catsch, 1962; Aaseth, 1983). The antagonists and the chelates produced are not themselves without toxic side effects, and should therefore not be administered therapeutically in mild cases of poisonings where removal from further exposure is sufficient to promote recovery. The use and misuse of chelation therapy are considered in greater detail later.

7.6 CHELATION THERAPY

Chelating agents are organic or inorganic compounds that can bind metal ions and form complex ring-like structures called chelates. Metal cations, for example, Ca^{2+}, Mg^{2+}, Hg^{2+}, Pb^{2+}, and Cd^{2+}, as well as transition metals like Mn, Cu, Fe, and Co may be chelated by exogenous (therapeutic) and endogenous chelating agents. An optimal therapeutic chelator should have high solubility in water, resistance to biotransformation, ability to reach the sites of metal deposition, and the capability to retain its chelating ability at the pH of body fluids, that is about 7.4 extracellularly and about 6.8 intracellularly. Renal ultrafiltrate may become significantly more acidic upon passage downward along the tubular system, giving rise to the chelate decomposition in urine. Ideally, the chelator should have low toxicity and the chelates formed should be inert and rapidly eliminated (Flora & Pachauri, 2010). Chelation is indicated in the treatment of metal poisoning, in the treatment of metal-storage diseases, in particular in Wilson's disease, in blood transfusion iron overload as in the thalassemia and sickle-cell anemias, and to aid the elimination of metallic radionuclides from the body. The pharmacology and therapeutic applications of chelating agents were reviewed by Catsch and Harmuth-Hoene (1976) and updated by Aaseth (1983), Andersen (1999), Andersen and Aaseth (2002), Andersen (2004) and Aaseth, Skaug, Cao, and Andersen (2015). An ideal chelator should bind selectively resulting in the chelation and sufficient elimination of a specific metal in its toxic form, without causing any adverse health effects or affecting the concentrations of essential elements (Smith, 2013). Hardly any chelators meet this criteria. The basic mechanism underlying chelation is that the therapeutic agent should possess electron donor groups showing a high affinity for the metal to be removed, thus releasing it from complexes with proteins or other endogenous ligands in a form in which it can be readily excreted. The effectiveness of therapeutic ligand exchange depends intraarterial (i.a.) on the following factors: (1) the relative stability constants for the metal–endogenous ligand and the metal–therapeutic ligand complexes, (2) the rate of ligand exchange, (3) the effective concentration of the agent in the region of the metal–endogenous ligand complex, and (4) the stability of the newly formed chelate.

The chelating agent should form complexes with the toxic metal that have much greater stability than those formed with physiologically essential metals such as calcium, zinc, or copper. Treatment is most effective if the chelating agent is given while the metal is still in the circulation or in the extracellular fluid compartment, because once intracellular, the metal is less accessible. Many chelating agents are appearing in an ionized form and, therefore, have limited ability to penetrate cell membranes.

Also, the solubility of the chelate in water and lipids, respectively, has to be considered. Water solubility facilitates the transport within blood and the excretion via the kidneys. A lipophilic chelator on the other hand can more easily pass the cellular membranes to chelate intracellular elements and has often a higher excretion via the bile (Sears, 2013). Account has to be taken that metal chelator effects may result in depletion of essential metals or to the redistribution of toxic metals to other tissues, for example, the brain (Andersen, 2004; Andersen & Aaseth, 2002).

7.6.1 Dimercaprol (BAL)—A Classic Agent, but Now Obsolete?

2,3-Dimercaptopropanol (dimercaprol, British AntiLewisite, BAL), now a classic chelator, was synthesized as a specific antagonist to the vesicant arsenical war gas Lewisite during World War II (Peters, Stocken, & Thompson, 1945; Carleton, Peters, & Thompson, 1948). It is a dithiol compound that successfully competes with protein sulfhydryl groups for arsenic compounds, and has also been used as antidote for other heavy metals by forming a stable chelate with them. Among other metals for which dimercaprol has been shown to possess chelating properties, mercury in inorganic form, antimony, arsenic, bismuth, and gold can be found (Andersen, 1999). In cases with acute lead encephalopathy and increased intracranial pressure, it has been advised to administer dimercaprol intramuscular (i.m.) combined with calcium ethylenediaminetetraacetic acid (EDTA) infusion, in an initial phase (Chisolm, 1968), but today this recommendation appears rather outdated (see later). The half-life of BAL is short, metabolism and excretion being complete within 4 h. BAL has unpleasant and sometimes alarming side effects when given in full dosage. One of the most consistent is a rise in blood pressure accompanied by tachycardia. Other untoward effects are nausea and vomiting, headache, burning sensations in the mouth and throat, with paresthesia of the hands, a feeling of constriction or pain in the chest, lacrimation, salivation, rhinorrhea, sweating, and abdominal pain accompanied by a feeling of anxiety. Because of its high toxicity, dimercaprol is now suited only for brief and initial treatment of acute and life-threatening intoxications (Mückter et al., 1997; Andersen & Aaseth, 2002). Due to the major drawbacks of dimercaprol such as small margin of safety, tendency to redistribute arsenic and other heavy metals to brain, and painful i.m. injections, its analogs DMPS and DMSA have now replaced dimercaprol in the treatment of most cases of poisoning (Flora & Pachauri, 2010; Aaseth et al., 2015).

In the few cases when dimercaprol is used, it is given by deep i.m. injection as a 5% solution in arachis oil. It is usually given in a dose of 2.5 mg/kg, every 4 h, for the first day(s) of an acute poisoning. Subsequently, the antidotal regimen should be changed to DMPS or DMSA. The drug BAL should be administered at a lower dosage to patients with impaired renal function. Dimercaprol is contraindicated for the treatment of cadmium poisoning and poisoning of both aryl- and alkylmercury compounds. Dimercaprol enhances the toxicity of selenium and tellurium, producing kidney damage, and is therefore contraindicated in poisoning by these metals (Amdur, 1958; Cerwenka & Cooper, 1961).

7.6.2 Sodium 2,3-Dimercaptopropane-1-Sulfonate (DMPS; Dimaval)—in Clinical Use

This water-soluble chemical analog of dimercaprol is an effective antidote for the treatment of several forms of heavy metal poisoning. It has a lower toxicity than dimercaprol. The agent was originally synthesized by Petrunkin (1956) and has for many years been used extensively as heavy metal antidote in Russia and during more recent years also in the Western world.

DMPS as well as its congener DMSA can increase the urinary excretion of copper and zinc. In therapeutic doses, however, this is not considered to be of clinical significance. Allergic side effects have been reported. The properties and uses of DMPS as well as of DMSA have been reviewed by Aposhian (1983). DMPS is effective in increasing metal excretion without causing severe adverse health effects in acute and chronic intoxication by organic and inorganic mercury, bismuth, arsenic, and chronic lead poisoning (Andersen, 1999; Aposhian et al., 1995; Aaseth et al., 2015).

DMPS (Dimaval) may be given orally or parenterally. It may be administered by continuous intravenous infusion, 20 mg/kg per day, in physiological saline or Ringer solutions during the first day after an acute intoxication. It can also be given intramuscularly as a 5% solution at the rate of 5 mg/kg three or four times during the first 24 h, two or three times on the second day, and once or twice on subsequent days. DMPS is mainly distributed extracellularly and to a small extent also intracellularly. In humans it is biotransformed to acyclic and cyclic disulfides and thereafter the drug and its metabolites are rapidly excreted from the body via urine. DMPS had a good treatment effect in one case of Wilson's disease where intolerance had developed to penicillamine and to triethylenetetramine, resulting in effective cupruresis (Walshe, 1984, 1985). In two other case reports by the same author, adverse health effects were observed. In experiments on animals, DMPS has prevented the lethal effects of a number of arsenic compounds. DMPS has been used in Eastern Europe in the treatment of arsenic poisoning in man. Therapy with DMPS gave a significant improvement of the clinical condition of patients with chronic arsenic intoxication due to intake of arsenic-contaminated drinking water, which affects millions of people in the West Bengal (Guha Mazumder et al., 2001). A treatment with DMPS combined with a good nutritious diet rich in proteins significantly reduced the symptoms of the patients.

DMPS is also the antidote of choice in polonium (Po) poisoning. As the murder of the former Russian spy, Alexander Litvinenko in 2006 shows, there is a need for potent agents to treat radiopolonium poisonings. The isotope ^{210}Po is a high-energy alpha emitter with a decay half-life of 138 days, and it is one of the most hazardous radioactive materials. Internal contamination with even minute doses can prove deadly. Its toxicity is caused by its radioactivity, not by its chemical properties. Treatment with a chelating agent is efficient only if administered early, preferably within the first hour after exposure. Intravenous DMPS is recommended for the first 2 days after ^{210}Po poisoning, followed by oral DMPS for the next days (Rencova, Volf, Jones, & Singh, 1994; Aaseth et al., 2015).

In the Soviet Union, DMPS has been used successfully in the treatment of chronic lead poisoning. DMPS may also have a major role in the treatment of alkylmercury poisoning. In a study of the relative effectiveness of DMPS compared to penicillamine, in the Iraqi outbreak of alkylmercury poisoning, DMPS was found to be the most effective agent, reducing the mean biologic half-life for mercury in blood from about 65 to 10 days (Clarkson et al., 1981). Adverse effects of treatment were not observed. The authors concluded that an accelerated excretion causing a reduction in blood mercury levels would be clinically useful if given before irreversible damage had occurred. DMPS has also been used for the treatment of inorganic mercury poisoning after the inhalation of mercury vapor or ingestion of mercuric oxide. It has been reported to be effective in increasing mercury excretion in urine (Dargan et al., 2003; Liu et al., 2011). In a study of a gold mining area in the Philippines, gold miners exposed to inorganic mercury were compared with a group of people living downstream, who ate fish containing considerable concentrations of methyl mercury (Böse-O'Reilly et al., 2003). In total 106 subjects were treated with oral DMPS 400 mg per day during a 2-week period. Despite the relatively short treatment period positive effects were observed in the metallic mercury exposed group as well as in the methyl mercury exposed group. Significant improvements were noted for Romberg test, tests for ataxia, pencil tapping, and visual perception. The majority of the patients reported a significant improvement in memory, sleeplessness, metallic taste in the mouth, fatigue, and anxiety. The only complication reported was an allergic skin rash in one patient, who was excluded from the trial (Böse-O'Reilly et al., 2003; Bernhoft, 2012). DMPS has also been effective for the treatment of inorganic mercury poisoning caused by the use of skin-lightening cosmetic products (Chan, 2011).

DMPS has been given as a diagnostic test for low-level mercury exposure, suggesting that urinary mercury after DMPS may be a better indicator of exposure than unchallenged urinary mercury excretion (Aposhian et al., 1995). However, the clinical use of such provocation tests have been questioned (Aaseth et al., 2015).

In conclusion, DMPS is now considered to be the optimal antidote for arsenic and inorganic mercury poisonings, whereas DMSA appears to be more effective in lead and organic mercury poisonings, but further studies in this field are justified (Aaseth, Jacobsen, Andersen, & Wickstrøm, 1995; Andersen, 1999).

7.6.3 Meso-2,3-Dimercaptosuccinic Acid (DMSA; Succimer)—Clinical Use and Misuse

Several reports from the Soviet Union, China, and the Western countries show the effectiveness and low toxicity of DMSA in the treatment of poisoning by arsenic, lead, and mercury (Andersen, 2004). This analog of dimercaprol is among the least toxic of the chelators. It may be given parenterally or orally in doses of 30 mg/kg per day for 5–7 days followed by 20 mg/kg per day for 1–3 weeks. The drug is 95% plasma protein bound, probably due to binding of one of its sulfhydryl groups to a cysteine residue on albumin, leaving the other SH available to chelate metals (Miller, 1998). DMSA is rapidly excreted in urine. Some 10–25% of an orally administered dose is excreted in urine, the major part within 24 h and most (>90%) as DMSA-cysteine disulfide conjugates (Bradberry & Vale, 2009). DMSA decreases the deposition of lead and also of methylmercury in the brain (Aaseth et al., 1995).

DMSA, which has a lower toxicity than DMPS, is usually the preferred antidote for severe and less severe lead poisoning, in children (Angle, 1993; Cao, Chen, Bottai, Caldwell, & Rogan, 2013) as well as in adults (Crinnion, 2011; Aaseth et al., 2015; Bradberry & Vale, 2009). It was registered in the United States in 1991 for the oral treatment of lead poisoning in children, which was a significant problem in poor population subgroups. Four lead-intoxicated children were treated with DMSA for five courses each lasting 10 days (Chisolm, 1992). After each course, the blood lead increased again, indicating the need for repeated chelation. The rebound in blood lead concentration that occurs after chelation courses is considered to be predominantly caused by mobilization of bone lead, necessitating the need for repeated chelation.

In a review paper, DMSA 30 mg/kg per day significantly increased urine lead excretion and significantly reduced blood lead levels in lead poisoned patients, although a substantial inter-individual variation was reported. Over a 5-day period, mean daily urine lead excretion exceeded baseline by between 5- and 20-fold, and blood lead levels decreased by up to 50% compared to baseline concentrations (Bradberry & Vale, 2009). Five lead-poisoned smelter workers were given DMSA in an increasing dosage from the first to the sixth day. A marked fall in blood lead concentration was accompanied by a significant increase in urinary lead and copper excretion but without effect on urinary calcium, iron, magnesium, or zinc excretion (Friedheim, Graziano, Popovac, Dragovic, & Kaul, 1978). Succimer-treated lead exposed children with low blood lead levels below 450 μg/L, aged 12–33 months, had a clear reduction of blood lead after one week of therapy (42%). In this study, DMSA produced a mean difference from placebo of 45 μg Pb/L during 6 months of follow-up and 27 μg Pb/L during 12 months. However, DMSA did not improve scores on test of cognition, behavior or neuropsychological function (Rogan et al., 2001). Apparently, chelation therapy is not indicated for children with blood Pb levels below 450 μg/L (2.2 μmol/L).

Although DMSA is effective for the treatment of lead intoxication, adverse effects have been reported. They include gastrointestinal discomfort, skin reaction, mild neutropenia, and elevated liver enzymes. A strong musculocutaneous reaction in one case of chronic lead poisoning (Grandjean, Jacobsen, & Jørgensen, 1991) and hemolytic anemia was reported in a worker with occupational lead exposure (Gerr, Frumkin, & Hodgins, 1994).

The efficacy of DMSA in binding and mobilizing mercury has been shown in a number of animal studies reviewed by Aposhian (1983) and Aaseth et al. (1995). The mobilization and removal of methylmercury by extracorporeal complexing hemodialysis with DMSA has given promising results in experiments on dogs (Kostyniak, 1982). In a study of children aged 12−33 months, DMSA treatment gave a modest reduction in organic mercury concentration after one week, and slowed or prevented the accumulation of organic mercury after multiple courses in 5 months (Cao et al., 2011). No effect was seen on the blood cadmium levels in the same group (Cao et al., 2013).

Both DMSA and DMPS have a therapeutic potential in cases of acute intoxication by arsenic and inorganic mercuric salts (Kosnett, 2013), although DMPS appears to be the most efficient agent in these latter poisonings. And the antidote needs to be administered early after the poisoning, preferably within minutes to hours. Contrary to BAL these agents do not redistribute arsenic or mercury to the brain.

Low-level mercury exposure in children might result from the addition of the antiseptic agent thiomersal in vaccines. Thiomersal is metabolized to ethylmercury in the human body. It has been claimed that this mercurial even in minute doses might lead to the serious medical condition of autism (Bernard, Enayati, Redwood, Roger, & Binstock, 2001). This hypothesis led to the proposal of mercury chelation with DMPS or DMSA as therapy for autism (Kidd, 2002). However, no peer-reviewed papers have reported mercury excess in blood, urine, or hair of subjects suffering from autism (Aschner & Walker, 2002; Wecker, Miller, Cochran, Dugger, & Johnson, 1985). Critical reviews have concluded that the scientific support for mercury chelation in autism is lacking (Davis et al., 2013; Crisponi et al., 2015).

7.6.4 Calcium Disodium Edetate ($CaNa_2EDTA$)—Clinical Use and Misuse

EDTA, another classic chelator, and related compounds are able to chelate many divalent and trivalent metals in vitro. $CaNa_2EDTA$ is a derivative of EDTA. Infusion of the sodium salt will chelate calcium from the body and hypocalcemic tetany may follow. However, the calcium disodium salt, calcium EDTA, has been used as a therapeutic agent, because it will bind lead with the displacement of calcium from the chelate. Thus, the $PbNa_2EDTA$ complex will be excreted from the body fluids leaving Ca behind. However, it has dangerous toxic side effects in the chelation of metals. Calcium EDTA is poorly absorbed from the gastrointestinal tract (<5%) and accordingly, it has to be given intravenously. It is distributed mainly in the extracellular fluid and is excreted rapidly by glomerular filtration, about 50% appearing in the urine within 1 h. The elimination half-life of the drug is 1.4–3 h in adults and it is entirely excreted within 24 h. Due to the toxic effects of calcium EDTA, the administration of the agent has to be monitored with care. Kidney is the critical organ. Unwanted side effects of the treatment of lead poisoning include a febrile reaction with headache, myalgia, nausea, and vomiting. Furthermore, EDTA may redistribute lead to the brain after acute or chronic lead exposure (Andersen, 2004). Lacrimation, nasal congestion, mucocutaneous lesions, glycosuria, hypotension, and ECG abnormalities have also been reported as well as allergic reactions (Wax, 2013). Prolonged treatment with calcium EDTA gives rise to depletion of magnesium and trace-metal depletion, the most marked being due to the excretion of zinc.

Chelation therapy with EDTA has been discussed as an alternative treatment for atherosclerotic cardiovascular diseases (Clarke, Clarke, & Mosher, 1955; Meltzer, Kitchell, & Palmon, 1961; Lamas et al., 2013). In a paper by Seely, Wu, and Mills, (2005), a systematic review of published articles in this field was undertaken. The authors concluded that the best current available evidence did not support the therapeutic use of EDTA chelation therapy in the treatment of cardiovascular disease. Similar results have been reported in review papers by Shrihari, Roy, Prabhakaran, and Reddy (2006) and Crisponi et al. (2015). It should be emphasized that EDTA treatment is associated with severe, life-threatening adverse effects. In one trial on possible antiatherogenic effect of EDTA, 6 patients of the experimental group showed clinical signs of potentially lethal hypocalcemia (Sloth-Nielsen et al., 1991), and several fatalities have been reported (Brown, Willis, Omalu, & Leiker, 2006; Baxter & Krenzelok, 2008). Furthermore, there have been reports about severe kidney damage after such chelation therapy (Nissel, 1986). The calcium chelate of EDTA (CaEDTA) has shown teratogenic effects (Catsch & Harmuth-Hoene, 1976) and produced abnormalities in pups of rats removed by cesarian section on day 21. Increases in several abnormalities (cleft palate, adactyly or syndactyly, abnormal rib or abnormal vertebrae) were observed with increased doses of CaEDTA. The incorporation of zinc in the chelate had a protective effect (Brownie & Aronson, 1984).

Many of the side effects of calcium EDTA have been ascribed to excessive chelation after administration of high doses over a short period of time. Because of its adverse effects, calcium EDTA is being progressively replaced by DMSA in the treatment of lead poisoning (Aposhian et al., 1995). In earlier studies, CaEDTA has also been used for the treatment of cases with manganese toxicity, showing neurotoxic symptoms resembling Parkinsonism (Andersen, 1999). Later case reports, however, indicate that another antidote, the tuberculostatic agent PAS (paraaminosalicylate), may be a more efficient neuroprotecting agent in manganese toxicity. However, this treatment must be administered early after exposure, before the appearance of irreversible changes (Jiang et al., 2006; Zheng et al., 2009).

7.6.5 Diethylenetriaminepentaacetic Acid (DTPA)—and Radionuclide Chelation

DTPA is another synthetic polyamino polycarboxylic acid with properties similar to those of EDTA. It also forms stable chelates with calcium. The calcium salt has been used to accelerate the elimination of plutonium and related actinide metals. The agent is mainly administered by intravenous or intramuscular routes—or by inhalation as it is poorly absorbed from the GI-tract. Because zinc depletion may occur during long-term administration, it has been suggested that the calcium DTPA should be replaced by zinc DTPA in the later stages of treatment (Taylor & Volf, 1980). As with all chelators, DTPA is most effective if administered shortly after exposure. Lipophilic derivatives of DTPA are being developed. One example is Puchel, which can be administered as an aerosol to decrease the lung concentration of inhaled carcinogenic plutonium oxide particles (Stradling, Stather, Ham, & Sumner, 1981). Plutonium and americium have, to some extent, been eliminated with DTPA given in a dose of about 1 g/day intravenously, in a few cases for long periods without adverse effect (Raymond & Smith, 1981; Fukuda, 2005). Whereas pulmonary insufflated DTPA was efficient to mobilize deposits of plutonium-239 from the lung, the most effective treatment for plutonium decorporation from the whole body was the early pulmonary delivery of DTPA supplemented by intravenous infusion of DTPA solution (Grémy, Tsapis, Bruel, Renault, & Van der Meeren, 2012). The parenteral DTPA-PAS (*p*-aminosalicylic acid) combination reduced the plutonium content in mouse liver and bone (Schubert, 1983). $CaNa_3DTPA$ is teratogenic due to its Mn and Zn depletion effect, and accordingly the agent is contraindicated during pregnancy, especially the administration of multiple doses (Flora & Pachauri, 2010).

7.6.6 Penicillamine (Cuprimine)—Old but Not Outdated

Dimethylcysteine, or penicillamine, is a monothiol derived from the hydrolytic degradation of penicillin. D-penicillamine has been used for several decades in oral chelation treatment. It has particularly high affinity for copper through its electron donor groups. It might also chelate iron, lead, mercury, and zinc, and to some extent increase the excretion of these metals in the urine. Penicillamine is well absorbed from the gastrointestinal tract (about 50% after oral supply) and the peak plasma concentration is observed between 1 and 4 h after oral intake. Its volume of distribution is close to that of extracellular water, and a part of a systemic dose forms mixed disulfides with serum albumin. The metabolism is insignificant, and the major part of a dose is rapidly excreted in urine as free D-penicillamine or the oxidized dimer. Its elimination half-life is in the range from 3 to more than 5 h (Netter, Bannwarth, Péré, & Nicolas, 1987). The most important side effects of penicillamine are acute sensitivity reactions manifested by fever, skin rashes, blood dyscrasias, and occasionally nephrotic syndrome with proteinuria. There is cross-sensitivity with penicillin, so subjects that are allergic to penicillin should not be given penicillamine. Penicillamine antagonizes pyridoxine, although clinical effects of such deficiency after treatment with D-penicillamine are unusual.

Penicillamine is given orally, before meals, in four divided doses at a rate of 0.5–1.5 g daily, although up to 5 g daily has been given without adverse health effects. The urine should be tested for protein, and a full blood count should be performed at weekly intervals, but when treatment continues for longer than 2–3 months, as in the management of Wilson's disease, these tests may then be performed monthly. In Wilson's disease, 500 mg penicillamine is given before meals three times a day. Once stability is attained, this may be reduced to 750 mg/day and continued indefinitely to maintain a negative copper balance. In children, 25 mg/kg is appropriate.

Penicillamine is also effective in the treatment of rheumatoid arthritis and related conditions. Its mode of action in these conditions is essentially unknown (Munthe, Jellum, & Aaseth, 1979).

7.6.7 Triethylenetetramine (Trientine, TETA)—Clinical Usefulness

TETA is a drug of choice for acute copper intoxications. It is mostly given perorally, although the gastrointestinal absorption is relatively poor. As less than 20% of an oral dose of ^{14}C - labeled TETA to rats was recovered in carcass and urine, a part of its action appears to involve a decreased intestinal copper absorption. Two major metabolites of TETA have been identified, N_1-acetyltriethylenetetramine and N_1N_{10}-diacetyltriethylenetetramine. The former metabolite is presumed to play a significant role for the molecular mechanisms by which TETA extracts copper from the body. After intravenous administration, half of the dose was rapidly excreted in urine, but a small fraction was recovered from feces indicating some biliary excretion (Gibbs & Walshe, 1986). Although trientine has been used in clinical situations for decades, many of its pharmacologic aspects have not been fully investigated, such as the exact fraction of absorption in humans and the extent of its presumed penetration across the blood–brain barrier. Trientine also appears to exert an anticancer effect, but the mechanism is unknown (Lu, 2010).

As evidence has grown for the effectiveness of trientine, with fewer side effects than penicillamine, trientine is by several experts regarded the first drug of choice for initial treatment of Wilson's disease (Andersen, 1999; Weiss et al., 2013). The recommended dosage for the treatment of Wilson's disease is 0.75–2 g/day (Flora & Pachauri, 2010).

7.6.8 Deferoxamine (DFO)—The Classical Iron Chelator

DFO is a chelating agent with a remarkable affinity for trivalent iron and less affinity for other metals. Thus it is a suitable chelating agent for the treatment of iron related diseases. It is poorly absorbed from the gastrointestinal tract, but given parenterally, it complexes with iron in a diffuse chelatable pool and is rapidly excreted as the red ferrioxamine, about two thirds through the kidneys and one third through the bile into feces. Deferoxamine may be given by the subcutaneous, intramuscular, or the intravenous route. Given perorally, it chelates iron remaining in the lumen of the gut, thereby preventing the iron absorption and detoxify the substance. It is the treatment of choice in acute iron poisoning, greatly reducing the mortality in children, provided it is given at an early stage. Its intravenous effectiveness also depends on the induction of forced diuresis, thus increasing the elimination of the ferrioxamine chelate. If oliguria develops, peritoneal dialysis or hemodialysis may be tried to aid elimination.

Deferoxamine has also proven to be efficient for the treatment of chronic iron overload after multiple blood transfusions. In thalassemia and sickle cell anemia, continuous subcutaneous infusion of DFO is a basic regimen, also given to young children on regular blood transfusion (DFO dose: 40 mg/kg, 8–12 h/day, 5 days/week). However, DFO is distributed mainly to the extracellular space, and has limited access to the iron deposits in heart and liver cells. Therefore, it is now often administered in combination with one of the new oral agents, deferiprone or deferasirox, to obtain a more efficient mobilization of intracellular deposits (Mourad et al., 2003). The iron overload in these patients causes damage primarily to the heart, but also to liver and other tissues. Cardiac disease is the primary cause of death in transfusional iron overload (Borgna-Pignatti et al., 2005). When monitoring the chelation treatment in these cases of siderosis, it is recommended to use cardiac MRI in addition to frequent determination of serum ferritin. This is because the iron-induced cardiomyopathy is clinically asymptomatic until late stages, when the prognosis is poor (Modell et al., 2008).

Long-term hemodialysis for chronic renal failure has been associated with the accumulation of aluminum in the brain, resulting from high aluminum content in the dialysis water supply causing encephalopathy. Deferoxamine has been used for the successful removal of aluminum in dialysis encephalopathy (Ackrill, Ralston, Day, & Hodge, 1980), resulting in clinical improvement. Deferoxamine raises serum aluminum to high levels and allows this to be removed by conventional dialysis techniques. Treatment with DFO has been shown to be beneficial for hemodialysis patients with aluminum associated bone disease (Smith, 2013).

In severe cases of iron poisoning with shock, DFO is given by slow intravenous infusion at a rate of not more than 15 mg/kg to a maximum of 80 mg/kg per 24 h. In the absence of shock, it may be given intramuscularly at a rate of 2 g for an adult and 1 g for a child every 12 h. Gastric lavage may be performed with 5 g DFO dissolved in 1 L of water, and 5–10 g deferoxamine in 50–100 mL water may be left in the stomach to chelate unabsorbed iron from the gut.

While being well tolerated, the rapid intravenous administration of DFO may cause transient hypotension with histamine-like or anaphylactic reactions. The drug should be used cautiously in patients with impaired renal function.

7.6.9 Deferiprone (Ferriprox)—An Oral Agent for Iron Detoxification

Deferiprone, 1, 2-dimethyl-3-hydroxypyrid-4-one, is effective for long-term iron chelation therapy of transfusional iron overload in thalassemia and sickle cell anemia. It is suitable for home treatment as it can be administered perorally (Kontoghiorghes, Pattichi, Hadjigavriel, & Kolnagou, 2000). In a study by Piga, Gaglioti, Fogliacco, and Tricta (2003) both mortality and worsening of cardiac dysfunction were significantly lower in patients treated with deferiprone than in patients treated with subcutaneous deferoxamine during an average 6-year follow-up period. This indicates that deferiprone is more effective in reducing cardiac iron compared to deferoxamine. Deferiprone together with deferoxamine in lower doses can be used in patients requiring lifelong chelation therapy (Mourad et al., 2003). This combination therapy has been shown to be very effective with regard to cardiac iron removal and the treatment of iron-related diseases (Kwiatkowski, 2011; Kolnagou, Kleanthous, & Kontoghiorghes, 2011). The usual dose of deferiprone is 75 mg/kg per day taken as tablets with about 8 h intervals. It is rapidly absorbed in the gastrointestinal tract and appears in serum few minutes after administration. The main excretion route is via kidneys, with a half-life of about 60 min. The elimination in urine is close to 100%, with the main species being free deferiprone. The acute toxicity of deferiprone is somewhat lower than that of deferoxamine (Flora & Pachauri, 2010). The iron excretion in urine after a dose of 75 mg/kg of deferiprone is comparable to that induced by deferoxamine at a dose of 50 mg/kg (Kwiatkowski, 2011). Main reported side effects include gastrointestinal symptoms, headache, and arthropathy. The most severe but rare complications of deferiprone treatment are transient agranulocytosis and neutropenia (Fig. 7.1).

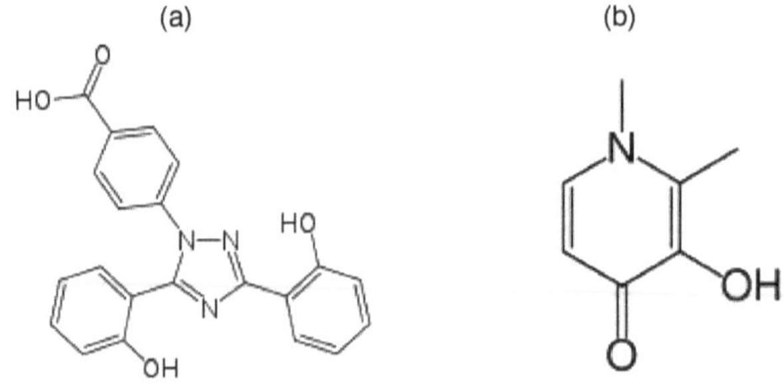

FIGURE 7.1 Chemical formulas of the oral iron chelating agents deferasirox (a) and deferiprone (b).

7.6.10 Deferasirox (Exjade)—A New Efficient Tablet for Iron Detoxification

A promising new alternative to deferoxamine and deferiprone is deferasirox (4-[3,5-bis(2-hydroxyphenyl)-1,2,4-triazol-1-yl]-benzoic acid (Exjade). This is an orally active tridentate chelator which binds iron in a 2:1 ratio. The drug has a rather selective affinity for iron and a minimal chelation of copper and zinc. Deferasirox efficiently and selectively mobilizes iron from liver and heart tissue, thereby facilitating the excretion of iron (Musallam & Taher, 2011). It can be given perorally, is rapidly absorbed and reaches the peak plasma level within 1–3 h after administration. The plasma half-life after a single oral dose in humans was about 10 h (range: 7–16 h) allowing a once a day dosing, of about two tablets of 500 mg to an adult individual (Piga et al., 2006). The deferasirox-iron chelate has a limited urinary excretion and is mainly excreted via bile into the feces.

Deferasirox has been investigated in several clinical trials (Nisbet-Brown et al., 2003). Adverse effects include gastrointestinal disturbances, nausea, vomiting, abdominal pain, skin rash, and nephrotoxicity (Kwiatkowski, 2011). The use of higher doses of deferasirox (maximum dose 40 mg/kg per day) will increase the iron excretion but also the toxic side effects. Although several nonrandomized trials suggest that deferasirox is effective to remove cardiac iron in patients with siderosis, randomized clinical trials are warranted to verify this observation (Xia, Zhang, Huang, & Jiang, 2013). As indicated from the meta-analysis by Xia et al. (2013), deferasirox seemed to have a reasonable safety margin compared with deferoxamine.

More effective, less toxic and less costly chelation therapies are available for the majority of patients by the use of deferiprone or the combination of deferiprone and deferoxamine (Kontoghiorghes, Kolnagou, Peng, Shah, & Aessopos, 2010).

7.6.11 Diethyldithiocarbamate (DDC)

DDC is a chelating agent that has been found to be efficient in the treatment of acute nickel carbonyl poisoning, significantly increasing the excretion of nickel in the urine and faeces (Sunderman, 1971). In moderately severe poisonings, DDC may be given orally initially at a rate of 50 mg/kg in divided doses. At the low pH of gastric juice, however, DDC is degraded to ethylamine and carbon disulfide. This reaction can be minimized by the concomitant administration of 2 g sodium bicarbonate by mouth. By forming lipophilic chelates with divalent nickel, DDC can reduce the nickel burden in the lungs. On the other hand, this complex has an affinity for lipid-rich tissues including the brain, and may therefore increase the nickel concentrations in the brain. Accordingly, DDC has been replaced by DMSA in such cases of poisoning. Thus, today DDC has no place in chelation therapy with the exception of nickel dermatitis (Barceloux, 1999). The disulfide form of DDC, disulfiram (Antabuse, Wyeth, PA) is a pharmacological agent against alcohol abuse. It can also be used for the treatment of nickel contact dermatitis. After absorption in the gut, disulfiram is metabolized into its monomeric form, DDC. The metabolite chelates with nickel, giving an increased concentration in blood and an enhanced excretion through urine and bile. This treatment has been reported to decrease the frequency and intensity of flare-ups in nickel-sensitized subjects with chronic relapsing contact dermatitis. (Tammaro, Narcisi, Persechino, Caperchi, & Gaspari, 2011).

7.6.12 Combinations of Chelating Agents

In thalassemic patients with siderosis recent studies have reported that combined treatment with deferoxamine and deferiprone at lower doses than the normal clinical ones efficiently removes iron from vulnerable organs including the heart (Kolnagou et al., 2011). Presumably, deferiprone can mobilize intracellular iron i.a. from cardiomyocytes and act as a shuttling agent, whereas deferoxamine predominantly operates extracellularly.

Deferasirox can also be combined with deferiprone in the treatment of iron overload (Totadri et al. 2015). This combination is preferable compared to the deferoxamine-deferiprone combination in β-thalassemia major patients, usually living in developing countries, due to the high costs of the parenteral deferoxamine infusions. And monotherapy with either deferiprone or deferasirox may not always attain optimal control, especially not in heavily iron-loaded thalassemic patients. The oral deferoxamine-deferiprone combination has been reported to be safe and efficacious in these patients (Totadri et al. 2015).

Coadministration of DMSA and its lipophilic monoisoamyl ester (MiA-DMSA) has been found to reduce arsenic-induced oxidative stress efficiently, and the combination gave lower arsenic concentrations in blood and soft tissues than mono-therapy (Mishra, Mehta, & Flora, 2008). Recently, it has been reported that combined administration of $CaNa_2EDTA$ and MiA-DMSA counteracts chronic lead toxicity in terms of altered levels of neurotransmitters, neurobehavioral changes, markers of apoptosis, and neuronal cell death (Flora, Saxena, & Mehta, 2007). However, the toxicity of this lipophilic DMSA derivative in clinical use is unknown (Mehta et al., 2002).

Combined treatment with EDTA and dimercaprol was previously recommended in acute lead poisoning in children with cerebral edema and/or encephalopathy or blood lead levels greater than 1000 μg/L (5 μmol/L), since the combination more effectively lowered blood lead levels than either agent alone (Chisolm, 1968). The acute lead encephalopathy that previously occurred frequently due to oral intake of lead based paint chips in infants, and led to high mortality is fortunately very rare today. An argument for the continued use of the BAL-EDTA is that EDTA operates in the extracellular space whereas BAL should enhance the efflux of lead from cells. Today, this argument seems obsolete, as DMSA, which in contrast to EDTA does not increase brain lead, is available as an alternative. The DMSA–EDTA combination was as good as the BAL-EDTA treatment to lower blood lead levels in poisoned children (Besunder, Super, & Anderson, 1997). Combined administration of DMSA and $CaNa_2EDTA$ in subjects with chronic lead poisoning caused a higher elimination of lead and an improvement of altered lead sensitive biochemical variables than treatment with Ca-EDTA alone (Flora, Bhattacharya, & Vijayaraghavan, 1995). Unfortunately, animal studies comparing the effect of BAL-EDTA with DMSA chelation in severe experimental lead intoxication are not available to our knowledge. Such studies would show whether DMSA is the superior antidote in all kinds of lead intoxication.

The possible therapeutic advantages of using combinations of chelating agents, with particular reference to aiding the elimination of cadmium and plutonium, are considered by Schubert (1983). Experimental observations in mice dosed with cadmium chloride indicated an additive protective effect using the two chelators DTPA and DMPS. Chelator combinations tested for their effectiveness in the elimination of plutonium have included DTPA with deferoxamine and EDTA together with a number of ligands. The EDTA-PAS (*p*-aminosalicylic acid) combination significantly reduced the plutonium content in mouse liver and bone.

The rationale in using two different complexing agents to produce a synergistic effect is that the first agent should be sufficiently lipophilic to mobilize the metal from intracellular binding sites and promote its release into the blood, whereas the second agent will promote ligand exchange to form an ionized chelate that can then be excreted into the urine.

7.7 EXPERIMENTAL CHELATION TREATMENT IN ATHEROSCLEROSIS AND IN ALZHEIMER DEMENTIA

7.7.1 Atherosclerosis

Chelation therapy with EDTA has been discussed as an alternative treatment for atherosclerotic cardiovascular diseases (Clarke et al., 1955; Meltzer et al., 1961; Lamas et al., 2013), although its therapeutic efficacy is not convincing. In a paper by Seely et al. (2005), a systematic review of published articles in this field was undertaken. The authors concluded that the best current available evidence did not support the therapeutic use of EDTA chelation therapy in the treatment of cardiovascular disease. Similar results have been reported in the review papers by Shrihari et al. (2006) and Crisponi et al. (2015). It should be emphasized that EDTA treatment is associated with severe, life-threatening adverse effects. In one trial on possible antiatherogenic effect of EDTA, six patients of the experimental group showed clinical signs of potentially lethal hypocalcemia (Sloth-Nielsen et al., 1991), and several fatalities have been reported (Brown et al., 2006; Baxter & Krenzelok, 2008). Furthermore, there have been reports about severe kidney damage after such chelation therapy (Nissel, 1986).

A reasonable assumption is, however, that EDTA may interfere with the catalytic activity of the angiotensin converting enzyme (ACE), since ACE is a metalloenzyme with zinc in its active site, and established ACE-inhibitors are widely used in modern cardiology.

The membrane-bound ACE-enzyme is a zinc-containing protein. In vitro, chelating agents abolish its activity by removing the metal ion to yield the inactive, metal-free apoenzyme. Addition of either Zn^{2+}, Co^{2+}, or Mn^{2+} to the apoenzyme generates an active metalloenzyme, whereas Fe^{2+}, Ni^{2+}, Cu^{2+}, Cd^{2+}, and Hg^{2+} fail to restore its activity. The protein binds Zn^{2+} more firmly than it does Co^{2+} or Mn^{2+}(Fig. 7.2).

An example of an established drug that can chelate zinc, copper, and some other metals is captopril (Jay, Cuéllar, Zamorano, Muñoz, & Gleason, 1991). Captopril inhibits the ACE-enzyme, and thus also inhibits the acceleration of heart decompensation and atherosclerosis. Other clinically used ACE-inhibitors with chelating properties are lisinopril and enalapril. Another conventionally used drug in the treatment of mild to severe congestive heart failure is carvedilol, usually described as a nonselective beta and alpha-1 receptor blocker. The molecule has oxygen donor groups that may bind iron, and the drug may act as an antioxidant. Several beta and calcium blockers may act as antioxidants (Zou, Li, Fan, & Wang, 2012).

Recent studies have shown that the thiol agent acetylcysteine given oral (p.o.) has an antiatherosclerotic effect, presumably by increasing the intracellular glutathione levels. Although this drug is almost exclusively used in chronic obstructive bronchitis today, its chelating potentials may widen its clinical usefulness (Cui et al., 2015).

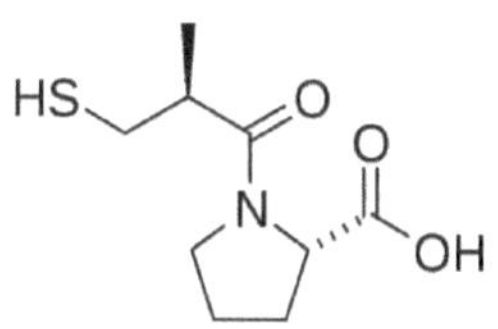

FIGURE 7.2 Chemical formula of captopril, an ACE-inhibitor (see text) with chelating properties, containing sulfur and oxygen donor groups. Captopril is used in clinical treatment of cardiac conditions such as congestive heart failure and after myocardial infarction.

Thus, several drugs with chelating properties are in routine use in cardiovascular and cerebrovascular diseases today. But the present authors consider disodium EDTA chelation therapy to be hazardous and contraindicated. Its use is ethically unjustified in modern cardiology.

7.7.2 Alzheimer's Disease

Preventive measures against Alzheimer's disease include a healthy lifestyle with adequate physical and mental activity and healthy food habits, which is also recommended in patients at risk of atherosclerotic diseases. However, here it is of particular interest that high levels of copper and iron are present in the insoluble beta-amyloid plaques in post-mortem brains from patients suffering from Alzheimer's disease (Castellani, Moreira, Perry, & Zhu, 2012; Ahuja, Dev, Tanwar, Selwal, & Tyagi, 2015). Thus, a pathological distribution of these essential trace elements appears to play a role in the misfolding and aggregation of amyloid precursor protein (APP) and presumably in the dementia progression (Guo et al., 2013). The toxicity of excessive amounts of iron is exemplified by the fact that increased amounts of iron will inhibit furin activity, which is important for the activation of secretases. Thus, lowered levels of furin may enhance the amyloidogenic pathway (Ward, Dexter, & Crichton, 2015). In addition, iron may modulate APP processing through the presence of a putative iron responsive element in APP-mRNA (Rogers et al., 2002). Early studies (Crapper McLachlan et al., 1991) showed that there was a significant reduction in the rate of decline of daily living skills in the 48 AD patients who received desferrioxamine (125 mg i.m. twice daily5 days/week for 24 months) when compared to AD patients receiving placebo. Despite such positive results, there have been no other clinical studies reported where any of the iron chelators have been investigated for their clinical efficacy in this disease.

Currently only one family of metal binding agents, PBT2 (5,7-dichloro-2-(dimethylamino)-methyl)-8-hydroxyquinoline) is in clinical trials for the treatment of Alzheimer's diseases. It mainly binds excesses copper and zinc and presumably iron in the brain, thereby diminishing the amount of amyloid plaque formation and relocating these metal ions to depleted cellular and neuronal compartments (Lannfelt et al., 2008).

7.8 MODIFICATION OF TOXIC EFFECTS OF METALS

Under this heading are included examples of therapeutic measures in metal poisoning that are directed toward a modification of the tissue response to the poison or to an alteration in the biochemical or metabolic state of the subject.

7.8.1 Modification of Inflammatory Response in Tissues

Chronic beryllium disease is characterized by an inflammatory response that is granulomatous in nature and that seems to result from a hypersensitive reaction in certain individuals (Stoeckle, Hardy, & Weber, 1969). The inflammatory process may be stopped, although not reversed, by adequate corticosteroid or azathioprine therapy (Salvator et al., 2013). This immunosuppressive treatment has resulted in a change in the clinical course of the disease with a reduction in symptoms and a favorable change in prognosis.

7.8.2 Modification of Biochemical Functions

Chronic manganese poisoning has pathological, biochemical, and clinical features that closely resemble those of Parkinson's disease, which, once established, becomes a permanent disabling occupational disorder. The neurochemical similarities between these two conditions were described by Cotzias, Papavasiliou, Ginos, Steck, and Duby (1971). This observation led to treatment trials with L-dopa in manganese-induced Parkinsonism showing positive results (Mena, Court, Fuenzalida, Papavasiliou, & Cotzias, 1970). In the majority of patients treated by L-dopa, hypokinesia and rigidity has been reduced, with improvement of postural reflexes and balance, although there was no evidence of a decreased body burden of manganese in the parkinsonian exminers treated in this way (Racette et al., 2001). Beneficial effects can be considered solely as a form of replacement therapy.

ACKNOWLEDGMENTS

The authors are indebted to Academic Press, Elsevier, and to the authors L. Gerhardsson and G. Kazantzis of Chapter 23 in *Handbook on the Toxicology of Metals*, 4th ed. (2014), G.F. Nordberg, B.A. Fowler, and M. Nordberg (Eds.), for permission to use portions of their chapter as a basis for the present text.

REFERENCES

Aaseth, J. (1983). Recent advance in the therapy of metal poisonings with chelating agents. *Human Toxicology*, *2*(2), 257–272.

Aaseth, J., Jacobsen, D., Andersen, O., & Wickstrøm, E. (1995). Treatment of mercury and lead poisonings with dimercaptosuccinic acid and sodium dimercaptopropanesulfonate. A review. *The Analyst*, *120*(3), 853–854.

Aaseth, J., Skaug, M. A., Cao, Y., & Andersen, O. (2015). Chelation in metal intoxication—principles and paradigms. *Journal of Trace Elements in Medicine and Biology*, *31*, 260–266.

Ackrill, P., Ralston, A. J., Day, J. P., & Hodge, K. C. (1980). Successful removal of aluminium from patient with dialysis encephalopathy. *The Lancet*, *316*(8196), 692–693.

Ahuja, A., Dev, K., Tanwar, R. S., Selwal, K. K., & Tyagi, P. K. (2015). Copper mediated neurological disorder: visions into amyotrophic lateral sclerosis, Alzheimer and Menkes disease. *Journal of Trace Elements in Medicine and Biology*, *29*, 11–23.

Amdur, M. L. (1958). Tellurium oxide; an animal study in acute toxicity. *AMA Archives of Industrial Health*, *17*(6), 665–667.

Andersen, O. (1999). Principles and recent developments in chelation treatment of metal intoxication. *Chemical Reviews*, *99*(9), 2683–2710.

Andersen, O. (2004). Chemical and biological considerations in the treatment of metal intoxications by chelating agents. *Mini Reviews in Medicinal Chemistry*, *4*(1), 11–21.

Andersen, O., & Aaseth, J. (2002). Molecular mechanisms of in vivo metal chelation: implications for clinical treatment of metal intoxications. *Environmental Health Perspectives*, *110*(Suppl. 5), 887–890.

Angle, C. R. (1993). Childhood lead poisoning and its treatment. *Annual Review of Pharmacology and Toxicology*, *33*(1), 409–434.

Aposhian, H. V. (1983). DMSA and DMPS-water soluble antidotes for heavy metal poisoning. *Annual Review of Pharmacology and Toxicology*, *23*(1), 193–215.

Aposhian, H. V., Maiorino, R. M., Gonzalez-Ramirez, D., Zuniga-Charles, M., Xu, Z., Hurlbut, K. M., & Aposhian, M. M. (1995). Mobilization of heavy metals by newer, therapeutically useful chelating agents. *Toxicology*, *97*(1–3), 23–38.

Aschner, M., & Walker, S. J. (2002). The neuropathogenesis of mercury toxicity. *Molecular Psychiatry*, *7*(Suppl. 2), S40–S41.

Bakir, F., Damluji, S. F., Amin-Zaki, L., Murtadha, M., Khalidi, A., Al-Rawi, N. Y., & Doherty, R. A. (1973). Methylmercury poisoning in Iraq. *Science*, *181*(4096), 230–241.

Barceloux, D. G. (1999). Nickel. *Journal of Toxicology: Clinical Toxicology*, *37*(2), 239–258.

Baxter, A. J., & Krenzelok, E. P. (2008). Pediatric fatality secondary to EDTA chelation. *Clinical Toxicology*, *46*(10), 1083–1084.

Bernard, S., Enayati, A., Redwood, L., Roger, H., & Binstock, T. (2001). Autism: a novel form of mercury poisoning. *Medical Hypotheses*, *56*(4), 462–471.

Bernhoft, R. A. (2012). Mercury toxicity and treatment: a review of the literature. *Journal of Environmental and Public Health*, *2012*, 460508.

Berning, J. (1975). Hypokalaemia of barium poisoning. *The Lancet*, *1*(7898), 110.

Besunder, J. B., Super, D. M., & Anderson, R. L. (1997). Comparison of dimercaptosuccinic acid and calcium disodium ethylenediaminetetraacetic acid versus dimercaptopropanol and ethylenediaminetetraacetic acid in children with lead poisoning. *The Journal of Pediatrics*, *130*(6), 966–971.

Borgna-Pignatti, C., Cappellini, M. D., De Stefano, P., Del Vecchio, G. C., Forni, G. L., Gamberini, M. R., & Cnaan, A. (2005). Survival and complications in thalassemia. *Annals of the New York Academy of Sciences*, *1054*(1), 40–47.

Bradberry, S., & Vale, A. (2009). Dimercaptosuccinic acid (succimer; DMSA) in inorganic lead poisoning. *Clinical Toxicology*, *47*(7), 617–631.

Brown, M. J., Willis, T., Omalu, B., & Leiker, R. (2006). Deaths resulting from hypocalcemia after administration of edetate disodium: 2003-2005. *Pediatrics*, *118*(2), e534–e536.

Brownie, C. F., & Aronson, A. L. (1984). Comparative effects of Ca-ethylenediaminetetraacetic acid (EDTA), ZnEDTA, and ZnCaEDTA in mobilizing lead. *Toxicology and Applied Pharmacology*, *75*(2), 167–172.

Böse-O'Reilly, S., Drasch, G., Beinhoff, C., Maydl, S., Vosko, M. R., Roider, G., & Dzaja, D. (2003). The Mt. Diwata study on the Philippines 2000—Treatment of mercury intoxicated inhabitants of a gold mining area with DMPS (2, 3-Dimercapto-1-propane-sulfonic acid, Dimaval®). *The Science of the Total Environment*, *307*(1–3), 71–82.

Cao, Y., Chen, A., Jones, R. L., Radcliffe, J., Dietrich, K. N., Caldwell, K. L., & Rogan, W. J. (2011). Efficacy of succimer chelation of mercury at background exposures in toddlers: a randomized trial. *The Journal of Pediatrics*, *158*(3), 480–485.

Cao, Y., Chen, A., Bottai, M., Caldwell, K. L., & Rogan, W. J. (2013). The impact of succimer chelation on blood cadmium in children with background exposures: a randomized trial. *The Journal of Pediatrics*, *163*(2), 598–600.

Carleton, A. B., Peters, R. A., & Thompson, R. H. S. (1948). The treatment of arsenical dermatitis with dimercaptopropanol (BAL). *The Quarterly Journal of Medicine*, *17*(65), 49–79.

Castellani, R. J., Moreira, P. I., Perry, G., & Zhu, X. (2012). The role of iron as a mediator of oxidative stress in Alzheimer disease. *Biofactors*, *38*(2), 133–138.

Catsch, A. (1962). Principles and trends in therapeutic removal of internally deposited radionuclides. *Health Physics*, *8*(6), 725–730.

Catsch, A., & Harmuth-Hoene, A. E. (1976). Pharmacology and therapeutic applications of agents used in heavy metal poisoning. *Pharmacology & Therapeutics. Part A: Chemotherapy, Toxicology and Metabolic Inhibitors*, *1*(1), 1–118.

Cerwenka, E. A., Jr., & Cooper, W. C. (1961). Toxicology of selenium and tellurium and their compounds. *Archives of Environmental Health*, *3*(2), 189–200.

Chan, T. Y. (2011). Inorganic mercury poisoning associated with skin-lightening cosmetic products. *Clinical Toxicology*, *49*(10), 886–891.

Chisolm, J. J. (1968). The use of chelating agents in the treatment of acute and chronic lead intoxication in childhood. *The Journal of Pediatrics*, *73*(1), 1–38.

Chisolm, J. J. (1992). BAL, EDTA DMSA and DMPS in the treatment of lead poisoning in children. *Journal of Toxicology: Clinical Toxicology*, *30*(4), 493–504.

Clarke, N. E., Clarke, C. N., & Mosher, R. E. (1955). The in vivo dissolution of metastatic calcium; an approach to atherosclerosis. *The American Journal of the Medical Sciences*, *229*(2), 142–149.

Clarkson, T. W., Small, H., & Norseth, T. (1973). Excretion and absorption of methyl mercury after polythiol resin treatment. *Archives of Environmental Health*, *26*(4), 173–176.

Clarkson, T. W., Magos, L., Cox, C., Greenwood, M. R., Amin-Zaki, L., Majeed, M. A., & Al-Damluji, S. F. (1981). Tests of efficacy of antidotes for removal of methylmercury in human poisoning during the Iraq outbreak. *The Journal of Pharmacology and Experimental Therapeutics*, *218*(1), 74–83.

Cotzias, G. C., Papavasiliou, P. S., Ginos, J., Steck, A., & Duby, S. (1971). Metabolic modification of Parkinson's disease and of chronic manganese poisoning. *Annual Review of Medicine*, *22*(1), 305–326.

Crapper McLachlan, D. R., Dalton, A. J., Kruck, T. P., Bell, M. Y., Smith, W. L., Kalow, W., & Andrews, D. F. (1991). Intramuscular desferrioxamine in patients with Alzheimer's disease. *The Lancet*, *337*(8753), 1304–1308.

Crinnion, W. J. (2011). EDTA redistribution of lead and cadmium into the soft tissues in a human with a high lead burden-should DMSA always be used to follow EDTA in such cases? *Alternative Medicine Review: A Journal of Clinical Therapeutics*, *16*(2), 109–112.

Crisponi, G., Nurchi, V. M., Lachowicz, J. I., Crespo-Alonso, M., Zoroddu, M. A., & Peana, M. F. (2015). Kill or cure: misuse of chelation therapy for human diseases. *Coordination Chemistry Reviews*, *284*, 278–285.

Cui, Y., Narasimhulu, C., Liu, L., Zhang, Q., Hao, H., Li, X., & Liu, Z. (2015). N-acetylcysteine prevents in vivo oxidation of native low-density lipoprotein. *The FASEB Journal*, *29*(Suppl. 1), 631.12.

Dargan, P. I., Giles, L. J., Wallace, C. I., House, I. M., Thomson, A. H., Beale, R. J., & Jones, A. L. (2003). Case report: severe mercuric sulphate poisoning treated with 2, 3-dimercaptopropane-1-sulphonate and haemodiafiltration. *Critical Care*, *7*(3), R1–R6.

Davis, T. N., O'Reilly, M., Kang, S., Lang, R., Rispoli, M., Sigafoos, J., & Mulloy, A. (2013). Chelation treatment for autism spectrum disorders: a systematic review. *Research in Autism Spectrum Disorders*, *7*(1), 49–55.

Dreisbach, R. H. (1983). *Handbook of poisoning; prevention, diagnosis and treatment* (11th ed.). Lange, Los Altos, CA: Lange Medical Publications.

Flora, S. J. S., Bhattacharya, R., & Vijayaraghavan, R. (1995). Combined therapeutic potential of meso-2, 3-dimercaptosuccinic acid and calcium disodium edetate on the mobilization and distribution of lead in experimental lead intoxication in rats. *Fundamental and Applied Toxicology*, *25*(2), 233–240.

Flora, S. J., Saxena, G., & Mehta, A. (2007). Reversal of lead-induced neuronal apoptosis by chelation treatment in rats: role of reactive oxygen species and intracellular Ca(2 +). *Journal of Pharmacology and Experimental Therapeutics*, *322*(1), 108–116.

Flora, S. J., & Pachauri, V. (2010). Chelation in metal intoxication. *International Journal of Environmental Research and Public Health*, *7*(7), 2745–2788.

Friedheim, E., Graziano, J. H., Popovac, D., Dragovic, D., & Kaul, B. (1978). Treatment of lead poisoning by 2 3-dimercaptosuccinic acid. *The Lancet*, *312*(8102), 1234–1236.

Fukuda, S. (2005). Chelating agents used for plutonium and uranium removal in radiation emergency medicine. *Current Medicinal Chemistry*, *12*(23), 2765–2770.

Gerhardsson, L., & Kazantzis, G. (2014). Diagnosis and treatment of metal poisoning: General aspects. In G. F. Nordberg, B. A. Fowler, & M. Nordberg (Eds.), *Handbook on the toxicology of metals* (pp. 487–505). Amsterdam, New York: Academic Press, Elsevier.

Gerr, F., Frumkin, H., & Hodgins, P. (1994). Hemolytic anemia following succimer administration in a glucose-6-phosphate dehydrogenase deficient patient. *Journal of Toxicology: Clinical Toxicology*, *32*(5), 569–575.

Gibbs, K. R., & Walshe, J. M. (1986). The metabolism of trientine: Animal studies. In I. H. Scheinberg, & J. M. Walshe (Eds.), *Orphan diseases and orphan drugs* (pp. 33–42). Manchester, UK: Manchester: University Press.

Grandjean, P., Jacobsen, I. A., & Jørgensen, P. J. (1991). Chronic lead poisoning treated with dimercaptosuccinic acid. *Pharmacology & Toxicology*, *68*(4), 266–269.

Grémy, O., Tsapis, N., Bruel, S., Renault, D., & Van der Meeren, A. (2012). Decorporation approach following rat lung contamination with a moderately soluble compound of plutonium using local and systemic Ca-DTPA combined chelation. *Radiation Research*, *178*(3), 217–223.

Guha Mazumder, D. N., De, B. K., Santra, A., Ghosh, N., Das, S., Lahiri, S., & Das, T. (2001). Randomized placebo-controlled trial of 2, 3-dimercapto-1-propanesulfonate (DMPS) in therapy of chronic arsenicosis due to drinking arsenic-contaminated water. *Journal of Toxicology: Clinical Toxicology*, *39*(7), 665–674.

Guo, C., Wang, P., Zhong, M. L., Wang, T., Huang, X. S., Li, J. Y., & Wang, Z. Y. (2013). Deferoxamine inhibits iron induced hippocampal tau phosphorylation in the Alzheimer transgenic mouse brain. *Neurochemistry International*, *62*(2), 165–172.

Jay, D., Cuéllar, A., Zamorano, R., Muñoz, E., & Gleason, R. (1991). Captopril does not scavenge superoxide: captopril prevents $O_2^{-\cdot}$ production by chelating copper. *Archives of Biochemistry and Biophysics*, *290*(2), 463–467.

Jiang, Y. M., Mo, X. A., Du, F. Q., Fu, X., Zhu, X. Y., Gao, H. Y., & Zheng, W. (2006). Effective treatment of manganese-induced occupational Parkinsonism with p-aminosalicylic acid: a case of 17-year follow-up study. *Journal of Occupational and Environmental Medicine/American College of Occupational and Environmental Medicine*, *48*(6), 644–649.

Kidd, P. M. (2002). Autism, an extreme challenge to integrative medicine. Part II: medical management. *Alternative Medicine Review*, *7*(6), 472–499.

Kolnagou, A., Kleanthous, M., & Kontoghiorghes, G. J. (2011). Efficacy, compliance and toxicity factors are affecting the rate of normalization of body iron stores in thalassemia patients using the deferiprone and deferoxamine combination therapy. *Hemoglobin*, *35*(3), 186–198.

Kontoghiorghes, G. J., Pattichi, K., Hadjigavriel, M., & Kolnagou, A. (2000). Transfusional iron overload and chelation therapy with deferoxamine and deferiprone (L1). *Transfusion Science*, *23*(3), 211–223.

Kontoghiorghes, G. J., Kolnagou, A., Peng, C. T., Shah, S. V., & Aessopos, A. (2010). Safety issues of iron chelation therapy in patients with normal range iron stores including thalassaemia, neurodegenerative, renal and infectious diseases. *Expert Opinion on Drug Safety*, *9*(2), 201–206.

Kosnett, M. J. (2013). The role of chelation in the treatment of arsenic and mercury poisoning. *Journal of Medical Toxicology*, *9*(4), 347–354.

Kostyniak, P. J. (1982). Mobilization and removal of methylmercury in the dog during extracorporeal complexing hemodialysis with 2, 3-dimercaptosuccinic acid (DMSA). *Journal of Pharmacology and Experimental Therapeutics*, *221*(1), 63–68.

Kwiatkowski, J. L. (2011). Management of transfusional iron overload–differential properties and efficacy of iron chelating agents. *Journal of Blood Medicine*, *2*, 135–149.

Lamas, G. A., Goertz, C., Boineau, R., Mark, D. B., Rozema, T., & Nahin, R. L. (2013). TACT Investigators Effect of disodium EDTA chelation regimen on cardiovascular events in patients with previous myocardial infarction: the TACT randomized trial. *Journal of the American Medical Association*, *309*(12), 1241–1250.

Lannfelt, L., Blennow, K., Zetterberg, H., Batsman, S., Ames, D., & Harrison, J. PBT2-201-Euro Study Group. (2008). Safety, efficacy, and biomarker findings of PBT2 in targeting Aβ as a modifying therapy for Alzheimer's disease: a phase IIa, double-blind, randomised, placebo-controlled trial. *The Lancet Neurology*, *7*(9), 779–786.

Liu, X. L., Wang, H. B., Sun, C. W., Xiong, X. S., Chen, Z., Li, Z. S., & Yang, G. (2011). The clinical analysis of mercury poisoning in 92 cases. *Zhonghua Nei Ke Za Zhi*, *50*(8), 687–689.

Lu, J. (2010). Triethylenetetramine pharmacology and its clinical applications. *Molecular Cancer Therapeutics*, *9*(9), 2458–2467.

Marx, J., Hockberger, R., Walls, R. (2014). *Rosen's Emergency Medicine-Concepts and Clinical Practice*, 2-Volume Set, 8th ed., Philadelphia, Pennsylvania: Elsevier Health Sciences.

Mehta, A., Kannan, G. M., Dube, S. N., Pant, B. P., Pant, S. C., & Flora, S. J. (2002). Haematological, hepatic and renal alterations after repeated oral or intraperitoneal administration of monoisoamyl DMSA. I. Changes in male rats. *Journal of Applied Toxicology*, *22*(6), 359–369.

Meltzer, L. E., Kitchell, J. R., & Palmon, F., Jr. (1961). The long term use, side effects, and toxicity of disodium ethylenediamine tetraacetic acid (EDTA). *American Journal of Medical Science*, *242*, 11–17.

Mena, I., Court, J., Fuenzalida, S., Papavasiliou, P. S., & Cotzias, G. C. (1970). Modification of chronic manganese poisoning. Treatment with L-dopa or 5-OH tryptophane. *The New England Journal of Medicine*, *282*(1), 5–10.

Miller, A. L. (1998). Dimercaptosuccinic acid (DMSA), a non-toxic, water-soluble treatment for heavy metal toxicity. *Alternative Medicine Review*, *3*(3), 199–207.

Mishra, D., Mehta, A., & Flora, S. J. (2008). Reversal of arsenic-induced hepatic apoptosis with combined administration of DMSA and its analogues in guinea pigs: role of glutathione and linked enzymes. *Chemical Research in Toxicology*, *21*(2), 400–407.

Modell, B., Khan, M., Darlison, M., Westwood, M. A., Ingram, D., & Pennell, D. J. (2008). Improved survival of thalassaemia major in the UK and relation to T2* cardiovascular magnetic resonance. *Journal of Cardiovascular Magnetic Resonance*, *10*, 42.

Mourad, F. H., Hoffbrand, A. V., Sheikh-Taha, M., Koussa, S., Khoriaty, A. I., & Taher, A. (2003). Comparison between desferrioxamine and combined therapy with desferrioxamine and deferiprone in iron overloaded thalassaemia patients. *British Journal of Haematology*, *121*(1), 187–189.

Munthe, E., Jellum, E., & Aaseth, J. (1979). Some aspects of the mechanism of action of penicillamine in rheumatoid arthritis. *Scandinavian Journal of Rheumatology*, *8*(S28), 6–12.

Musallam, K. M., & Taher, A. T. (2011). Deferiprone or deferasirox for cardiac siderosis in beta-thalassemia major. *Haematologica*, *96*(2), e5–e6.

Mückter, H., Liebl, B., Reichl, F. X., Hunder, G., Walther, U., & Fichtl, B. (1997). Are we ready to replace dimercaprol (BAL) as an arsenic antidote? *Human & Experimental Toxicology*, *16*(8), 460–465.

Nisbet-Brown, E., Olivieri, N. F., Giardina, P. J., Grady, R. W., Neufeld, E. J., Séchaud, R., & Nathan, D. G. (2003). Effectiveness and safety of ICL670 in iron-loaded patients with thalassaemia: a randomised, double-blind, placebo-controlled, dose-escalation trial. *The Lancet*, *361*(9369), 1597–1602.

Netter, P., Bannwarth, B., Péré, P., & Nicolas, A. (1987). Clinical pharmacokinetics of D-penicillamine. *Clinical Pharmacokinetics*, *13*(5), 317–333.

Nissel, H. (1986). Arteriosclerosis and chelate therapy. *Wiener Medizinische Wochenschrift*, *136*(21–22), 586–588.

Pearce, J. (1994). Studies of any toxicological effects of Prussian blue compounds in mammals—a review. *Food and Chemical Toxicology*, *32*(6), 577–582.

Peters, R. A., Stocken, L. A., & Thompson, R. H. (1945). British anti-lewisite (BAL). *Nature*, *156*, 616–619.

Petrunkin, V. E. (1956). Synthesis and properties of dimercapto derivatives of alkylsulfonic acids. *Ukrainskii Khimicheskii Zhurnal*, *22*, 603–611.

Piga, A., Gaglioti, C., Fogliacco, E., & Tricta, F. (2003). Comparative effects of deferiprone and deferoxamine on survival and cardiac disease in patients with thalassemia major: a retrospective analysis. *Haematologica*, *88*(5), 489–496.

Piga, A., Galanello, R., Forni, G. L., Cappellini, M. D., Origa, R., Zappu, A., & Alberti, D. (2006). Randomized phase II trial of deferasirox (Exjade, ICL670), a once-daily, orally-administered iron chelator, in comparison to deferoxamine in thalassemia patients with transfusional iron overload. *Haematologica*, *91*(7), 873–880.

Racette, B. A., McGee-Minnich, L., Moerlein, S. M., Mink, J. W., Videen, T. O., & Perlmutter, J. S. (2001). Welding-related parkinsonism: clinical features, treatment, and pathophysiology. *Neurology*, *56*(1), 8–13.

Raymond, K. N., & Smith, W. L. (1981). Actinide-specific sequestering agents and decontamination applications. In J. B. Goodenough et al.,(Ed.), *Structure and bonding* (pp. 159–186). Berlin, Heidelberg: Springer-Verlag.

Rencova, J., Volf, V., Jones, M. M., & Singh, P. K. (1994). Decorporation of polonium from rats by new chelating agents. *Radiation Protection Dosimetry*, *53*(1–4), 311–313.

Rogers, J. T., Randall, J. D., Cahill, C. M., Eder, P. S., Huang, X., Gunshin, H., & Gullans, S. R. (2002). An iron-responsive element type II in the 5′-untranslated region of the Alzheimer's amyloid precursor protein transcript. *Journal of Biological Chemistry*, *277*(47), 45518–45528.

Rogan, W. J., Dietrich, K. N., Ware, J. H., Dockery, D. W., Salganik, M., Radcliffe, J., & Rhoads, G. G. (2001). The effect of chelation therapy with succimer on neuropsychological development in children exposed to lead. *The New England Journal of Medicine*, *344*(19), 1421–1426.

Salvator, H., Gille, T., Hervé, A., Bron, C., Lamberto, C., & Valeyre, D. (2013). Chronic beryllium disease: azathioprine as a possible alternative to corticosteroid treatment. *The European Respiratory Journal*, *41*(1), 234–236.

Schubert, J. (1983). In S. Bibudhandra (Ed.), *Biological aspects of metals and metal related diseases* (pp. 27–907). New York: Raven Press.

Sears, M. E. (2013). Chelation: harnessing and enhancing heavy metal detoxification—a review. *The Scientific World Journal*, *2013*, 219840.

Seely, D. M., Wu, P., & Mills, E. J. (2005). EDTA chelation therapy for cardiovascular disease: a systematic review. *BMC Cardiovascular Disorders*, *5*(1), 32.

Shrihari, J. S., Roy, A., Prabhakaran, D., & Reddy, K. S. (2006). Role of EDTA chelation therapy in cardiovascular diseases. *National Medical Journal of India*, *19*(1), 24–26.

Smith, S. W. (2013). The role of chelation in the treatment of other metal poisonings. *Journal of Medical Toxicology*, *9*(4), 355–369.

Sloth-Nielsen, J., Guldager, B., Mouritzen, C., Lund, E. B., Egeblad, M., Nørregaard, O., & Jelnes, R. (1991). Arteriographic findings in EDTA chelation therapy on peripheral arteriosclerosis. *The American Journal of Surgery*, *162*(2), 122–125.

Stoeckle, J. D., Hardy, H. L., & Weber, A. L. (1969). Chronic beryllium disease. Long-term follow-up of sixty cases and selective review of the literature. *The American Journal of Medicine*, *46*(4), 545–561.

Stradling, G. N., Stather, J. W., Ham, S. E., & Sumner, S. A. (1981). The use of Puchel and DTPA for removing 238 PuO2 from the lungs of hamsters. *Health Physics*, *41*(2), 387–391.

Sunderman, F. W., Sr. (1971). The treatment of acute nickel carbonyl poisoning with sodium diethyldithiocarbamate. *Annals of Clinical Research*, *3*(3), 182–185.

Tammaro, A., Narcisi, A., Persechino, S., Caperchi, C., & Gaspari, A. (2011). Topical and systemic therapies for nickel allergy. *Dermatitis*, *22*(5), 251–255.

Taylor, D. M., & Volf, V. (1980). Oral chelation treatment of injected 241Am or 239Pu in rats. *Health Physics*, *38*(2), 147–158.

Totadri, S., Bansal, D., Bhatia, P., Attri, S. V., Trehan, A., & Marwaha, R. K. (2015). The deferiprone and deferasirox combination is efficacious in iron overloaded patients with β-thalassemia major: A prospective, single center, open-label study. *Pediatric Blood & Cancer*, *62*(9), 1592–1596.

Vale, J. A., & Meredith, T. J. (1981). *Poisoning diagnosis and treatment*. London: Update Books.

Walshe, J. M. (1984). Copper: its role in the pathogenesis of liver disease. *Seminars in Liver Disease*, *4*(3), 252–263.

Walshe, J. M. (1985). Unithiol in Wilson's disease. *British Medical Journal*, *290*(6469), 673–674.

Ward, R. J., Dexter, D. T., & Crichton, R. R. (2015). Neurodegenerative diseases and therapeutic strategies using iron chelators. *Journal of Trace Elements in Medicine and Biology*, *31*, 267–273.

Wax, P. M. (2013). Current use of chelation in American health care. *Journal of Medical Toxicology*, *9*(4), 303–307.

Wecker, L., Miller, S. B., Cochran, S. R., Dugger, D. L., & Johnson, W. D. (1985). Trace element concentrations in hair from autistic children. *Journal of Mental Deficiency Research*, *29*(Pt 1), 15–22.

Weiss, K. H., Thurik, F., Gotthardt, D. N., Schäfer, M., Teufel, U., & Wiegand, F. EUROWILSON Consortium. (2013). Efficacy and safety of oral chelators in treatment of patients with Wilson disease. *Clinical Gastroenterology and Hepatology*, *11*(8), 1028–1035.

Xia, S., Zhang, W., Huang, L., & Jiang, H. (2013). Comparative efficacy and safety of deferoxamine, deferiprone and deferasirox on severe thalassemia: a meta-analysis of 16 randomized controlled trials. *PloS One*, *8*(12), e82662.

Zheng, W., Jiang, Y. M., Zhang, Y., Jiang, W., Wang, X., & Cowan, D. M. (2009). Chelation therapy of manganese intoxication with para-aminosalicylic acid (PAS) in Sprague–Dawley rats. *Neurotoxicology*, *30*(2), 240–248.

Zou, J., Li, Y., Fan, H. Q., & Wang, J. G. (2012). Effects of dihydropyridine calcium channel blockers on oxidized low-density lipoprotein induced proliferation and oxidative stress of vascular smooth muscle cells. *BMC Research Notes*, *5*(1), 168.

Chapter 8

Conclusions and Guidelines for Future Research

Guido Crisponi, Ole Andersen, Jan Aaseth

Chapter Outline

8.1 CONCLUSIONS ON CLINICAL CHELATION TREATMENT AND INDICATIONS OF IMPORTANT RESEARCH NEEDS

Metal toxicity represents a worldwide major health problem, both in developed and in emerging countries. Multiple etiological factors are concerned, including environmental, occupational, iatrogenic, and genetic ones. The research efforts invested in further development in the treatment of metal overexposures in acute and chronic poisonings, including radionuclides exposures and iron and copper overload diseases, have resulted both in effective clinical achievements and in the advancement of scientific knowledge. Nonetheless, these achievements are still inadequate to effectively counteract metal induced diseases, and a joint effort of chemical, biochemical, pathological, and clinical researchers might be appropriate to solve the related clinical problems, supported by large investments by central governments and international health organizations.

The evaluation of the clinical effectiveness and safety of chelating agents is difficult as few data from adequate clinical studies are available. Much of our present conclusive evaluation, therefore, has still to be based on the data from animal studies.

Chemical studies can be of great help in the design of chelating agents for a specific target metal ion, by choosing proper coordinating groups correctly assembled. Quantum chemical calculations nowadays help in the choice among different potential structures of the chelating groups around the target metal ion, and chemical simulation software programs are available for a reliable evaluation of

Chelation Therapy in the Treatment of Metal Intoxication. http://dx.doi.org/10.1016/B978-0-12-803072-1.00008-0

the fundamental properties that determine the behavior of a drug in vivo. These methods thus allow the selection of molecules with the best potential properties to act as a chelating agent. These are then synthesized and the stability constants with the target toxic metal ion, and with the competing essential metal ions, evaluated. These thermodynamic properties are only indicative of effectiveness in vivo and they serve as guidance for the following cellular and animal studies, saving money and time expended on surely ineffective molecules. The ligands with good thermodynamic properties and good bioavailability parameters surely deserve to be addressed to animal studies. A systematic procedure based on the chemical and animal studies will identify the best candidates for clinically useful chelating agents. The studies of the group of Bergeron (Bergeron, Wiegand, McManis, & Bharti, 2014) starting from desferrithiocin to the effective desferitazole can be paradigmatic of this kind of approach. Nonetheless safety in use can never be judged from this type of data. Extrapolation from animal studies to humans must always be viewed with caution and undertaken with care. In this respect the studies on the pyridoxal isonicotinoyl hydrazone (PIH) are exemplificative: while PIH, and its analogues, demonstrated effective in the excretion of iron in a number of animal models, only a modest excretion resulted in clinical trials (Hider, 2014). However, since in acute metal poisonings clinicians must always choose the treatment believed to be optimal, comparative analysis of the efficacy of chelating agents can be performed only in animal studies.

A critical issue in metal toxicity is the distribution of metals or metalloids into the target organ(s), and the influence of the chelation agent on this distribution. An example is lead which is stored in the skeleton but the brain is an important target organ, usually referred to as the *critical organ.* Chelation therapy should ideally aim at removing lead from the critical organ or at least prevent further deposition in the critical organ by lowering blood lead. Certainly the treatment should not redistribute lead from the skeleton into the brain, as has been demonstrated with dimercaprol and calcium ethylenediaminetetraacetate therapy. The ability of dimercaprol to cause unwanted redistribution of metals into the brain is linked to the lipophilic character of its chelates. This has led to the development of the water-soluble analogs dimercapto-propane sulfonate (DMPS) and dimercaptosuccinic acid (DMSA), both of which forming water-soluble chelates. These latter agents may take over as "universal" antidotes for metals with high electronegativity (Hg, Pb, etc.) as they are effective in several types of poisoning of these metals, which are often classified as sulfur-seekers. Metal ions (electron pair acceptors, "Lewis acids") and chelator ligands (electron pair donors, "Lewis bases") form complexes determined by their softness-hardness character. Generally, hard metal ions form stable complexes with hard donors, while soft metal ions form stable complexes with soft donor ligands (Table 8.1). For a detailed discussion of the soft-hard classification of metal ions (electron acceptors) and complexing ligands (electron donors) in biological systems, the reader is referred to Nieboer and Richardson (1980), and to the fundamental papers of Pearson (1963, 1968a, 1968b).

TABLE 8.1 Classification of Metal Ions, and of Coordinating Groups, as a Function of Their Hard, Soft or Intermediate Nature (see chapter: Chelating Agents as Therapeutic Compounds—Basic Principles)

Metal ions			Coordinating groups		
Hard	Intermediate	Soft	Hard	Intermediate	Soft
Be^{2+}, Mg^{2+}, Ca^{2+}, Sr^{2+}, Mn^{2+}, Al^{3+}, Ga^{3+}, Cr^{3+}, Fe^{3+}, Sn^{4+}, $(CH_3)_2Sn^{2+}$, UO_2^{2+}, VO^{2+}	Fe^{2+}, Co^{2+}, Ni^{2+}, Cu^{2+}, Zn^{2+}, Pb^{2+}, Sn^{2+}	Cu^{+}, Ag^{+}, Au^{+}, Hg^{+}, Pd^{2+}, Cd^{2+}, Pt^{2+}, Hg^{2+}, CH_3Hg^{+}, Pt^{4+}	H_2O, OH^{-}, F^{-}, $RCOO^{-}$, RO^{-},	RNH_2	R_2S, RSH, RS^{-}, R-Se^{-}

Softness itself favors formation of stable complexes through covalent forces. In popular terms, softness is related to the deformability of the outer electron shell as well as to the size of the ionization energy and thus related to the propensity to form covalent bonds.

Various authors have developed hardness/softness describers: Nieboer and Richardson (1980) used the covalent index, $X_m{}^2r$, where X_m is the electronegativity of the ions, to describe softness. The rationale is that X_m is related to the empty frontier orbital energy of a metal ion, and this parameter indicates the ability of the ion to accept electrons and form covalent bonds. $X_m{}^2r$ increases with increasing softness, its values for Be^{++} and Hg^{++} are 0.84 and 4.10, respectively. Z^2/r, where Z is the ion's formal charge and r is the crystal ion's radius, was used by Weast (1977–1978) to describe hardness, its values for Be^{++} and Hg^{++} are 9.09 and 3.63, respectively.

DMSA and DMPS have gained more general acceptance among clinicians during the recent decades, undoubtedly improving the management of many human metal intoxications. However, clinical case reports still emerge where acute metal poisonings were treated with BAL despite this chelator's inferiority to DMSA or DMPS. This is odd since DMPS and DMSA are available as cheaper and more stable preparations for both oral and parenteral use with lower toxicities and less side effects and without increasing the brain deposition of metals.

Poisoning with "hard" metals, also classified as oxygen-seekers, for example, transuranic elements (U, Pu, Am, etc.), including also aluminum and iron, may be treated with calcium or zinc salts of EDTA and DTPA. However, deposits of Al or Fe are more efficiently removed by deferoxamine (DFO) combined with deferiprone (L1) or deferasirox. The extensive occurrence of iron overload diseases related to hemoglobinopathies mainly in Southern

Europe, Africa and the near and far-off Asia led pharmaceutical industries to large investments, resulted in excellent outcomes regarding the drugs in use and the route of their administration. The related research has greatly improved the knowledge on the role of iron and of chelators in living organisms, and a variety of features of the greatest utility in chelation therapy are now clarified, as the target organs of chelators, the thermodynamic and kinetic competition with endogenous ligands, the metabolism, and the factors affecting oral absorption and bioavailability.

It should be emphasized here that the management of acute metal poisoning usually requires emergency resuscitative procedures, although first aid treatment may need to be started in the work or home environment. Careful diagnostics, and clinical and laboratory evaluation of the therapy is of crucial importance. Preliminary recommendations for the use of chelating agents may be briefly summarized as follows (Table 8.2):

- Desferal for aluminum compounds, L1, and deferasirox are potential alternative chelators.
- Desferal for acute poisoning by iron compounds, L1, and deferasirox are potential chelators.
- DMPS for acute and chronic poisonings by arsenic compounds, presumably selenium supplement as adjuvant.
- DMSA for acute and chronic poisonings by lead compounds.
- DMPS for inorganic mercury compounds including mercury vapor, DMSA may be superior for organic mercury compounds.
- Triethylenetetramine (trien) for copper overload, with D-penicillamine (DPA) as a second choice.

The classic chelators DPA, BAL, and EDTA have been used generally for decades in acute poisoning by several metals, but they are today outdated for most uses and even contraindicated in some situations. DMSA and DMPS, originally developed in the previous Soviet Union and in China, have been licensed since several decades also in the Western World and are taking over. Moreover, the relatively new oral agents, deferiprone and deferasirox have been adopted into clinical use in cases of siderosis, after several clinical trials (see chapter: Chelating Therapy in Metal Storage Diseases), and the two agents may be combined for in-home treatment in thalassemia cases with excessive iron deposits. Such treatment may be lifesaving and improve the quality of life for hundreds of thousands of people worldwide in the numerous cases with siderosis due to thalassemia or sickle cell anemia (see chapter: Chelating Therapy in Metal Storage Diseases). It has nevertheless to be underlined that, despite the ascertained utility of desferal and deferasirox in thalassemia patients, the high cost prevents their use by the large part of patients, not only in developing countries. The development of chelating agents accessible to all the patients constitutes thus an impelling issue.

TABLE 8.2 Representative Toxic and Essential Divalent Metal Ions Ordered According to Their HSAB Character, and Clinically Approved Chelating Agents Effective in Acute or Chronic Animal (A) or Human (H) Poisonings (see chapter: Chelation Treatment During Acute and Chronic Metal Overexposures—Experimental and Clinical Studies)

HS character	Metal ion	Acute poisoning	Chronic poisoning	Remark
Hard	Be^{++}	CaEDTA (A)	Tiron (A)	
	Sr^{++}	CaEDTA (A), Ca salts (A)	Ca salts (A)	
Intermediate	Ni^{++}	CaEDTA (A), DMSA (A)	DDC (H)	
	Fe^{++}	PB (A), DTPA (A), DFO (A, H)	DFO (A, H), deferiprone (A, H), DFX (A, H)	
	Co^{++}	CaDTPA (A), DMSA (A)	CaEDTA (H)	BAL contraindicated
	Mn^{++}	PAS (A,H), DTPA (A)	DTPA (A), PAS (A, H)	
	Zn^{++}	DMSA (A), DTPA (A), EDTA (H)		DDC contraindicated
Soft	Cd^{++}	DTPA (A), DMSA (A), DMPS (A)	Carbodithioate and DMSA esters (A)	BAL and DDC contraindicated
	Cu^{+}	DMPS or DMSA (A)	Trien or DPA (H)	BAL, DDC and EDTA contraindicated
	Pb^{++}	DMSA (A, H), BAL/EDTA? (H)	DMSA (A, H)	
	Hg^{++}	DMPS (A, H), DMSA (A)	DMPS (H), DMSA (H)	BAL contraindicated

PAS, para-aminosalicylate; DFO, deferoxamine; Tiron, disodium 4,5-dihydroxy-1,3-benzenedisulfonate; DFX, deferasirox.

8.2 GUIDELINES FOR FUTURE RESEARCH

Millions of people world-wide suffer from metal overload with disabling and life-shortening outcomes, not only iron overload in thalassemia and sickle cell anemia, but also arsenic toxicity in contaminated areas.

Other metal poisonings including radionuclides also present future challenges, where development of oral chelation treatment or inhalation treatment instead of parenteral treatment with the zinc or calcium salts of DTPA would be of enormous potential in case of mass poisonings due to major accidents or acts of terrorism. The development of combinations of chelating agents that can also mobilize aged intracellular metal deposits offers possible future development of potent treatment regimens that may provide improved clinical usefulness. An example in current use is the small molecule of deferiprone that appears to act as a "shuttling agent" converting intracellularly deposited iron into a diffusible form, followed by extracellularly scavenging of iron by DFO for transportation into urine. New *oral iron chelators*, now in clinical trials in cases of siderosis, may provide improved clinical possibilities in thalassemia and related disorders (Bergeron et al., 2014; Hider, 2014; Hider et al., 2015). In such cases, combinations of orally administered chelators might also represent therapeutic advances by accelerating both intracellular removal and excretion into bile or urine, for example, in thalassemic siderosis (Totadri et al., 2015).

Oral poisoning with iron supplements is among the most frequent poisonings in children below 6 years of age. Orally administered DFO appears to inhibit GI absorption, while additional treatment with L1 or deferasirox may act as potential adjuvants. Animal studies have however indicated that oral Prussian blue or oral CaDTPA are even better than DFO to inhibit iron absorption, and studies to explore this approach clinically should have high priority.

Another metal with affinity to oxygen or nitrogen ligands is manganese. Recent studies (Zhen et al., 2009) indicate that intravenous (i.v.) administration of paraaminosalicylate (PAS) is superior in removing neurotoxic manganese deposits in brain, but further studies are of utmost importance to assess the clinical antidotal role of this originally tuberculostatic agent.

In many reviews on the use of chelating agents in acute metal poisoniong, questions of initiation of chelation treatment while exposure still occurs are raised. Such questions can be answered by well planned animal studies. In many cases, the chelate formed, for example, in the gastrointesinal tract is absorbed far less than the metal itself, so in these cases early chelation may be beneficial.

Arsenic contaminated drinking water affects the health of numerous people. A few, small epidemiological studies have demonstrated that DMPS chelation combined with supply of nonarsenic contaminated water results in clinical alleviation of arsenicosis. Due to the million-number of people affected by arsenicosis in Asia and South America, this treatment should be further evaluated. It is not possible to supply clean water to such population sizes, so animal studies to clarify if chelation during continued As exposure would be beneficial or harmful, should have high priority. Combinations of DMPS (Aposhian et al., 2000) and selenite (Alexander & Aaseth, 1985) may enhance the excretion or detoxification of most toxic arsenical metabolites, in particular the toxic monomethylated As(III)-metabolite. Further research is important to explore this approach. Another selenium compound, selenoneine, found in tuna fish, has appeared to be an efficient antidote against methyl mercury poisoning (Yamashita, Yabu, & Yamashita, 2010). This analog of ergothioneine has yet not been studied in cases of inorganic or elemental mercury overexposure.

Combination of a water soluble chelator, for example, DMPS or mercaptodextran (Aaseth, 1973) with a lipophilic "shuttling" chelator, for example, monoisoamyl-DMSA (MiADMSA) or even minor amounts of BAL to facilitate the conversion of intracellular metal into a diffusible chelate for subsequent rapid urinary elimination, might represent a potential advance in the therapy of aged mercury deposits (Bhadauria & Flora, 2004). Also, combinations using the early synthesized water soluble BAL-glucoside, has been insufficiently studied (Gilman, Allen, Philips, & John, 1946).

In addition, careful diagnostics of metal overexposure is crucial. Thus, the development of new diagnostic tools, including advanced imaging techniques, which can be used more safely than the traditional EDTA test for lead exposure are of importance.

Still, further knowledge is needed in several basic research areas within the field of in vivo chelation of metals, and call for studies, for example:

- Molecular mechanisms of action of clinically important chelators.
- Intracellular and extracellular chelation in relation to mobilization of aged metal deposits and removal of toxic metal from sensitive organs, for example, brain and heart.
- Improved removal of toxic metal deposits characterizing some neurodegenerative diseases, for example, Wilson's disease and NBIAs (neurodegeneration with brain iron accumulation).
- Effects of chelators on metal biokinetics, during continued exposure to the metal, particularly reduction of intestinal metal uptake.
- Studies on combined chelation treatment with lipophilic and hydrophilic chelators.
- Minimization of the mobilization of essential trace elements during long-term chelation.
- Fetotoxic and teratogenic effects of chelators.
- Further development of orally active chelators.
- Development of less toxic and orally administrable chelators for chronic chelation treatment of diseases due to metal storage.

Especially the two last points, continued development of orally administrable chelating agents for efficient, nontoxic mobilization on home-patient basis over extended time periods (even life-long chelation) of aged deposits of toxic metal amounts, for example, iron, arsenic, copper, and cadmium will probably be a main future research issue. Also appropriate animal experimental comparison of the efficacies of new and old chelators in acute intoxications using relevant exposure routes, that is, oral administration of relevant species of the metals, as well as inhalation of Hg vapor, is a prerequisite for out-phasing the old chelators in uses where a more effective alternative is now available. Thus, if BAL were suggested as a new drug today, it would probably not be approved for clinical use. The advent of the more efficient and safe drugs DMSA and DMPS, has provided a state, where BAL most likely should be made unavailable as a drug.

REFERENCES

Aaseth, J. (1973). The effect of mercaptodextran on distribution and toxicity of mercury in mice. *Acta Pharmacologica Et Toxicologica*, *32*(6), 430–441.

Alexander, J., & Aaseth, J. (1985). Excretion of arsenic in rat bile: a role of complexing ligands containing sulphur or selenium. *Nutrition Research*, *1*, S515–S519.

Aposhian, H. V., Zheng, B., Aposhian, M. M., Le, X. C., Cebrian, M. E., Cullen, W., Zakharyan, R. A., Ma, M., Dart, R. C., Cheng, Z., Andrewes, P., Yip, L., O'Malley, G. F., Maiorino, R. M., Van Voorhies, W., Healy, S. M., & Titcomb, A. (2000). DMPS-arsenic challenge test. II. Modulation of arsenic species, including monomethylarsonous acid (MMA(III)), excreted in human urine. *Toxicology and Applied Pharmacology*, *165*(1), 74–83.

Bergeron, R. J., Wiegand, J., McManis, J. S., & Bharti, N. (2014). Desferrithioc: a search for clinically effective iron chelators. *Journal of Medicinal Chemistry*, *57*, 9259–9291.

Bhadauria, S., & Flora, S. J. S. (2004). Arsenic induced inhibition of δ-aminolevulinate dehydratase activity in rat blood and its response to meso 2,3-dimercaptosuccinic acid and monoisoamyl DMSA. *Biomedical Environmental Sciences*, *17*, 101–108.

Gilman, A., Allen, R. P., Philips, F. S., & John, E. S. (1946). Clinical uses of 2, 3-dimercaptopropanol (BAL). X. The treatment of acute systemic mercury poisoning in experimental animals with BAL, thiosorbitol and BAL glucoside. *The Journal of Clinical Investigation*, *25*(4), 549–556.

Hider, R. C. (2014). Recent developments centered on orally active iron chelators. *Thalassemia Reports*, *4*(2), 20–27.

Hider, R. C., Kong, X., Abbate, V., Harland, R., Conlon, K., & Luker, T. (2015). Deferitazole, a new orally active iron chelator. *Dalton Transactions*, *44*(11), 5197–5204.

Nieboer, E., & Richardson, D. H. S. (1980). The replacement of the nondescript term "heavy metals" by a biologically and chemically significant classification of metal ions. *Environmental Pollution*, *1*, 3–26.

Pearson, R. G. (1963). Hard and soft acids and bases. *Journal of the American Chemical Society*, *85*, 3533–3539.

Pearson, R. G. (1968a). Hard and soft acids and bases, HSAB part 1: fundamental principles. *Journal of Chemical Education*, *45*, 581–587.

Pearson, R. G. (1968b). Hard and soft acids and bases, HSAB, Part II: underlying theories. *Journal of Chemical Education*, *45*, 643–648.

Totadri, S., Bansal, D., Bhatia, P., Attri, S. V., Trehan, A., & Marwaha, R. K. (2015). The deferiprone and deferasirox combination is efficacious in iron overloaded patients with β-thalassemia major: A prospective, single center, open-label study. *Pediatric Blood & Cancer*, *62*(9), 1592–1596.

Yamashita, Y., Yabu, T., & Yamashita, M. (2010). Discovery of the strong antioxidant selenoneine in tuna and selenium redox metabolism. *World Journal of Biological Chemistry*, *1*(5), 144–150.

Weast, R. C. (Ed.). (1977–1978). *CRC handbook of chemistry and physics*. Cleveland: CRC Press.

Zhen, W., Jiang, Y. M., Zhang, Y., Jiang, W., Wang, X., & Cowan, D. M. (2009). Chelation therapy of manganese intoxication with para-aminosalicylic acid (PAS) in Sprague–Dawley rats. *Neurotoxicology*, *30*(2), 240–248.

Subject Index

A

B

C

G

H

I

N

O

Q

R

U

FSC
www.fsc.org
MIX
Papier | Fördert
gute Waldnutzung
FSC® C083411

Kolibri 360 GmbH
Ferdinand-Jühlke-Straße 7
99095 Erfurt, Deutschland
produktsicherheit@kolibri360.de